I0055633

Type 1 Diabetes

Advances in Understanding and Treatment 100 Years after the Discovery of Insulin

SECOND EDITION

A subject collection from *Cold Spring Harbor Perspectives in Medicine*

OTHER SUBJECT COLLECTIONS FROM *COLD SPRING HARBOR PERSPECTIVES IN MEDICINE*

Cancer Metabolism: Historical Landmarks, New Concepts, and Opportunities
Modeling Cancer in Mice
Breast Cancer: From Fundamental Biology to Therapeutic Strategies
Aging: Geroscience as the New Public Health Frontier, Second Edition
Retinal Disorders: Genetic Approaches to Diagnosis and Treatment, Second Edition
Combining Human Genetics and Causal Inference to Understand Human Disease and Development
Lung Cancer: Disease Biology and Its Potential for Clinical Translation
Influenza: The Cutting Edge
Leukemia and Lymphoma: Molecular and Therapeutic Insights
Addiction, Second Edition
Hepatitis C Virus: The Story of a Scientific and Therapeutic Revolution
The PTEN Family
Metastasis: Mechanism to Therapy
Genetic Counseling: Clinical Practice and Ethical Considerations
Bioelectronic Medicine
Function and Dysfunction of the Cochlea: From Mechanisms to Potential Therapies
Next-Generation Sequencing in Medicine
Prostate Cancer
RAS and Cancer in the 21st Century

SUBJECT COLLECTIONS FROM *COLD SPRING HARBOR PERSPECTIVES IN BIOLOGY*

Glia, Second Edition
Speciation
The Biology of Lipids: Trafficking, Regulation, and Function, Second Edition
Synthetic Biology and Greenhouse Gases
Wound Healing: From Bench to Bedside
The Endoplasmic Reticulum, Second Edition
Sex Difference in Brain and Behavior
Regeneration
The Nucleus, Second Edition
Auxin Signaling: From Synthesis to Systems Biology, Second Edition
Stem Cells: From Biological Principles to Regenerative Medicine
Heart Development and Disease
Cell Survival and Cell Death, Second Edition
Calcium Signaling, Second Edition
Engineering Plants for Agriculture
Protein Homeostasis, Second Edition
Translation Mechanisms and Control
Cytokines
Circadian Rhythms

Type 1 Diabetes

Advances in Understanding and Treatment 100 Years after the Discovery of Insulin

SECOND EDITION

A subject collection from *Cold Spring Harbor Perspectives in Medicine*

EDITED BY

Jeffrey A. Bluestone
Sonoma Biotherapeutics

Kevan C. Herold
Yale School of Medicine

Lori Sussel
University of Colorado Anschutz Medical Center

CSH PRESS

COLD SPRING HARBOR LABORATORY PRESS
Cold Spring Harbor, New York • www.cshlpress.org

Type 1 Diabetes: Advances in Understanding and Treatment 100 Years after the Discovery of Insulin, Second Edition

A subject collection from *Cold Spring Harbor Perspectives in Medicine*
Articles online at www.cshperspectives.org

Executive Editor	Richard Sever
Project Supervisor	Barbara Acosta
Editorial Assistant	Danett Gil
Permissions Administrator	Carol Brown
Production Editor	Diane Schubach
Production Manager/Cover Designer	Denise Weiss
Publisher	John Inglis

Front cover artwork: Confocal images of islets of Langerhans from NOD mice. Immune cells are stained in red and insulin is in green. Cell nuclei are stained with 4′,6-diamidino-2-phenylindole (DAPI). Cover design by Maria Exposito Roncon and Ana Lledo Delgado with images courtesy of Noah Biru.

Library of Congress Cataloging-in-Publication Data

Names: Bluestone, Jeffrey A., editor. | Herold, Kevan C., 1956- editor. |Sussel, Lori, 1963- editor.
Title: Type 1 diabetes : advances in understanding and treatment 100 years after the discovery of insulin / edited by Jeffrey A. Bluestone, Kevan C. Herold and Lori Sussel.
Other titles: Type 1 diabetes (Bluestone) | Type one diabetes | Cold Spring Harbor perspectives in medicine.
Description: Second edition. | Cold Spring Harbor, New York : Cold Spring Harbor Laboratory Press, [2025] | Series: A subject collection from Cold Spring Harbor perspectives in medicine | Includes bibliographical references and index. | Summary: "Type 1 diabetes is caused by destruction of pancreatic cells that produce insulin and affects millions of individuals worldwide. Celebrating the 100th year of the discovery of insulin, this book reviews advances, our understanding of the pathology of type 1 diabetes and its environmental and genetic triggers, the role of the immune system, and novel therapeutic approaches" Provided by publisher.
Identifiers: LCCN 2024029639 (print) | LCCN 2024029640 (ebook) | ISBN 9781621825074 (hardcover) | ISBN 9781621825081 (epub)
Subjects: Diabetes Mellitus, Type 1--etiology | Autoantibodies | Diabetes Mellitus, Type 1--drug therapy | Collected Work
Classification: LCC RC660.4 (print) | LCC RC660.4 (ebook) | NLM WK 5 | DDC 616.4/622--dc23/eng/20241114
LC record available at https://lccn.loc.gov/2024029639
LC ebook record available at https://lccn.loc.gov/2024029640

Contents

Preface

IN 1919, ELIZABETH EVANS HUGHES, then an 11-year-old girl, was diagnosed with juvenile diabetes. At that time, the diagnosis was a death sentence, and few people lived for more than weeks or months after the diagnosis. The greatest toll was on children, who succumbed rapidly because the source of insulin, pancreatic β cells, had been destroyed. Ms. Hughes survived with a starvation diet, consuming no more than 500 kcal per day combined with severe restrictions of her activity and the constant presence of a nurse by her side who continually monitored her body's processes and every gram of food consumed. In referring to the prognosis at the time, Elliot Joslin noted that "we literally starved the child and adult with the faint hope that something new in treatment would appear...." In 1922, that "most improbable" scientific breakthrough happened—Frederick Banting and Charles Best discovered insulin and, with the help of James Collip, purified the protein. Through her family's contact (she was the daughter of the Governor of New York) and her mother's pleading, Elizabeth became one of the first recipients of insulin in the first clinical trial. At the time she received insulin, her weight had declined from 75 lb at diagnosis to 45 lb. With insulin injections, she rapidly regained weight and recovered her life. Ultimately, Elizabeth attended college and had children. She became an advocate and devoted her philanthropic work to support education and lived a joyful life, particularly enjoying reading—her sole pleasure after her diagnosis. She died at the age of 73. Banting and Best won the Nobel Prize in 1923, and Banting, Best, and Collip shared the patent for insulin, which they sold to the University of Toronto for one dollar.

For the next 100 years, the treatment of diabetes, subsequently termed insulin-dependent and eventually type 1 diabetes (T1D), consisted of diet and chronic insulin injections. Although T1D is treatable, the inability to effectively control glucose levels remains a challenge and long-term complications remain a serious concern, even today. In the 1970s, investigators identified features of immunity associated with diabetes such as immune cell infiltration into the islets of Langerhans in those who died with diabetes. As the clinical features of T1D were distinguished from the more common type 2 diabetes (T2D), T1D was recognized as an immune-mediated disease. Two transformational studies in the 1980s, one conducted in the United States led by George Eisenbarth, and the other in France led by Jean-Francois Bach, showed that treatment with the immunosuppressive drug cyclosporine reversed diabetes, documenting the key role of autoimmunity in the pathogenesis of the disease. These results accelerated investigations into the immune, genetic, and environmental causes of the disease, including a role for β cells in their own demise. Insights gained from both murine and human studies led to deeper characterization of T1D as a model of antigen-driven autoimmune diseases, and discoveries in basic immunology and other fields, such as cancer immunobiology, led to a deeper understanding of the immunologic dysregulation that underlies T1D.

This book is the second in the *Cold Spring Harbor Perspectives in Medicine* series devoted to T1D. The chapters describe discoveries that have advanced our theories of T1D pathogenesis, spanning immunologic, genetic, and environmental research contributions to understanding of both disease susceptibility and pathogenesis. The book also reviews details of the role β cells play in T1D, how they interact with the immune system, and how this contributes to the disease. Finally, multiple chapters bridge the gap between the fundamental research and clinical studies aimed at prevention and treatment.

Chapter 1 (Herold and Krischer) provides an overview of the pathogenesis of T1D. Immune (autoantibodies) and metabolic (dysglycemia) markers have led to the concept of disease stages, pre- and post-insulin dependence, which represent mileposts in its progression. These disease features and serum biomarkers are critical individual patient features that define the disease course (termed endotypes) and potentially responses to immune therapies. This chapter and Chapter 2 by Hyöty et al. describe how environmental insults may enhance disease via innate and adaptive immune mechanisms but, as importantly, may prevent disease progression (the "hygiene hypothesis"), potentially explaining the increasing rates of T1D in past decades particularly in westernized countries.

As described by Nepom in Chapter 3, T1D represents a failure of normal immune tolerance. The failures leading to disease in innate and adaptive immune pathways are discussed in Chapters 10 and 11 by Smith et al. and Bertrand et al., respectively. Relevant naturally occurring genetic mutations are discussed in Chapters 4 (Chamberlain et al.) and 13 (Kang and Youngblood) as well as induced breakdown of tolerance following immunotherapies to treat cancer (Quandt et al., Chapter 16). Our concepts of the pathogenesis, diagnosis, and biomarkers of immunotherapy successes in T1D have been advanced with the use of new technologies and tools as described in Chapter 15 by Long and Linsley. The authors discuss how biomarkers of immune responses, especially in the setting of immune perturbations with biologics, can help to identify targets for treatment and mechanisms that are central to disease.

Multiple chapters in the book focus on T cells, which are thought to be the effectors that cause β-cell killing. Unlike immune responses elicited by viral infections, transplanted organs or other conventional challenges, autoimmunity displays specific characteristics such as chronic exposure to antigens, tissue specificity, and slow progression. Features that distinguish T cells that respond to autoantigens include stem-cell-like properties, as described in chapters by Kang and Youngblood and Schietinger et al. (Chapter 12) and may provide clues to why they are difficult to eliminate. Moreover, it is not just peptides produced by β cells in healthy individuals, but neoantigens to which tolerance has not been induced may be involved. These are discussed in Chapter 14 by Delong and Nakayama, while autoantigen therapies are described in Chapter 19 by Peakman and Santamaria.

Further disease insights have come from the study of tissues from animal models (Serreze et al., Chapter 5) and humans (Kusmartseva et al., Chapter 9). In addition to increasing our understanding of T1D pathogenesis, these efforts have identified cross talk between the target tissue (β cells) and immune cells that may lead to activation of immune cells and β-cell death. Samassa et al. (Chapter 6) focus on the communication between these systems and how they influence each other. Bhushan and Thompson (Chapter 7) speak to the internal and external stresses that instigate the process on both sides, while Hansen et al. (Chapter 8) delve into the question of whether the β cells or the immune system becomes dysfunctional first.

These advances in our understanding of the pathobiology of T1D have driven progress in development of treatments to change the course of the disease, as reviewed by Tatovic and Dayan (Chapter 18). Nepom (Chapter 3) describes how the breakdown and repair of immune tolerance has been achieved with novel therapeutics that "rebalance" the immune system. The approaches include using regulatory T cells, as described by Muller et al. (Chapter 17), and antigen-specific immune therapies (Delong and Nakayama, Chapter 14, and Peakman and Santamaria, Chapter 19) building on the discoveries of the targets of immune cells. This is an ideal therapeutic approach because of their specificity for T1D. Islet transplantation and restoring β-cell function, especially without the need for chronic immune suppression, represents the ultimate cure for T1D and is discussed by Kieffer et al. (Chapter 21).

Based on the work of many researchers and multiple national and international networks, such as TrialNet, DAISY, TEDDY, DIPP, and BABYDIAB in the Eisenbarth model of T1D progression, the disease initiates before any clinical presentation. This suggests that patients can benefit from treatments before they present with severe metabolic derangement. In 2015, 96 years after Edith Hughes' diagnosis, another girl, a 10-year-old, whose sister had insulin-dependent T1D, was found to have multiple autoantibodies and impaired glucose tolerance that suggested a 75% risk of progressing to clinical T1D within 5 years. She also enrolled in a clinical trial, but this time the trial was with teplizumab to test whether the diagnosis of T1D might be delayed or prevented. Over the next nearly 9 years, without diabetes, she went to school without the need for a special diet, glucose monitoring, or insulin injections, and she danced, skied, traveled, and sailed. She went to the prom with her peers. She never set foot in the school nurse's office. She was eventually diagnosed with T1D not by clinical presentation with acute metabolic deterioration but through biochemical findings from a glucose tolerance test and free of insulin treatment. The story of the development and FDA approval of teplizumab to treat individuals at high risk of developing T1D, has changed the course of T1D—it is the first approved drug since insulin. The long journey beginning in preclinical studies and the hurdles that were overcome in development before its final approval after 30 years are discussed by Chatenoud et al. (Chapter 20).

We are in a new era for treatment, prevention, and eradication of T1D. Therapies are now more specific and seek immune modulation rather than immune suppression, which makes treatment safer and more acceptable, particularly for children. Finally, we are on the path to replace β cells even in those in whom they have been destroyed.

Jeffrey A. Bluestone
Kevan C. Herold
Lori Sussel

The Pathogenesis of Type 1 Diabetes

Kevan C. Herold[1] and Jeffrey P. Krischer[2]

[1]Departments of Immunobiology and Internal Medicine, Yale University, New Haven, Connecticut 06519, USA
[2]Department of Internal Medicine, University of South Florida, Tampa, Florida 33602, USA
Correspondence: Kevan.herold@yale.edu

Type 1 diabetes (T1D) is a chronic autoimmune disease with a metabolic outcome. Studies over the past decades, have identified the contributions of genetics, environmental factors, and disorders of innate and adaptive immunity that collectively cause β-cell killing. The risk for T1D can be genetically identified but genotypes alone do not identify factors that lead to disease progression. The incidence of T1D has been increasing in the past few decades, which may be due to reduced exposure to infections and other environmental factors that can reduce autoimmunity (hygiene hypothesis). Once initiated, the disease pathogenesis progresses through stages that have been defined on the bases of immunologic (i.e., autoantibodies) and metabolic markers (glucose tolerance). The stages only loosely capture the risk for the time to diagnosis of disease, do not directly reflect disease activity, and there may be variance in the rate of progression within stages. In a general way, the stages can be used to identify patients at risk in whom interventions may be considered to modulate progression. This was achieved with the approval of teplizumab, a humanized anti-CD3 monoclonal antibody, for delaying the diagnosis of T1D.

Over the decades since the discovery of insulin in 1922, there have been many advances in methods to replace insulin and to do so in as near a normal physiologic pattern as possible. These advances have involved new formulations of insulin with kinetics that allow more precise dosing for activity and meals, glucose monitors and continuous glucose monitoring, and delivery of insulin by continuous subcutaneous infusions. However, even when used optimally, they do not fully recapitulate the homeostasis that is achieved with pancreatic β cells, and the majority of patients, particularly children, do not achieve the standards of care that are needed to avoid the long-term complications of the disease (Foster et al. 2019). Moreover, the uptake of these technologies has not been universal and in addition to cost, the need for continuous attention to metabolic management and its imperfections represent a lifelong burden. In addition, there is a cost in human life: For children diagnosed with type 1 diabetes (T1D), there is a 10- to 13-year loss of life expectancy even in Western countries and as much as 49 years elsewhere in the world (Gregory et al. 2022).

Insulitis in the pancreas of patients who died with diabetes was originally described more than 100 years ago. Autoantibodies that recognized the islets of Langerhans in a patient diagnosed

Cite this article as *Cold Spring Harb Perspect Med* doi: 10.1101/cshperspect.a041623

with diabetes mellitus with autoimmune polyendocrine deficiencies suggested an immune cause of these endocrinopathies (Bottazzo et al. 1974). Subsequently, activated cytotoxic T lymphocytes and other immune cells were found infiltrating the pancreas of a 12-year-old who succumbed to new-onset T1D, and indicated an immune mechanism may account for the disease (Bottazzo et al. 1985). Other immune biomarkers of the autoimmune process were identified, including antibodies against the surfaces of β cells, which were ultimately found to recognize glutamic acid decarboxylase 65 (GAD65) (Baekkeskov et al. 1990). In this review, we discuss the increasing incidence of T1D in genetically susceptible individuals and the possible contribution of environmental factors to these rates, often attributed to reduced exposures to infectious agents (i.e., the "hygiene hypothesis"). We then discuss the immunologic basis for the disease beginning with the genetic underpinnings and initiation of autoimmunity. Autoantibodies are the most frequently used biomarkers of autoimmunity, and we present how these serologic and metabolic measures define disease risk. The recognition that T1D is a progressive autoimmune disease has led to the development of clinical studies to intervene prevent the progression. Most recently, this resulted in the approval of teplizumab, a humanized FcR nonbinding anti-CD3ε mAb, for the delay of clinical T1D diagnosis.

TYPE 1 DIABETES IS A CHRONIC AUTOIMMUNE DISEASE THAT OCCURS IN PATIENTS WITH A SUSCEPTIBLE GENETIC BACKGROUND

There are 143 regions of the genome that are associated with susceptibility for T1D, comprising nearly 60 independent candidate genes (Robertson et al. 2021). HLA molecules are the most significant, most likely because of their ability to shape the immune repertoire—more than 90% of patients express HLA-DR3 and/or DR4. The HLA locus accounts for 40%–50% of the familial predisposition. The high-risk HLA-peptide complex is speculated to enable the development of autoreactive diabetogenic T cells and the differentiation of regulatory T cells. In addition to central T-cell tolerance in the thymus, most likely mediated by these HLA genes as well as others such as PTPN22, there are also failures of central B-cell tolerance, which has been identified through the findings of autoreactive B cells (Kinnunen et al. 2013).

Genetic risk scores (GRSs) using microarray chips with defined alleles can improve the prediction of T1D in the general population and relatives of patients. These genetic tools are useful for identifying populations that are at increased risk and those in whom more immunologic and metabolic testing might be considered. The Illumina ImmunoChip for genotyping was shown to improve the prediction of risk for progression in autoantibody + individuals and may, therefore, identify those who should be evaluated more closely with metabolic studies (Redondo et al. 2018a). The GRS may also be useful in evaluating patients from diverse backgrounds and as a first approach for screening the general population (Bonifacio et al. 2018; Oram et al. 2022; Redondo et al. 2024).

There are also several examples of autoimmune diabetes that have developed because of mutations involving single genes that affect immune cell development, regulation, and activation that have suggested disease mechanisms. These examples (e.g., APS-1 or AIRE gene mutations, X-linked neonatal diabetes mellitus, enteropathy and endocrinopathy syndrome [IPEX] and FOXP3 or IL-2 receptor gene mutations, and others) have shown how mutations that affect the development and functions of immune cells can lead to autoimmune diabetes (Anderson et al. 2005; Roth et al. 2018; Chaimowitz et al. 2020). More common polymorphisms (e.g., PTPN22, CTLA-4) may also affect immune cell development and function (Steck and Rewers 2011).

THE INCIDENCE OF T1D HAS BEEN INCREASING SUGGESTING THAT ENVIRONMENTAL FACTORS ARE AT PLAY

Most individuals who develop clinical T1D do not have a relative with the disease. Even among identical twins, the concordance rate is <50% and among the concordant twins, the time of clinical diagnosis varies widely (Redondo et al. 2008; Triolo et al. 2019). The SEARCH for Diabetes in Youth Study has prospectively identified individuals <age 20 with physician-diagnosed T1D. In 2002–2012, the incidence, using 2-year moving averages, increased from 19.5/100,000 to 21.7/100,000 representing an annual increase of 1.8%/year (Mayer-Davis et al. 2017). Modeling studies have projected continued increases. Gregory et al. (2022) suggested that prevalent cases in 2040 will be 60%–107% higher than in 2021 with the greatest increases in resource-limited countries. These projected increased rates suggest that acquired or environmental factors are involved, and there are several potential mechanisms related to responses to infectious agents that may explain these findings (Fig. 1). In a recent study, the relationship between Epstein–Barr virus (EBV) and multiple sclerosis (MS) was postulated to involve a mechanism of cross-reactivity between EBV EBNA1 and GlialCAM (Lanz et al. 2022). Likewise, in a longitudinal analysis, a very strong relationship between EBV infection and MS was found (Bjornevik et al. 2022). Indeed, some observational studies have suggested similar relationships between enteroviruses and T1D (Dotta et al. 2007; Krogvold et al. 2015; Nekoua et al. 2022).

However, infectious agents can also suppress allergic and autoimmune disorders. In 2002, Bach suggested that the increased rates of both autoimmune and allergic diseases are best explained by the decline of infections (i.e., the "hygiene hypothesis") (Bach 2002; Bach and Chatenoud 2012). The inverse relationships between intestinal infections as well as measles, mumps, and rheumatic fever and autoimmune diseases are striking. An illustration of the significant effect of exposure to environmental factors is seen in the rate of autoimmune diabetes among inbred nonobese diabetic (NOD) mice. In this most commonly used inbred murine model of T1D, spontaneous hyperglycemia develops in up to 75% of female mice by 30 weeks of age when the mice are housed in clean environments, whereas with conventional housing the rates rarely exceed 50%. Interestingly, more recent data have highlighted the interactions between

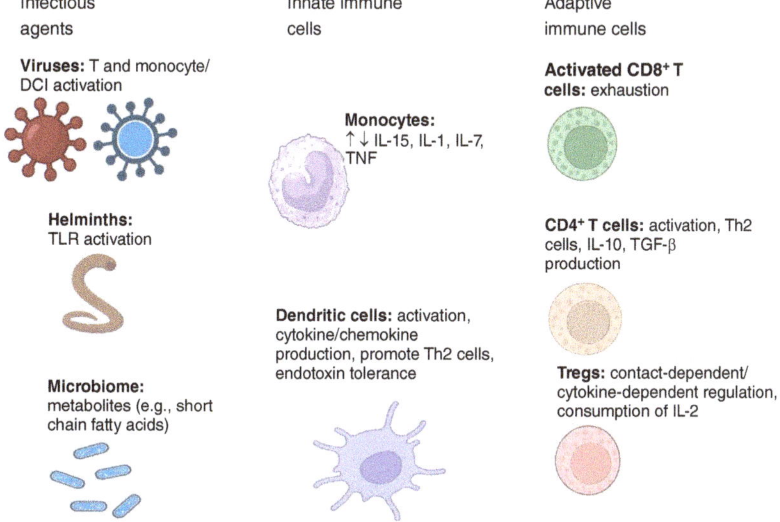

Figure 1. Infectious agents and the hygiene hypothesis. Exposure to viruses, bacteria (including the microbiome), and helminths has been postulated to reduce the development of autoimmune diseases. There are a number of mechanisms that may be involved, including nonspecific activation of T cells after viral exposure, enhancing sex steroid production or short-chain fatty acids that may have direct effects on Tregs, activation of Toll-like receptors (TLRs) by lipopolysaccharide (LPS) that is produced by bacteria or helminths, effects on antigen presentation including stimulation of immune inhibitor ligands such as IL-10 or TGF-β.

environmental factors and innate immune signaling in triggering disease in these mice. MyD88-deficient NOD mice do not develop spontaneous diabetes when housed in a clean specific pathogen-free environment. However, germ-free MyD88-negative NOD mice develop robust diabetes, and colonization of these germ-free MyD88-negative NOD mice with a defined microbial consortium attenuates T1D (Wen et al. 2008). The rate of diabetes is about half in male mice compared to female mice, and a parallel mechanism described how commensal microbes may be responsible for increased serum testosterone that may protect male NOD mice from diabetes. It is also possible that microbiota can produce short-chain fatty acids that can affect Tregs (Brown et al. 2011; Markle et al. 2013; Kim 2018).

Similar examples of the effect of environmental factors have been observed in human communities and provide some insight into causative and protective mechanisms. The TEDDY study was designed to prospectively identify environmental factors that may be associated with progression to T1D by carefully following 8777 genetically at-risk individuals, including offspring of parents with T1D, for the relationship between acquired infections and other exposures and the acquisition of autoantibodies or diagnosis of T1D. Gastrointestinal infections and Norwalk virus exposure in the first year of life were associated with the development of insulin autoantibodies (IAAs); however, the relationship was reversed if infection occurred in the second year of life. Likewise, there was a different transcriptional immune response to enteroviruses in children under the age of 6 years, but not in children who later developed islet autoimmunity (Lin et al. 2023). Other epidemiologic data support a modulating effect of environmental factors such as socioeconomic status, place of residence (across a north/south gradient), childhood infections, sunlight, and pollutants. When comparing the gut microbiome among three genetically similar communities (Finnish, Estonian, and Russian) at the same latitude, the rates of T1D varied five- to sixfold (lowest in Russia, highest in Finland) (Vatanen et al. 2016). The characteristics of the microbiomes differ among these three communities: *Bacteroides dorei* and other Bacteroides species that are highly abundant in Finland and Estonia produce lipopolysaccharide (LPS) that inhibits the immunostimulatory activity of *Escherichia coli* LPS. LPS from *B. dorei* does not protect NOD mice from autoimmune diabetes. These investigators suggest that the LPS from *B. dorei* inhibits the activation of immune cells by LPS from *E. coli* that would otherwise result in "endotoxin tolerance," an older concept that was ascribed to a protein in rabbit sera that could confer tolerance to pyrogenic endotoxin (Kim and Watson 1965). A more recent example suggests how viral infections in humans can establish new immunological set-points that affect future immune responses in an antigen-agnostic manner that are affected by the host's immunologic state. Male individuals who had recovered from COVID-19 had coordinately higher innate, influenza-specific plasmablast, and antibody responses after vaccination compared with healthy male and female individuals who had recovered from COVID-19. The effects of the prior COVID-19 infection were associated with higher IL-15 responses after vaccination and before vaccination, an increased frequency of memory $CD8^+$ T cells (Sparks et al. 2023). Likewise, prior SARS-CoV-2 infection was associated with inflammatory cytokine profiles in patients with tuberculosis (TB) or other respiratory diseases (Cottam et al. 2023) and helminth infections have been ascribed to skewing toward Th2 responses (Méndez-Samperio 2016; Redondo et al. 2018a,b).

DATA FROM ANIMAL MODELS AND CLINICAL STUDIES HAVE DEVELOPED A GENERAL MODEL OF DISEASE PATHOGENESIS FIRST IDENTIFIED IN HUMANS BY THE PRESENCE OF AUTOANTIBODIES AND AUTOANTIGEN REACTIVE T CELLS

Insights into the earliest changes in the pancreas have been based on NOD mouse studies. Single-cell analysis showed that $CD8^+$ and $CD4^+$ T cells infiltrate early and there is a stepwise activation program of resident macrophages that acquire a proinflammatory state (Ferris et al. 2017).

This description of local events, largely dependent on inflammatory macrophages, may contribute to the patchy nature of insulitis that has been observed in animal models and in patients; islets that are heavily infiltrated with immune cells can be found next to islets that are free of inflammatory cells. Other studies have localized changes to the secondary lymph nodes, including antigen presentation and even the differentiation of effector T cells from a stem-like cell pool that then migrates to the islets (Tang et al. 2006; Gearty et al. 2022). The factor(s) that trigger the conversion from stem-like to effector T cells are not clear. They may even be nonspecific, but disease progression may be limited to individuals who harbor an autoreactive repertoire or whose β cells produce inflammatory cytokines and chemokines that can drive recruitment of the immune cells to the islets (e.g., CXCL10) (Christen et al. 2003; Ejrnaes et al. 2005; Rhode et al. 2005).

With the unchecked feedforward cycle of inflammation, there are changes in β cells over time that involve the production of neoantigens such as hybrid peptides, posttranslational modifications, defective ribosomal initiation products (DRIPs), and others (Delong et al. 2016; Kracht et al. 2017; Yang et al. 2022). Therefore, the antigens that are recognized by adaptive immune cells at the diagnosis of T1D may not be those responsible for its initiation. Interestingly, and consistent with the inflammatory events in the pancreas as initiators of islet autoimmunity, it has been observed that the volume of the pancreas may decline during the disease progression (Campbell-Thompson et al. 2019). The basis for this anatomical change has not been identified but could reflect scarring from inflammation, reduced vascular supply, or even involvement of the exocrine pancreas in the local inflammation.

AUTOANTIBODIES SERVE AS BIOMARKERS OF ADAPTIVE AUTOIMMUNITY

Genetic factors identify those at risk for developing autoimmunity and subsequently T1D, but are not useful in identifying the time of initiation or disease process. Because there is only access to peripheral blood in humans, measures of these proposed mechanisms are only possible through the detection of autoantibodies and antigen-reactive T cells in the serum and peripheral blood. Autoreactive $CD4^+$ and $CD8^+$ T cells can be detected in the peripheral blood of patients following the diagnosis of disease but also before diagnosis. These cells are reactive to peptides from autoantigens such as proinsulin, GAD65, IGRP, and others as well as modified peptides, presented by T1D risk alleles (Arif et al. 2004, 2014, 2017, 2022; Gonzalez-Duque et al. 2018; Mitchell et al. 2021). However, there is not a clear threshold that can be used to identify the destructive mechanisms occurring in the pancreas using qualitative and quantitative measurements of autoreactive T cells in the peripheral blood (Arif et al. 2014; Culina et al. 2018; Ogura et al. 2018). Furthermore, the effects of biologics that target T and B cells and inflammatory mediators such as TNF-α in animal models and patients provide strong evidence for the roles of multiple subsets of immune cells in causing the disease progression (Mastrandrea et al. 2009; Jacobsen et al. 2020; Quattrin et al. 2020).

More often, the assessment of autoantibodies is used to predict disease risk. The presence of two or more autoantibodies identifies the initiation of pathogenic autoimmunity and patients who will ultimately develop T1D (Ziegler et al. 2013). These autoantibodies recognize autoantigens that are expressed by β cells. Curiously, the number of different biochemical autoantibodies rather than the titer of the autoantibodies is most closely associated with risk. Individuals in whom only a single autoantibody is detected do not have a higher risk than those with no autoantibodies.

Individuals who have autoantibodies at a younger age are more likely to progress, and progress more rapidly, than older individuals with the same autoantibody profile. The autoantibodies that are first discovered are tempered by age, and increased age at autoantibody detection is inversely related to the rate of progression. Most commonly, the first-appearing autoantibody in young children is IAAs, whereas, after age 5, glutamic acid decarboxylase autoantibodies (GADAs) appear first and the incidence of

IAA-first declines significantly (Fig. 2). The type of the first-appearing autoantibody defines a distinct endotype in terms of genetics (IAA-first associated with DR4, GADA-first associated with DR3), transcriptomics (IAA-first associated with natural killer [NK]-cell expansion not seen in GADA-first) and rates of disease progression (Battaglia et al. 2020).

The incidence of T1D remains constant through the second decade of life and mirrors the incidence of GADA-first autoimmunity. The autoantibodies to IA2 or ZnT8 rarely appear as single antibodies, but the rate of progression from autoimmunity to T1D is markedly higher when they appear with either IAA or GADA.

Using autoantibody detection to identify the risk of diabetes is not without limitations. The autoantibodies are not direct reflections of β-cell killing, and therefore, even when adjusting for the age of detection of autoantibodies, the rate of progression to abnormal glucose tolerance and T1D is highly variable. The autoantibodies may be found for months or even years before deterioration in glucose tolerance. While the modulating effects of age on disease progression are thought to reflect differences in immune responses between younger and older individuals, there may also be age-related differences in β cells between younger and older individuals. For example, stressed β cells have impaired processing of proinsulin and release a disproportionate amount of the prohormone compared to insulin or C-peptide (Sims et al. 2019). The ratio of proinsulin:C-peptide is increased in younger patients at risk for T1D (Sims et al. 2023). Environmental exposures have been associated with conversion to autoantibody positivity. In the TEDDY study, respiratory viruses and enteroviruses were associated with the subsequent risk of autoimmunity ($P < 0.001$) (Lönnrot et al. 2017; Lin et al. 2023). For both environmental exposure and genetics, additional analyses are needed to characterize that risk in terms of diabetes sensitivity and specificity over a defined period or at a defined age. Typically, a marker of high sensitivity has a higher false-positive rate

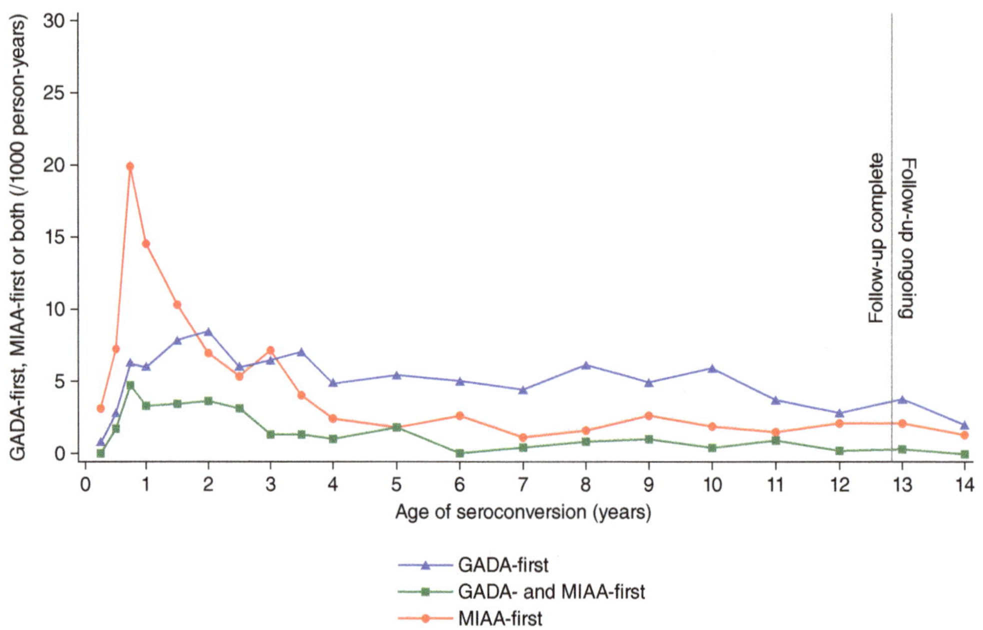

Figure 2. Incidence of islet autoantibody detection by age and type of autoantibody. The data are from the TEDDY study of relatives with and without a diabetes-affected first-degree member in children 0–15 years of age (N= 8776). The autoantibody incidence rate was lower among children without a diabetes-affected family member, but the pattern of appearance was exactly the same.

 Cite this article as *Cold Spring Harb Perspect Med* doi: 10.1101/cshperspect.a041623

(lower specificity), and these factors need to be included in consideration of autoantibody screening strategies and potential interventions to interdict the disease process. Finally, it is worth recognizing that while the presence of multiple autoantibodies has 35%–50% T1D risk over 5 years and overall ~80% over their lifetime, it still means that 50% or more of individuals would not progress during a 5-year treatment period or 20% over their lifetime if left untreated.

Importantly, there are no differences between the risk or rates of progression of first-degree relatives of an individual affected with T1D and individuals with no family history (Ziegler et al. 2020). This finding, based on screening young children in the general population in Bavaria Germany, suggests that the large body of published work in a population of first-degree relatives is generalizable to the general population even though T1D incidence is significantly higher among first-degree relatives. These investigators screened with autoantibodies and found an autoantibody prevalence rate of 0.31% of the 90,632 children. This suggests that general population screening might be considered (Sims et al. 2022). To limit the number of individuals who undergo autoantibody screening, other groups have first screened for T1D risk genotypes and measured autoantibodies in those with the highest GRS.

STAGES OF DIABETES

A practical approach has been adopted to define progression through the prediabetes period into "stages" based on the detection of autoantibodies and metabolic function, which are measurements that can be used in clinical practice (Insel et al. 2015). Those who have two or more biochemical autoantibodies but normal response to an oral glucose tolerance test are classified as having stage 1 T1D. Among relatives with two or more positive autoantibodies, the 5-year progression rate to clinical T1D is 45% (Insel et al. 2015). When there is progression and impairment in glucose tolerance, indicating progressive loss of β-cell function, stage 2 T1D and the risk of progression to clinical T1D is ~50% in 2 years or 75% in 5 years. Of note, the clinical criteria for the definitions of this stage have had different definitions: For purposes of identifying individuals at high risk for the clinical diagnosis of T1D, TrialNet has used fasting, 2 hours, and intermediate glucose levels above the threshold diagnosis during a standard OGTT, whereas the ADA criteria rely on fasting and 2-hour glucose or HbA1c levels (American Diabetes Association Professional Practice Committee 2022). The evidence of the reduced β-cell mass is confirmed from clinical studies that have used these stages as enrollment criteria in prevention trials (Fig. 3). These definitions provided "mile markers" on the road to clinical T1D among those at high risk. They also serve as intermediate endpoints for clinical trials designed to interdict the disease process (Russell et al. 2023).

Stage 3 T1D refers to the fulfillment of the clinical diagnostic criteria for diabetes (American Diabetes Association Professional Practice Committee 2022). Most individuals who present with stage 3 T1D are not identified before their diagnosis and between 30% and 50% of patients present with severe metabolic decompensation —diabetic ketoacidosis (DKA). A clear benefit from identifying those with earlier stages of

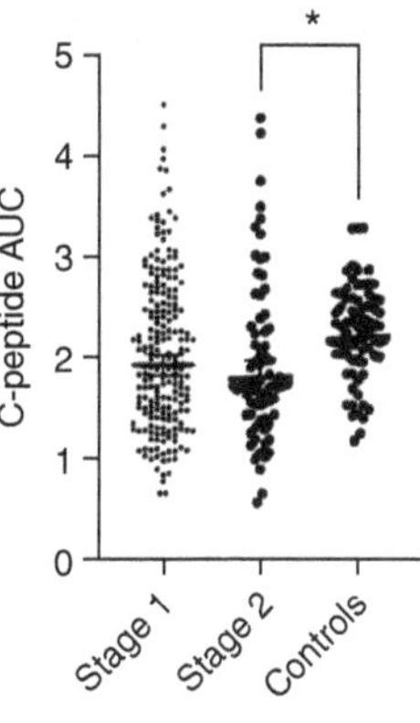

Figure 3. Stimulated C-peptide area under the curve (AUC) to oral glucose tolerance tests in patients with preclinical type 1 diabetes (T1D). Patients enrolled in a trial with stage 1 T1D (from the TrialNet TN18 study), stage 2 T1D (from the TrialNet TN10 study), or matched autoantibody controls underwent OGTTs ($P < 0.05$ by ANOVA). (Figure based on data in Herold et al. 2019 and Russell et al. 2023.)

T1D is the avoidance of DKA, which has a 4.5% mortality (Ramphul and Joynauth 2020).

PROGRESSION OF DIABETES AFTER CLINICAL DIAGNOSIS

Despite the metabolic decompensation that results in the diagnosis, the majority of patients with stage 3 T1D still retain significant levels of endogenous β-cell function (Steele et al. 2004; Greenbaum et al. 2012). Most patients have a stimulated C-peptide level of at least 0.2 pmol/mL, which has been shown to represent a threshold with reduced risk of secondary end-organ complications if the level can be maintained (Palmer et al. 2004).

Provocative tests are used to assess β-cell function. Before the diagnosis, the response is measured during an oral glucose tolerance test by the levels of C-peptide that is cosecreted with insulin by pancreatic β cells. After the clinical diagnosis, a mixed meal tolerance test is more frequently used, which uses a liquid meal with protein and carbohydrate to enhance β-cell responses. Clinical trials generally use the area under the C-peptide response curve as a trackable measure.

For most patients, there is a progressive decline in function over time. In the first 2 years after the diagnosis, this rate has been estimated, from control participants in TrialNet studies, using a mixed meal tolerance test, to be −0.0245 pmol/mL/month (95% CI −0.0271 to −0.0215) in the first 12 months and −0.0079 pmol/mL/month (−0.0113 to −0.0050) in month 12–24 (Greenbaum et al. 2012). As in the prediagnosis period, the rate of decline varies by age and is slower for those >age 21 but with variance across all ages. Overall, at 2 years after diagnosis, 12% of patients ($n = 191$) had <7.5% decline in the stimulated C-peptide response compared to the time of diagnosis. In the Joslin Medalist Study, which is a follow-up of patients with T1D of more than 50-year duration, detectable C-peptide levels were found in 67.4% of patients. However, other studies have confirmed a more universal decline (Keenan et al. 2010). Data from the EDIC trial, that has followed 944 patients from the Diabetes Control and Complications Trial (DCCT) for an average of 35 years, showed that only 1.2% had a stimulated C-peptide level of at least 0.2 pmol/mL. An additional 100 patients (10.5%) had some detectable C-peptide response. Any detectable C-peptide response (i.e., >0.03 pmol/mL) is of clinical value. In the EDIC study, detectable C-peptide was associated with a reduced risk of severe hypoglycemia (adjusted odds ratio = 0.35, $P < 0.0001$) (Gubitosi-Klug et al. 2021). Similar rates of progression and protection from severe hypoglycemia were seen in the Scottish Diabetes Research Network Type 1 Bioresource (SDRNT1BIO) cohort of 6076 people with T1D (Jeyam et al. 2021).

There is little evidence of sustained spontaneous recovery of β cells after the diagnosis with stage 3 T1D. Within weeks after clinical presentation, there may be a transient improvement in β-cell function (i.e., the "honeymoon") but the decline in function then continues in a near-linear manner following a pattern that was established before the clinical diagnosis. With modeling studies, these parameters have been used to predict the loss of C-peptide with time in any individual patient. This quantitative response (QR) can be used to identify early signs of effective therapies and with fewer subjects than with standardized randomized placebo-controlled trials (Bundy et al. 2020; Ylescupidez et al. 2023; Pribitzer et al. 2024). In patients treated with immune therapies, the magnitude of the improvement during the honeymoon is exaggerated but in most cases, a decline follows. At later times after the diagnosis, the improvement in β-cell function is rarely seen although a report of treatment of patients age 25 and ∼1 year after clinical diagnosis with T1D with ATG did show improvement in stimulated C-peptide levels. At 6 months after ATG treatment, there was an 11.3% improvement in the area under the curve (AUC) (Haller et al. 2015).

IMPLICATIONS OF STUDIES ON DISEASE INITIATION AND PROGRESSION FOR CLINICAL STUDIES—STILL MORE WORK TO BE DONE

The recognition that T1D is a progressive disease in which the ongoing process can be identified has opened up the opportunity to intervene before and even after the diagnosis (these studies are described in Tatovic and Dayan 2024). The investigations of disease mechanisms suggest appropriate targets for therapies, but also have identified features that have not been addressed and require consideration for the design of future clinical studies. First, the effects of age and variability even with age adjustment complicate the design of prevention studies and require sample sizes that are larger than those needed to evaluate drug treatment effects in patients with new-onset T1D. For example, in the recently completed trial of abatacept in patients with ≥2+ autoantibodies but without glucose intolerance (i.e., stage 1 T1D, see below) (TN18), the median time to progression to glucose intolerance in the placebo treatment arm ($n = 111$) was 71.5 months but in those that progressed ($n = 45$) the time until glucose intolerance varied widely (range 5.3–100.5 months) (Russell et al. 2023). Even in those who have >2+ autoantibodies and glucose intolerance, the median time to diagnosis with clinical T1D is 27.7 months ($n = 32$) and in those who do progress ($n = 28$), the time varied (range 2.4–85.5 months) (Sims et al. 2021).

Second, by the time that these serologic markers can be identified in the peripheral blood, antigen presentation, and activation of immune cells have been established. Arresting an ongoing activated immune response is more challenging than primary prevention, and it requires intervention in young individuals. Genetic screening alone cannot determine the timing of the initiation of autoimmunity. Therefore, agents to be considered before stage 1 disease need to be safe with extended efficacy.

Third, the finding of endotypes may reflect different disease mechanisms or other features that require a personalized approach to therapies. The TEDDY study has shown that individuals presenting with IAA show an expansion of NK cells, which is not found in those who present with GADA as their first-appearing autoantibody (Krischer et al. 2019). In addition, the B-cell infiltrates that are found more in children than adults and the differences in immunologic markers between endotypes even raise the possibility of a different pathogenic mechanism (Smith et al. 2020). Therefore, not all therapies are likely to be effective in all patients. Identifying the clinical and mechanistic differences among these endotypes is ongoing and may be aided by the analysis of the responses of individuals to immune perturbations by therapies. These investigations may improve the matching of specific agents for individual patients.

Fourth, we do not have a way of measuring the active autoimmune process directly in islets, and, therefore, to date, endpoints have required clinical outcomes that require extended follow-up. As discussed above, autoantibodies are markers of immune priming but themselves do not destroy β cells. Several groups have developed methods for the analysis of antigen-specific T cells and have postulated that these cells can mediate β-cell killing. The effectiveness of anti-T-cell drugs such as teplizumab and ATG supports this contention. The absence of a direct measure of disease activity has practical consequences since T-cell and even other therapies have been shown to be most effective when the disease process is active. If there is reactivation of autoreactive cells, combinations of or even repeated therapies will be needed.

CONCLUSIONS

Data from multiple disciplines over the past four decades that includes preclinical studies in murine models analysis of human samples from blood and from the pancreas at the time of death and results from clinical studies have established T1D as an autoimmune disease leading to metabolic failure of β cells. Genetic studies have identified high risk and other genes that are linked to the disease but the factors that initiate disease in those at genetic risk remain uncertain. The reduced exposure to viral and bacterial infections and improvement in living conditions, particularly among developed countries, are consistent with the central tenet of the "hygiene hypothesis," which suggests that exposure to environmental pathogens may lead to reduced autoimmunity. The chronicity of β-cell killing and multiple targets of the autoimmune response that evolve over time suggest there is a dynamic process between the target (β) and immune cells.

Biologic markers of patients at risk can identify T1D before clinical presentation. The combination of metabolic and immune testing can determine risk, but the actual rate of disease progression and the pathologic activity is not directly measured. Nonetheless, these tools have enabled the approval of the first successful treatment to delay T1D onset in patients at risk with teplizumab.

ACKNOWLEDGMENTS

Supported by grants U01DK106993, R01DK057 846, and R01DK129523.

REFERENCES

Reference is also in this subject collection.

American Diabetes Association Professional Practice Committee. 2022. Classification and diagnosis of diabetes. *Diabetes Care* **45:** S17–S38. doi:10.2337/dc22-S002

Anderson MS, Venanzi ES, Chen Z, Berzins SP, Benoist C, Mathis D. 2005. The cellular mechanism of Aire control of T cell tolerance. *Immunity* **23:** 227–239. doi:10.1016/j.immuni.2005.07.005

Arif S, Tree TI, Astill TP, Tremble JM, Bishop AJ, Dayan CM, Roep BO, Peakman M. 2004. Autoreactive T cell responses show proinflammatory polarization in diabetes but a regulatory phenotype in health. *J Clin Invest* **113:** 451–463. doi:10.1172/JCI19585

Arif S, Leete P, Nguyen V, Marks K, Nor NM, Estorninho M, Kronenberg-Versteeg D, Bingley PJ, Todd JA, Guy C, et al. 2014. Blood and islet phenotypes indicate immunological heterogeneity in type 1 diabetes. *Diabetes* **63:** 3835–3845. doi:10.2337/db14-0365

Arif S, Gibson VB, Nguyen V, Bingley PJ, Todd JA, Guy C, Dunger DB, Dayan CM, Powrie J, Lorenc A, et al. 2017. β-Cell specific T-lymphocyte response has a distinct inflammatory phenotype in children with type 1 diabetes compared with adults. *Diabet Med* **34:** 419–425. doi:10.1111/dme.13153

Arif S, Yusuf N, Domingo-Vila C, Liu YF, Bingley PJ, Peakman M. 2022. Evaluating T cell responses prior to the onset of type 1 diabetes. *Diabet Med* **39:** e14860. doi:10.1111/dme.14860

Bach JF. 2002. The effect of infections on susceptibility to autoimmune and allergic diseases. *N Engl J Med* **347:** 911–920. doi:10.1056/NEJMra020100

Bach JF, Chatenoud L. 2012. The hygiene hypothesis: an explanation for the increased frequency of insulin-dependent diabetes. *Cold Spring Harb Perspect Med* **2:** a007799. doi:10.1101/cshperspect.a007799

Baekkeskov S, Aanstoot HJ, Christgau S, Reetz A, Solimena M, Cascalho M, Folli F, Richter-Olesen H, De Camilli P. 1990. Identification of the 64K autoantigen in insulin-dependent diabetes as the GABA-synthesizing enzyme glutamic acid decarboxylase. *Nature* **347:** 151–156. doi:10.1038/347151a0

Battaglia M, Ahmed S, Anderson MS, Atkinson MA, Becker D, Bingley PJ, Bosi E, Brusko TM, DiMeglio LA, Evans-Molina C, et al. 2020. Introducing the endotype concept to address the challenge of disease heterogeneity in type 1 diabetes. *Diabetes Care* **43:** 5–12. doi:10.2337/dc19-0880

Bjornevik K, Cortese M, Healy BC, Kuhle J, Mina MJ, Leng Y, Elledge SJ, Niebuhr DW, Scher AI, Munger KL, et al. 2022. Longitudinal analysis reveals high prevalence of Epstein–Barr virus associated with multiple sclerosis. *Science* **375:** 296–301. doi:10.1126/science.abj8222

Bonifacio E, Beyerlein A, Hippich M, Winkler C, Vehik K, Weedon MN, Laimighofer M, Hattersley AT, Krumsiek J, Frohnert BI, et al. 2018. Genetic scores to stratify risk of developing multiple islet autoantibodies and type 1 diabetes: a prospective study in children. *PLoS Med* **15:** e1002548. doi:10.1371/journal.pmed.1002548

Bottazzo GF, Florin-Christensen A, Doniach D. 1974. Islet-cell antibodies in diabetes mellitus with autoimmune polyendocrine deficiencies. *Lancet* **304:** 1279–1283. doi:10.1016/S0140-6736(74)90140-8

Bottazzo GF, Dean BM, McNally JM, MacKay EH, Swift PG, Gamble DR. 1985. In situ characterization of autoimmune phenomena and expression of HLA molecules in the pancreas in diabetic insulitis. *N Engl J Med* **313:** 353–360. doi:10.1056/NEJM198508083130604

Brown CT, Davis-Richardson AG, Giongo A, Gano KA, Crabb DB, Mukherjee N, Casella G, Drew JC, Ilonen J, Knip M, et al. 2011. Gut microbiome metagenomics analysis suggests a functional model for the development of autoimmunity for type 1 diabetes. *PLoS ONE* **6:** e25792. doi:10.1371/journal.pone.0025792

Bundy BN, Krischer JP; Type 1 Diabetes TrialNet Study Group. 2020. A quantitative measure of treatment response in recent-onset type 1 diabetes. *Endocrinol Diabetes Metab* **3:** e00143. doi:10.1002/edm2.143

Campbell-Thompson ML, Filipp SL, Grajo JR, Nambam B, Beegle R, Middlebrooks EH, Gurka MJ, Atkinson MA, Schatz DA, Haller MJ. 2019. Relative pancreas volume is reduced in first-degree relatives of patients with type 1 diabetes. *Diabetes Care* **42:** 281–287. doi:10.2337/dc18-1512

Chaimowitz NS, Ebenezer SJ, Hanson IC, Anderson M, Forbes LR. 2020. STAT1 gain of function, type 1 diabetes, and reversal with JAK inhibition. *N Engl J Med* **383:** 1494–1496. doi:10.1056/NEJMc2022226

Christen U, McGavern DB, Luster AD, von Herrath MG, Oldstone MB. 2003. Among CXCR3 chemokines, IFN-γ-inducible protein of 10 kDa (CXC chemokine ligand (CXCL) 10) but not monokine induced by IFN-γ (CXCL9) imprints a pattern for the subsequent development of autoimmune disease. *J Immunol* **171:** 6838–6845. doi:10.4049/jimmunol.171.12.6838

Cottam A, Manneh IL, Gindeh A, Sillah AK, Cham O, Mendy J, Barry A, Coker EG, Daffeh GK, Badjie S, et al. 2023. The impact of prior SARS-CoV-2 infection on host inflammatory cytokine profiles in patients with TB or other respiratory diseases. *Front Immunol* **14:** 1292486. doi:10.3389/fimmu.2023.1292486

Culina S, Lalanne AI, Afonso G, Cerosaletti K, Pinto S, Sebastiani G, Kuranda K, Nigi L, Eugster A, Østerbye T, et al. 2018. Islet-reactive $CD8^+$ T cell frequencies in the pancreas, but not in blood, distinguish type 1 diabetic patients from healthy donors. *Sci Immunol* **3:** eaao4013. doi:10.1126/sciimmunol.aao4013

Delong T, Wiles TA, Baker RL, Bradley B, Barbour G, Reisdorph R, Armstrong M, Powell RL, Reisdorph N, Kumar N, et al. 2016. Pathogenic CD4 T cells in type 1 diabetes recognize epitopes formed by peptide fusion. *Science* **351:** 711–714. doi:10.1126/science.aad2791

Dotta F, Censini S, van Halteren AG, Marselli L, Masini M, Dionisi S, Mosca F, Boggi U, Muda AO, Prato SD, et al. 2007. Coxsackie B4 virus infection of β cells and natural killer cell insulitis in recent-onset type 1 diabetic patients. *Proc Natl Acad Sci* **104:** 5115–5120. doi:10.1073/pnas.0700442104

Ejrnaes M, Videbaek N, Christen U, Cooke A, Michelsen BK, von Herrath M. 2005. Different diabetogenic potential of autoaggressive CD8⁺ clones associated with IFN-γ-inducible protein 10 (CXC chemokine ligand 10) production but not cytokine expression, cytolytic activity, or homing characteristics. *J Immunol* **174:** 2746–2755. doi:10.4049/jimmunol.174.5.2746

Ferris ST, Zakharov PN, Wan X, Calderon B, Artyomov MN, Unanue ER, Carrero JA. 2017. The islet-resident macrophage is in an inflammatory state and senses microbial products in blood. *J Exp Med* **214:** 2369–2385. doi:10.1084/jem.20170074

Foster NC, Beck RW, Miller KM, Clements MA, Rickels MR, DiMeglio LA, Maahs DM, Tamborlane WV, Bergenstal R, Smith E, et al. 2019. State of type 1 diabetes management and outcomes from the T1D exchange in 2016-2018. *Diabetes Technol Ther* **21:** 66–72. doi:10.1089/dia.2018.0384

Gearty SV, Dündar F, Zumbo P, Espinosa-Carrasco G, Shakiba M, Sanchez-Rivera FJ, Socci ND, Trivedi P, Lowe SW, Lauer P, et al. 2022. An autoimmune stem-like CD8 T cell population drives type 1 diabetes. *Nature* **602:** 156–161. doi:10.1038/s41586-021-04248-x

Gonzalez-Duque S, Azoury ME, Colli ML, Afonso G, Turatsinze JV, Nigi L, Lalanne AI, Sebastiani G, Carré A, Pinto S, et al. 2018. Conventional and neo-antigenic peptides presented by β cells are targeted by circulating naïve CD8⁺ T cells in type 1 diabetic and healthy donors. *Cell Metab* **28:** 946–960.e6. doi:10.1016/j.cmet.2018.07.007

Greenbaum CJ, Beam CA, Boulware D, Gitelman SE, Gottlieb PA, Herold KC, Lachin JM, McGee P, Palmer JP, Pescovitz MD, et al. 2012. Fall in C-peptide during first 2 years from diagnosis: evidence of at least two distinct phases from composite type 1 diabetes TrialNet data. *Diabetes* **61:** 2066–2073. doi:10.2337/db11-1538

Gregory GA, Robinson TIG, Linklater SE, Wang F, Colagiuri S, de Beaufort C, Donaghue KC; International Diabetes Federation Diabetes Atlas Type 1 Diabetes in Adults Special Interest Group; Magliano DJ, Maniam J, et al. 2022. Global incidence, prevalence, and mortality of type 1 diabetes in 2021 with projection to 2040: a modelling study. *Lancet Diabetes Endocrinol* **10:** 741–760. doi:10.1016/S2213-8587(22)00218-2

Gubitosi-Klug RA, Braffett BH, Hitt S, Arends V, Uschner D, Jones K, Diminick L, Karger AB, Paterson AD, Roshandel D, et al. 2021. Residual β cell function in long-term type 1 diabetes associates with reduced incidence of hypoglycemia. *J Clin Invest* **131:** e143011. doi:10.1172/JCI143011

Haller MJ, Gitelman SE, Gottlieb PA, Michels AW, Rosenthal SM, Shuster JJ, Zou B, Brusko TM, Hulme MA, Wasserfall CH, et al. 2015. Anti-thymocyte globulin/G-CSF treatment preserves β cell function in patients with established type 1 diabetes. *J Clin Invest* **125:** 448–455. doi:10.1172/JCI78492

Herold KC, Bundy BN, Long SA, Bluestone JA, DiMeglio LA, Dufort MJ, Gitelman SE, Gottlieb PA, Krischer JP, Linsley PS, et al. 2019. An anti-CD3 antibody, teplizumab, in relatives at risk for type 1 diabetes. *N Engl J Med* **381:** 603–613. doi:10.1056/NEJMoa1902226

Insel RA, Dunne JL, Atkinson MA, Chiang JL, Dabelea D, Gottlieb PA, Greenbaum CJ, Herold KC, Krischer JP, Lernmark A, et al. 2015. Staging presymptomatic type 1 diabetes: a scientific statement of JDRF, the Endocrine Society, and the American Diabetes Association. *Diabetes Care* **38:** 1964–1974. doi:10.2337/dc15-1419

Jacobsen LM, Bundy BN, Greco MN, Schatz DA, Atkinson MA, Brusko TM, Mathews CE, Herold KC, Gitelman SE, Krischer JP, et al. 2020. Comparing β cell preservation across clinical trials in recent-onset type 1 diabetes. *Diabetes Technol Ther* **22:** 948–953. doi:10.1089/dia.2020.0305

Jeyam A, Colhoun H, McGurnaghan S, Blackbourn L, McDonald TJ, Palmer CNA, McKnight JA, Strachan MWJ, Patrick AW, Chalmers J, et al. 2021. Clinical impact of residual C-peptide secretion in type 1 diabetes on glycemia and microvascular complications. *Diabetes Care* **44:** 390–398. doi:10.2337/dc20-0567

Keenan HA, Sun JK, Levine J, Doria A, Aiello LP, Eisenbarth G, Bonner-Weir S, King GL. 2010. Residual insulin production and pancreatic β-cell turnover after 50 years of diabetes: Joslin Medalist Study. *Diabetes* **59:** 2846–2853. doi:10.2337/db10-0676

Kim CH. 2018. Microbiota or short-chain fatty acids: which regulates diabetes? *Cell Mol Immunol* **15:** 88–91. doi:10.1038/cmi.2017.57

Kim YB, Watson DW. 1965. Modification of host responses to bacterial endotoxins. II. Passive transfer of immunity to bacterial endotoxin with fractions containing 19S antibodies. *J Exp Med* **121:** 751–759. doi:10.1084/jem.121.5.751

Kinnunen T, Chamberlain N, Morbach H, Cantaert T, Lynch M, Preston-Hurlburt P, Herold KC, Hafler DA, O'Connor KC, Meffre E. 2013. Specific peripheral B cell tolerance defects in patients with multiple sclerosis. *J Clin Invest* **123:** 2737–2741. doi:10.1172/JCI68775

Kracht MJ, van Lummel M, Nikolic T, Joosten AM, Laban S, van der Slik AR, van Veelen PA, Carlotti F, de Koning EJ, Hoeben RC, et al. 2017. Autoimmunity against a defective ribosomal insulin gene product in type 1 diabetes. *Nat Med* **23:** 501–507. doi:10.1038/nm.4289

Krischer JP, Liu X, Vehik K, Akolkar B, Hagopian WA, Rewers MJ, She JX, Toppari J, Ziegler AG, Lernmark A, et al. 2019. Predicting islet cell autoimmunity and type 1 diabetes: an 8-year TEDDY study progress report. *Diabetes Care* **42:** 1051–1060. doi:10.2337/dc18-2282

Krogvold L, Edwin B, Buanes T, Frisk G, Skog O, Anagandula M, Korsgren O, Undlien D, Eike MC, Richardson SJ, et al. 2015. Detection of a low-grade enteroviral infection in the islets of langerhans of living patients newly diagnosed with type 1 diabetes. *Diabetes* **64:** 1682–1687. doi:10.2337/db14-1370

Lanz TV, Brewer RC, Ho PP, Moon JS, Jude KM, Fernandez D, Fernandes RA, Gomez AM, Nadj GS, Bartley CM, et al. 2022. Clonally expanded B cells in multiple sclerosis bind EBV EBNA1 and GlialCAM. *Nature* **603:** 321–327. doi:10.1038/s41586-022-04432-7

Lin J, Moradi E, Salenius K, Lehtipuro S, Häkkinen T, Laiho JE, Oikarinen S, Randelin S, Parikh HM, Krischer JP, et al. 2023. Distinct transcriptomic profiles in children prior to the appearance of type 1 diabetes-linked islet autoantibodies and following enterovirus infection. *Nat Commun* **14:** 7630. doi:10.1038/s41467-023-42763-9

Lönnrot M, Lynch KF, Elding Larsson H, Lernmark A, Rewers MJ, Torn C, Burkhardt BR, Briese T, Hagopian WA, She JX, et al. 2017. Respiratory infections are temporally associated with initiation of type 1 diabetes autoimmunity: the TEDDY study. *Diabetologia* **60:** 1931–1940. doi:10.1007/s00125-017-4365-5

Markle JG, Frank DN, Mortin-Toth S, Robertson CE, Feazel LM, Rolle-Kampczyk U, von Bergen M, McCoy KD, Macpherson AJ, Danska JS. 2013. Sex differences in the gut microbiome drive hormone-dependent regulation of autoimmunity. *Science* **339:** 1084–1088. doi:10.1126/science.1233521

Mastrandrea L, Yu J, Behrens T, Buchlis J, Albini C, Fourtner S, Quattrin T. 2009. Etanercept treatment in children with new-onset type 1 diabetes: pilot randomized, placebo-controlled, double-blind study. *Diabetes Care* **32:** 1244–1249. doi:10.2337/dc09-0054

Mayer-Davis EJ, Lawrence JM, Dabelea D, Divers J, Isom S, Dolan L, Imperatore G, Linder B, Marcovina S, Pettitt DJ, et al. 2017. Incidence trends of type 1 and type 2 diabetes among youths, 2002-2012. *N Engl J Med* **376:** 1419–1429. doi:10.1056/NEJMoa1610187

Méndez-Samperio P. 2016. Molecular events by which dendritic cells promote Th2 immune protection in helmith infection. *Infect Dis (Lond)* **48:** 715–720. doi:10.1080/23744235.2016.1194529

Mitchell AM, Alkanani AA, McDaniel KA, Pyle L, Waugh K, Steck AK, Nakayama M, Yu L, Gottlieb PA, Rewers MJ, et al. 2021. T-cell responses to hybrid insulin peptides prior to type 1 diabetes development. *Proc Natl Acad Sci* **118:** e2019129118. doi:10.1073/pnas.2019129118

Nekoua MP, Alidjinou EK, Hober D. 2022. Persistent coxsackievirus B infection and pathogenesis of type 1 diabetes mellitus. *Nat Rev Endocrinol* **18:** 503–516. doi:10.1038/s41574-022-00688-1

Ogura H, Preston-Hurlburt P, Perdigoto AL, Amodio M, Krishnaswamy S, Clark P, Yu H, Egli D, Fouts A, Steck AK, et al. 2018. Identification and analysis of islet antigen-specific $CD8^+$ T cells with T cell libraries. *J Immunol* **201:** 1662–1670. doi:10.4049/jimmunol.1800267

Oram RA, Sharp SA, Pihoker C, Ferrat L, Imperatore G, Williams A, Redondo MJ, Wagenknecht L, Dolan LM, Lawrence JM, et al. 2022. Utility of diabetes type-specific genetic risk scores for the classification of diabetes type among multiethnic youth. *Diabetes Care* **45:** 1124–1131. doi:10.2337/dc20-2872

Palmer JP, Fleming GA, Greenbaum CJ, Herold KC, Jansa LD, Kolb H, Lachin JM, Polonsky KS, Pozzilli P, Skyler JS, et al. 2004. C-peptide is the appropriate outcome measure for type 1 diabetes clinical trials to preserve β-cell function: report of an ADA workshop, 21-22 October 2001. *Diabetes* **53:** 250–264. doi:10.2337/diabetes.53.1.250

Pribitzer S, O'Rourke C, Ylescupidez A, Smithmyer M, Bender C, Speake C, Lord S, Greenbaum CJ. 2024. Beyond stages: predicting individual time dependent risk for type 1 diabetes. *J Clin Endocrinol Metab* doi:10.1210/clinem/dgae292

Quattrin T, Haller MJ, Steck AK, Felner EI, Li Y, Xia Y, Leu JH, Zoka R, Hedrick JA, Rigby MR, et al. 2020. Golimumab and β-cell function in youth with new-onset type 1 diabetes. *N Engl J Med* **383:** 2007–2017. doi:10.1056/NEJMoa2006136

Ramphul K, Joynauth J. 2020. An update on the incidence and burden of diabetic ketoacidosis in the U.S. *Diabetes Care* **43:** e196–e197. doi:10.2337/dc20-1258

Redondo MJ, Jeffrey J, Fain PR, Eisenbarth GS, Orban T. 2008. Concordance for islet autoimmunity among monozygotic twins. *N Engl J Med* **359:** 2849–2850. doi:10.1056/NEJMc0805398

Redondo MJ, Geyer S, Steck AK, Sharp S, Wentworth JM, Weedon MN, Antinozzi P, Sosenko J, Atkinson M, Pugliese A, et al. 2018a. A type 1 diabetes genetic risk score predicts progression of islet autoimmunity and development of type 1 diabetes in individuals at risk. *Diabetes Care* **41:** 1887–1894. doi:10.2337/dc18-0087

Redondo MJ, Steck AK, Pugliese A. 2018b. Genetics of type 1 diabetes. *Pediatr Diabetes* **19:** 346–353. doi:10.1111/pedi.12597

Redondo MJ, Harrall KK, Glueck DH, Tosur M, Uysal S, Muir A, Atkinson EG, Shapiro MR, Yu L, Winter WE, et al. 2024. Diabetes study of children of diverse ethnicity and race: study design. *Diabetes Metab Res Rev* **40:** e3744. doi:10.1002/dmrr.3744

Rhode A, Pauza ME, Barral AM, Rodrigo E, Oldstone MB, von Herrath MG, Christen U. 2005. Islet-specific expression of CXCL10 causes spontaneous islet infiltration and accelerates diabetes development. *J Immunol* **175:** 3516–3524. doi:10.4049/jimmunol.175.6.3516

Robertson CC, Inshaw JRJ, Onengut-Gumuscu S, Chen WM, Santa Cruz DF, Yang H, Cutler AJ, Crouch DJM, Farber E, Bridges SL, et al. 2021. Fine-mapping, *trans*-ancestral and genomic analyses identify causal variants, cells, genes and drug targets for type 1 diabetes. *Nat Genet* **53:** 962–971. doi:10.1038/s41588-021-00880-5

Roth TL, Puig-Saus C, Yu R, Shifrut E, Carnevale J, Li PJ, Hiatt J, Saco J, Krystofinski P, Li H, et al. 2018. Reprogramming human T cell function and specificity with non-viral genome targeting. *Nature* **559:** 405–409. doi:10.1038/s41586-018-0326-5

Russell WE, Bundy BN, Anderson MS, Cooney LA, Gitelman SE, Goland RS, Gottlieb PA, Greenbaum CJ, Haller MJ, Krischer JP, et al. 2023. Abatacept for delay of type 1 diabetes progression in stage 1 relatives at risk: a randomized, double-masked, controlled trial. *Diabetes Care* **46:** 1005–1013. doi:10.2337/dc22-2200

Sims EK, Bahnson HT, Nyalwidhe J, Haataja L, Davis AK, Speake C, DiMeglio LA, Blum J, Morris MA, Mirmira RG, et al. 2019. Proinsulin secretion is a persistent feature of type 1 diabetes. *Diabetes Care* **42:** 258–264. doi:10.2337/dc17-2625

Sims EK, Bundy BN, Stier K, Serti E, Lim N, Long SA, Geyer SM, Moran A, Greenbaum CJ, Evans-Molina C, et al. 2021. Teplizumab improves and stabilizes β cell function in antibody-positive high-risk individuals. *Sci Transl Med* **13:** eabc8980. doi:10.1126/scitranslmed.abc8980

Sims EK, Besser REJ, Dayan C, Geno Rasmussen C, Greenbaum C, Griffin KJ, Hagopian W, Knip M, Long AE, Martin F, et al. 2022. Screening for type 1 diabetes in the general population: a status report and perspective. *Diabetes* **71:** 610–623. doi:10.2337/dbi20-0054

Sims EK, Geyer SM, Long SA, Herold KC. 2023. High proinsulin:C-peptide ratio identifies individuals with stage 2 type 1 diabetes at high risk for progression to clinical diagnosis and responses to teplizumab treatment. *Diabetologia* **66:** 2283–2291. doi:10.1007/s00125-023-06003-5

Smith MJ, Cambier JC, Gottlieb PA. 2020. Endotypes in T1D: B lymphocytes and early onset. *Curr Opin Endocrinol Diabetes Obes* **27:** 225–230. doi:10.1097/MED.0000000000000547

Sparks R, Lau WW, Liu C, Han KL, Vrindten KL, Sun G, Cox M, Andrews SF, Bansal N, Failla LE, et al. 2023. Influenza vaccination reveals sex dimorphic imprints of prior mild COVID-19. *Nature* **614:** 752–761. doi:10.1038/s41586-022-05670-5

Steck AK, Rewers MJ. 2011. Genetics of type 1 diabetes. *Clin Chem* **57:** 176–185. doi:10.1373/clinchem.2010.148221

Steele C, Hagopian WA, Gitelman S, Masharani U, Cavaghan M, Rother KI, Donaldson D, Harlan DM, Bluestone J, Herold KC. 2004. Insulin secretion in type 1 diabetes. *Diabetes* **53:** 426–433. doi:10.2337/diabetes.53.2.426

Tang Q, Adams JY, Tooley AJ, Bi M, Fife BT, Serra P, Santamaria P, Locksley RM, Krummel MF, Bluestone JA. 2006. Visualizing regulatory T cell control of autoimmune responses in nonobese diabetic mice. *Nat Immunol* **7:** 83–92. doi:10.1038/ni1289

* Tatovic D, Dayan C. 2024. Clinical immunologic interventions for the treatment of type 1 diabetes. *Cold Spring Harb Perspect Med* doi:10.1101/cshperspect.a041597

Triolo TM, Fouts A, Pyle L, Yu L, Gottlieb PA, Steck AK; Type 1 Diabetes TrialNet Study Group. 2019. Identical and nonidentical twins: risk and factors involved in development of islet autoimmunity and type 1 diabetes. *Diabetes Care* **42:** 192–199. doi:10.2337/dc18-0288

Vatanen T, Kostic AD, d'Hennezel E, Siljander H, Franzosa EA, Yassour M, Kolde R, Vlamakis H, Arthur TD, Hämäläinen AM, et al. 2016. Variation in microbiome LPS immunogenicity contributes to autoimmunity in humans. *Cell* **165:** 842–853. doi:10.1016/j.cell.2016.04.007

Wen L, Ley RE, Volchkov PY, Stranges PB, Avanesyan L, Stonebraker AC, Hu C, Wong FS, Szot GL, Bluestone JA, et al. 2008. Innate immunity and intestinal microbiota in the development of type 1 diabetes. *Nature* **455:** 1109–1113. doi:10.1038/nature07336

Yang ML, Horstman S, Gee R, Guyer P, Lam TT, Kanyo J, Perdigoto AL, Speake C, Greenbaum CJ, Callebaut A, et al. 2022. Citrullination of glucokinase is linked to autoimmune diabetes. *Nat Commun* **13:** 1870. doi:10.1038/s41467-022-29512-0

Ylescupidez A, Bahnson HT, O'Rourke C, Lord S, Speake C, Greenbaum CJ. 2023. A standardized metric to enhance clinical trial design and outcome interpretation in type 1 diabetes. *Nat Commun* **14:** 7214. doi:10.1038/s41467-023-42581-z

Ziegler AG, Rewers M, Simell O, Simell T, Lempainen J, Steck A, Winkler C, Ilonen J, Veijola R, Knip M, et al. 2013. Seroconversion to multiple islet autoantibodies and risk of progression to diabetes in children. *J Am Med Assoc* **309:** 2473–2479. doi:10.1001/jama.2013.6285

Ziegler AG, Kick K, Bonifacio E, Haupt F, Hippich M, Dunstheimer D, Lang M, Laub O, Warncke K, Lange K, et al. 2020. Yield of a public health screening of children for islet autoantibodies in Bavaria, Germany. *J Am Med Assoc* **323:** 339–351. doi:10.1001/jama.2019.21565

Environmental Factors in Type 1 Diabetes

Heikki Hyöty,[1,2,3] Jutta E. Laiho,[1] and Suvi M. Virtanen[4,5,6,7]

[1]Faculty of Medicine and Health Technology, Tampere University, Tampere 33520, Finland
[2]Fimlab Laboratories, Tampere 33520, Finland
[3]Department of Pediatrics, Tampere University Hospital, Tampere 33520, Finland
[4]Department of Public Health, Finnish Institute for Health and Welfare, Helsinki FI 00271, Finland
[5]Unit of Health Sciences, Faculty of Social Sciences, Tampere University, Tampere 33520, Finland
[6]Tampere University Hospital, Wellbeing Services County of Pirkanmaa, Tampere 33520, Finland
[7]Center for Child Health Research, Tampere University and Tampere University Hospital, Tampere 33520, Finland

Correspondence: heikki.hyoty@tuni.fi

The contribution of environmental factors to the pathogenesis of type 1 diabetes is considered substantial, but their identification has turned out to be challenging. Large prospective studies are crucial for reliable identification of environmental risk and protective factors. However, only few large prospective birth cohort studies have been carried out. Enterovirus infections have shown quite consistent risk association with the initiation of islet autoimmunity (IA) across these studies. Also, certain dietary factors have been consistently associated with IA risk, omega-3 fatty acids inversely, and childhood cow's milk intake directly. However, the mechanisms of these associations are not fully understood, and possible causality has not been confirmed. Clinical trial programs with enterovirus vaccines and antiviral drugs are in progress to evaluate the causality of enterovirus association. The only nutritional primary prevention randomized trial, TRIGR, did not find a difference between weaning to extensively hydrolyzed versus conventional cow's milk–based infant formula.

While the genetic background of type 1 diabetes (T1D) is well characterized, the environmental triggers of the disease remain unknown. Still, several lines of evidence indirectly suggest that environmental factors play an important role in the disease pathogenesis. This knowledge gap is markedly hindering the understanding of the pathogenetic mechanisms of T1D. The flip side of this fact is that the research on environmental factors offers an opportunity to take an impactful progress leap in the field and to develop preventive and curative treatments for the disease, particularly if some major environmental triggers can be identified. During the last decades, large international research consortia have been established to identify such environmental triggers, and they have already generated some good candidates for fu-

Cite this article as *Cold Spring Harb Perspect Med* doi: 10.1101/cshperspect.a041590

ture research. However, the causality has not yet been proven for any of them. Currently, clinical trials testing the effect of the elimination of the key candidate factors on T1D risk are in progress. Such clinical trials, together with studies on the underlying mechanisms, are now needed for proof or disproof of causality.

EVIDENCE FOR ENVIRONMENTAL INFLUENCE IN TYPE 1 DIABETES

Genetic factors contribute significantly to an individual's susceptibility for T1D. More than 90 different genetic loci modulate the risk (Redondo et al. 2023). Human leukocyte antigen (HLA) genes have the major effect of representing ~50% of the genetic risk. However, only a part of genetically susceptible individuals will develop T1D, and the concordance rate even among identical twins is relatively low (25%–50%) (Lee and Hwang 2019). This has drawn attention to the role of environmental factors, and the identification of factors either decreasing or increasing the disease risk is considered a major goal in the current research landscape. This parallels the ongoing expansion of exposomic research in noncommunicable diseases emphasizing the need to identify the environmental factors that contribute to their pathogenesis (Wild 2012).

The fact that the incidence of T1D has rapidly increased in many countries (DIAMOND Project Group 2006) strongly speaks for the role of the environment since the genetic pool cannot significantly change in such a short time. In parallel, the proportion of T1D patients with the highest HLA-defined genetic risk has decreased suggesting an increasing environmental impact in the pathogenesis of T1D (Hermann et al. 2003). Additional evidence has been obtained from studies showing marked differences in T1D incidence between different populations. For example, Finns have the highest incidence of T1D in the world, and, for example, when compared to the neighboring Karelian population with a similar genetic background, the incidence there is markedly lower (Kondrashova et al. 2013). The Finnish and Karelian children live in contrasting environments, which is reflected by significantly different exposure to many infections (e.g., *Helicobacter pylori*), different composition of gut microbiome, and different gene expression profiles in cord blood.

Overall, the existing evidence clearly points out that the impact of environmental factors is substantial. Assuming that the environmental factors are the main underlying cause of the increasing incidence of T1D, it has been estimated that 80% of T1D could be preventable by actions targeting these environmental factors (Hyöty 2016). Table 1 summarizes the evidence suggesting the role of the environment and the main characteristics of potential environmental risk factors.

Table 1. Role of environmental factors in the pathogenesis of human type 1 diabetes (T1D)

Indicators of environmental influence
Rapid increase in T1D incidence
Low concordance rate in identical twins
Marked difference in T1D incidence between populations with quite similar genetic background
Footprints of causative environmental factors
Common already at early age: important contribution to the marked islet autoimmunity (IA) peak <1 year of age (particularly autoantibodies against insulin [IAA] first autoantibody pattern)
Have been around for decades: the early IA peak has been seen in children studied over the past decades
Common in different populations: the early IA peak occurs in different countries
Impact and penetrance are increasing: both the incidence of T1D and the proportion of patients with lower genetic risk have increased during the past decades
Are not included in the national vaccination programs: even the national vaccination programs with high coverage have not led to a clear decrease in T1D incidence

The Nature of Environmental Factors that Could Modulate the Risk of T1D

Certain chemicals, such as streptozotocin and *N*-3-pyridylmethyl-*N*′-4-nitrophenyl urea (Vacor) rodenticide, and viruses (e.g., encephalomyocarditis virus) selectively damage β cells in rodents leading to diabetes (Yoon 1990). On the other hand, certain infections can prevent or attenuate (Tracy et al. 2010) and dietary factors (e.g., fermentable fibers) strengthen the β-cell damaging process in the NOD mouse model, which spontaneously develops β-cell damage via immunological mechanisms (Toivonen et al. 2014). Even though one of these factors, the rat poison Vacor, has inevitably caused T1D also in humans (Prosser and Karam 1978), the identification of environmental causes of human T1D has turned out to be challenging.

Several reasons have hindered the identification of environmental triggers of T1D (Table 2). One important challenge is that the exposures to some environmental factors such as infections may last only a few days and occur long before T1D, making them difficult to trace at the time when T1D is diagnosed. Also, the critical exposure period in relation to the onset of the disease process is unknown. The incidence of islet autoantibody seroconversion peaks already at the age of 1–3 years (Krischer et al. 2015; Mikk et al. 2020), suggesting that in many cases these exposures happen early in life and possibly already in utero. The complexity is further increased by the fact that the time from the autoantibody appearance to the diagnosis of T1D varies greatly, ranging from some weeks to even decades. Both risk and protective factors may exist, and they may have interactions with each other that are difficult to explore. There can also be a major necessary risk factor (necessary cause of T1D) or sufficient risk factors that can cause the disease but can be replaced by other risk, protective, or modulating factors (Fig. 1). Critical risk factors may be common, but with a low penetrance. This is the case when almost everyone is exposed but only a fraction of the exposed develops T1D. Critical risk factors may also be rare but with a high penetrance when a higher proportion of those exposed will develop T1D. In the case where the causative factor is so common that almost everyone is exposed, its identification is extremely difficult in observation studies due to the lack of a representative control group. A good example comes from the case of celiac disease and its causative factor. The role of gluten was discovered during World War II in the Netherlands when people suffering from celiac disease–related symptoms experienced an improvement in their disease (van Berge-Henegouwen and Mulder 1993). Once the war was over their symptoms reappeared. This was related to the unintended intervention (wheat consumption decreased dramatically during World War II) that led to the identification of gluten as a causative factor of celiac disease. In normal conditions, almost everyone is exposed to gluten and this association would have remained unidentified in case-control studies.

This complexity is further increased if environmental triggers interact with T1D risk genes. For example, *IFIH1* codes for an innate immune system receptor that recognizes nucleic acids of

Table 2. Challenges in the identification of environmental causes of type 1 diabetes (T1D)

T1D is relatively rare and therefore large sample sizes and long follow-ups are needed in prospective etiological studies making them expensive
Critical exposure periods and lag times to the outcomes are largely unknown with the exception that at least one significant exposure period exists early in life (before the age of 1 year, including the in utero period)
Several risk and protective factors may exist, and they may have mutual interactions and interactions with host genes, making the identification of the true causal factor(s) challenging
Possible effect of confounding factors is difficult to eliminate even in large prospective observational studies
Intervention trials are needed to obtain a final proof for causality; these are expensive and it takes a long time to document the effect of intervention on islet autoimmunity (IA) or T1D risk

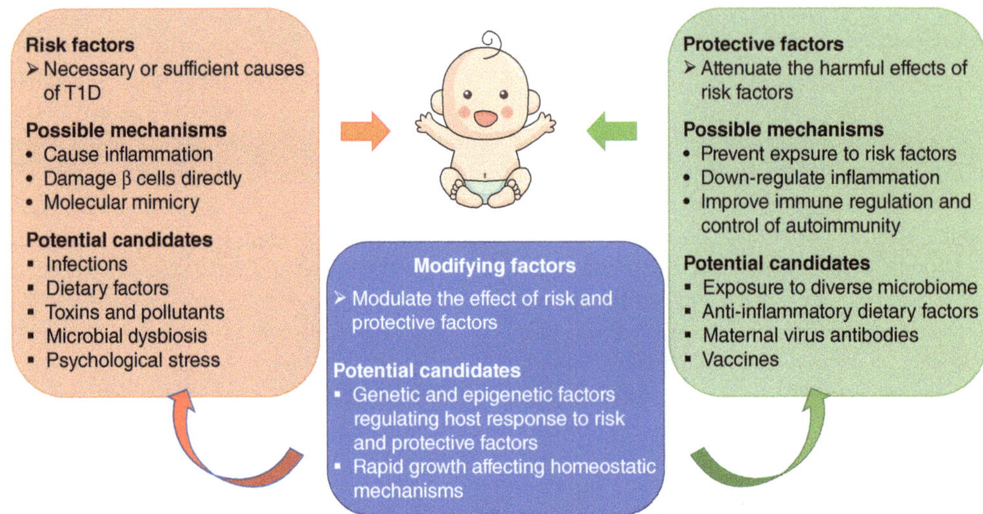

Figure 1. The balance between risk and protective factors determines the risk of type 1 diabetes (T1D). These factors can have complex mutual interactions, which creates a challenge for studies aiming at the identification of the causative risk factors. The elimination of such risk factors would offer an opportunity to develop efficient prevention of T1D as shown in other chronic diseases (e.g., prevention of cervical cancer by papillomavirus vaccine).

enterovirus, one possible risk factor for T1D. T1D-associated *IFIH1* single-nucleotide polymorphisms (SNPs) have been associated with the presence of enterovirus in white blood cells (Sioofy-Khojine et al. 2022) and with the intensity of innate immune system activation during the infection (Domsgen et al. 2016; Gorman et al. 2017). Also, other T1D risk genes (e.g., *CXADR*, *FUT2*, and *TYK2*) are known to modulate the course of virus infections (Blanter et al. 2019). Other examples include certain polymorphisms in vitamin D receptor modifying the association between vitamin D and the appearance of islet autoimmunity (IA) (Norris et al. 2018).

In summary, individual combinations of exposures to both risk and protective environmental factors and their interactions with the host genetic background contribute to the risk of T1D (Fig. 1). In other words, exposure to a risk factor may not lead to T1D in those individuals who have been exposed to protective environmental factors and/or who have a protective genetic setup. For example, these "protective" signatures may include efficient regulation of harmful immune responses that can be induced by the triggering agents in susceptible individuals or specific mutations in receptor molecules that mediate the effects of environmental factors.

Candidate Environmental Factors in Human T1D

Several environmental factors have been reported to be associated with T1D but only few of them have repeatedly shown this association in large-scale prospective studies carried out in different populations. About 30 years ago, cow's milk proteins were suggested as triggers since early exposure to these proteins and short breastfeeding were found to be associated with T1D (Virtanen et al. 1991; Åkerblom et al. 1993). Increased antibody levels against cow's milk proteins were found in subjects with T1D in case-control design studies. Also, investigations in animal models of immune-mediated diabetes supported the hypothesis. The evidence was compelling enough to start a large international double-blind randomized clinical trial (trial to reduce insulin-dependent diabetes mellitus in the genetically at risk [TRIGR] study) to evaluate whether the use of extensively hydrolyzed infant formula as compared to conventional cow's milk–based formula during the first 6–8 months of life could reduce the risk of T1D. The intervention showed that the risk of IA or T1D did not differ between children weaned to hydrolysate and conventional formula (Knip et al. 2014; Writing Group for the TRIGR Study Group et al. 2018). The TRIGR study pointed out the importance of well-designed rigid intervention trials in the evaluation of the causal role of environmental factors that have been associated with T1D in observational studies. Several prospective cohort studies including TRIGR suggest a direct link between cow's milk consumption during childhood and the risk of IA and T1D (Virtanen et al. 1998; Lampousi et al. 2021; Niinistö et al. 2024), suggesting that there can be some yet unidentified risk-modifying factors that link to cow's milk exposure. Milk processing seems not to play a major role (Koivusaari et al. 2020). In TRIGR trials, cow's milk antibody levels in cord blood and early childhood were directly associated with IA and T1D risk (Niinistö et al. 2024).

Currently, enteroviruses are among the main candidates for environmental risk factors of T1D. Infections with these viruses have been repeatedly connected with T1D in large prospective cohorts in children with genetically increased risk of T1D or studies carried on pancreas tissue (Foulis et al. 1990; Richardson et al. 2009; Krogvold et al. 2015; Hyöty 2016; Vehik et al. 2019). Another important group of candidates possibly protecting from islet immunity are omega-3 fatty acids (Norris et al. 2007; Niinistö et al. 2017, 2021; Díaz Ludovico et al. 2023; Hakola et al. 2023). In addition, active research is currently focusing on other virus infections (e.g., SARS-CoV-2, gastroenteritis), exposures to certain dietary compounds (e.g., probiotics, vitamins C and D, gluten-containing cereals, oats, dietary fibers, fruits, berries, vegetables) (Mattila et al. 2020, 2021, 2024; Lampousi et al. 2021), environmental toxicants (e.g., endocrine disruptors), metabolic activity of microbiome, psychological stress, lack of mobility, rapid growth, and weight gain (Nucci et al. 2021).

Recently, several reports have suggested an increase in T1D incidence during the COVID-19 pandemic. These findings are based on the analysis of T1D incidence before and during the pandemic (Zhang et al. 2022; Kashfi et al. 2023). It has also been shown that SARS-CoV-2 can spread to the pancreas and infect both endocrine and exocrine cells (Wang et al. 2023; Poma et al. 2024). Only one prospective study where SARS-CoV-2 infections have been diagnosed by laboratory assays has been published—it showed no association between SARS-CoV-2 infections and the development of IA or T1D (Krischer et al. 2023). One recent study suggested that the observed increase in T1D incidence could be a consequence of lockdown and physical distancing rather than a direct effect of SARS-CoV-2 infection (Knip et al. 2023)—the dramatic decrease in common infections during the lockdown period may have changed the balance of the immune system favoring the progression of IA to T1D.

The existing evidence and ongoing research on these factors are described below, focusing particularly on virus infections and dietary factors.

THE IMPORTANCE OF PROSPECTIVE STUDIES

Large prospective cohort studies play a key role in the identification of environmental factors that are associated with increased or decreased risk of T1D. The international TEDDY study and the Finnish Diabetes Prediction and Prevention (DIPP) study are the largest birth cohort studies carried out so far to evaluate the etiopathogenesis of T1D. Other prospective studies include DAISY, TRIGR, ENDIA, MIDIA, and BabyDiab. The main findings on the role of environmental factors in these prospective studies are summarized below.

The TEDDY Study

The Environmental Determinants of Diabetes in the Young (TEDDY) study has been designed to identify environmental factors that could play a role in the pathogenesis of T1D (TEDDY Study

Group 2007). It is a prospective birth-cohort study, which has screened newborn infants for HLA alleles that confer increased risk for T1D in three study sites in the United States and in three study sites in Europe since 2004. The children with increased genetic risk were invited to a follow-up that begins at the age of 3 months and lasts until the age of 15 years. More than 8667 children have been in the follow-up and, so far, 451 have developed clinical stage 3 T1D, and 522 have turned persistently positive for multiple islet autoantibodies (stage 1 T1D). Study end points include the development of persistent confirmed IA defined by the appearance of at least one biochemical islet autoantibody and clinical T1D. A comprehensive series of blood, stool, and other biological samples as well as questionnaire data have been collected every 3–6 months during the follow-up allowing detailed analyses of the role of environmental factors in the initiation of IA and in its progression to different stages of T1D (stages 1–3 of T1D).

The TEDDY study has used a wide panel of technologies to identify various kinds of exposures and correlated them with the risk of developing IA and T1D. This includes detailed questionnaires about infections, medications, dietary factors, and psychological stress, as well as detailed genotyping of study participants by ImmunoChip and TEDDY-T1D ExomChip. Childhood diet was assessed by 3 days of food records at 3- to 6-month intervals. The food composition databases that were used in the food data processing were harmonized for foods and nutrients (Uusitalo et al. 2013; Joslowski et al. 2017). Infections have been recorded by detailed questionnaires and classified using the international ICD10 coding system (Lönnrot et al. 2015). In addition, TEDDY has carried out several nested case-control studies for both study end points using various biomarkers and different omics technologies and analyzed the whole microbiome (bacteriome, fungi, and virome) from stool and other samples (Rewers et al. 2018).

Infectious Agents in the TEDDY Study

One of the main findings of TEDDY has been the association between enterovirus infections and the appearance of IA by analyzing the virome of longitudinal stool samples. Out of the 621 different viral taxa representing 96 genera of known eukaryotic viruses and 57 genera of bacteriophage, enteroviruses belonging to *Enterovirus B* species were associated with an increased risk of IA (Vehik et al. 2019). Even though this association has already been documented in previous studies, the TEDDY study found that IA-associated enterovirus infections were prolonged, suggesting that the clearance of infections was delayed. This fits with previous observations, indicating that a low-grade persisting enterovirus infection in the pancreatic islets may contribute to the development of T1D (Lloyd et al. 2022; Nekoua et al. 2022). In addition to enteroviruses, TEDDY virome analyses showed that some other viruses are associated with IA. Adenovirus C infections (species C causing respiratory illness) before the age of 6 months were associated with a decreased risk of IA, whereas with Adenovirus F (species F causing gastroenteritis), the number of positive samples showed a weak increased risk for IA. Certain Adenovirus C and Enterovirus B (coxsackie B viruses [CVBs]) viruses use the same receptor (coxsackie and adenovirus receptor [CAR]), which may result in competition in receptor binding and explain the protective effect of Adenovirus C. Questionnaire data showed that febrile common cold–type respiratory infections were associated with increased risk of IA (Lönnrot et al. 2017). This could link to the risk association between Enterovirus B and IA since the common cold is the most frequent symptom of Enterovirus B infections. In addition, gastroenteritis either increased or decreased the risk of IA, depending on the age of infection and type of first appearing autoantibody, and this phenomenon correlated with the detection of norovirus in the stools (Lönnrot et al. 2023). TEDDY was among the first studies showing that the autoantigen specificity of the first appearing autoantibodies can distinguish two subtypes of T1D, which are characterized by a different genetic background and the age when the IA begins. Enterovirus was mainly associated with IA, which begins with the appearance of autoantibodies against insulin (IAA) (first subtype) (Lernmark et al. 2023), which is in line with previous findings from the

DIPP study (see DIPP study below). Bacteriome was characterized by 16S sequencing and fungal populations by ITS2 sequencing from stool samples. The microbiome maturated gradually by the age of 30 months after which it reached a stable phase. Receipt of breast milk was the most significant factor associated with the microbiome structure. Birth mode, geographical location, and presence of siblings and furry pets at home also influenced the microbiome. Although some interesting trends were seen, the abundance or diversity of different bacterial or fungal species showed no clear T1D-associated patterns (Stewart et al. 2018; Auchtung et al. 2022). However, the microbiomes of control children contained more genes that were related to the production of short-chain fatty acids that have been shown to have anti-inflammatory properties (Vatanen et al. 2018). Cesarean section was found to increase slightly the progression of IA to T1D (Singh et al. 2024) being in line with the previously reported modest association between cesarean section and T1D (Stene and Gale 2013). On the other hand, antibiotic use was not associated with IA (Kemppainen et al. 2017).

The analysis of SARS-CoV-2 antibodies in the TEDDY cohort showed no association between SARS-CoV-2 infections and the appearance of IA or T1D (Krischer et al. 2023). However, TEDDY was able to study this association only among relatively old children (teens) as the recruitment to the study occurred during 2004–2010, long before the pandemic. Thus, prospective studies that have followed young children through the pandemic are clearly needed to get the final answer.

In conclusion, the findings from the TEDDY study support previous studies showing an association between enterovirus infections and initiation of IA. In addition, the TEDDY study identified adenoviruses and noroviruses as potential new T1D-associated agents.

Dietary Factors in the TEDDY Study

TEDDY has shown for the first time in a prospective setting that early probiotic supplementation and plasma ascorbic acid concentration during childhood are associated with decreased (Uusitalo et al. 2016; Mattila et al. 2020) and protein intake with increased risk of IA (Aronsson et al. 2023). Interestingly, the inverse association of probiotics with IA was only seen among genetically high-risk children. Association of plasma ascorbate with IA was observed particularly for the IAA first outcome and that of protein intake with GADA first.

TEDDY suggests that higher vitamin D status may protect from IA, particularly in children with certain vitamin D receptor genotypes (Norris et al. 2018). Erythrocyte omega-3 fatty acid, eicosapentaenoic acid (EPA) and docosapentaenoic acid (DPA), status in infancy and that of conjugated linoleic acid in childhood were associated with lower and some saturated and monounsaturated fatty acids with higher risk of IA (Niinistö et al. 2017). In line with the previous findings (Niinistö et al. 2017), omega-3 polyunsaturated fatty acids may protect particularly from the development of insulin autoimmunity. Of note is that α-linolenic acid (ALA) and linolic acid (LA) status were inversely associated with IA in non-breastfed children only.

Higher energy intake is associated with a higher body mass index, which in turn is associated with the development of IA. Protein intake showed a direct association with GADA development (Aronsson et al. 2023). Child's higher intake of pyridoxine and vitamin B_{12} was associated with a decreased risk of IAA first and that of riboflavin with an increased risk of GADA first (Hakola et al. 2024). Iron intake's association with IAA first was modified with gene variants affecting iron absorption and cellular release while a U-shaped relationship was seen between iron intake and GADA first (Thorsen et al. 2023).

TEDDY findings suggest that the introduction of gluten to children older than 9 months of age as compared to younger age is associated with an increased risk of IA and IAA (Uusitalo et al. 2018). In TEDDY we also found that early probiotic exposure modified the association between infant feeding and IA so that early introduction of solid foods was associated with IAA first and multiple autoantibodies solely among children with the highest genetic risk and no probiotic exposure (Uusitalo et al. 2023). The introduction of extensively hydrolyzed infant formula before the age of 7 days as compared to non-hydrolyzed cow's milk–based formula showed an increased risk of IA (Hummel et al. 2017). Weight z-score at 12 months was associated with an increased risk of IA and IAA and GADA first.

In conclusion, TEDDY has found novel dietary candidates for the development of IA, diet–gene interactions, and associations between dietary factors and different disease subtypes.

The DIPP Study

The Finnish Diabetes Prediction and Prevention (DIPP) study screens newborn infants for HLA-defined genetic susceptibility for T1D in three centers in Finland and invites children with increased risk to a prospective observation beginning from birth. The study began in 1994 and is still recruiting. More than 24,000 children have participated in the follow-up, and >1500 have developed IA and >600 have developed T1D. Questionnaire data and blood and hair samples have been collected every 3–12 months (including cord blood) and stool samples monthly. In addition, an asthma and allergy study was performed at the age of 5, and maternal first trimester pregnancy serum is available through the Finnish biobank system. DIPP study has carried out several studies on the possible role of environmental factors in the pathogenesis of T1D focusing particularly on infections, microbiome, and dietary factors.

Infectious Agents in the DIPP Study

One of the most important research lines deals with virus infections. DIPP has carried out virome-wide sequence analyses from stool samples and diagnosed specific virus infections using polymerase chain reaction (PCR) and serology. The main observation has been the association between enterovirus infections, particularly coxsackie B group infections, and initiation of IA (Hyöty 2016). This association has been found in a series of studies based on the detection of enterovirus RNA from stool, peripheral blood mononuclear cells (PBMCs), and serum, and by analyzing enterovirus antibodies from serum (Honkanen et al. 2017). This association is linked to postnatal infections that preceded the appearance of IA. A large systematic screening of neutralizing antibodies against >40 different enterovirus types suggested that particularly coxsackie B serotypes modulated the risk of IA (Laitinen et al. 2014). Interestingly, also enterovirus infections during pregnancy showed a risk association suggesting that in some cases in utero exposures could already play a role (Viskari et al. 2012). DIPP study also made a new discovery suggesting that CVB infections are associated particularly with one main subtype of T1D, which is characterized by the appearance of autoantibodies against insulin as the first sign of β-cell autoimmunity (Sioofy-Khojine et al. 2018). This subtype differs from the other T1D subtype, characterized by the appearance of autoantibodies first against GAD65, for the predisposing HLA alleles (HLA-DR4 vs. HLA-DR3) and other susceptibility genes as well as the age of autoantibody seroconversion (IAA seroconversions already show a sharp peak at the age of 6–9 months while GADA seroconversions appear later with no clear age-related peaks). These differences suggest that different pathogenetic paths lead to these two T1D subtypes and CVBs may contribute particularly to the IAA first subtype. In addition, the DIPP study found a tendency for more frequent prolonged enterovirus infections in children who later developed IA than in control children (Honkanen et al. 2017), a phenomenon that was discovered in the TEDDY study (see above). Other tested viruses, including rotavirus, respiratory syncytial virus, influenza A virus, cytomegalovirus (CMV), and adenovirus were not associated with initiation of IA (Lempainen et al. 2012) but early CMV infection was associated with slower progression of IA to T1D.

Some changes were observed in the composition of gut bacteriome (e.g., abundance of *Bacteroides dorei* and *vulgatus*) in children who developed IA compared to control children, but the results varied between the two studies done, and further studies are needed to understand the significance of these changes (Davis-Richardson et al. 2014). Interestingly, children who had an indoor dog at home had a decreased risk of IA and T1D, suggesting that exposure to an environmental microbiome could play a role in T1D (Virtanen et al. 2014). This was also supported by a study that was based on satellite data, showing that DIPP children whose homes were located in agricultural environments had a decreased risk of IA and T1D (Nurminen et al. 2021). These results are in line with the biodiversity hypothesis suggesting that the exposure to environmental microbial biodiversity can improve the regulation of the immune system and decrease the risk of immune-mediated diseases (Haahtela et al. 2021).

In summary, the DIPP study was the first prospective study showing an association between enterovirus infections and initiation of IA. This finding contributed to the expansion of studies addressing the role of viruses in T1D and to the ongoing development of a new vaccine against T1D-associated enterovirus types (Hyöty et al. 2018; Dunne et al. 2019).

Dietary Factors in the DIPP Study

DIPP study has analyzed maternal diet during pregnancy and lactation by a validated food frequency questionnaire (Erkkola et al. 2001) and child's diet with repeated 3-day food records and structured questionnaires. Food record data corresponded well with biomarker measurements (Uusitalo et al. 2013; Prasad et al. 2018). Consumption of certain food items during pregnancy was associated with the risk of IA or T1D in the offspring: low-fat margarines, berries, and coffee were inversely associated with the development of IA (Virtanen et al. 2011), and fresh milk and cheese with T1D, while the consumption of sour milk was associated with increased disease risk (Niinistö et al. 2014). During lactation, maternal consumption of red meat and meat products was associated with an increased risk of IA and T1D and vegetable oils with an increased risk of IA (Niinistö et al. 2015). No conclusive associations between maternal fatty acid intake and risk of IA/T1D in the offspring were found during pregnancy or lactation (Niinistö et al. 2014, 2015). Maternal intake of gluten-containing cereals, oats, gluten, and dietary fiber during pregnancy or lactation was not associated with IA or T1D (Hakola et al. 2024). This contradicts the findings from the Danish birth cohort, where gluten intake was associated with an increased risk of T1D (Antvorskov et al. 2018). No relationships were found between the intake of several antioxidant vitamins and minerals during pregnancy and the risk of IA in the offspring (Uusitalo et al. 2008b). Neither was maternal vitamin D intake during pregnancy associated with child's IA or T1D (Marjamäki et al. 2010). Maternal iron, nitrate, or nitrite intake during pregnancy was not related to the risk of IA or T1D (Mattila et al. 2020, 2021).

Breastfeeding has been inconsistently associated with IA/T1D (Lampousi et al. 2021). In the DIPP study, breastfeeding showed an inverse relationship with the risk of IA (particularly IAA first subtype) (Niinistö et al. 2017). In line with this, the early age at introduction of solid foods was associated with an increased risk of IA (Hakola et al. 2018). The mechanism of possible protective effect of breastfeeding is not known. It could be mediated by multiple factors including maternal virus antibodies in breast milk, which can protect the child from infections, and cytokines, which can modulate the child's immune system, effect on microbiota, or diminished exposure to other foods.

The analyses of food consumption in childhood showed that cruciferous vegetables and berries associate inversely, while dairy products, gluten-containing cereals (wheat, rye), oats, and fruits associate directly with the risk of IA, T1D, and/or progression from IA to T1D (Hakola et al. 2019; Syrjälä et al. 2019; Koivusaari et al. 2020; Mattila et al. 2024). Also, fish and meat intake showed weak inverse and direct associations with IA, respectively (Syrjälä et al. 2019). In addition, total fat, monounsaturated fatty acid, and omega-3 fatty acid intake were inversely associated with IA (Hakola et al. 2023). In line with this, the analysis of child's serum fatty acid concentrations revealed that several polyunsaturated omega-3 fatty acids were inversely associated with IAA first outcome (Niinistö et al. 2017). Polyunsaturated docosahexaenoic acid showed also an inverse association with IA but only among non-breastfed children (Niinistö et al. 2017). Serum palmitoleic, *cis*-vaccenic

Table 3. Summary of findings from prospective studies on the possible role of environmental factors in the pathogenesis of type 1 diabetes (T1D)

	Prospective cohort						
	DIPP	TEDDY	TRIGR	DiMe sibling cohort	DAISY	MIDIA	BabyDiab and Babydiet
Study design	Birth cohort with increased human leukocyte antigen (HLA)-conferred genetic risk for T1D in Finland and case-control series nested within the cohort	Birth cohort with increased HLA-conferred genetic risk for T1D in four countries and case-control series nested within the cohort	Birth cohort with increased HLA-conferred genetic risk of T1D, first-degree relatives with T1D in 15 countries, and case-control series nested within the cohort	Follow-up cohort of siblings of T1D patients in Finland and case-control series within the cohort	Cohort of children with increased genetic risk of T1D and a case-cohort nested within the cohort	Birth cohort with increased HLA-conferred genetic risk for T1D in Norway and case-control series nested within the cohort	Birth cohorts with increased HLA-conferred genetic risk of T1D, first-degree relatives with T1D in Germany, and nested case-control series nested within the cohort
Enterovirus	Series of studies; risk association with islet autoimmunity (IA) found by serology and virus detection in serum, peripheral blood mononuclear cells (PBMCs) and stools	Risk association with IA found by analyzing the whole stool virome; prolonged infections a risk factor	Risk association with IA found by serology	Risk association with IA and T1D found by serology and virus detection in serum	Risk association with progression of IA to T1D found by virus detection in serum	Risk trend with IA found by virus detection in blood but reversed causality possible	No association found with IA by serology or virus detection in stools

Continued

Table 3. *Continued*

	Prospective cohort						
	DIPP	TEDDY	TRIGR	DiMe sibling cohort	DAISY	MIDIA	BabyDiab and Babydiet
Omega-3 fatty acids	Child's total omega-3 fatty acid intake associated with decreased IA risk; serum DHA at 3 months of age associated with decreased IA risk; serum eicosapentaenoic acid (EPA) at 3 and 6 months and DHA at 6 months associated with decreased and serum α-linolenic acid (ALA) at 3 months with increased IAA first risk	Erythrocyte EPA and DHA at 3 months of age-associated decreased risk of IA	Cord blood DPA associated with decreased IA risk		Omega-3 fatty acid intake and erythrocyte content associated with decreased risk of IA		
Dairy consumption	Higher dairy intake associated with increased IA risk		Frequent milk consumption after infancy associated with an increased risk of IA and T1D	Higher milk intake associated with increased IA and T1D risk	Higher cow's milk protein intake associated with increased IA risk in children with low/moderate risk HLA-DR genotypes and with progression from IA to T1D		

See the text for references.

(DIPP) Diabetes Prediction and Prevention, (TEDDY) The Environmental Determinants of Diabetes in the Young, (TRIGR) trial to reduce insulin-dependent diabetes mellitus in the genetically at risk, (DiMe) Childhood Diabetes in Finland, (DAISY) Diabetes Autoimmunity Study in the Young, (MIDIA) Environmental Triggers of Type 1 Diabetes.

acid, and pentadecanoic acid levels were also associated with decreased risk of IA (Niinistö et al. 2017). Direct associations were detected with some saturated fatty acids in childhood (Virtanen et al. 2010; Niinistö et al. 2017). Serum α- and γ-tocopherol (Uusitalo et al. 2008a) and carotenoid concentrations (Prasad et al. 2011) were not associated with IA. Child's vitamin D status at birth or in childhood was not associated with IA or T1D in the DIPP study (Mäkinen et al. 2016, 2019). In DIPP, higher fecal human β-defensin-2 (HBD2) at 1 year of age was associated with IA risk. Interestingly, child's dietary higher fat intake and lower dietary fiber, potassium, and magnesium intake were related to higher HBD2 (Salo et al. 2024).

Omega-3 fatty acids have immunological effects and may, for example, reduce inflammation or improve protection against infections, which could explain their inverse association with IA (Hakola et al. 2022). TRIGR findings also indicate that fatty acids may have immunomodulatory potential in the early phase of disease development (Niinistö et al. 2022).

To conclude, DIPP has produced several novel dietary risk and protective candidates for IA and T1D. Several nutritionally important foods in young child's diet such as cow's milk, cereals, and fruits have been linked to increased and cruciferous vegetables and berries with decreased risk of IA/T1D and warrant confirmation or rejection by other studies. Environmental chemical exposures could be one common denominator for milk, cereals, and fruits, as well as for dietary fiber.

Conclusion from Prospective Studies

The largest prospective studies (DIPP and TEDDY) have identified certain viruses and dietary factors as the most feasible candidates for risk and protective factors in T1D (Table 3). Based on the combined findings from these studies, enteroviruses and omega-3 fatty acids are prime candidates for triggers and protective factors. When put in a larger context, other prospective studies (e.g., TRIGR and MIDIA studies) have also found similar associations in relation to these two candidates (Table 3). Also, findings from prospective cohort studies on cow's milk intake are consistent (Wahlberg et al. 2005). Many dietary findings await confirmation or rejection. In some studies, these viral and dietary factors have been associated predominantly with the IAA first subtype of T1D (Niinistö et al. 2017), which may offer new opportunities to identify environmentally induced disease pathways. Both DIPP and TEDDY studies suggested that among enteroviruses, particularly the species B enteroviruses, including CVBs, show association with the development of IA.

However, there are also important knowledge gaps that still need to be studied in large prospective cohorts. For example, even though certain toxicants are known to damage β cells and cause diabetes in animal models, and one of them (Vacor) also in humans (McGlinchey et al. 2020), prospective studies are lacking. Other important questions relate to possible interactions between different risk and protective factors, and interactions between these factors and the host susceptibility factors. Large prospective studies and joint data analyses in multiple cohorts are probably needed to identify such interactions.

STUDIES OF PANCREAS TISSUE

Possible presence of environmental factors in the pancreas tissue of T1D patients has been considered as a putative sign of their role in the development of β-cell damage. The largest studies have been done in the nPOD (USA) and the Exeter Archival Diabetes Biobank (UK) pancreas collections, which include pancreas tissues from cadaver organ donors with T1D (and from controls) and patients who have died after the onset of T1D, respectively. In addition, the Norwegian DiViD study collected pancreas biopsies from living newly diagnosed T1D patients. These studies have mainly focused on the detection of different viruses in the pancreas of T1D patients. Virome-wide analyses (random primer sequencing) have been used to detect a wide range of viruses, but they have not found T1D-associated viruses. In contrast, targeted detection of enterovirus RNA and proteins using immunohistochemistry, proteomics, and RT-PCR has identified enterovirus in the pancreas in the majority of T1D patients and autoantibody-positive individuals, and significantly more frequently than in control subjects (Fig. 2; Richardson and Morgan 2018). The findings support a low-grade persisting-type infection, similar to that previously reported in enterovirus-linked cardiomyopathies (Bouin et al. 2019). Immunohistochemistry has shown that the enterovirus VP1 protein is almost exclusively located in β cells. This parallels the observation that the receptor that coxsackie B group enteroviruses use to enter the cell (CAR) is strongly expressed in β cells, particularly in insulin secretory granules (Ifie et al. 2018).

HOW ENVIRONMENTAL FACTORS COULD EXPLAIN THE INCREASE IN T1D INCIDENCE

The identification of T1D-associated environmental factors opens the opportunity to study how they could explain the increasing incidence of T1D. The main hypotheses proposed to explain the increase in T1D incidence either assume that the incidence of potential risk factors has increased in the population during the past decades, or the incidence of protective factors has decreased, or both. In addition, an inverse correlation may exist between the incidence of risk factor and the disease, as shown previously in polio paralysis.

Hygiene hypothesis was originally developed to explain the increase in allergic diseases, but it has been expanded to cover also other immune-mediated diseases. The original hypothesis was based on the observation that the children who have an older sibling had a lower risk of allergy compared to first-born children (Strachan 1989). Since older siblings are an important source of infections in the family, the hygiene hypothesis proposed that increasing hygiene has led to a decrease in early childhood infections, which, in turn, shifted the balance of the immune system in a way that favors the breakdown of immune tolerance to allergens. Recently, the biodiversity hypothesis extended this idea to all microbial exposures including exposure to environmental microbial diversity (Haahtela 2019). Biodiversity hypothesis sug-

A

Fulminant acute CVB-infection

Islets are full of EV VP1-protein

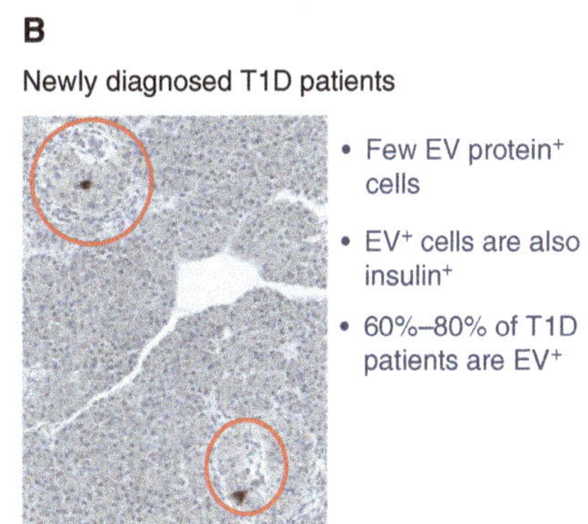

Figure 2. Detection of enterovirus VP1 protein in the pancreas by immunohistochemistry. (*A, left*) VP1 staining (brown color) in the pancreas taken from a nondiabetic child who died of coxsackievirus B3 (CVB3) infection (The Exeter Archival Diabetes Biobank collection) (Morgan et al. 2022). (Figure courtesy of Prof. Sarah Richardson and Noel Morgan, University of Exeter, UK; Exeter Archival Diabetes Biobank) Several islets and many islet cells express VP1 (marked by red circles), a pattern that fits with a fulminant CVB infection in the islets. (*B, right*) Similar staining of pancreas biopsy taken from a living newly diagnosed type 1 diabetes (T1D) patient (staining by Dr. Jutta Laiho from a pancreas sample of the DiViD study). (Figure courtesy of Prof. Knut Dahl-Jörgensen, University of Oslo, Norway; DiViD study described in Krogvold et al. 2015.) It represents a typical pattern in T1D patients showing only few infected cells. This pattern fits with a low-grade possibly persisting infection and the fact that also the amount of enterovirus RNA is extremely low in the pancreas of T1D patients.

gests that the modern urban lifestyle has decreased our contacts to nature and its biodiversity, leading to decreased stimulation of the immune system. This, in turn, leads to poor immune regulation and an inability to control immune responses that target autoantigens, allergens, or commensal intestinal bacteria. Thus, the biodiversity hypothesis could explain the increase that has happened simultaneously in several immune-mediated diseases including T1D, celiac disease, multiple sclerosis disease, atopic diseases, and inflammatory bowel diseases. Several lines of evidence support the biodiversity hypothesis in allergy, but it has not been widely studied in T1D. However, the findings from the DIPP study have generated some support showing that having a dog in the family or living in an agricultural environment is associated with a decreased risk of IA (Virtanen et al. 2014; Nurminen et al. 2021).

Another hypothesis, the polio hypothesis, suggests that a change in the population dynamics of enterovirus infections may contribute to the increasing incidence of T1D (Viskari et al. 2000). The name of this hypothesis stems from the experience of polio epidemics, which began to become more common after the end of the nineteenth century. Polio paralysis is caused by three enterovirus serotypes, polioviruses 1–3, which infect motor neurons in the central nervous system leading to a flaccid paralysis of muscles that are innervated by these neurons. Polio paralysis was rare until large epidemics started to occur after the end of the nineteenth century peaking in large epidemics in the 1950s in the United States and in Scandinavian countries. The reason for the increase in polio paralysis was a change in the dynamics of infections: Increasing hygiene level broke the fecal–oral transmission chains and infections became less frequent. This led to a delay in the child's first infection, which more often occurred at the time when maternal poliovirus antibodies had disappeared from the child's circulation. Before that time, almost everyone was infected by poliovirus, and, in many cases, the first infection came before the age of 6 months when maternal antibodies in the blood prevented the spread of the virus to the central nervous system. However, the child still got a superficial mucosal infection, which served as a natural vaccination against later infections. Decreasing antibody levels in the mother further decreased the protection of the child. Polio hypothesis suggests that this same phenomenon happens now in T1D since certain other enterovirus serotypes have been linked to T1D. The Polio hypothesis got support from studies showing that enterovirus infections have become less common and maternal enterovirus antibody levels have decreased (Viskari et al. 2005) at the same time when the incidence of T1D has increased. In addition, enterovirus antibodies are less common in Finland, which has the highest incidence of T1D, as compared to lower incidence countries (Viskari et al. 2005).

In addition to these key hypotheses, other hypotheses have been proposed. For example, an increase in pollutants and radiation has been proposed. Increased energy intake can lead to obesity and rapid growth in childhood increasing the burden of insulin-producing cells in the pancreas (accelerator hypothesis) (Gorus et al. 2002; Fourlanos et al. 2008). Industrial food processing has introduced several changes in the composition of our diet.

HOW TO PROVE CAUSALITY FOR ENVIRONMENTAL CAUSES OF TYPE 1 DIABETES?

Proving causality is one of the biggest challenges in medical research. Different criteria of causality, including the widely used Bradford Hill criteria (e.g., strength of association, consistency, specificity, temporality, dose–response, plausibility, coherence, experiment, analogy), have been used to assess causality of observed associations (Shimonovich et al. 2021). There is no simple way to prove causality, but clearly, the strongest possible evidence is to show that the elimination of the suspected trigger leads to a decrease in the disease incidence. In modern medical research, this usually requires randomized clinical trials. Other important aspects include the strength and consistency of the association observed in observational studies, the time relationship between the exposure and the initiation of the pathogenetic process, and the understanding of the molecular mechanisms of this process. Based on historical experience, it usually takes decades from the first documentation of associations between environmental trigger and the disease until causality has been proven and there are causative treatments available.

The biggest randomized clinical trial carried out so far to evaluate the role of environmental triggers of T1D aimed at confirming the causality of the association observed between early exposure to cow's milk proteins and increased risk of T1D. This study, TRIGR, recruited 2159 children from 15 countries during 2002–2007. The results showed that extensively hydrolyzed infant formula that did not contain intact cow's milk proteins was not able to reduce the risk of T1D as compared to conventional cow's milk–based formula in a rigid double-blind trial setting with good dietary compliance (Knip et al. 2014; Writing Group for the TRIGR Study Group et al. 2018; Virtanen et al. 2021).

Currently, the association between enterovirus infections and T1D is considered as an important target for clinical trials with vaccines and antiviral drugs (Dunne et al. 2019). An ongoing trial program aims at developing a vaccine against T1D-associated enterovirus types. This multivalent vaccine, PRV-101, includes five CVB serotypes and it recently successfully passed the first-in-human phase 1 trial (PROVENT trial) (Hyöty et al. 2018, 2024). The ultimate goal is to test whether this vaccine, when given during the first months of life, can decrease the risk of IA. Another recent clinical trial tested whether a 6-month treatment with a combination of two antiviral drugs, pleconaril and ribavirin, can preserve β-cell function in newly diagnosed T1D patients (DiViD Intervention trial) (Krogvold et al. 2023). The aim was to eradicate possible persisting enterovirus infection from the pancreas. The β-cell function (C-peptide secretion) showed better preservation in patients who received the treatment compared to the placebo group. The effect was significant but relatively modest. It was also accompanied by a decrease in HbA1c levels. Further trials are needed to confirm this finding and the possible clinical benefits of this treatment. Thus, the tested vaccine and antiviral drug regimens seem to be applicable in further clinical trials to proof or disproof causality of enterovirus–T1D association. Intervention trials that evaluate the impact of other environmental factors are also in progress. These include the BabyDiab study, which tested whether delayed introduction of gluten could reduce the risk of IA. No clear effect was found (Beyerlein et al. 2014). Another example is the SINT1A trial (NCT04769037), which investigates whether giving the probiotic *Bifidobacterium infantis* can prevent the development of T1D in children with increased risk for the disease. In addition, the AVANT1A trial is testing whether a SARS-CoV-2 vaccination during the first year of life can reduce the incidence of IA and T1D (www.helmholtz-munich.de/en/idf/studies/avant1a-study).

Mechanisms of enterovirus–T1D association have been studied in a number of studies. As described above, infection of β cells and viral persistence in these cells is the prevailing concept (Fig. 3). The role of aberrant host immune response is currently actively studied as well as viral interaction with T1D-associated immune response genes. For example, HLA genes modulate the course of many virus infections and one study showed that children who carry T1D-associated HLA-DR3 or -DR4 haplotypes have stronger antibody responses to enterovirus than children who carry protective HLA-DR2 haplotype (Sadeharju et al. 2003). HLA may also determine whether a putative cross-reactive mimicry epitope in viral and host proteins is recognized by the immune system of certain individuals. Other important research targets are *CXADR* (CAR receptor), *IFIH1* (innate immune system receptor recognizing enterovirus RNA), and *TYK2* (key regulator of innate immune responses) as SNPs in these genes linked to T1D risk. Enteroviruses may also cause epigenetic changes (e.g., DNA methylation), which could influence the function of β cells or the immune system, or viruses may cause posttranslational modifications in β-cell proteins making them more recognizable for autoreactive T cells (Akhbari et al. 2020). However, despite the actively ongoing research to proof causality, this goal has not yet been reached for any of the candidates for environmental triggers of T1D.

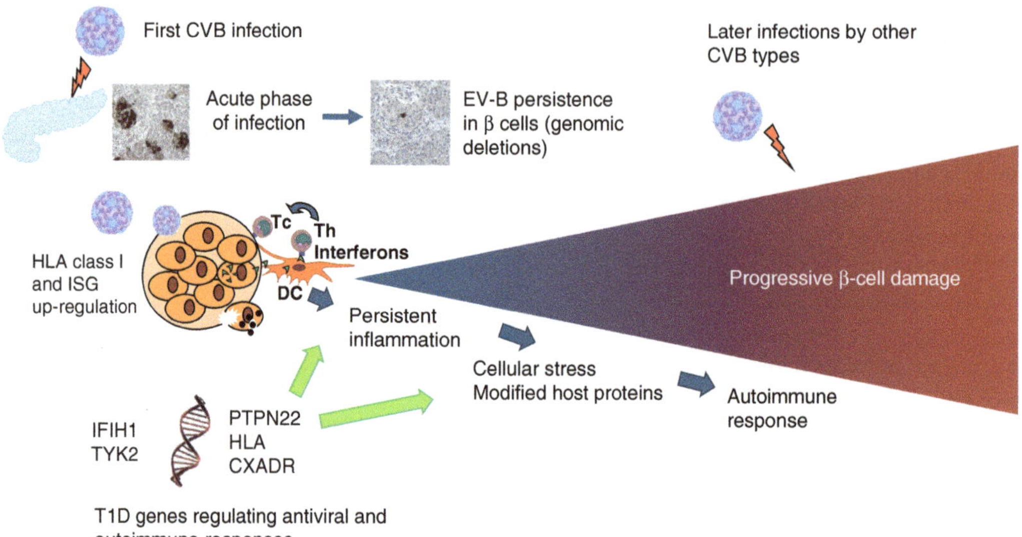

Figure 3. Hypothetical model of how coxsackie B virus (CVB) infection could cause β-cell damage and type 1 diabetes (T1D). CVB infection spreads to the pancreas via blood or intestinal lymphatic system. Infection of β cells begins before the other islet cells since β cells strongly express coxsackie and adenovirus receptor (CAR) and their antiviral innate immune system response is weaker. Acute infection in β cells leads to secretion of type 1 interferons, which renders the other islet cells resistant to the virus and limits the infection to β cells. The replication of the virus in β cells gradually decreases due to the antiviral immune response and the virus turns to a terminally deleted and slowly replicating form. This kind of terminally deleted CVB persists in β cells causing long-term inflammation and posttranslational changes in β-cell proteins eventually leading to islet autoimmunity. (EV-B) Enterovirus B, (HLA) human leukocyte antigen, (ISG) interferon-stimulated gene, (DC) dendritic cell. (Figure modified from Hyöty et al. 2018; © 2018 The Author(s). Published by Taylor and Francis Group.)

CONCLUDING REMARKS

Even though the influence of the environment in the pathogenesis of T1D is considered important, the huge number of different environmental exposures makes the identification of causal risk and protective factors challenging. Currently, enterovirus infections are among the prime candidates for environmental triggers of T1D, but also several other candidates exist and should be studied further. The identification of causative environmental factors would open possibilities to prevent the development of T1D and to develop curative treatments. This is demonstrated by the impact of the discovery of causative environmental factors in other diseases (e.g., the discovery of gluten as the cause of celiac disease and the discovery of *H. pylori* as a causative agent in gastritis and gastric cancer). Thus, it is important to fully explore the potential of the main candidates of environmental triggers of T1D and carry out intervention studies to evaluate the causality. At the same time, new candidates should be sought by carrying our large prospective studies and by facilitating the use of already existing data by joint international collaboration efforts.

COMPETING INTEREST STATEMENT

H.H. is a shareholder and member of the board of Vactech Ltd, which develops vaccines against picornaviruses. No other potential conflicts of interest relevant to this article were reported.

ACKNOWLEDGMENTS

Since this article focuses on the results from the two largest prospective birth cohort studies, DIPP and TEDDY studies, we wish to express our special gratitude to the steering groups and all our other coinvestigators in these studies. In addition, the leadership and all our other collaborators in the nPOD virus study group are gratefully acknowledged for good collaboration and for sharing their interest in the role of viruses and other factors in the pathogenesis of T1D. The preparation of this article was supported by funding from the ENT1DEP project (Enterovirus-linked Type 1 Diabetes Exposed—Mechanisms and Prevention), which is funded by the Horizon Europe Research and innovation program of the European Union under Grant Agreement 101136259 (H.H.), the Research Council of Finland (grant 339922 to S.M.V.), and Päivikki and Sakari Sohlberg's Foundation grant (J.E.L.).

REFERENCES

Åkerblom HK, Savilahti E, Saukkonen TT, Paganus A, Virtanen SM, Teramo K, Knip M, Ilonen J, Reijonen H, Karjalainen J, et al. 1993. The case for elimination of cow's milk in early infancy in the prevention of type 1 diabetes: the Finnish experience. *Diabetes Metab Rev* **9:** 269–278. doi:10.1002/dmr.5610090407

Akhbari P, Richardson SJ, Morgan NG. 2020. Type 1 diabetes: interferons and the aftermath of pancreatic β-cell enteroviral infection. *Microorganisms* **8:** 1419. doi:10.3390/microorganisms8091419

Antvorskov JC, Halldorsson TI, Josefsen K, Svensson J, Granström C, Roep BO, Olesen TH, Hrolfsdottir L, Buschard K, Olsen SF. 2018. Association between maternal gluten intake and type 1 diabetes in offspring: national prospective cohort study in Denmark. *BMJ* **362:** k3547. doi:10.1136/bmj.k3547

Aronsson CA, Tamura R, Vehik K, Uusitalo U, Yang J, Haller MJ, Toppari J, Hagopian W, McIndoe RA, Rewers MJ, et al. 2023. Dietary intake and body mass index influence the risk of islet autoimmunity in genetically at-risk children: a mediation analysis using the TEDDY cohort. *Pediatr Diabetes* **2023:** 3945064. doi:10.1155/2023/3945064

Auchtung TA, Stewart CJ, Smith DP, Triplett EW, Agardh D, Hagopian WA, Ziegler AG, Rewers MJ, She JX, Toppari J, et al. 2022. Temporal changes in gastrointestinal fungi and the risk of autoimmunity during early childhood: the TEDDY study. *Nat Commun* **13:** 3151. doi:10.1038/s41467-022-30686-w

Beyerlein A, Chmiel R, Hummel S, Winkler C, Bonifacio E, Ziegler AG. 2014. Timing of gluten introduction and islet autoimmunity in young children: updated results from the BABYDIET study. *Diabetes Care* **37:** e194–e195. doi:10.2337/dc14-1208

Blanter M, Sork H, Tuomela S, Flodström-Tullberg M. 2019. Genetic and environmental interaction in type 1 diabetes: a relationship between genetic risk alleles and molecular traits of enterovirus infection? *Curr Diab Rep* **19:** 82. doi:10.1007/s11892-019-1192-8

Bouin A, Gretteau PA, Wehbe M, Renois F, N'Guyen Y, Lévêque N, Vu MN, Tracy S, Chapman NM, Bruneval P, et al. 2019. Enterovirus persistence in cardiac cells of patients with idiopathic dilated cardiomyopathy is linked to 5′ terminal genomic RNA-deleted viral populations with viral-encoded proteinase activities. *Circulation* **139:** 2326–2338. doi:10.1161/CIRCULATIONAHA.118.035966

Davis-Richardson AG, Ardissone AN, Dias R, Simell V, Leonard MT, Kemppainen KM, Drew JC, Schatz D, Atkinson MA, Kolaczkowski B, et al. 2014. *Bacteroides dorei* dominates gut microbiome prior to autoimmunity in Finnish children at high risk for type 1 diabetes. *Front Microbiol* **5:** 678. doi:10.3389/fmicb.2014.00678

DIAMOND Project Group. 2006. Incidence and trends of childhood type 1 diabetes worldwide 1990–1999. *Diabet Med* **23:** 857–866. doi:10.1111/j.1464-5491.2006.01925.x

Díaz Ludovico I, Sarkar S, Elliott E, Virtanen SM, Erlund I, Ramanadham S, Mirmira RG, Metz TO, Nakayasu ES. 2023. Fatty acid-mediated signaling as a target for developing type 1 diabetes therapies. *Expert Opin Ther Targets* **27:** 793–806. doi:10.1080/14728222.2023.2259099

Domsgen E, Lind K, Kong L, Hühn MH, Rasool O, van Kuppeveld F, Korsgren O, Lahesmaa R, Flodström-Tullberg M. 2016. An IFIH1 gene polymorphism associated with risk for autoimmunity regulates canonical antiviral defence pathways in Coxsackievirus infected human pancreatic islets. *Sci Rep* **6:** 39378. doi:10.1038/srep39378

Dunne JL, Richardson SJ, Atkinson MA, Craig ME, Dahl-Jørgensen K, Flodström-Tullberg M, Hyöty H, Insel RA, Lernmark Å, Lloyd RE, et al. 2019. Rationale for enteroviral vaccination and antiviral therapies in human type 1 diabetes. *Diabetologia* **62:** 744–753. doi:10.1007/s00125-019-4811-7

Erkkola M, Karppinen M, Javanainen J, Räsänen L, Knip M, Virtanen SM. 2001. Validity and reproducibility of a food frequency questionnaire for pregnant Finnish women. *Am J Epidemiol* **154:** 466–476. doi:10.1093/aje/154.5.466

Foulis AK, Farquharson MA, Cameron SO, McGill M, Schönke H, Kandolf R. 1990. A search for the presence of the enteroviral capsid protein VP1 in pancreases of patients with type 1 (insulin-dependent) diabetes and pancreases and hearts of infants who died of coxsackieviral myocarditis. *Diabetologia* **33:** 290–298. doi:10.1007/BF00403323

Fourlanos S, Harrison LC, Colman PG. 2008. The accelerator hypothesis and increasing incidence of type 1 diabetes. *Curr Opin Endocrinol Diabetes Obes* **15:** 321–325. doi:10.1097/MED.0b013e3283073a5a

Gorman JA, Hundhausen C, Errett JS, Stone AE, Allenspach EJ, Ge Y, Arkatkar T, Clough C, Dai X, Khim S, et al. 2017. The A946T variant of the RNA sensor IFIH1 mediates an interferon program that limits viral infection but increases the risk for autoimmunity. *Nat Immunol* **18:** 744–752. doi:10.1038/ni.3766

Gorus FK, Weets I, Pipeleers DG. 2002. To: T.J. Wilkin (2001) The accelerator hypothesis: weight gain as the missing link between type I and type II diabetes. Diabetologia 44: 914–921. *Diabetologia* **45:** 288–289; author reply 289. doi:10.1007/s00125-001-0724-2

Haahtela T. 2019. A biodiversity hypothesis. *Allergy* **74:** 1445–1456. doi:10.1111/all.13763

Haahtela T, Alenius H, Lehtimäki J, Sinkkonen A, Fyhrquist N, Hyöty H, Ruokolainen L, Mäkelä MJ. 2021. Immunological resilience and biodiversity for prevention of allergic diseases and asthma. *Allergy* **76:** 3613–3626. doi:10.1111/all.14895

Hakola L, Takkinen HM, Niinistö S, Ahonen S, Nevalainen J, Veijola R, Ilonen J, Toppari J, Knip M, Virtanen SM. 2018. Infant feeding in relation to the risk of advanced islet autoimmunity and type 1 diabetes in children with increased genetic susceptibility: a cohort study. *Am J Epidemiol* **187:** 34–44. doi:10.1093/aje/kwx191

Hakola L, Miettinen ME, Syrjälä E, Åkerlund M, Takkinen HM, Korhonen TE, Ahonen S, Ilonen J, Toppari J, Veijola R, et al. 2019. Association of cereal, gluten, and dietary fiber intake with islet autoimmunity and type 1 diabetes. *JAMA Pediatr* **173:** 953–960. doi:10.1001/jamapediatrics.2019.2564

Hakola L, Oikarinen M, Niinistö S, Cuthbertson D, Lehtonen J, Puustinen L, Sioofy-Khojine AB, Honkanen J, Knip M, Krischer JP, et al. 2022. Serum 25-hydroxyvitamin D and fatty acids in relation to the risk of microbial infections in children: the TRIGR Divia study. *Clin Nutr* **41:** 2729–2739. doi:10.1016/j.clnu.2022.10.017

Hakola L, Vuorinen AL, Takkinen HM, Niinistö S, Ahonen S, Rautanen J, Peltonen EJ, Nevalainen J, Ilonen J, Toppari J, et al. 2023. Dietary fatty acid intake in childhood and the risk of islet autoimmunity and type 1 diabetes: the DIPP birth cohort study. *Eur J Nutr* **62:** 847–856. doi:10.1007/s00394-022-03035-2

Hakola L, Mramba LK, Uusitalo U, Andrén Aronsson C, Hummel S, Niinistö S, Erlund I, Yang J, Rewers MJ, Akolkar B, et al. 2024. Intake of B vitamins and the risk of developing islet autoimmunity and type 1 diabetes in the TEDDY study. *Eur J Nutr* **63:** 1329–1338. doi:10.1007/s00394-024-03346-6

Hermann R, Knip M, Veijola R, Simell O, Laine AP, Åkerblom HK, Groop PH, Forsblom C, Pettersson-Fernholm K, Ilonen J, et al. 2003. Temporal changes in the frequencies of HLA genotypes in patients with type 1 diabetes—indication of an increased environmental pressure? *Diabetologia* **46:** 420–425. doi:10.1007/s00125-003-1045-4

Honkanen H, Oikarinen S, Nurminen N, Laitinen OH, Huhtala H, Lehtonen J, Ruokoranta T, Hankaniemi MM, Lecouturier V, Almond JW, et al. 2017. Detection of enteroviruses in stools precedes islet autoimmunity by several months: possible evidence for slowly operating mechanisms in virus-induced autoimmunity. *Diabetologia* **60:** 424–431. doi:10.1007/s00125-016-4177-z

Hummel S, Beyerlein A, Tamura R, Uusitalo U, Andrén Aronsson C, Yang J, Riikonen A, Lernmark Å, Rewers MJ, Hagopian WA, et al. 2017. First infant formula type and risk of islet autoimmunity in the environmental determinants of diabetes in the young (TEDDY) study. *Diabetes Care* **40:** 398–404. doi:10.2337/dc16-1624

Hyöty H. 2016. Viruses in type 1 diabetes. *Pediatr Diabetes* **17:** 56–64. doi:10.1111/pedi.12370

Hyöty H, Leon F, Knip M. 2018. Developing a vaccine for type 1 diabetes by targeting coxsackievirus B. *Expert Rev Vaccines* **17:** 1071–1083. doi:10.1080/14760584.2018.1548281

Hyöty H, Kääriäinen S, Laiho JE, Comer GM, Tian W, Härkönen T, Lehtonen JP, Oikarinen S, Puustinen L, Snyder M, et al. 2024. Safety, tolerability and immunogenicity of PRV-101, a multivalent vaccine targeting coxsackie B viruses (CVBs) associated with type 1 diabetes: a double-blind randomised placebo-controlled phase I trial. *Diabetologia* **67:** 811–821. doi:10.1007/s00125-024-06092-w

Ifie E, Russell MA, Dhayal S, Leete P, Sebastiani G, Nigi L, Dotta F, Marjomäki V, Eizirik DL, Morgan NG, et al. 2018. Unexpected subcellular distribution of a specific isoform of the Coxsackie and adenovirus receptor, CAR-SIV, in human pancreatic β cells. *Diabetologia* **61:** 2344–2355. doi:10.1007/s00125-018-4704-1

Joslowski G, Yang J, Aronsson CA, Ahonen S, Butterworth M, Rautanen J, Norris JM, Virtanen SM, Uusitalo U; TEDDY Study Group. 2017. Development of a harmonized food grouping system for between-country comparisons in the TEDDY study. *J Food Compost Anal* **63:** 79–88. doi:10.1016/j.jfca.2017.07.037

Kashfi K, Anbardar N, Asadipooya A, Asadipooya K. 2023. Type 1 diabetes and COVID-19: a literature review and possible management. *Int J Endocrinol Metab* **21:** e139768. doi:10.5812/ijem-139768

Kemppainen KM, Vehik K, Lynch KF, Larsson HE, Canepa RJ, Simell V, Koletzko S, Liu E, Simell OG, Toppari J, et al. 2017. Association between early-life antibiotic use and the risk of islet or celiac disease autoimmunity. *JAMA Pediatr* **171:** 1217–1225. doi:10.1001/jamapediatrics.2017.2905

Knip M, Åkerblom HK, Becker D, Dosch HM, Dupre J, Fraser W, Howard N, Ilonen J, Krischer JP, Kordonouri O, et al. 2014. Hydrolyzed infant formula and early β-cell autoimmunity: a randomized clinical trial. *JAMA* **311:** 2279–2287. doi:10.1001/jama.2014.5610

Knip M, Parviainen A, Turtinen M, But A, Härkönen T, Hepojoki J, Sironen T, Iheozor-Ejiofor R, Uğurlu H, Saksela K, et al. 2023. SARS-CoV-2 and type 1 diabetes in children in Finland: an observational study. *Lancet Diabetes Endocrinol* **11:** 251–260. doi:10.1016/S2213-8587(23)00041-4

Koivusaari K, Syrjälä E, Niinistö S, Takkinen HM, Ahonen S, Åkerlund M, Korhonen TE, Toppari J, Ilonen J, Peltonen J, et al. 2020. Consumption of differently processed milk products in infancy and early childhood and the risk of islet autoimmunity. *Br J Nutr* **124:** 173–180. doi:10.1017/S0007114520000744

Kondrashova A, Seiskari T, Ilonen J, Knip M, Hyöty H. 2013. The "hygiene hypothesis" and the sharp gradient in the incidence of autoimmune and allergic diseases between Russian Karelia and Finland. *APMIS* **121:** 478–493. doi:10.1111/apm.12023

Krischer JP, Lynch KF, Schatz DA, Ilonen J, Lernmark Å, Hagopian WA, Rewers MJ, She JX, Simell OG, Toppari J, et al. 2015. The 6 year incidence of diabetes-associated autoantibodies in genetically at-risk children: the TEDDY study. *Diabetologia* **58:** 980–987. doi:10.1007/s00125-015-3514-y

Krischer JP, Lernmark Å, Hagopian WA, Rewers MJ, McIndoe R, Toppari J, Ziegler AG, Akolkar B; TEDDY Study Group. 2023. SARS-CoV-2—no increased islet autoimmunity or type 1 diabetes in teens. *N Engl J Med* **389:** 474–475. doi:10.1056/NEJMc2216477

Krogvold L, Edwin B, Buanes T, Frisk G, Skog O, Anagandula M, Korsgren O, Undlien D, Eike MC, Richardson SJ, et al. 2015. Detection of a low-grade enteroviral infection in the islets of langerhans of living patients newly diagnosed with type 1 diabetes. *Diabetes* **64:** 1682–1687. doi:10.2337/db14-1370

Krogvold L, Mynarek IM, Ponzi E, Mørk FB, Hessel TW, Roald T, Lindblom N, Westman J, Barker P, Hyöty H, et al. 2023. Pleconaril and ribavirin in new-onset type 1 diabetes: a phase 2 randomized trial. *Nat Med* **29:** 2902–2908. doi:10.1038/s41591-023-02576-1

Laitinen OH, Honkanen H, Pakkanen O, Oikarinen S, Hankaniemi MM, Huhtala H, Ruokoranta T, Lecouturier V, André P, Harju R, et al. 2014. Coxsackievirus B1 is associated with induction of β-cell autoimmunity that portends type 1 diabetes. *Diabetes* **63:** 446–455. doi:10.2337/db13-0619

Lampousi AM, Carlsson S, Löfvenborg JE. 2021. Dietary factors and risk of islet autoimmunity and type 1 diabetes: a systematic review and meta-analysis. *EBioMedicine* **72:** 103633. doi:10.1016/j.ebiom.2021.103633

Lee HS, Hwang JS. 2019. Genetic aspects of type 1 diabetes. *Ann Pediatr Endocrinol Metab* **24:** 143–148. doi:10.6065/apem.2019.24.3.143

Lempainen J, Tauriainen S, Vaarala O, Mäkelä M, Honkanen H, Marttila J, Veijola R, Simell O, Hyöty H, Knip M, et al. 2012. Interaction of enterovirus infection and cow's milk-based formula nutrition in type 1 diabetes-associated autoimmunity. *Diabetes Metab Res Rev* **28:** 177–185. doi:10.1002/dmrr.1294

Lernmark Å, Akolkar B, Hagopian W, Krischer J, McIndoe R, Rewers M, Toppari J, Vehik K, Ziegler AG; TEDDY Study Group. 2023. Possible heterogeneity of initial pancreatic islet β-cell autoimmunity heralding type 1 diabetes. *J Intern Med* **294:** 145–158. doi:10.1111/joim.13648

Lloyd RE, Tamhankar M, Lernmark Å. 2022. Enteroviruses and type 1 diabetes: multiple mechanisms and factors? *Annu Rev Med* **73:** 483–499. doi:10.1146/annurev-med-042320-015952

Lönnrot M, Lynch K, Larsson HE, Lernmark Å, Rewers M, Hagopian W, She JX, Simell O, Ziegler AG, Akolkar B, et al. 2015. A method for reporting and classifying acute infectious diseases in a prospective study of young children: TEDDY. *BMC Pediatr* **15:** 24. doi:10.1186/s12887-015-0333-8

Lönnrot M, Lynch KF, Elding Larsson H, Lernmark Å, Rewers MJ, Törn C, Burkhardt BR, Briese T, Hagopian WA, She JX, et al. 2017. Respiratory infections are temporally associated with initiation of type 1 diabetes autoimmunity: the TEDDY study. *Diabetologia* **60:** 1931–1940. doi:10.1007/s00125-017-4365-5

Lönnrot M, Lynch KF, Rewers M, Lernmark Å, Vehik K, Akolkar B, Hagopian W, Krischer J, McIndoe RA, Toppari J, et al. 2023. Gastrointestinal infections modulate the risk for insulin autoantibodies as the first-appearing autoantibody in the TEDDY study. *Diabetes Care* **46:** 1908–1915. doi:10.2337/dc23-0518

Mäkinen M, Mykkänen J, Koskinen M, Simell V, Veijola R, Hyöty H, Ilonen J, Knip M, Simell O, Toppari J. 2016. Serum 25-hydroxyvitamin D concentrations in children progressing to autoimmunity and clinical type 1 diabetes. *J Clin Endocrinol Metab* **101:** 723–729. doi:10.1210/jc.2015-3504

Mäkinen M, Löyttyniemi E, Koskinen M, Vähä-Mäkilä M, Siljander H, Nurmio M, Mykkänen J, Virtanen SM, Simell O, Hyöty H, et al. 2019. Serum 25-hydroxyvitamin D concentrations at birth in children screened for HLA-DQB1 conferred risk for type 1 diabetes. *J Clin Endocrinol Metab* **104:** 2277–2285. doi:10.1210/jc.2018-02094

Marjamäki L, Niinistö S, Kenward MG, Uusitalo L, Uusitalo U, Ovaskainen ML, Kronberg-Kippilä C, Simell O, Veijola R, Ilonen J, et al. 2010. Maternal intake of vitamin D during pregnancy and risk of advanced β cell autoimmunity and type 1 diabetes in offspring. *Diabetologia* **53:** 1599–1607. doi:10.1007/s00125-010-1734-8

Mattila M, Erlund I, Lee HS, Niinistö S, Uusitalo U, Andrén Aronsson C, Hummel S, Parikh H, Rich SS, Hagopian W, et al. 2020. Plasma ascorbic acid and the risk of islet autoimmunity and type 1 diabetes: the TEDDY study. *Diabetologia* **63:** 278–286. doi:10.1007/s00125-019-05028-z

Mattila M, Hakola L, Niinistö S, Tapanainen H, Takkinen HM, Ahonen S, Ilonen J, Toppari J, Veijola R, Knip M, et al. 2021. Maternal vitamin C and iron intake during pregnancy and the risk of islet autoimmunity and type 1 diabetes in children: a birth cohort study. *Nutrients* **13:** 928. doi:10.3390/nu13030928

Mattila M, Takkinen HM, Peltonen EJ, Vuorinen AL, Niinistö S, Metsälä J, Ahonen S, Åkerlund M, Hakola L, Toppari J, et al. 2024. Fruit, berry, and vegetable consumption and the risk of islet autoimmunity and type 1 diabetes in children—the Type 1 Diabetes Prediction and Prevention birth cohort study. *Am J Clin Nutr* **119:** 537–545. doi:10.1016/j.ajcnut.2023.12.014

McGlinchey A, Sinioja T, Lamichhane S, Sen P, Bodin J, Siljander H, Dickens AM, Geng D, Carlsson C, Duberg D, et al. 2020. Prenatal exposure to perfluoroalkyl substances modulates neonatal serum phospholipids, increasing risk of type 1 diabetes. *Environ Int* **143:** 105935. doi:10.1016/j.envint.2020.105935

Mikk ML, Pfeiffer S, Kiviniemi M, Laine AP, Lempainen J, Härkönen T, Toppari J, Veijola R, Knip M, Ilonen J, et al. 2020. HLA-DR-DQ haplotypes and specificity of the initial autoantibody in islet specific autoimmunity. *Pediatr Diabetes* **21:** 1218–1226. doi:10.1111/pedi.13073

Morgan NG, Richardson SJ, Powers AC, Saunders DC, Brissova M. 2022. Images from the Exeter archival diabetes biobank now accessible via pancreatlas. *Diabetes Care* **45:** e174–e175. doi:10.2337/dc22-1613

Nekoua MP, Alidjinou EK, Hober D. 2022. Persistent coxsackievirus B infection and pathogenesis of type 1 diabetes mellitus. *Nat Rev Endocrinol* **18:** 503–516. doi:10.1038/s41574-022-00688-1

Niinistö S, Takkinen HM, Uusitalo L, Rautanen J, Nevalainen J, Kenward MG, Lumia M, Simell O, Veijola R, Ilonen J, et al. 2014. Maternal dietary fatty acid intake during pregnancy and the risk of preclinical and clinical type 1 diabetes in the offspring. *Br J Nutr* **111:** 895–903. doi:10.1017/S0007114513003073

Niinistö S, Takkinen HM, Uusitalo L, Rautanen J, Vainio N, Ahonen S, Nevalainen J, Kenward MG, Lumia M, Simell O, et al. 2015. Maternal intake of fatty acids and their food sources during lactation and the risk of preclinical and clinical type 1 diabetes in the offspring. *Acta Diabetol* **52:** 763–772. doi:10.1007/s00592-014-0673-0

Niinistö S, Takkinen HM, Erlund I, Ahonen S, Toppari J, Ilonen J, Veijola R, Knip M, Vaarala O, Virtanen SM. 2017. Fatty acid status in infancy is associated with the risk of type 1 diabetes-associated autoimmunity. *Diabetologia* **60:** 1223–1233. doi:10.1007/s00125-017-4280-9

Niinistö S, Erlund I, Lee HS, Uusitalo U, Salminen I, Aronsson CA, Parikh HM, Liu X, Hummel S, Toppari J, et al. 2021. Children's erythrocyte fatty acids are associated with the risk of islet autoimmunity. *Sci Rep* **11:** 3627. doi:10.1038/s41598-021-82200-9

Niinistö S, Miettinen ME, Cuthbertson D, Honkanen J, Hakola L, Autio R, Erlund I, Arohonka P, Vuorela A, Härkönen T, et al. 2022. Associations between serum fatty acids and immunological markers in children developing islet autoimmunity-the TRIGR nested case-control study. *Front Immunol* **13:** 858875. doi:10.3389/fimmu.2022.858875

Niinistö S, Cuthbertson D, Miettinen ME, Hakola L, Nucci A, Korhonen TE, Hyöty H, Krischer JP, Vaarala O, Knip M, et al. 2024. High levels of immunoglobulin G against cow's milk proteins and frequency of cow milk consumption are associated with the development of islet autoimmunity and type 1 diabetes. *J Nutr* **154:** 2493–2500. doi:10.1016/j.tjnut.2024.06.005

Norris JM, Yin X, Lamb MM, Barriga K, Seifert J, Hoffman M, Orton HD, Barón AE, Clare-Salzler M, Chase HP, et al. 2007. Omega-3 polyunsaturated fatty acid intake and islet autoimmunity in children at increased risk for type 1 diabetes. *JAMA* **298:** 1420–1428. doi:10.1001/jama.298.12.1420

Norris JM, Lee HS, Frederiksen B, Erlund I, Uusitalo U, Yang J, Lernmark Å, Simell O, Toppari J, Rewers M, et al. 2018. Plasma 25-hydroxyvitamin D concentration and risk of islet autoimmunity. *Diabetes* **67:** 146–154. doi:10.2337/db17-0802

Nucci AM, Virtanen SM, Cuthbertson D, Ludvigsson J, Einberg U, Huot C, Castano L, Aschemeier B, Becker DJ, Knip M, et al. 2021. Growth and development of islet autoimmunity and type 1 diabetes in children genetically at risk. *Diabetologia* **64:** 826–835. doi:10.1007/s00125-020-05358-3

Nurminen N, Cerrone D, Lehtonen J, Parajuli A, Roslund M, Lönnrot M, Ilonen J, Toppari J, Veijola R, Knip M, et al. 2021. Land cover of early-life environment modulates the risk of type 1 diabetes. *Diabetes Care* **44:** 1506–1514. doi:10.2337/dc20-1719

Poma AM, Basolo A, Alì G, Bonuccelli D, Di Stefano I, Conti M, Mazzetti P, Sparavelli R, Vignali P, Macerola E, et al. 2024. SARS-CoV-2 spread to endocrine organs is associated with obesity: an autopsy study of COVID-19 cases. *Endocrine* **83:** 110–117. doi:10.1007/s12020-023-03518-0

Prasad M, Takkinen HM, Nevalainen J, Ovaskainen ML, Alfthan G, Uusitalo L, Kenward MG, Veijola R, Simell O, Ilonen J, et al. 2011. Are serum α- and β-carotene concentrations associated with the development of advanced β-cell autoimmunity in children with increased genetic susceptibility to type 1 diabetes? *Diabetes Metab* **37:** 162–167. doi:10.1016/j.diabet.2010.10.002

Prasad M, Takkinen HM, Uusitalo L, Tapanainen H, Ovaskainen ML, Alfthan G, Erlund I, Ahonen S, Åkerlund M, Toppari J, et al. 2018. Carotenoid intake and serum concentration in young Finnish children and their relation with fruit and vegetable consumption. *Nutrients* **10:** 1533. doi:10.3390/nu10101533

Prosser PR, Karam JH. 1978. Diabetes mellitus following rodenticide ingestion in man. *JAMA* **239:** 1148–1150. doi:10.1001/jama.1978.03280390044019

Redondo MJ, Onengut-Gumuscu S, Gaulton KJ. 2023. Genetics of type 1 diabetes. In *Diabetes in America* (ed. Lawrence JM, Casagrande SS, Herman WH, Wexler DJ, Cefalu WT), National Institute of Diabetes and Digestive and Kidney Diseases, Bethesda, Maryland.

Rewers M, Hyöty H, Lernmark Å, Hagopian W, She JX, Schatz D, Ziegler AG, Toppari J, Akolkar B, Krischer J. 2018. The Environmental Determinants of Diabetes in the Young (TEDDY) study: 2018 update. *Curr Diab Rep* **18:** 136. doi:10.1007/s11892-018-1113-2

Richardson SJ, Morgan NG. 2018. Enteroviral infections in the pathogenesis of type 1 diabetes: new insights for therapeutic intervention. *Curr Opin Pharmacol* **43:** 11–19. doi:10.1016/j.coph.2018.07.006

Richardson SJ, Willcox A, Bone AJ, Foulis AK, Morgan NG. 2009. The prevalence of enteroviral capsid protein vp1 immunostaining in pancreatic islets in human type 1 diabetes. *Diabetologia* **52:** 1143–1151. doi:10.1007/s00125-009-1276-0

Sadeharju K, Knip M, Hiltunen M, Akerblom HK, Hyöty H. 2003. The HLA-DR phenotype modulates the humoral immune response to enterovirus antigens. *Diabetologia* **46:** 1100–1105. doi:10.1007/s00125-003-1157-x

Salo TEI, Hakola L, Niinistö S, Takkinen HM, Ahonen S, Puustinen L, Ilonen J, Toppari J, Veijola R, Hyöty H, et al. 2024. Gut inflammation markers, diet, and risk of islet autoimmunity in Finnish children—a nested case-control study. *J Nutr* **154:** 2244–2254. doi:10.1016/j.tjnut.2024.05.015

Shimonovich M, Pearce A, Thomson H, Keyes K, Katikireddi SV. 2021. Assessing causality in epidemiology: revisiting Bradford Hill to incorporate developments in causal thinking. *Eur J Epidemiol* **36:** 873–887. doi:10.1007/s10654-020-00703-7

Singh T, Weiss A, Vehik K, Krischer J, Rewers M, Toppari J, Lernmark Å, Hagopian W, Akolkar B, Bonifacio E, et al. 2024. Caesarean section and risk of type 1 diabetes. *Diabetologia* **67:** 1582–1587. doi:10.1007/s00125-024-06176-7

Sioofy-Khojine AB, Lehtonen J, Nurminen N, Laitinen OH, Oikarinen S, Huhtala H, Pakkanen O, Ruokoranta T, Hankaniemi MM, Toppari J, et al. 2018. Coxsackievirus B1 infections are associated with the initiation of insulin-driven autoimmunity that progresses to type 1 diabetes. *Diabetologia* **61:** 1193–1202. doi:10.1007/s00125-018-4561-y

Sioofy-Khojine AB, Richardson SJ, Locke JM, Oikarinen S, Nurminen N, Laine AP, Downes K, Lempainen J, Todd JA, Veijola R, et al. 2022. Detection of enterovirus RNA in peripheral blood mononuclear cells correlates with the presence of the predisposing allele of the type 1 diabetes risk gene IFIH1 and with disease stage. *Diabetologia* **65:** 1701–1709. doi:10.1007/s00125-022-05753-y

Stene LC, Gale EA. 2013. The prenatal environment and type 1 diabetes. *Diabetologia* **56:** 1888–1897. doi:10.1007/s00125-013-2929-6

Stewart CJ, Ajami NJ, O'Brien JL, Hutchinson DS, Smith DP, Wong MC, Ross MC, Lloyd RE, Doddapaneni H, Metcalf GA, et al. 2018. Temporal development of the gut microbiome in early childhood from the TEDDY study. *Nature* **562:** 583–588. doi:10.1038/s41586-018-0617-x

Strachan DP. 1989. Hay fever, hygiene, and household size. *BMJ* **299:** 1259–1260. doi:10.1136/bmj.299.6710.1259

Syrjälä E, Nevalainen J, Peltonen J, Takkinen HM, Hakola L, Åkerlund M, Veijola R, Ilonen J, Toppari J, Knip M, et al. 2019. A joint modeling approach for childhood meat, fish and egg consumption and the risk of advanced islet autoimmunity. *Sci Rep* **9:** 7760. doi:10.1038/s41598-019-44196-1

TEDDY Study Group. 2007. The Environmental Determinants of Diabetes in the Young (TEDDY) study: study design. *Pediatr Diabetes* **8:** 286–298. doi:10.1111/j.1399-5448.2007.00269.x

Thorsen SU, Liu X, Kataria Y, Mandrup-Poulsen T, Kaur S, Uusitalo U, Virtanen SM, Norris JM, Rewers M, Hagopian W, et al. 2023. Interaction between dietary iron intake and genetically determined iron overload: risk of islet autoimmunity and progression to type 1 diabetes in the TEDDY study. *Diabetes Care* **46:** 1014–1018. doi:10.2337/dc22-1359

Toivonen RK, Emani R, Munukka E, Rintala A, Laiho A, Pietilä S, Pursiheimo JP, Soidinsalo P, Linhala M, Eerola E, et al. 2014. Fermentable fibres condition colon microbiota and promote diabetogenesis in NOD mice. *Diabetologia* **57:** 2183–2192. doi:10.1007/s00125-014-3325-6

Tracy S, Drescher KM, Jackson JD, Kim K, Kono K. 2010. Enteroviruses, type 1 diabetes and hygiene: a complex relationship. *Rev Med Virol* **20:** 106–116. doi:10.1002/rmv.639

Uusitalo L, Nevalainen J, Niinistö S, Alfthan G, Sundvall J, Korhonen T, Kenward MG, Oja H, Veijola R, Simell O, et al. 2008a. Serum α- and γ-tocopherol concentrations and risk of advanced β cell autoimmunity in children with HLA-conferred susceptibility to type 1 diabetes mellitus. *Diabetologia* **51:** 773–780. doi:10.1007/s00125-008-0959-2

Uusitalo L, Uusitalo U, Ovaskainen ML, Niinistö S, Kronberg-Kippilä C, Marjamäki L, Ahonen S, Kenward MG, Knip M, Veijola R, et al. 2008b. Sociodemographic and lifestyle characteristics are associated with antioxidant intake and the consumption of their dietary sources during pregnancy. *Public Health Nutr* **11:** 1379–1388. doi:10.1017/S1368980008003522

Uusitalo L, Nevalainen J, Salminen I, Ovaskainen ML, Kronberg-Kippilä C, Ahonen S, Niinistö S, Alfthan G, Simell O, Ilonen J, et al. 2013. Fatty acids in serum and diet—a canonical correlation analysis among toddlers. *Matern Child Nutr* **9:** 381–395. doi:10.1111/j.1740-8709.2011.00374.x

Uusitalo U, Liu X, Yang J, Aronsson CA, Hummel S, Butterworth M, Lernmark Å, Rewers M, Hagopian W, She JX, et al. 2016. Association of early exposure of probiotics and islet autoimmunity in the TEDDY study. *JAMA Pediatr* **170:** 20–28. doi:10.1001/jamapediatrics.2015.2757

Uusitalo U, Lee HS, Andrén Aronsson C, Vehik K, Yang J, Hummel S, Silvis K, Lernmark Å, Rewers M, Hagopian W, et al. 2018. Early infant diet and islet autoimmunity in the TEDDY study. *Diabetes Care* **41:** 522–530. doi:10.2337/dc17-1983

Uusitalo U, Mramba LK, Aronsson CA, Vehik K, Yang J, Hummel S, Lernmark Å, Rewers M, Hagopian W, McIndoe R, et al. 2023. HLA genotype and probiotics modify the association between timing of solid food introduction and islet autoimmunity in the TEDDY study. *Diabetes Care* **46:** 1839–1847. doi:10.2337/dc23-0417

van Berge-Henegouwen GP, Mulder CJ. 1993. Pioneer in the gluten free diet: Willem-Karel Dicke 1905–1962, over 50 years of gluten free diet. *Gut* **34:** 1473–1475. doi:10.1136/gut.34.11.1473

Vatanen T, Franzosa EA, Schwager R, Tripathi S, Arthur TD, Vehik K, Lernmark Å, Hagopian WA, Rewers MJ, She JX, et al. 2018. The human gut microbiome in early-onset type 1 diabetes from the TEDDY study. *Nature* **562:** 589–594. doi:10.1038/s41586-018-0620-2

Vehik K, Lynch KF, Wong MC, Tian X, Ross MC, Gibbs RA, Ajami NJ, Petrosino JF, Rewers M, Toppari J, et al. 2019. Prospective virome analyses in young children at increased genetic risk for type 1 diabetes. *Nat Med* **25:** 1865–1872. doi:10.1038/s41591-019-0667-0

Virtanen SM, Räsänen L, Aro A, Lindström J, Sippola H, Lounamaa R, Toivanen L, Tuomilehto J, Åkerblom HK. 1991. Infant feeding in Finnish children less than 7 yr of age with newly diagnosed IDDM. Childhood Diabetes in Finland Study Group. *Diabetes Care* **14:** 415–417. doi:10.2337/diacare.14.5.415

Virtanen SM, Hyppönen E, Läärä E, Vähäsalo P, Kulmala P, Savola K, Räsänen L, Aro A, Knip M, Åkerblom HK. 1998. Cow's milk consumption, disease-associated autoantibodies and type 1 diabetes mellitus: a follow-up study in siblings of diabetic children. Childhood Diabetes in Finland Study Group. *Diabet Med* **15:** 730–738.<730::AID-DIA646>3.0.CO;2-C

Virtanen SM, Niinistö S, Nevalainen J, Salminen I, Takkinen HM, Kääriä S, Uusitalo L, Alfthan G, Kenward MG, Veijola R, et al. 2010. Serum fatty acids and risk of advanced β-cell autoimmunity: a nested case-control study among children with HLA-conferred susceptibility to type I diabetes. *Eur J Clin Nutr* **64:** 792–799. doi:10.1038/ejcn.2010.75

Virtanen SM, Uusitalo L, Kenward MG, Nevalainen J, Uusitalo U, Kronberg-Kippilä C, Ovaskainen ML, Arkkola T, Niinistö S, Hakulinen T, et al. 2011. Maternal food consumption during pregnancy and risk of advanced β-cell autoimmunity in the offspring. *Pediatr Diabetes* **12:** 95–99. doi:10.1111/j.1399-5448.2010.00668.x

Virtanen SM, Takkinen HM, Nwaru BI, Kaila M, Ahonen S, Nevalainen J, Niinistö S, Siljander H, Simell O, Ilonen J, et al. 2014. Microbial exposure in infancy and subsequent appearance of type 1 diabetes mellitus-associated autoantibodies: a cohort study. *JAMA Pediatr* **168:** 755–763. doi:10.1001/jamapediatrics.2014.296

Virtanen SM, Cuthbertson D, Nucci AM, Hyytinen M, Ormisson A, Salonen M, Turrini T, Cummings EA, Bradley B, Tanner-Blasiar M, et al. 2021. Dietary compliance in a randomized double-blind infant feeding trial during infancy aiming at prevention of type 1 diabetes. *Food Sci Nutr* **9:** 4221–4231. doi:10.1002/fsn3.2389

Viskari HR, Koskela P, Lönnrot M, Luonuansuu S, Reunanen A, Baer M, Hyöty H. 2000. Can enterovirus infections explain the increasing incidence of type 1 diabetes? *Diabetes Care* **23:** 414–416. doi:10.2337/diacare.23.3.414

Viskari H, Ludvigsson J, Uibo R, Salur L, Marciulionyte D, Hermann R, Soltesz G, Füchtenbusch M, Ziegler AG, Kondrashova A, et al. 2005. Relationship between the incidence of type 1 diabetes and maternal enterovirus antibodies: time trends and geographical variation. *Diabetologia* **48:** 1280–1287. doi:10.1007/s00125-005-1780-9

Viskari H, Knip M, Tauriainen S, Huhtala H, Veijola R, Ilonen J, Simell O, Surcel HM, Hyöty H. 2012. Maternal enterovirus infection as a risk factor for type 1 diabetes in the exposed offspring. *Diabetes Care* **35:** 1328–1332. doi:10.2337/dc11-2389

Wahlberg J, Fredriksson J, Nikolic E, Vaarala O, Ludvigsson J, ABIS-Study Group. 2005. Environmental factors related to the induction of β-cell autoantibodies in 1-yr-old healthy children. *Pediatr Diabetes* **6:** 199–205. doi:10.1111/j.1399-543X.2005.00129.x

Wang Y, Guo H, Wang G, Zhai J, Du B. 2023. COVID-19 as a trigger for type 1 diabetes. *J Clin Endocrinol Metab* **108:** 2176–2183. doi:10.1210/clinem/dgad165

Wild CP. 2012. The exposome: from concept to utility. *Int J Epidemiol* **41:** 24–32. doi:10.1093/ije/dyr236

Writing Group for the TRIGR Study Group; Knip M, Åkerblom HK, Al Taji E, Becker D, Bruining J, Castano L, Danne T, de Beaufort C, Dosch HM, et al. 2018. Effect of hydrolyzed infant formula vs conventional formula on risk of type 1 diabetes: the TRIGR randomized clinical trial. *JAMA* **319:** 38–48. doi:10.1001/jama.2017.19826

Yoon JW. 1990. The role of viruses and environmental factors in the induction of diabetes. *Curr Top Microbiol Immunol* **164:** 95–123. doi:10.1007/978-3-642-75741-9_6

Zhang T, Mei Q, Zhang Z, Walline JH, Liu Y, Zhu H, Zhang S. 2022. Risk for newly diagnosed diabetes after COVID-19: a systematic review and meta-analysis. *BMC Med* **20:** 444. doi:10.1186/s12916-022-02656-y

Breakdown and Repair of Peripheral Immune Tolerance in Type 1 Diabetes

Gerald T. Nepom

Benaroya Research Institute, Seattle, Washington 98101, USA

Correspondence: jnepom@benaroyaresearch.org

Failures in peripheral immune tolerance mechanisms create a permissive environment for autoimmune diabetes initiation and disease progression. Biomarker analyses provide tools that allow recognition of this loss of tolerance, reflecting a serial acquisition of pathogenic characteristics causally linked to islet β-cell dysfunction and death. Autoimmune effector cell activation and expansion, ineffective immune regulation, and tissue response to injury during active disease each represent challenges to homeostasis; however, they also represent targets for therapeutic intervention, with the potential for restoration of tolerance. Limited success in recent clinical trials demonstrates that tolerance in type 1 diabetes (T1D) is achievable, but currently occurs in few subjects and is not durable in most. Combining therapeutic agents to rebuild multiple immune components to restore tolerance, particularly addressing both effector and regulatory T-cell dysfunction, is needed.

Perspectives on immune tolerance in type 1 diabetes (T1D) reflect our understanding of key checkpoints in pathogenesis that determine susceptibility, disease progression, and resistance to therapy. At each of these three steps, immunological outcomes either promote immune activation or immune regulation, and the balance defines whether tolerance prevails. By viewing these checkpoints from the perspective of genetic enablers (susceptibility), environmental triggers (progression), and homeostatic controllers (including response to therapy), a framework emerges that provides a useful paradigm for aligning stages of T1D pathogenesis with prospects for restoration of homeostasis and immune tolerance.

SUSCEPTIBILITY

The principal enablers of T1D are genetic traits that generate a potential for aberrant autoreactivity to islet autoantigens. Most of the genes known to be associated with T1D are involved in immune responses (Concannon et al. 2009), and the two most important of these genes, HLA and INS, are directly mechanistically linked to establishing a peripheral immune repertoire with potential autoreactivity: The HLA genetic association is attributable to specific HLA class II genes, notably HLA-DQB1*0302, which acts as a restriction element for autoreactive CD4 T-cell recognition through presentation of islet-derived peptides binding to either *cis-* (DQA1*0301/DQB1*0302)

Cite this article as *Cold Spring Harb Perspect Med* doi: 10.1101/cshperspect.a041596

or *trans*- (DQA1*0201/DQB1*0302) class II HLA-DQ8 molecules encoded by particular HLA-DR4 or HLA-DR3/4 haplotypes (Nepom and Erlich 1991; Nepom and Kwok 1998; Chow et al. 2019). The INS genetic association with T1D is attributable to allelic variation in the INS promoter region, which corresponds to differential expression of proinsulin in thymic tissue (Pugliese et al. 1997), and this correlates with the frequency of peripheral insulin-specific CD4 T cells, in which lower thymic expression of INS corresponds to higher autoreactive potential (Durinovic-Belló et al. 2010), presumably due to inefficient negative selection during T-cell maturation.

Notably, neither of these genetic traits, or even the combination of the two, is fully penetrant for T1D clinical outcome. Nondiabetic individuals with these same genes also have a peripheral repertoire populated by autoreactive CD4 T cells with the same specificity, indicating that while these genes confer the potential for disease, they are not sufficient. In this sense, the susceptibility genes are mechanistically responsible for creating a potentially autoreactive host environment, fertile ground for subsequent immune activation events via environmental triggers that enable disease progression. Precedent for this type of environmental interaction with genetic susceptibility is found in other immunologic diseases, which show the types of triggering events that can initiate a break in tolerance. For example, in rheumatoid arthritis, the combination of a history of smoking in individuals carrying the HLA-DR0401 susceptibility genes synergizes for the development of anti-ACPA autoantibodies, a precursor to progressive autoimmune rheumatic disease, apparently due to the up-regulation of PAD enzymes in the lung from chronic smoke irritation (Klareskog et al. 2011; Gravallese and Firestein 2023). Another example is seen in the food allergy to peanuts, in which a specific HLA-DQA allele and a genetic variant of MALT1 are associated with sensitization and progression to allergy, respectively (Huffaker et al. 2023). Intriguingly, in this latter example, the same HLA association modifies the likelihood that oral antigen immunotherapy will be successful, consistent with the notion that a very specific antigen–HLA interaction leads to antigen presentation for immune responses that can be pathogenic or tolerogenic, depending on clinical context (Kanchan et al. 2022).

At this initial stage of disease susceptibility, predisposition is hard-wired into an individual's background, and is challenging to target for tolerogenic therapies. In the NOD mouse, which displays a class II molecule (IAg7) structurally similar to DQ8, the introduction of a modified class II transgene (Singer et al. 1998) or selective breeding with nonsusceptible haplotypes in heterozygous animals (Wicker et al. 1995) is sufficient to prevent spontaneous progression to diabetes. HLA-DQ0602 may have a similar role in protection from T1D in humans, since it is negatively associated with disease incidence, particularly in children (Kockum et al. 1995). Distinct physicochemical properties of the class II molecule encoded by this protective allele have been described that suggest a potential role in enhanced negative selection of T cells (Ettinger et al. 2000). However, feasible ways to manipulate the islet peptide–HLA interaction to recapitulate a tolerance outcome that alters the frequency or fate of the peripheral autoreactive CD4T cells are daunting and will require novel forms of intervention. Potential examples include attempts to interfere with the DQ8–peptide interface (Ostrov et al. 2018) or to enhance thymic negative selection directly via specific antigen exposure (Atibalentja et al. 2009), but there are relatively few therapeutic efforts to tolerize at this very early step in pathogenesis compared to a multitude of therapeutic initiatives aimed at the next step, when activation, expansion, and regulation of the immune response coalesce in a progressive autoreactivity that results in clinically evident disease.

PROGRESSION

Since autoreactive T cells with islet specificity are found in all genetically susceptible individuals, what are the characteristics that represent a loss of tolerance leading to disease progression in some, but not all? Which of these offer opportunities or specific molecular targets for tolerogenic therapy?

One fundamental observation was the finding that the age of onset and rate of progression to T1D can be markedly different among identical twins (Redondo et al. 2008). This simple but significant concept indicates that control of disease progression is a potent homeostatic system and provides a rationale for comparisons between T1D and genetically matched non-T1D subjects to identify indicators and potential control points for tolerance. These types of studies identify numerous T-cell characteristics, which correspond to a loss of tolerance, such as the acquisition of markers indicating in vivo activation (e.g., CD38; Yang et al. 2017) or chronic activation (e.g., Kv1.3; Beeton et al. 2006), an apparent deficit in functional regulatory T cells (Long et al. 2010; Hull et al. 2017) or the inability of effector T cells to respond to regulation (Schneider et al. 2008), expansions in potentially inflammatory subsets (Arif et al. 2017), oligoclonal expansions of autoreactive cells (Cerosaletti et al. 2017), or the prevalence of stem cell memory T cells (Abdelsamed et al. 2020). Studies focused on a similar stem-like CD8T cell in the NOD mouse model of autoimmune diabetes have identified a distinct TCF1^{hi} phenotype with a key role as a self-renewing progenitor cell for generating and replenishing effector autoimmune T cells responsible for β-cell destruction (Gearty et al. 2022).

Each of these T-cell characteristics represent properties of autoreactive immune activity that occur during loss of tolerance, and therefore they are potentially useful biomarkers for monitoring disease status. In other cases, it is the loss of a T-cell phenotype, such as T-cell exhaustion, that indicates an effector response associated with more rapid disease progression (Wiedeman et al. 2020). This constellation of autoimmune characteristics presents both an opportunity and a challenge. The opportunity is to use the properties of the acquired marker(s) as therapeutic targets, for example using depletional agents directed to acquired activation markers, providing support for Tregs through cell therapy or IL-2 administration, enhancing T-cell exhaustion (e.g., with teplizumab, a Mab against CD3; Long et al. 2016), deviating immune programming away from Th17 using anti-IL-6 or anti-IL-6R, etc. As discussed in the next section, many of these therapeutic strategies have been advanced into clinical trials, but successful tolerance has been elusive, with modest success in a limited number of individuals. Each of these features of disease progression is likely a downstream consequence of autoreactive activation, making successful tolerance somewhat refractory to single drug strategies without addressing root causes or addressing multiple targets.

There have been many analyses that use epidemiologic or observational investigational tools to study the apparent breakdown of tolerance in early T1D. Particularly notable are longitudinal cohort studies monitoring genetically susceptible children who acquire evidence of immune activation usually documented by the appearance of islet autoantibodies (Ziegler et al. 2003; Lynch et al. 2018; Vatanen et al. 2018; Krischer et al. 2022). One of the recurring observations is the association of various enteroviral or rotaviral infections with disease progression (Hyöty et al. 1995; Honeyman et al. 2010; Honkanen et al. 2017). While often interpreted as evidence for molecular mimicry between viral and islet antigens, alternative explanations such as generalized inflammation from tissue cell death (Horwitz et al. 1998), indirect effects mediated through altered microbiome, or interference with systemic regulatory responses are also reasonable possibilities. Another type of induced breakdown of tolerance leading to autoimmune diabetes is seen occasionally in cancer patients treated with immune checkpoint inhibitors (ICIs), which directly demonstrates a role for T-cell costimulation checkpoints in maintaining homeostasis, although the comparability of ICI-induced diabetes and T1D has been questioned (Perdigoto et al. 2022; Quandt et al. 2024).

The time between the initial production of autoantibodies against islet antigens and the onset of dysglycemia is highly variable, a window of opportunity not only for intervention to restore tolerance but also a time frame in which disease amplifiers may arise that escape tolerogenic mechanisms. In this context, T-cell recognition of posttranslationally modified islet proteins (PTM antigens) is particularly interesting. Proposed to be products of transpeptidation reactions in islet granules (Wang et al. 2019; Reed and Kappler 2021) or defective ribosomal translation (Kracht et al. 2017) or enzymatic modification (McGinty et al. 2014), the presence of activation and memory properties of peripheral T cells reactive to PTM antigens (Nguyen et al. 2023) indicates an intriguing amplification mechanism associated with disease progression consistent with the hypothesis that a lack of thymic negative selection has led to a peripheral repertoire biased toward de novo activation, moving the immune response in a pathogenic direction. Whether these PTM modifications actually initiate disease is not clear, but since islet stress appears to foster transpeptidation and enzymatic PTM, it is plausible that a neoantigenic T-cell response to PTM antigens acts as an important amplifier of anti-islet immunity that can potentially bypass and overcome underlying tolerance mechanisms, thereby contributing to disease progression.

Direct comparisons between these immune parameters associated with T1D progression in humans with the disease course in murine models of autoimmune diabetes are rare, in part due to the differences between cells recovered from peripheral blood in humans versus lymph nodes and spleen in rodents. In addition, major differences (von Herrath and Nepom 2009) between the most common murine model (NOD strain of mice) and human pathophysiology, such as a strong gender effect on penetrance in NOD but not humans and accumulation of peri-insulitic infiltrates of lymphocytes immediately before rapid destruction of islets in NOD but not seen in the nPOD catalog of human pancreatic pathology specimens, are two such examples. Thus, although there may be a few cases of human T1D that are pathophysiologically similar to the NOD mouse, they are certainly not common, reflected in the large list of therapeutic interventions that interfere with disease progression in the NOD but have failed in human trials, including heat shock proteins, various insulin-related antigens, immune adjuvants, and others (Shoda et al. 2005). In spite of these differences, some general concepts from mouse models regarding mechanisms of disease remain useful for translational applications. One such concept is the importance of genetic background for influencing tolerance. Although the disease in the NOD mouse is highly penetrant, extensive backcrossing onto other strains has identified multiple disease-associated genetic loci (Wicker et al. 2005), most of which provide relative protection against spontaneous diabetes. Examples that have translated well to humans include IL-2 and CTLA4, where relevant pathways were implicated in murine models and conform to regulatory pathways in human immunobiology that influence the progression of T1D. In this way, efforts to understand disease protective mechanisms in mice are candidates for investigation in humans. Another concept that translates well between murine and human diabetes is the generation of PTM antigens in the islet. As discussed above, multiple types of PTM are associated with T1D progression, and this understanding developed in human diabetes as a direct consequence of the discovery of transpeptidase-generated "hybrid antigens" in the BDC2.4 model of murine NOD diabetes (Baker et al. 2019).

Perhaps the highest utility of murine models is in generating concepts that, although differing in detail from human immunology, nevertheless suggest novel pathways and strategies with tolerogenic potential. Anti-CD3 monoclonal antibody therapy for T1D was initially developed based on efficacy in the NOD mouse (Herold et al. 1992; Chatenoud et al. 1994), but the resulting high degree of durable efficacy is not fully recapitulated in humans, where the response is more heterogeneous, and a minority of treated subjects show long-term clinical remission (Perdigoto et al. 2019). Another example is the report that genetic deletion of regulatory T cells in mice is sufficient to allow spontaneous polyclonal self-reactive follicular T cells to expand (Lee et al. 2023), reiterating the importance of FOXP3-positive regulatory T cells to control autoimmunity (Spence et al. 2018; Sakaguchi et al. 2023) and lending support to efforts to increase robust regulatory T cells as a tolerogenic, or at least homeostatic maintenance, therapy in humans (Dong et al. 2021). Another example that led to a direct translational strategy was the demonstration in the NOD mouse that the therapeutic benefit of anti-CD3 given in a suboptimal dose could be enhanced by coadministration of an oral bacterial carrier encoding IL-10 alongside proinsulin

(Cook et al. 2020), an experiment that was recapitulated in a phase 1 clinical trial (Mathieu et al. 2024).

Two of the important features of T1D disease progression that are difficult to recapitulate in murine models are the complexity of an outbred population and diverse environmental elements including microbiome, diet, and infections that influence immunologic development and maturation. An overly literal translation of murine models, particularly the NOD mouse, can lead to viewing T1D as a single disease pathway, overlooking the heterogeneous nature of immune responses that occur in people. In this regard, lessons can be learned from other autoimmune diseases, such as systemic lupus erythematosus and rheumatoid arthritis, which differ from T1D in many respects but which show how diverse immune responses and environmental interactions can converge to manifest as particular diseases, and in the process identify therapeutic targets. For example, a general theme in lupus pathogenesis is an inappropriate response to intra- or extracellular nucleic acids that trigger intracellular signals and sensors leading to exuberant immune activation, which, when accompanied by a failure of regulation, leads to progressive immune-mediated pathology (Accapezzato et al. 2023). In rheumatoid arthritis, an important causal pathway appears to be an inappropriate response to pathogens that elicit neutrophil TRAPs involving citrullination defense mechanisms that, when accompanied by a failure of regulation, lead to immune responses to PTM antigens and progressive pathology (Gravallese and Firestein 2023). The analogous paradigm in T1D allows for diverse triggering events from environmental stimuli in the context of genetic susceptibility, which elicit exuberant immune activation when there is a failure of regulation, a simple recipe for loss of tolerance and immunopathology that converges in a final common pathway of islet cell destruction. From this perspective, peripheral tolerance mechanisms that protect from tissue damage represent the last bulwark against disease progression, in which therapeutic restoration of tolerance requires not only boosting these regulatory elements but also negating the exuberant autoimmune responses, in parallel.

RESTORATION OF HOMEOSTASIS

Does the loss of tolerance in T1D indicate defects in immune regulation or defective overactivation? As summarized above, biomarker, phenotypic, and functional studies indicate that both are closely linked to disease progression. Indeed, a large body of evidence from clinical trials and observational studies indicates that therapeutic interventions that address only one but not the other are insufficient to restore tolerance (Huffaker et al. 2021; Nepom 2022). One of the notable features of immunomodulatory clinical trials in T1D is that multiple therapeutic strategies have shown similar transient clinical outcomes. For example, partial preservation of C-peptide secretion occurs following various anti-T-cell (e.g., teplizumab, alefacept, ATG), anti-B-cell (e.g., rituximab), anti-cytokine (e.g., golimumab), or costimulatory blockade (e.g., abatacept) therapies (Herold et al. 2013; Orban et al. 2014; Pescovitz et al. 2014; Rigby et al. 2015, 2023; Haller et al. 2018). Relapse, as measured by the rate of C-peptide loss, occurs in most subjects for each of these agents. In the clinical trials of teplizumab and alefacept, however, between 10% and 30% of treated subjects displayed a more durable response, and focusing on the immune system characteristics in those individuals provides additional lessons for understanding peripheral tolerance.

A key observation is that therapies directed against T cells, unless they spare the regulatory T-cell compartment, are insufficient for tolerance when therapy is discontinued. This has actually been appreciated since the initial studies of cyclosporine as a potential therapy in T1D, which showed durable remission in a minority of treated subjects (Papoz et al. 1990) and is reinforced by the description of recurrent T1D in subjects who received pancreatic transplants, in spite of receiving potent anti-rejection immunosuppression (Burke et al. 2015). Both teplizumab and alefacept are more selective with respect to T-cell inhibition, and although each was initially developed with depletional or antagonistic activity expected, it is now recognized that their unanticipated agonist activity-inducing exhaustion-like properties in effector T-cell populations are the dominant phenotypic correlate of clinical response (Linsley and Long 2019; Diggins et al. 2021). Importantly, neither of these drugs reduce regulatory T-cell numbers or function, and thus they somewhat fortuitously impact both effector and regulatory arms of the immune system in a favorable direction.

Although a tolerogenic strategy of ablating, deviating, or anergizing the effector response while at the same time boosting regulatory responses seems like a simple equation, there are significant challenges ahead. One issue is recognition of the importance of heterogeneity in the early stages of the pathogenic sequence leading to T1D. As discussed above, it is likely that multiple pathways are variably activated in the progression to a pathogenic state of immune activation, raising the possibility that the type of tolerogenic therapy may need to be tailored for targeting particular pathways in different individuals (Linsley et al. 2021). The concept of disease "endotypes" is intended in part to address this issue (Battaglia et al. 2020), and may help explain why fairly small numbers of patients respond to different particular types of immune therapies such as anti-cytokines, costimulatory blockade, B-cell depletion, etc. A second issue is concern about the durability of regulatory responses that are based on immunologic plasticity—the concept that the immune response is well adapted to change phenotype in response to external cues. For example, the demonstration that IL-6 exposure strongly influences the development of Th17 cells versus Treg cells suggested that tissue inflammation could be a strong barrier to enhancing regulation (Bettelli et al. 2008), a concept that was validated in preclinical model systems documenting the evolution of "ex-Treg" cells from a regulatory to a potentially pathogenic phenotype (Zhou et al. 2009). This type of reprogramming of regulatory cells toward pathogenic characteristics is an issue that clouds prospects for regulatory cell therapy, and may require combination therapy with anti-inflammatory agents, deletion or inhibition of effector responses, and/or manipulation of the regulatory cells to be refractory to reprogramming, perhaps requiring gene editing or molecular engineering strategies.

Figure 1 shows the accumulation of defects in immune tolerance that cascade during the course of T1D disease onset, and indicates opportunities for targeted tolerance therapies. While genetic predisposition for autoreactivity is not amenable to direct revision, inadequate tolerance functions attributed to those genes are potential therapeutic targets. Preventing loss of tolerance at a very early stage may involve modifying environmental stimuli or remodeling the developing immune repertoire to interfere with autoantigen sensitization of naive autoreactive T cells. NOD mouse colonies can be protected from autoimmune diabetes using dietary, microbiome, or housing changes, observations that have been recognized for decades, providing rationale for efforts to find ways to modify those types of environmental stimuli in susceptible populations (Chapman et al. 2012). More targeted approaches that aspire to directly modify the selection and expansion of autoreactive T cells by modifying the peptide–MHC interaction during T-cell development are also potential ways to create an immune system refractory to breakdown of tolerance, by lowering the peripheral population of autoantigen-specific T cells and thus creating a higher barrier to initial immune activation. The evolution from T1D predisposition to progression is marked by activation and expansion of immune reactivities to islet antigens, offering a variety of opportunities for restoration of tolerance. Indeed, it is not the specific recognition of autoantigens that dictates pathogenic outcomes, it is the type of immune sequelae that follow such recognition events, with a multitude of nonpathogenic possibilities. Antigen recognition in a format that encourages deletion, deviation, anergy, or exhaustion of effector T cells is, therefore, a primary goal of many therapeutic strategies. Several tolerization strategies use different ways of delivering autoantigens for antigen presentation, considering localization to pancreata or lymph nodes, use of various or multiple islet antigens, and linking such autoantigens to ligands or functional tethering molecules to favor immune deletion or deviation of responses, for example by targeting antigen presentation in the liver or via tolerogenic dendritic cells. Since this phase of developing autoimmunity is characterized by antigen determinant spreading, it is also a time in which therapies

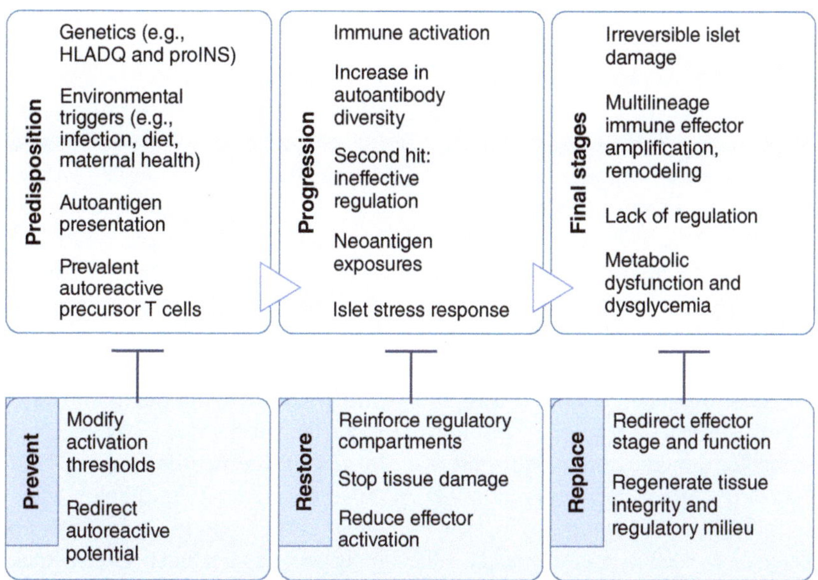

Figure 1. The serial loss of tolerance in type 1 diabetes (T1D): opportunities for intervention. The establishment and perpetuation of defective peripheral immune tolerance in T1D is a cumulative process, illustrated as an evolution in three phases. First is the generation of a peripheral immune T-cell repertoire that is prone to autoimmunity, in which the predisposition for a loss of tolerance is genetically controlled and reflected in an increased frequency of autoreactive naiveperipheral T cells. Expansion of these autoreactive cells can be a result of antigen-specific or nonspecific environmental factors that represent a transition from a potentially autoimmune to an autoimmune-prone T-cell repertoire. Next is the activation of these autoreactive cells, which occurs in the peripheral immune system coincident with a failure of regulatory constraints, the "second hit" in unleashing pathogenic effector immune responses. In this phase, the spreading of the immune response occurs through the recruitment of B cells driving autoantibody production and additional antigen presentation, expansion to additional tissue antigens, and recognition of neoantigens generated from posttranslationally modified target proteins. Islet cell damage is accompanied by a β-cell stress response that further amplifies immune activity. A final phase is the confluence of multiple activated immune cell types and inflammatory pathways, which, in the absence of effective counterregulation, reflects unrestrained pathogenic autoimmunity without tolerogenic barriers. Immune defects that accumulate during this serial loss of tolerance identify pathways and targets for potential therapy designed to restore homeostasis. Opportunities for this type of mechanism-informed therapeutic intervention strategy are indicated in the lower panels, either preventing initial loss of tolerance, restoring tolerance capacity through rebalancing of regulatory and effector compartments, or replacing tolerogenic potential through multilineage immune reconstruction. As discussed in the text, a combination of therapeutic strategies is needed to address the extent and diversity of failed tolerance mechanisms during these phases of disease.

designed to interfere with intercellular collaboration, such as T-cell interactions with B cells and/or with dendritic cells, are most promising. In particular, addressing both T-cell and B-cell tolerization may be most effective to interfere with this early expansion of antigen breadth, potentially inhibiting the spreading of autoreactivity to other islet antigens and PTM antigens. Recent studies of disease-associated B cells in T1D identify peripheral anergic autoreactive B cells (B_{ND}) that are potentially tolerant, although this appears to be reversible in a subset of cells ($B_{ND}2$) that directly contribute to pathogenesis (Stensland et al. 2023). Insight into the role of these cells in antigen presentation to autoreactive T cells could enable targeted therapeutics to help sustain a tolerogenic response. Interfering with stress pathways that favor PTM formation, potentially including inhibition of PAD enzymes (Barasa and Thompson 2023), may also have a role at this stage of the disease. These types of therapeutic strategies interfering with antigen-specific effector responses may be difficult later in disease progression, a time when multiple islet antigens are recognized as targets and when tissue inflammation is robust.

Selective interference with autoreactive effector cells, however, is insufficient for tolerance in the context of progressive autoimmunity, as evidenced by recurrent islet cell loss after discontinuation of depletional therapies, discussed in the previous section and summarized elsewhere (Smilek et al. 2014; Nepom 2022). Targeting effector responses during this phase of immune expansion and disease progression must be accompanied by efforts to enhance regulatory immune systems essential for durable immune homeostasis. Generating or reinforcing regulatory immune activity in the context of T1D progression, however, is challenged by several conundrums: (1) is it sufficient to boost regulatory T-cell responses to a particular islet antigen, or is it necessary to have regulatory specificity for multiple antigens; (2) will naturally occurring regulatory T cells, if boosted in numbers, be sufficient to control autoimmunity, or is it necessary to engineer stability and functional robustness into such cells; (3) will the islet microenvironment inflammatory profile of cytokines and chemokines obviate desired regulatory activity; and (4) is it necessary to use sequential therapies, first abrogating pathogenic effector responses to have a hospitable opportunity for therapies that support regulatory dominance? These are fundamental questions that lack suitable preclinical T1D models, and pose a challenge to conventional clinical trial designs. Novel "umbrella" or other adaptive trial designs (Woodcock and LaVange 2017) may be helpful for testing various options in an efficient manner, and/or a multidrug approach (Skyler 2015), perhaps modeled after the decades-old transformational "reverse the pyramid" strategy in rheumatoid arthritis (Wilske and Healey 1989), in which therapy starts with multiple agents combined, followed by selective withdrawal of individual components to assess durable tolerance.

The last panel in Figure 1 addresses the daunting task of reestablishing tolerance in the context of a raging autoimmune response, in which there are multiple types of activated immune cells, tissue inflammation, and innate immune catalysts all simultaneously converging on β-cell damage and destruction. Regenerating insulin secretory capacity, tissue integrity, and establishing a regulatory environment in the islets is likely to require a comprehensive approach to therapy that silences immune system effector responses, supports β-cell recovery to minimize a tissue stress response, and creates a robust regulatory network to prevent recurrent pathology. Notably, although some antigen-specific T-cell effectors and regulatory cells and some autoantibody specificities have been well-studied, very little is known about the tissue response in vivo. In particular, the role of the tissue environment in driving the pathogenesis of T1D and resistance to tolerization therapy may be critical and may differ among individuals due to underlying genetic variation or β-cell fitness. The findings in T1D clinical trials that anti-TNF monoclonal antibody therapy, but not anti-IL-1 or anti-IL-6R monoclonals, result in partial improvements in β-cell function is currently a conundrum (Moran et al. 2013; Greenbaum et al. 2021; Rigby et al. 2023) but an indication that there are opportunities to target both innate and adaptive immune pathways and explore potential synergistic effects. Even less is known about alternative stress-induced responses, including the neuronal interface with islet cells, that may prove to have a role in perpetuating disease or the tissue response to therapy.

CONCLUDING REMARKS

Immune tolerance in T1D is achievable, as evidenced by well-documented examples of the successful rescue of β cells in the early stages of the disease, with durable retention of islet function. When this occurs in the context of immune therapies such as teplizumab and alefacept, it is accompanied by functional and phenotypic changes in the peripheral immune response that are likely responsible for success. In other words, changes in peripheral immunity reflect and functionally arrest the pathogenic loss of β-cell function. However, this desirable result currently occurs infrequently, with most therapeutic outcomes being short-lived and not having durable effects on disease progression. Better understanding of the relationship between tissue-localized immune responses in the islet and those that are measured in the periphery may help improve tolerization success, which likely will require insight into innate immune pathways and other non-T-cell components perpetuating autoimmunity. Expanding the frequency of success and addressing the widespread clinical need requires using an entire toolbox of immune tolerance mechanisms and exploring novel combinations of therapeutic targets, simultaneously abrogating pathogenic effector responses and boosting homeostatic regulatory immunity.

ACKNOWLEDGMENTS

It takes a village. Many colleagues and organizations are responsible for the studies summarized in this article, and I am grateful for their collaboration. Concepts reflected here have been refined through many discussions at the Immune Tolerance Network, National Institutes of Health (NIH), TrialNet, JDRF, DiabetesUK, FOCIS, and elsewhere. Special acknowledgment goes to my coinvestigators at the Benaroya Research Institute, without whom this article, and knowledge in the field, would be much smaller. I apologize for any shortcomings in citations to original work in the field; as a Perspectives article, this is necessarily limited, and not intended to be a comprehensive metaanalysis or review.

REFERENCES

**Reference is also in this subject collection.*

Abdelsamed HA, Zebley CC, Nguyen H, Rutishauser RL, Fan Y, Ghoneim HE, Crawford JC, Alfei F, Alli S, Ribeiro SP, et al. 2020. β-Cell-specific CD8$^+$ T cells maintain stem cell memory-associated epigenetic programs during type 1 diabetes. *Nat Immunol* **21:** 578–587. doi:10.1038/s41590-020-0633-5

Accapezzato D, Caccavale R, Paroli MP, Gioia C, Nguyen BL, Spadea L, Paroli M. 2023. Advances in the pathogenesis and treatment of systemic lupus erythematosus. *Int J Mol Sci* **24:** 6578. doi:10.3390/ijms24076578

Arif S, Gibson VB, Nguyen V, Bingley PJ, Todd JA, Guy C, Dunger DB, Dayan CM, Powrie J, Lorenc A, et al. 2017. β-Cell specific T-lymphocyte response has a distinct inflammatory phenotype in children with type 1 diabetes compared with adults. *Diabet Med* **34:** 419–425. doi:10.1111/dme.13153

Atibalentja DF, Byersdorfer CA, Unanue ER. 2009. Thymus-blood protein interactions are highly effective in negative selection and regulatory T cell induction. *J Immunol* **183:** 7909–7918. doi:10.4049/jimmunol.0902632

Baker RL, Jamison BL, Haskins K. 2019. Hybrid insulin peptides are neo-epitopes for CD4 T cells in autoimmune diabetes. *Curr Opin Endocrinol Diabetes Obes* **26:** 195–200. doi:10.1097/MED.0000000000000490

Barasa L, Thompson PR. 2023. Protein citrullination: inhibition, identification and insertion. *Philos Trans R Soc Lond B Biol Sci* **378:** 20220240. doi:10.1098/rstb.2022.0240

Battaglia M, Ahmed S, Anderson MS, Atkinson MA, Becker D, Bingley PJ, Bosi E, Brusko TM, DiMeglio LA, Evans-Molina C, et al. 2020. Introducing the endotype concept to address the challenge of disease heterogeneity in type 1 diabetes. *Diabetes Care* **43:** 5–12. doi:10.2337/dc19-0880

Beeton C, Wulff H, Standifer NE, Azam P, Mullen KM, Pennington MW, Kolski-Andreaco A, Wei E, Grino A, Counts DR, et al. 2006. Kv1.3 channels are a therapeutic target for T cell-mediated autoimmune diseases. *Proc Natl Acad Sci* **103:** 17414–17419. doi:10.1073/pnas.0605136103

Bettelli E, Korn T, Oukka M, Kuchroo VK. 2008. Induction and effector functions of T_H17 cells. *Nature* **453:** 1051–1057. doi:10.1038/nature07036

Burke GW III, Vendrame F, Virdi SK, Ciancio G, Chen L, Ruiz P, Messinger S, Reijonen HK, Pugliese A. 2015. Lessons from pancreas transplantation in type 1 diabetes: recurrence of islet autoimmunity. *Curr Diab Rep* **15:** 121. doi:10.1007/s11892-015-0691-5

Cerosaletti K, Barahmand-Pour-Whitman F, Yang J, DeBerg HA, Dufort MJ, Murray SA, Israelsson E, Speake C, Gersuk VH, et al. 2017. Single-cell RNA sequencing reveals expanded clones of islet antigen-reactive CD4$^+$ T cells in peripheral blood of subjects with type 1 diabetes. *J Immunol* **199:** 323–335. doi:10.4049/jimmunol.1700172

Chapman NM, Coppieters K, von Herrath M, Tracy S. 2012. The microbiology of human hygiene and its impact on type 1 diabetes. *Islets* **4:** 253–261. doi:10.4161/isl.21570

Chatenoud L, Thervet E, Primo J, Bach JF. 1994. Anti-CD3 antibody induces long-term remission of overt autoimmunity in nonobese diabetic mice. *Proc Natl Acad Sci* **91:** 123–127. doi:10.1073/pnas.91.1.123

Chow IT, Gates TJ, Papadopoulos GK, Moustakas AK, Kolawole EM, Notturno RJ, McGinty JW, Torres-Chinn N, James EA, Greenbaum C, et al. 2019. Discriminative T cell recognition of cross-reactive islet-antigens is associated with HLA-DQ8 transdimer-mediated autoimmune diabetes. *Sci Adv* **5:** eaaw9336. doi:10.1126/sciadv.aaw9336

Concannon P, Rich SS, Nepom GT. 2009. Genetics of type 1A diabetes. *N Engl J Med* **360:** 1646–1654. doi:10.1056/NEJMra0808284

Cook DP, Cunha JPMCM, Martens PJ, Sassi G, Mancarella F, Ventriglia G, Sebastiani G, Vanherwegen AS, Atkinson MA, Van Huynegem K, et al. 2020. Intestinal delivery of proinsulin and IL-10 via *Lactococcus lactis* combined with low-dose anti-CD3 restores tolerance outside the window of acute type 1 diabetes diagnosis. *Front Immunol* **11:** 1103. doi:10.3389/fimmu.2020.01103

Diggins KE, Serti E, Muir V, Rosasco M, Lu T, Balmas E, Nepom G, Long SA, Linsley PS. 2021. Exhausted-like CD8$^+$ T cell phenotypes linked to C-peptide preservation in alefacept-treated T1D subjects. *JCI Insight* **6:** e142680. doi:10.1172/jci.insight.142680

Dong S, Hiam-Galvez KJ, Mowery CT, Herold KC, Gitelman SE, Esensten JH, Liu W, Lares AP, Leinbach AS, Lee M, et al. 2021. The effect of low-dose IL-2 and Treg adoptive cell therapy in patients with type 1 diabetes. *JCI Insight* **6:** e147474. doi:10.1172/jci.insight.147474

Durinovic-Belló I, Wu RP, Gersuk VH, Sanda S, Shilling HG, Nepom GT. 2010. Insulin gene VNTR genotype associates with frequency and phenotype of the autoimmune response to proinsulin. *Genes Immun* **11:** 188–193. doi:10.1038/gene.2009.108

Ettinger RA, Liu AW, Nepom GT, Kwok WW. 2000. β57-Asp plays an essential role in the unique SDS stability of HLA-DQA1*0102/DQB1*0602 αβ protein dimer, the class II MHC allele associated with protection from insulin-dependent diabetes mellitus. *J Immunol* **165:** 3232–3238. doi:10.4049/jimmunol.165.6.3232

Gearty SV, Dündar F, Zumbo P, Espinosa-Carrasco G, Shakiba M, Sanchez-Rivera FJ, Socci ND, Trivedi P, Lowe SW, Lauer P, et al. 2022. An autoimmune stem-like CD8T cell population drives type 1 diabetes. *Nature* **602:** 156–161. doi:10.1038/s41586-021-04248-x

Gravallese EM, Firestein GS. 2023. Rheumatoid arthritis—common origins, divergent mechanisms. *N Engl J Med* **388:** 529–542. doi:10.1056/NEJMra2103726

Greenbaum CJ, Serti E, Lambert K, Weiner LJ, Kanaparthi S, Lord S, Gitelman SE, Wilson DM, Gaglia JL, Griffin KJ, et al. 2021. IL-6 receptor blockade does not slow β cell loss in new-onset type 1 diabetes. *JCI Insight* **6:** e150074. doi:10.1172/jci.insight.150074

Haller MJ, Schatz DA, Skyler JS, Krischer JP, Bundy BN, Miller JL, Atkinson MA, Becker DJ, Baidal D, DiMeglio LA, et al. 2018. Low-dose anti-thymocyte globulin (ATG) preserves β-cell function and improves HbA_{1c} in new-onset type 1 diabetes. *Diabetes Care* **41:** 1917–1925. doi:10.2337/dc18-0494

Herold KC, Bluestone JA, Montag AG, Parihar A, Wiegner A, Gress RE, Hirsch R. 1992. Prevention of autoimmune diabetes with nonactivating anti-CD3 monoclonal antibody. *Diabetes* **41:** 385–391. doi:10.2337/diab.41.3.385

Herold KC, Gitelman SE, Ehlers MR, Gottlieb PA, Greenbaum CJ, Hagopian W, Boyle KD, Keyes-Elstein L, Aggarwal S, Phippard D, et al. 2013. Teplizumab (anti-CD3 mAb) treatment preserves C-peptide responses in patients with new-onset type 1 diabetes in a randomized controlled trial: metabolic and immunologic features at baseline identify a subgroup of responders. *Diabetes* **62:** 3766–3774. doi:10.2337/db13-0345

Honeyman MC, Stone NL, Falk BA, Nepom G, Harrison LC. 2010. Evidence for molecular mimicry between human T cell epitopes in rotavirus and pancreatic islet autoantigens. *J Immunol* **184:** 2204–2210. doi:10.4049/jimmunol.0900709

Honkanen H, Oikarinen S, Nurminen N, Laitinen OH, Huhtala H, Lehtonen J, Ruokoranta T, Hankaniemi MM, Lecouturier V, Almond JW, et al. 2017. Detection of enteroviruses in stools precedes islet autoimmunity by several months: possible evidence for slowly operating mechanisms in virus-induced autoimmunity. *Diabetologia* **60:** 424–431. doi:10.1007/s00125-016-4177-z

Horwitz MS, Bradley LM, Harbertson J, Krahl T, Lee J, Sarvetnick N. 1998. Diabetes induced by Coxsackie virus: initiation by bystander damage and not molecular mimicry. *Nat Med* **4:** 781–785. doi:10.1038/nm0798-781

Huffaker MF, Sanda S, Chandran S, Chung SA, St Clair EW, Nepom GT, Smilek DE. 2021. Approaches to establishing tolerance in immune mediated diseases. *Front Immunol* **12:** 744804. doi:10.3389/fimmu.2021.744804

Huffaker MF, Kanchan K, Bahnson HT, Baloh C, Lack G, Nepom GT, Mathias RA. 2023. Incorporating genetics in identifying peanut allergy risk and tailoring allergen immunotherapy: a perspective on the genetic findings from the LEAP trial. *J Allergy Clin Immunol* **151:** 841–847. doi:10.1016/j.jaci.2022.12.819

Hull CM, Peakman M, Tree TIM. 2017. Regulatory T cell dysfunction in type 1 diabetes: what's broken and how can we fix it? *Diabetologia* **60:** 1839–1850. doi:10.1007/s00125-017-4377-1

Hyöty H, Hiltunen M, Knip M, Laakkonen M, Vähäsalo P, Karjalainen J, Koskela P, Roivainen M, Leinikki P, Hovi T, et al. 1995. A prospective study of the role of coxsackie B and other enterovirus infections in the pathogenesis of IDDM. Childhood Diabetes in Finland (DiMe) Study Group. *Diabetes* **44:** 652–657. doi:10.2337/diab.44.6.652

Kanchan K, Shankar G, Huffaker MF, Bahnson HT, Chinthrajah RS, Sanda S, Manohar M, Ling H, Paschall JE, Toit GD, et al. 2022. HLA-associated outcomes in peanut oral immunotherapy trials identify mechanistic and clinical determinants of therapeutic success. *Front Immunol* **13:** 941839. doi:10.3389/fimmu.2022.941839

Klareskog L, Malmström V, Lundberg K, Padyukov L, Alfredsson L. 2011. Smoking, citrullination and genetic variability in the immunopathogenesis of rheumatoid arthritis. *Semin Immunol* **23:** 92–98. doi:10.1016/j.smim.2011.01.014

Kockum I, Sanjeevi CB, Eastman S, Landin-Olsson M, Dahlquist G, Lernmark A. 1995. Population analysis of protection by HLA-DR and DQ genes from insulin-dependent diabetes mellitus in Swedish children with insulin-dependent diabetes and controls. *Eur J Immunogenet* **22:** 443–465. doi:10.1111/j.1744-313x.1995.tb00282.x

Kracht MJ, van Lummel M, Nikolic T, Joosten AM, Laban S, van der Slik AR, van Veelen PA, Carlotti F, de Koning EJ, Hoeben RC, et al. 2017. Autoimmunity against a defective ribosomal insulin gene product in type 1 diabetes. *Nat Med* **23:** 501–507. doi:10.1038/nm.4289

Krischer JP, Liu X, Lernmark Å, Hagopian WA, Rewers MJ, She JX, Toppari J, Ziegler AG, Akolkar B; TEDDY Study Group. 2022. Predictors of the initiation of islet autoimmunity and progression to multiple autoantibodies and clinical diabetes: the TEDDY study. *Diabetes Care* **45:** 2271–2281. doi:10.2337/dc21-2612

Lee V, Rodriguez DM, Ganci NK, Zeng S, Ai J, Chao JL, Walker MT, Miller CH, Klawon DEJ, Schoenbach MH, et al. 2023. The endogenous repertoire harbors self-reactive $CD4^+$ T cell clones that adopt a follicular helper T cell-like phenotype at steady state. *Nat Immunol* **24:** 487–500. doi:10.1038/s41590-023-01425-0

Linsley PS, Long SA. 2019. Enforcing the checkpoints: harnessing T-cell exhaustion for therapy of T1D. *Curr Opin Endocrinol Diabetes Obes* **26:** 213–218. doi:10.1097/MED.0000000000000488

Linsley PS, Greenbaum CJ, Nepom GT. 2021. Uncovering pathways to personalized therapies in type 1 diabetes. *Diabetes* **70:** 831–841. doi:10.2337/db20-1185

Long SA, Cerosaletti K, Bollyky PL, Tatum M, Shilling H, Zhang S, Zhang ZY, Pihoker C, Sanda S, Greenbaum C, et al. 2010. Defects in IL-2R signaling contribute to diminished maintenance of FOXP3 expression in $CD4^{+}CD25^{+}$ regulatory T-cells of type 1 diabetic subjects. *Diabetes* **59:** 407–415. doi:10.2337/db09-0694

Long SA, Thorpe J, DeBerg HA, Gersuk V, Eddy J, Harris KM, Ehlers M, Herold KC, Nepom GT, Linsley PS. 2016. Partial exhaustion of CD8 T cells and clinical response to teplizumab in new-onset type 1 diabetes. *Sci Immunol* **1:** eaai7793. doi:10.1126/sciimmunol.aai7793

Lynch KF, Lee HS, Törn C, Vehik K, Krischer JP, Larsson HE, Haller MJ, Hagopian WA, Rewers MJ, She JX, et al. 2018. Gestational respiratory infections interacting with offspring HLA and CTLA-4 modifies incident β-cell autoantibodies. *J Autoimmun* **86:** 93–103. doi:10.1016/j.jaut.2017.09.005

Mathieu C, Wiedeman A, Cerosaletti K, Long SA, Serti E, Cooney L, Vermeiren J, Caluwaerts S, Van Huynegem K, Steidler L, et al. 2024. A first-in-human, open-label phase 1b and a randomised, double-blind phase 2a clinical trial in recent-onset type 1 diabetes with AG019 as monotherapy and in combination with teplizumab. *Diabetologia* **67:** 27–41. doi:10.1007/s00125-023-06014-2

McGinty JW, Chow IT, Greenbaum C, Odegard J, Kwok WW, James EA. 2014. Recognition of posttranslationally modified GAD65 epitopes in subjects with type 1 diabetes. *Diabetes* **63:** 3033–3040. doi:10.2337/db13-1952

Moran A, Bundy B, Becker DJ, DiMeglio LA, Gitelman SE, Goland R, Greenbaum CJ, Herold KC, Marks JB, Raskin P, et al. 2013. Interleukin-1 antagonism in type 1 diabetes of recent onset: two multicentre, randomised, double-blind, placebo-controlled trials. *Lancet* **381:** 1905–1915. doi:10.1016/S0140-6736(13)60023-9

Nepom GT. 2022. Synergistic targeting of immunologic pathways to empower durable tolerance therapies. *Front Immunol* **13:** 962177. doi:10.3389/fimmu.2022.962177

Nepom GT, Erlich H. 1991. MHC class-II molecules and autoimmunity. *Annu Rev Immunol* **9:** 493–525. doi:10.1146/annurev.iy.09.040191.002425

Nepom GT, Kwok WW. 1998. Molecular basis for HLA-DQ associations with IDDM. *Diabetes* **47:** 1177–1184. doi:10.2337/diab.47.8.1177

Nguyen H, Arribas-Layton D, Chow IT, Speake C, Kwok WW, Hessner MJ, Greenbaum CJ, James EA. 2023. Characterizing T cell responses to enzymatically modified β cell neo-epitopes. *Front Immunol* **13:** 1015855. doi:10.3389/fimmu.2022.1015855

Orban T, Bundy B, Becker DJ, Dimeglio LA, Gitelman SE, Goland R, Gottlieb PA, Greenbaum CJ, Marks JB, Monzavi R, et al. 2014. Costimulation modulation with abatacept in patients with recent-onset type 1 diabetes: follow-up 1 year after cessation of treatment. *Diabetes Care* **37:** 1069–1075. doi:10.2337/dc13-0604

Ostrov DA, Alkanani A, McDaniel KA, Case S, Baschal EE, Pyle L, Ellis S, Pöllinger B, Seidl KJ, Shah VN, et al. 2018. Methyldopa blocks MHC class II binding to disease-specific antigens in autoimmune diabetes. *J Clin Invest* **128:** 1888–1902. doi:10.1172/JCI97739

Papoz L, Lenegre F, Hors J, Assan R, Vague P, Tchobroutsky G, Passa P, Charbonnel B, Mirouze J, Feutren G, et al. 1990. Probability of remission in individuals in early adult insulin dependent diabetic patients. Results from the Cyclosporine Diabetes French Study Group. *Diabete Metab* **16:** 303–310.

Perdigoto AL, Preston-Hurlburt P, Clark P, Long SA, Linsley PS, Harris KM, Gitelman SE, Greenbaum CJ, Gottlieb PA, Hagopian W, et al. 2019. Treatment of type 1 diabetes with teplizumab: clinical and immunological follow-up after 7 years from diagnosis. *Diabetologia* **62:** 655–664. doi:10.1007/s00125-018-4786-9

Perdigoto AL, Deng S, Du KC, Kuchroo M, Burkhardt DB, Tong A, Israel G, Robert ME, Weisberg SP, Kirkiles-Smith N, et al. 2022. Immune cells and their inflammatory mediators modify β cells and cause checkpoint inhibitor-induced diabetes. *JCI Insight* **7:** e156330. doi:10.1172/jci.insight.156330

Pescovitz MD, Greenbaum CJ, Bundy B, Becker DJ, Gitelman SE, Goland R, Gottlieb PA, Marks JB, Moran A, Raskin P, et al. 2014. B-lymphocyte depletion with rituximab and β-cell function: two-year results. *Diabetes Care* **37:** 453–459. doi:10.2337/dc13-0626

Pugliese A, Zeller M, Fernandez A Jr, Zalcberg LJ, Bartlett RJ, Ricordi C, Pietropaolo M, Eisenbarth GS, Bennett ST, Patel DD. 1997. The insulin gene is transcribed in the human thymus and transcription levels correlated with allelic variation at the INS VNTR-IDDM2 susceptibility locus for type 1 diabetes. *Nat Genet* **15:** 293–297. doi:10.1038/ng0397-293

* Quandt Z, Perdigoto A, Anderson MS, Herold KC. 2024. Checkpoint inhibitor-induced autoimmune diabetes: an autoinflammatory disease. *Cold Spring Harb Perspect Med* doi:10.1101/cshperspect.a041603

Redondo MJ, Jeffrey J, Fain PR, Eisenbarth GS, Orban T. 2008. Concordance for islet autoimmunity among monozygotic twins. *N Engl J Med* **359:** 2849–2850. doi:10.1056/NEJMc0805398

Reed BK, Kappler JW. 2021. Hidden in plain view: discovery of chimeric diabetogenic CD4 T cell neo-epitopes. *Front Immunol* **12:** 669986. doi:10.3389/fimmu.2021.669986

Rigby MR, Harris KM, Pinckney A, DiMeglio LA, Rendell MS, Felner EI, Dostou JM, Gitelman SE, Griffin KJ, Tsalikian E, et al. 2015. Alefacept provides sustained clinical and immunological effects in new-onset type 1 diabetes patients. *J Clin Invest* **125:** 3285–3296. doi:10.1172/JCI81722

Rigby MR, Hayes B, Li Y, Vercruysse F, Hedrick JA, Quattrin T. 2023. Two-year follow-up from the T1GER study: continued off-therapy metabolic improvements in children and young adults with new-onset T1D treated with golimumab and characterization of responders. *Diabetes Care* **46:** 561–569. doi:10.2337/dc22-0908

Sakaguchi S, Kawakami R, Mikami N. 2023. Treg-based immunotherapy for antigen-specific immune suppression and stable tolerance induction: a perspective. *Immunother Adv* **3:** ltad007. doi:10.1093/immadv/ltad007

Schneider A, Rieck M, Sanda S, Pihoker C, Greenbaum C, Buckner JH. 2008. The effector T cells of diabetic subjects are resistant to regulation via $CD4^{+}FOXP3^{+}$ regulatory T cells. *J Immunol* **181:** 7350–7355. doi:10.4049/jimmunol.181.10.7350

Shoda LK, Young DL, Ramanujan S, Whiting CC, Atkinson MA, Bluestone JA, Eisenbarth GS, Mathis D, Rossini AA, Campbell SE, et al. 2005. A comprehensive review of interventions in the NOD mouse and implications for translation. *Immunity* **23:** 115–126. doi:10.1016/j.immuni.2005.08.002

Singer SM, Tisch R, Yang XD, Sytwu HK, Liblau R, McDevitt HO. 1998. Prevention of diabetes in NOD mice by a mutated I-Ab transgene. *Diabetes* **47:** 1570–1577. doi:10.2337/diabetes.47.10.1570

Skyler JS. 2015. Prevention and reversal of type 1 diabetes—past challenges and future opportunities. *Diabetes Care* **38:** 997–1007. doi:10.2337/dc15-0349

Smilek DE, Ehlers MR, Nepom GT. 2014. Restoring the balance: immunotherapeutic combinations for autoimmune disease. *Dis Model Mech* **7:** 503–513. doi:10.1242/dmm.015099

Spence A, Purtha W, Tam J, Dong S, Kim Y, Ju CH, Sterling T, Nakayama M, Robinson WH, Bluestone JA, et al. 2018. Revealing the specificity of regulatory T cells in murine autoimmune diabetes. *Proc Natl Acad Sci* **115:** 5265–5270. doi:10.1073/pnas.1715590115

Stensland ZC, Magera CA, Broncucia H, Gomez BD, Rios-Guzman NM, Wells KL, Nicholas CA, Rihanek M, Hunter MJ, Toole KP, et al. 2023. Identification of an anergic BND cell–derived activated B cell population (BND2) in young-onset type 1 diabetes patients. *J Exp Med* **220:** e20221604. doi:10.1084/jem.20221604

Vatanen T, Franzosa EA, Schwager R, Tripathi S, Arthur TD, Vehik K, Lernmark Å, Hagopian WA, Rewers MJ, She JX, et al. 2018. The human gut microbiome in early-onset type 1 diabetes from the TEDDY study. *Nature* **562:** 589–594. doi:10.1038/s41586-018-0620-2

von Herrath M, Nepom GT. 2009. Animal models of human type 1 diabetes. *Nat Immunol* **10:** 129–132. doi:10.1038/ni0209-129

Wang Y, Sosinowski T, Novikov A, Crawford F, White J, Jin N, Liu Z, Zou J, Neau D, Davidson HW, et al. 2019. How C-terminal additions to insulin B-chain fragments create superagonists for T cells in mouse and human type 1 diabetes. *Sci Immunol* **4:** eaav7517. doi:10.1126/sciimmunol.aav7517

Wicker LS, Todd JA, Peterson LB. 1995. Genetic control of autoimmune diabetes in the NOD mouse. *Annu Rev Immunol* **13:** 179–200. doi:10.1146/annurev.iy.13.040195.001143

Wicker LS, Clark J, Fraser HI, Garner VE, Gonzalez-Munoz A, Healy B, Howlett S, Hunter K, Rainbow D, Rosa RL, et al. 2005. Type 1 diabetes genes and pathways shared by humans and NOD mice. *J Autoimmun* **25**(Suppl)**:** 29–33. doi:10.1016/j.jaut.2005.09.009

Wiedeman AE, Muir VS, Rosasco MG, DeBerg HA, Presnell S, Haas B, Dufort MJ, Speake C, Greenbaum CJ, Serti E, et al. 2020. Autoreactive CD8$^+$ T cell exhaustion distinguishes subjects with slow type 1 diabetes progression. *J Clin Invest* **130:** 480–490. doi:10.1172/JCI126595

Wilske KR, Healey LA. 1989. Remodeling the pyramid—a concept whose time has come. *J Rheumatol* **16:** 565–567.

Woodcock J, LaVange LM. 2017. Master protocols to study multiple therapies, multiple diseases, or both. *N Engl J Med* **377:** 62–70. doi:10.1056/NEJMra1510062

Yang J, Wen X, Xu H, Torres-Chinn N, Speake C, Greenbaum CJ, Nepom GT, Kwok WW. 2017. Antigen-specific T cell analysis reveals that active immune responses to β cell antigens are focused on a unique set of epitopes. *J Immunol* **199:** 91–96. doi:10.4049/jimmunol.1601570

Zhou X, Bailey-Bucktrout S, Jeker LT, Bluestone JA. 2009. Plasticity of CD4$^+$ FoxP3$^+$ T cells. *Curr Opin Immunol* **21:** 281–285. doi:10.1016/j.coi.2009.05.007

Ziegler AG, Schmid S, Huber D, Hummel M, Bonifacio E. 2003. Early infant feeding and risk of developing type 1 diabetes-associated autoantibodies. *J Am Med Assoc* **290:** 1721–1728. doi:10.1001/jama.290.13.1721

Monogenic Type 1 Diabetes: A High Yield Pool in Which to Discover New Mechanisms and Candidate Therapeutics for Type 1 Diabetes

Chester E. Chamberlain,[1] Michael S. German,[1] Louis H. Philipson,[2] and Mark S. Anderson[1]

[1]Diabetes Center, University of California, San Francisco, San Francisco, California 94143, USA

[2]Kovler Diabetes Center, University of Chicago Pritzker School of Medicine, Chicago, Illinois 60201, USA

Correspondence: chester.chamberlain@ucsf.edu; mark.anderson@ucsf.edu

Rare monogenic forms of disease provide a unique opportunity to understand novel pathways in human biology. With the rapid advances in genomics and next-generation sequencing, we now have the tools to interrogate the genomes of patients on a large scale to identify candidate genes in patients with rare monogenic forms of type 1 diabetes (T1D). These cases are more likely to represent genetic defects in critical pathways of immune tolerance, and the study of these patients provides a high-yield pool in which to discover new mechanisms of disease in T1D. These studies are also expected to have high translational impact for the T1D community by helping to identify at-risk individuals and provide compelling candidate targets for prevention and treatment.

Type 1 diabetes (T1D) is an autoimmune disease characterized by an immune-mediated destruction of pancreatic β cells. The pathogenesis of T1D involves both a mix of genetic and environmental factors and extensive work on the genetics of disease has helped identify a wide number of common variants that contribute to disease risk. The majority of genetic risk maps to the polymorphic human leukocyte antigen (HLA) locus with a number of alleles that confer high to moderate risk and even some alleles that confer disease protection. In addition to this major locus, the rapid evolution of using genome-wide association studies (GWAS) on large numbers of patients in the last two decades has helped reveal a wide number of common variants that confer weaker genetic risk. These non-HLA common variants generally map to genes that operate in the immune system but mechanistic dissection of these variants has been challenging given their weak influence and that the majority of variants map to noncoding regions that alter gene expression. An alternative approach to harness genetics to help unlock T1D disease pathogenesis is to examine and identify rare coding variants in patients with monogenic forms of T1D.

Although monogenic forms of T1D are rare, rapid advances in high-throughput DNA sequencing have helped expand the identification of coding genetic variants that confer significant risk for T1D. In this review, we will cover known

Cite this article as *Cold Spring Harb Perspect Med* doi: 10.1101/cshperspect.a041601

monogenic forms of T1D and how this has helped provide insights into T1D pathogenesis.

DEFINITION

It has been long known that there are many monogenic types of diabetes that are linked to genetic variants that confer strong genetic risk for triggering diabetes. Mature onset diabetes of the young (MODY) and neonatal diabetes are classic examples of a group of disorders that are linked to coding genetic variants that confer strong risk for diabetes; however, these cases do not generally involve an autoimmune mechanism (Salguero et al. 2023). T1D is generally characterized by the presence of islet autoantibodies and relative insulin deficiency at the time of diagnosis (Quattrin et al. 2023). Here, we define monogenic T1D as a patient with diabetes with (1) the clinical evidence of T1D with islet autoantibodies and insulin deficiency along with (2) an identifiable rare genetic mutation in a single gene that is linked to disease. In the case of the latter, additional evidence for causality is needed. In this case, linkage of deleterious mutations in multiple affected family members along with the identification of similar mutations and phenotype in multiple families is one component for evidence. Second, it is evidence for a biological effect conferred by the genetic mutation. As will be outlined below, monogenic T1D is now linked to both homozygous mutations and also heterozygous mutations. Interestingly, in the case of the latter, these can be linked to both gain-of-function (GOF) mutations or dominant-negative mutations on one allele.

IMMUNE DYSREGULATION AND MONOGENIC T1D

In most types of monogenic T1D, the disease occurs in the context of a major dysregulation of the immune system and most patients present with other features. These other features frequently included other autoimmune features (i.e., autoimmune hypothyroidism, autoimmune cytopenias) and somewhat paradoxically infectious disease susceptibility. With the expanding recognition of this picture, investigators have started using a working definition of inborn errors of immunity (IEI) to refer to this broad group of monogenic disorders. There over several hundred defined IEI disorders (Tangye et al. 2021) with a fraction linked to a T1D phenotype in some patients. Overall, IEIs frequently involve selected immune deficiencies but also have increased frequency of allergy susceptibility, inflammatory disease features, and autoimmunity.

Despite this complexity, it remains that insights provided by monogenic T1D have provided some mechanistic insights to pathways in the immune system that help control immune tolerance to the pancreatic islets. Here, we will discuss individual monogenic T1D disorders and their link to thymic central tolerance (*AIRE*), T regulatory cell function (*FOXP3, IL2RA, CTLA4, LRBA*), peripheral tolerance (*PDCD1*), and JAK/STAT signaling (*STAT3* and *STAT1*).

CENTRAL TOLERANCE

APS1/AIRE

Autoimmune polyglandular syndrome type 1 (APS1, OMIM #240300) is a monogenic disorder that maps to a defect in the *autoimmune regulator* (*AIRE*) gene (Husebye et al. 2018). The disease classically manifests as an autosomal recessive disorder and patients typically develop an array of organ-specific autoimmune features. Patients frequently develop hypoparathyroidism, adrenal insufficiency, and mucocutaneous candidiasis susceptibility, but in addition to these major features they can manifest many other autoimmune diseases, including T1D in ~10%–15% of all subjects (Husebye and Anderson 2010). The defective gene in the disorder was originally identified in 1997 by a positional cloning effort using linkage and was termed AIRE based on the clinical picture of APS1 (Finnish-German APECED Consortium 1997; Nagamine et al. 1997). Subsequent studies have come to determine that AIRE is mainly expressed in the thymus where it exerts control on T-cell tolerance by providing a means to present "self" to the developing T-cell repertoire (Anderson et al. 2002). AIRE is highly expressed in specialized antigen-presenting cells in the medulla of the thymus dubbed medullary thymic epithelial cells (mTECs), within which AIRE acts like a transcriptional activator to promote the promiscuous expression of a wide array of self-proteins that include islet-specific proteins like insulin (Anderson et al. 2002). In this case, this display system helps ensure that the wide array of self is presented to developing T cells and those T cells that have specificity for such proteins are then deleted or removed from the immune repertoire (Anderson et al. 2005; DeVoss et al. 2006).

Interestingly, among the self-proteins that AIRE helps promote expression of in mTECs is insulin (Anderson et al. 2002). GWAS and candidate gene studies have previously identified common variants in the promoter region of the insulin gene that are linked to T1D susceptibility (Bell et al. 1984; Barrett et al. 2009; Robertson et al. 2021). The common risk variant is associated with weaker expression in the thymus (Pugliese et al. 1997; Vafiadis et al. 1997). Also, mechanistic data gleaned from studies of the NOD mouse model show that insulin is the major epitope for autoimmune diabetes (Nakayama et al. 2005) and AIRE deficiency causes defects in the negative selection of insulin-specific T cells (Smith et al. 2024). Together, these findings provide a working framework for how the thymus plays a key role in setting the stage for T1D susceptibility by helping rid the immune system of T cells with this specificity.

GENETIC T REGULATORY CELL DISORDERS

IPEX/FOXP3

Immune polyendocrinopathy X-linked (IPEX; OMIM #304790) is an X-linked disorder in which affected males typically present early in life with a constellation of inflammatory and autoimmune features (Powell et al. 1982; Wildin et al. 2002). Common clinical features include an inflammatory rash, colitis, autoimmune thyroiditis, and T1D. T1D can often present in the first year of life in these patients and is frequently accompanied by the presence of T1D autoantibodies. The defective gene in the disorder, Forkhead Box P3 (FOXP3), was mapped in the early 2000s in an analogous spontaneous mouse model termed Scurfy (Brunkow et al. 2001). Such mice are typically affected by colitis, multiple immune infiltrated tissues, and a wasting disease that is X-linked (Lyon et al. 1990). Using this framework, FOXP3 as the candidate genetic defect for IPEX was explored and proven to be correct (Bennett et al. 2001; Wildin et al. 2001). FOXP3 is a forkhead domain family transcription factor whose expression maps specifically to a key population of $CD4^+$ $CD25^+$ T cells called T regulatory cells (Tregs) (Fontenot et al. 2003; Hori et al. 2003; Khattri et al. 2003). Tregs are a suppressive population of T cells that help control and prevent autoimmune responses in tissues through a combination of different factors (Sakaguchi et al. 2020). The identification of FOXP3 helped further refine and define this important population of T cells and defects in the function of these cells are linked to both T1D (Lawson et al. 2008; Schneider et al. 2008) and also in the development of diabetes in the NOD mouse model of T1D (D'Alise et al. 2008). Furthermore, Tregs are also being explored as a potential therapeutic for the treatment of autoimmune diseases like T1D with approaches that include ex vivo expansion (Bluestone et al. 2015) and also targeting of growth factors like IL-2 to preferentially expand these cells in vivo (Dong et al. 2021).

IPEX typically presents with a number of challenging autoimmune and inflammatory disorders and affected boys succumb to disease early in life if not treated. Currently, the mainstay of treatment is allogeneic bone marrow transplantation with many treated patients showing remarkable clinical improvement (Barzaghi et al. 2018). There are now efforts underway to utilize genetic editing of bone marrow cells to restore FOXP3 expression and function as an alternative method for therapy (Hippen et al. 2011; Bluestone et al. 2015).

Recently, we identified a familial group of males that developed T1D a bit later than typical IPEX patients that harbored a unique splice variant in FOXP3 (Hwang et al. 2018). These affected males did not manifest some of the other classic features of IPEX like the colitis and rash. Thus, this study helps provide evidence that even partial defects in FOXP3 can help promote the development of T1D. Indeed, such data are also bolstered by studies in the NOD mouse model of T1D where partial defects in FOXP3 appear to accelerate the development of T1D (Darce et al. 2012; Leon et al. 2023).

CD25 Deficiency/IL2RA

After the identification of FOXP3 in the IPEX syndrome, there was identification of families with children with a similar phenotype that included early-onset T1D and inflammation but harbored a different genetic defect. The clue was provided by the fact that in these families' inheritance was not X-linked but rather autosomal recessive. Here, the defect mapped to the IL2RA gene (Sharfe et al. 1997; Caudy et al. 2007; Goudy et al. 2013; Bezrodnik et al. 2014) that encodes CD25, which is highly expressed on Tregs, also encodes the high-affinity component of the IL-2 receptor (Sakaguchi et al. 1995). Patients with loss of function of IL2RA (OMIM #606367) also have been shown to have a major defect in Treg function, and the mainstay of therapy is also allogeneic bone marrow transplantation (Vignoli et al. 2019). There are also efforts underway to develop genetic editing methods in hematopoietic cells to correct the IL2RA defect (Shy et al. 2023). Furthermore, this work also underscores the importance of IL-2 as a maintenance factor for Tregs, and there are currently multiple efforts underway to design methods to selectively expand Tregs with low-dose IL-2 (Hartemann et al. 2013; Rosenzwajg et al. 2015; Yu et al. 2015) or IL-2 muteins (Hernandez et al. 2022). Also, the success of these therapeutic approaches in the NOD mouse model (Trotta et al. 2018; Khoryati et al. 2020; Ward et al. 2020), coupled with GWAS studies that genetically link IL2RA and T1D (Robertson et al. 2021), suggest that these therapeutic approaches may also apply to the broader T1D patient population.

IDAIL/CTLA4

Cytotoxic T-lymphocyte-associated 4 (CTLA4) haploinsufficiency has been recently described as distinct immune dysregulation syndrome (OMIM #616100). The disease has variable penetrance, and patients that are affected will frequently manifest autoimmune cytopenias, hypogammaglobinemia, and multiple organ immune infiltrates (Kuehn et al. 2014; Schubert et al. 2014). T1D is enriched in these patients with an incidence of ~5% (Mancuso et al. 2023). CTLA4 is an inhibitory receptor constitutively expressed on Tregs (Wing et al. 2008) and also on effector T cells after they become activated (Krummel and Allison 1996). It engages with the costimulatory molecules CD80 and CD86 on antigen-presenting cells and compete with another costimulatory activating molecule on T cells called CD28 (Qureshi et al. 2011). Interestingly, GWAS studies have also linked common variants in the region of the CTLA4 gene to T1D susceptibility (Nistico et al. 1996; Ueda et al. 2003). Assessment of CTLA4 haploinsufficient patients have suggested that at least in part they harbor a defect in Treg function and current treatment is being used with CTLA4-Ig (abatacept), which also binds to CD80/CD86 (Orban et al. 2014).

CVID8/LRBA

Common variable immunodeficiency-8 (CVID8) with autoimmunity is caused by homozygous mutations in the lipopolysaccharide-responsive, beige-like anchor protein (LRBA) gene (OMIM #614700). Deficiency in LRBA has been recently described in which patients typically develop enteropathy, lung infiltrates, hypogammaglobulinemia, and autoimmune disease that frequently includes T1D (Alangari et al. 2012; Lopez-Herrera et al. 2012; Charbonnier et al. 2015; Lo et al. 2015; Schreiner et al. 2016; Johnson et al. 2017; Kardelen et al. 2021). The syndrome does appear to have some clinical overlap with CTLA4 haploinsufficiency (Catak et al. 2022). Interestingly, LRBA appears to be a key protein involved in the intracellular trafficking of CTLA4, which recycles between endosomes and the cell surface of T cells (Linsley et al. 1996). Indeed, affected patients show evidence of decreased cell surface expression of CTLA4, which is similar to what is observed in CTLA4 haploinsufficiency (Lo et al. 2015: Hou et al. 2017). Again, altered Treg function likely contributes to disease (Alangari et al. 2012) and patients can be successfully treated with allogeneic hematopoietic stem cell transplantation (Seidel et al. 2018; Kiykim et al. 2019; Tesch et al. 2020). Like CTLA4 haploinsufficiency, these patients are also treated with CTLA4-Ig (abatacept) with good clinical responses (Lo et al. 2015; Lanz et al. 2021; Taghizade et al. 2023).

PERIPHERAL TOLERANCE DEFECTS

Recently, a single case of a boy with the early development of T1D, autoimmune thyroiditis, and idiopathic arthritis was described in a consanguineous family and this child harbored deficiency in PDCD1 (PD1; OMIM #600244) (Ogishi et al. 2021). PD1 is an inhibitory molecule expressed on T cells after they have become activated (Ishida et al. 1992; Agata et al. 1996; Vibhakar et al. 1997) and binds to its ligands PDL1 (Freeman et al. 2000) and/or PDL2 (Latchman et al. 2001) on antigen-presenting cells. Interestingly, there is now widespread use of blocking antibodies to PD1 and its ligands for cancer immune therapy (Pardoll 2012). Here, the treatment helps reinvigorate exhausted T cells to attack tumors and a fraction of patients treated with this drug develop autoimmune diabetes as a complication (Stamatouli et al. 2018). In addition, treatment of prediabetic NOD mice with PD1 blockade results in the rapid development of T1D (Ansari et al. 2003). This data in sum indicates that this is a key tolerance pathway for controlling autoimmunity in the islets.

JAK/STAT PATHWAY DEFECTS

A collection of patients has now been identified with unique heterozygous point mutations in signal transducer and activator of transcription 3 (STAT3) that confer GOF activity (STAT3 GOF disease; OMIM #615952). Here, patients typically manifest with autoimmune cytopenias, lung infiltrates, and short stature. Approximately 20% of patients also develop T1D (Mancuso et al. 2023). STAT proteins are in a family that help transduce signaling from cell surface cytokine and hormone receptors to the cell nucleus, where they can go on to activate transcriptional gene activation (Villarino et al. 2017). There are seven distinct STAT proteins and they individually map to certain cytokine family members. In the case of STAT3, major cytokines that are involved in this pathway include IL-6, IL-21, and IL-22 (Villarino et al. 2017). GOF mutations in STAT3 can thus confer constitutive and excessive cytokine signaling during T-cell differentiation, and there has been a notion that the defect in these patients when related to T1D is in excessive Th17 differentiation over Treg differentiation (Fabbri et al. 2019). This comes from work with naive T cells wherein differentiation in the presence of IL-6 promotes Th17 cell development and the presence of IL-6 inhibits TGF-β-induced Treg development (Bettelli et al. 2006; Mangan et al. 2006; Veldhoen et al. 2006). Recent work in a NOD mouse model of STAT3 GOF disease suggests that perhaps a distinct mechanism is in play that promotes T1D (Warshauer et al. 2021). Here, NOD mice with the presence of the STAT3 GOF mutation in the germline indeed develop an accelerated form of T1D; however, Treg numbers are expanded and within the islets is actually an expansion of CD8 T cells that would otherwise be exhausted. Indeed, transfer of islet-specific CD8 T cells with the STAT3 GOF mutation into NOD hosts also developed accelerated diabetes. Thus, it appears that the mutation here is altering the induction of CD8 T-cell exhaustion, and indeed similar findings have been described in these patients and in a distinct mouse model of the disease (Masle-Farquhar et al. 2022).

In addition to STAT3 GOF disease, there is also recognition that patients with STAT1 GOF mutations also harbor an increased risk for T1D. STAT1 GOF disease (OMIM #614162) is typically characterized by the development of frequent sinopulmonary infections, mucocutaneous candidiasis, and autoimmunity including T1D. The STAT1 protein is linked to several cytokines, including IFNγ, IL-12, and IL-27 (Boisson-Dupuis et al. 2012). Here, the mechanism by which candida susceptibility is conferred is through excessive γ interferon signaling in T cells (Th1-like cells), which in and of itself can inhibit the differentiation of IL-17-producing T cells (Th17 cells) (Okada et al. 2020). Th17 cells now appear to be crucial in protecting against mucocutaneous candida infections as patients with defects in the IL-17 receptor (Ling et al. 2015) and those treated with IL-17 blocking antibodies can frequently develop candida (Lebwohl et al. 2015; van de Kerkhof et al. 2016). Treatment of patients with this disorder is typically with a JAK inhibitor (JAKi) (Forbes et al. 2018). JAK family members work in concert with STAT proteins to regulate signaling and the JAK pathway has proven to be amenable to targeting by chemical inhibition (O'Shea et al. 2015). Recently, a single male patient with STAT1 GOF disease and T1D was described that started on JAKi 21 months after the diagnosis of T1D. This patient responded well to therapy with improvement of the recurrent infections and candida but, in addition, this patient had a remarkable event of the reversal of his T1D (Chaimowitz et al. 2020). In addition, there has now been completion of a clinical trial with a JAKi in new-onset T1D with evidence for a delay in the decay of C-peptide of these patients similar to other immune therapies like teplizumab (Waibel et al. 2023). Of interest will be to determine how the JAKi reversed diabetes in the single-patient case but also slowed T1D in the clinical trial. Taken together, this data shows the potential power and insights that could come from careful observations of rare patients with monogenic T1D.

PERSPECTIVES AND SUMMARY

As with any complex disease, the genetic contribution to T1D varies between patients and is distributed across a spectrum of disease variants that span between rare, high-impact alleles that cause Mendelian disease and more common alleles of low impact that elevate disease risk (Fig. 1; Manolio et al. 2009).

Interestingly, we and others have found that the genes associated with rare and common T1D disease variants share common biological pathways, suggesting that the knowledge, tools, and therapies developed for monogenic T1D will also benefit patients with the more common polygenic T1D (Warshauer et al. 2020; Robertson et al. 2021; Rutsch et al. 2021). Also, as next-generation sequencing becomes part of T1D evaluation and standard care, the insights gained from studying monogenic T1D are expected to help care providers better predict the natural course of disease, provide more personalized therapies, and eventually provide a customized cure.

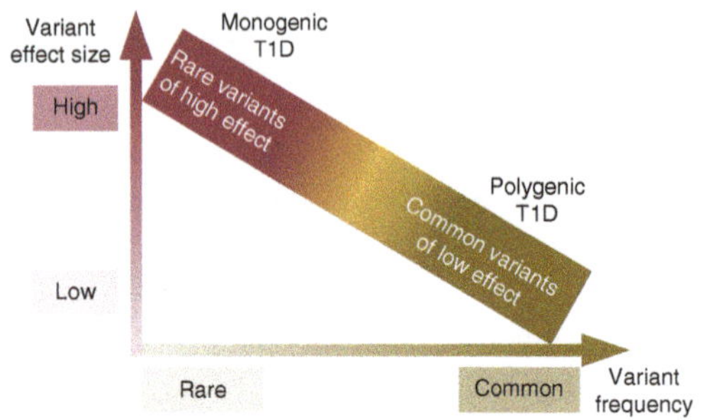

Figure 1. Spectrum of genetic disease variants in type 1 diabetes (T1D). T1D disease variants span between rare alleles that cause Mendelian disease and more common alleles of low impact. Genes associated with rare and common T1D disease variants share common biological pathways, suggesting that the knowledge, tools, and therapies developed for rare monogenic T1D will also benefit patients with more common polygenic T1D.

ACKNOWLEDGMENTS

This work was supported by the Leona M. and Harry B. Helmsley Charitable Trust (G-2018PG-T1D018, G-2003-04376, G-2404-06823), and the National Institute of Diabetes and Digestive and Kidney Diseases of the National Institutes of Health (NIH) (R01-DK-104942, P30-DK-020595, T32DK007418).

REFERENCES

Agata Y, Kawasaki A, Nishimura H, Ishida Y, Tsubata T, Yagita H, Honjo T. 1996. Expression of the PD-1 antigen on the surface of stimulated mouse T and B lymphocytes. *Int Immunol* **8:** 765–772. doi:10.1093/intimm/8.5.765

Alangari A, Alsultan A, Adly N, Massaad MJ, Kiani IS, Aljebreen A, Raddaoui E, Almomen AK, Al-Muhsen S, Geha RS, et al. 2012. LPS-responsive beige-like anchor (LRBA) gene mutation in a family with inflammatory bowel disease and combined immunodeficiency. *J Allergy*

Clin Immunol **130:** 481–488.e482. doi:10.1016/j.jaci.2012.05.043

Anderson MS, Venanzi ES, Klein L, Chen Z, Berzins SP, Turley SJ, von Boehmer H, Bronson R, Dierich A, Benoist C, et al. 2002. Projection of an immunological self shadow within the thymus by the aire protein. *Science* **298:** 1395–1401. doi:10.1126/science.1075958

Anderson MS, Venanzi ES, Chen Z, Berzins SP, Benoist C, Mathis D. 2005. The cellular mechanism of Aire control of T cell tolerance. *Immunity* **23:** 227–239. doi:10.1016/j.immuni.2005.07.005

Ansari MJ, Salama AD, Chitnis T, Smith RN, Yagita H, Akiba H, Yamazaki T, Azuma M, Iwai H, Khoury SJ, et al. 2003. The programmed death-1 (PD-1) pathway regulates autoimmune diabetes in nonobese diabetic (NOD) mice. *J Exp Med* **198:** 63–69. doi:10.1084/jem.20022125

Barrett JC, Clayton DG, Concannon P, Akolkar B, Cooper JD, Erlich HA, Julier C, Morahan G, Nerup J, Nierras C, et al. 2009. Genome-wide association study and meta-analysis find that over 40 loci affect risk of type 1 diabetes. *Nat Genet* **41:** 703–707. doi:10.1038/ng.381

Barzaghi F, Amaya Hernandez LC, Neven B, Ricci S, Kucuk Y, Bleesing JJ, Nademi Z, Slatter MA, Ulloa ER, Shcherbina A, et al. 2018. Long-term follow-up of IPEX syndrome patients after different therapeutic strategies: an international multicenter retrospective study. *J Allergy Clin Immunol* **141:** 1036–1049.e5. doi:10.1016/j.jaci.2017.10.041

Bell GI, Horita S, Karam JH. 1984. A polymorphic locus near the human insulin gene is associated with insulin-dependent diabetes mellitus. *Diabetes* **33:** 176–183. doi:10.2337/diab.33.2.176

Bennett CL, Christie J, Ramsdell F, Brunkow ME, Ferguson PJ, Whitesell L, Kelly TE, Saulsbury FT, Chance PF, Ochs HD. 2001. The immune dysregulation, polyendocrinopathy, enteropathy, X-linked syndrome (IPEX) is caused by mutations of FOXP3. *Nat Genet* **27:** 20–21. doi:10.1038/83713

Bettelli E, Carrier Y, Gao W, Korn T, Strom TB, Oukka M, Weiner HL, Kuchroo VK. 2006. Reciprocal developmental pathways for the generation of pathogenic effector TH17 and regulatory T cells. *Nature* **441:** 235–238. doi:10.1038/nature04753

Bezrodnik L, Caldirola MS, Seminario AG, Moreira I, Gaillard MI. 2014. Follicular bronchiolitis as phenotype associated with CD25 deficiency. *Clin Exp Immunol* **175:** 227–234. doi:10.1111/cei.12214

Bluestone JA, Buckner JH, Fitch M, Gitelman SE, Gupta S, Hellerstein MK, Herold KC, Lares A, Lee MR, Li K, et al. 2015. Type 1 diabetes immunotherapy using polyclonal regulatory T cells. *Sci Transl Med* **7:** 315ra189. doi:10.1126/scitranslmed.aad4134

Boisson-Dupuis S, Kong XF, Okada S, Cypowyj S, Puel A, Abel L, Casanova JL. 2012. Inborn errors of human STAT1: allelic heterogeneity governs the diversity of immunological and infectious phenotypes. *Curr Opin Immunol* **24:** 364–378. doi:10.1016/j.coi.2012.04.011

Brunkow ME, Jeffery EW, Hjerrild KA, Paeper B, Clark LB, Yasayko SA, Wilkinson JE, Galas D, Ziegler SF, Ramsdell F. 2001. Disruption of a new forkhead/winged-helix protein, scurfin, results in the fatal lymphoproliferative disorder of the scurfy mouse. *Nat Genet* **27:** 68–73. doi:10.1038/83784

Catak MC, Akcam B, Bilgic Eltan S, Babayeva R, Karakus IS, Akgun G, Baser D, Bulutoglu A, Bayram F, Kasap N, et al. 2022. Comparing the levels of CTLA-4-dependent biological defects in patients with LRBA deficiency and CTLA-4 insufficiency. *Allergy* **77:** 3108–3123. doi:10.1111/all.15331

Caudy AA, Reddy ST, Chatila T, Atkinson JP, Verbsky JW. 2007. CD25 deficiency causes an immune dysregulation, polyendocrinopathy, enteropathy, X-linked-like syndrome, and defective IL-10 expression from CD4 lymphocytes. *J Allergy Clin Immunol* **119:** 482–487. doi:10.1016/j.jaci.2006.10.007

Chaimowitz NS, Ebenezer SJ, Hanson IC, Anderson M, Forbes LR. 2020. STAT1 gain-of-function, type 1 diabetes, and reversal with JAK Inhibition. *N Engl J Med* **383:** 1494–1496. doi:10.1056/NEJMc2022226

Charbonnier LM, Janssen E, Chou J, Ohsumi TK, Keles S, Hsu JT, Massaad MJ, Garcia-Lloret M, Hanna-Wakim R, Dbaibo G, et al. 2015. Regulatory T-cell deficiency and immune dysregulation, polyendocrinopathy, enteropathy, X-linked-like disorder caused by loss-of-function mutations in LRBA. *J Allergy Clin Immunol* **135:** 217–227.e9. doi:10.1016/j.jaci.2014.10.019

D'Alise AM, Auyeung V, Feuerer M, Nishio J, Fontenot J, Benoist C, Mathis D. 2008. The defect in T-cell regulation in NOD mice is an effect on the T-cell effectors. *Proc Natl Acad Sci* **105:** 19857–19862. doi:10.1073/pnas.0810713105

Darce J, Rudra D, Li L, Nishio J, Cipolletta D, Rudensky AY, Mathis D, Benoist C. 2012. An N-terminal mutation of the Foxp3 transcription factor alleviates arthritis but exacerbates diabetes. *Immunity* **36:** 731–741. doi:10.1016/j.immuni.2012.04.007

DeVoss J, Hou Y, Johannes K, Lu W, Liou GI, Rinn J, Chang H, Caspi RR, Fong L, Anderson MS. 2006. Spontaneous autoimmunity prevented by thymic expression of a single self-antigen. *J Exp Med* **203:** 2727–2735. doi:10.1084/jem.20061864

Dong S, Hiam-Galvez KJ, Mowery CT, Herold KC, Gitelman SE, Esensten JH, Liu W, Lares AP, Leinbach AS, Lee M, et al. 2021. The effect of low-dose IL-2 and Treg adoptive cell therapy in patients with type 1 diabetes. *JCI Insight* **6:** e147474. doi:10.1172/jci.insight.147474

Fabbri M, Frixou M, Degano M, Fousteri G. 2019. Type 1 diabetes in STAT protein family mutations: regulating the Th17/Treg equilibrium and beyond. *Diabetes* **68:** 258–265. doi:10.2337/db18-0627

Finnish-German APECED Consortium. 1997. An autoimmune disease, APECED, caused by mutations in a novel gene featuring two PHD-type zinc-finger domains. *Nat Genet* **17:** 399–403. doi:10.1038/ng1297-399

Fontenot JD, Gavin MA, Rudensky AY. 2003. Foxp3 programs the development and function of $CD4^+$ $CD25^+$ regulatory T cells. *Nat Immunol* **4:** 330–336. doi:10.1038/ni904

Forbes LR, Vogel TP, Cooper MA, Castro-Wagner J, Schussler E, Weinacht KG, Plant AS, Su HC, Allenspach EJ, Slatter M, et al. 2018. Jakinibs for the treatment of immune dysregulation in patients with gain-of-function signal transducer and activator of transcription 1 (STAT1) or

STAT3 mutations. *J Allergy Clin Immunol* **142:** 1665–1669. doi:10.1016/j.jaci.2018.07.020

Freeman GJ, Long AJ, Iwai Y, Bourque K, Chernova T, Nishimura H, Fitz LJ, Malenkovich N, Okazaki T, Byrne MC, et al. 2000. Engagement of the PD-1 immunoinhibitory receptor by a novel B7 family member leads to negative regulation of lymphocyte activation. *J Exp Med* **192:** 1027–1034. doi:10.1084/jem.192.7.1027

Goudy K, Aydin D, Barzaghi F, Gambineri E, Vignoli M, Mannurita SC, Doglioni C, Ponzoni M, Cicalese MP, Assanelli A, et al. 2013. Human IL2RA null mutation mediates immunodeficiency with lymphoproliferation and autoimmunity. *Clin Immunol* **146:** 248–261. doi:10.1016/j.clim.2013.01.004

Hartemann A, Bensimon G, Payan CA, Jacqueminet S, Bourron O, Nicolas N, Fonfrede M, Rosenzwajg M, Bernard C, Klatzmann D. 2013. Low-dose interleukin 2 in patients with type 1 diabetes: a phase 1/2 randomised, double-blind, placebo-controlled trial. *Lancet Diabetes Endocrinol* **1:** 295–305. doi:10.1016/S2213-8587(13)70113-X

Hernandez R, Põder J, LaPorte KM, Malek TR. 2022. Engineering IL-2 for immunotherapy of autoimmunity and cancer. *Nat Rev Immunol* **22:** 614–628. doi:10.1038/s41577-022-00680-w

Hippen KL, Merkel SC, Schirm DK, Nelson C, Tennis NC, Riley JL, June CH, Miller JS, Wagner JE, Blazar BR. 2011. Generation and large-scale expansion of human inducible regulatory T cells that suppress graft-versus-host disease. *Am J Transplant* **11:** 1148–1157. doi:10.1111/j.1600-6143.2011.03558.x

Hori S, Nomura T, Sakaguchi S. 2003. Control of regulatory T cell development by the transcription factor *Foxp3*. *Science* **299:** 1057–1061. doi:10.1126/science.1079490

Hou TZ, Verma N, Wanders J, Kennedy A, Soskic B, Janman D, Halliday N, Rowshanravan B, Worth A, Qasim W, et al. 2017. Identifying functional defects in patients with immune dysregulation due to LRBA and CTLA-4 mutations. *Blood* **129:** 1458–1468. doi:10.1182/blood-2016-10-745174

Husebye ES, Anderson MS. 2010. Autoimmune polyendocrine syndromes: clues to type 1 diabetes pathogenesis. *Immunity* **32:** 479–487. doi:10.1016/j.immuni.2010.03.016

Husebye ES, Anderson MS, Kämpe O. 2018. Autoimmune polyendocrine syndromes. *N Engl J Med* **378:** 1132–1141. doi:10.1056/NEJMra1713301

Hwang JL, Park SY, Ye H, Sanyoura M, Pastore AN, Carmody D, Del Gaudio D, Wilson JF, Hanis CL, Liu X, et al. 2018. *FOXP3* mutations causing early-onset insulin-requiring diabetes but without other features of immune dysregulation, polyendocrinopathy, enteropathy, X-linked syndrome. *Pediatr Diabetes* **19:** 388–392. doi:10.1111/pedi.12612

Ishida Y, Agata Y, Shibahara K, Honjo T. 1992. Induced expression of PD-1, a novel member of the immunoglobulin gene superfamily, upon programmed cell death. *EMBO J* **11:** 3887–3895. doi:10.1002/j.1460-2075.1992.tb05481.x

Johnson MB, De Franco E, Lango Allen H, Al Senani A, Elbarbary N, Siklar Z, Berberoglu M, Imane Z, Haghighi A, Razavi Z, et al. 2017. Recessively inherited *LRBA* mutations cause autoimmunity presenting as neonatal diabetes. *Diabetes* **66:** 2316–2322. doi:10.2337/db17-0040

Kardelen AD, Kara M, Güller D, Ozturan EK, Abali ZY, Ceylaner S, Kıykim A, Cantez S, Torun SH, Poyrazoglu S, et al. 2021. LRBA deficiency: a rare cause of type 1 diabetes, colitis, and severe immunodeficiency. *Hormones (Athens)* **20:** 389–394. doi:10.1007/s42000-020-00257-z

Khattri R, Cox T, Yasayko SA, Ramsdell F. 2003. An essential role for Scurfin in $CD4^+CD25^+$ T regulatory cells. *Nat Immunol* **4:** 337–342. doi:10.1038/ni909

Khoryati L, Pham MN, Sherve M, Kumari S, Cook K, Pearson J, Bogdani M, Campbell DJ, Gavin MA. 2020. An IL-2 mutein engineered to promote expansion of regulatory T cells arrests ongoing autoimmunity in mice. *Sci Immunol* **5:** 50. doi:10.1126/sciimmunol.aba5264

Kiykim A, Ogulur I, Dursun E, Charbonnier LM, Nain E, Cekic S, Dogruel D, Karaca NE, Cogurlu MT, Bilir OA, et al. 2019. Abatacept as a long-term targeted therapy for LRBA deficiency. *J Allergy Clin Immunol Pract* **7:** 2790–2800.e15. doi:10.1016/j.jaip.2019.06.011

Krummel MF, Allison JP. 1996. CTLA-4 engagement inhibits IL-2 accumulation and cell cycle progression upon activation of resting T cells. *J Exp Med* **183:** 2533–2540. doi:10.1084/jem.183.6.2533

Kuehn HS, Ouyang W, Lo B, Deenick EK, Niemela JE, Avery DT, Schickel JN, Tran DQ, Stoddard J, Zhang Y, et al. 2014. Immune dysregulation in human subjects with heterozygous germline mutations in *CTLA4*. *Science* **345:** 1623–1627. doi:10.1126/science.1255904

Lanz AL, Riester M, Peters P, Schwerd T, Lurz E, Hajji MS, Rohlfs M, Ley-Zaporozhan J, Walz C, Kotlarz D, et al. 2021. Abatacept for treatment-refractory pediatric CTLA4-haploinsufficiency. *Clin Immunol* **229:** 108779. doi:10.1016/j.clim.2021.108779

Latchman Y, Wood CR, Chernova T, Chaudhary D, Borde M, Chernova I, Iwai Y, Long AJ, Brown JA, Nunes R, et al. 2001. PD-L2 is a second ligand for PD-1 and inhibits T cell activation. *Nat Immunol* **2:** 261–268. doi:10.1038/85330

Lawson JM, Tremble J, Dayan C, Beyan H, Leslie RD, Peakman M, Tree TI. 2008. Increased resistance to $CD4^+$ CD25hi regulatory T cell-mediated suppression in patients with type 1 diabetes. *Clin Exp Immunol* **154:** 353–359. doi:10.1111/j.1365-2249.2008.03810.x

Lebwohl M, Strober B, Menter A, Gordon K, Weglowska J, Puig L, Papp K, Spelman L, Toth D, Kerdel F, et al. 2015. Phase 3 studies comparing brodalumab with ustekinumab in psoriasis. *N Engl J Med* **373:** 1318–1328. doi:10.1056/NEJMoa1503824

Leon J, Chowdhary K, Zhang W, Ramirez RN, André I, Hur S, Mathis D, Benoist C. 2023. Mutations from patients with IPEX ported to mice reveal different patterns of FoxP3 and Treg dysfunction. *Cell Rep* **42:** 113018. doi:10.1016/j.celrep.2023.113018

Ling Y, Cypowyj S, Aytekin C, Galicchio M, Camcioglu Y, Nepesov S, Ikinciogullari A, Dogu F, Belkadi A, Levy R, et al. 2015. Inherited IL-17RC deficiency in patients with chronic mucocutaneous candidiasis. *J Exp Med* **212:** 619–631. doi:10.1084/jem.20141065

Linsley PS, Bradshaw J, Greene J, Peach R, Bennett KL, Mittler RS. 1996. Intracellular trafficking of CTLA-4 and focal localization towards sites of TCR engagement. *Immunity* **4:** 535–543. doi:10.1016/S1074-7613(00)80480-X

Lo B, Zhang K, Lu W, Zheng L, Zhang Q, Kanellopoulou C, Zhang Y, Liu Z, Fritz JM, Marsh R, et al. 2015. Autoimmune disease. Patients with LRBA deficiency show CTLA4 loss and immune dysregulation responsive to abatacept therapy. *Science* **349:** 436–440. doi:10.1126/science.aaa1663

Lopez-Herrera G, Tampella G, Pan-Hammarström Q, Herholz P, Trujillo-Vargas CM, Phadwal K, Simon AK, Moutschen M, Etzioni A, Mory A, et al. 2012. Deleterious mutations in LRBA are associated with a syndrome of immune deficiency and autoimmunity. *Am J Hum Genet* **90:** 986–1001. doi:10.1016/j.ajhg.2012.04.015

Lyon MF, Peters J, Glenister PH, Ball S, Wright E. 1990. The scurfy mouse mutant has previously unrecognized hematological abnormalities and resembles Wiskott–Aldrich syndrome. *Proc Natl Acad Sci* **87:** 2433–2437. doi:10.1073/pnas.87.7.2433

Mancuso G, Bechi Genzano C, Fierabracci A, Fousteri G. 2023. Type 1 diabetes and inborn errors of immunity: complete strangers or two sides of the same coin? *J Allergy Clin Immunol* **151:** 1429–1447. doi:10.1016/j.jaci.2023.03.026

Mangan PR, Harrington LE, O'Quinn DB, Helms WS, Bullard DC, Elson CO, Hatton RD, Wahl SM, Schoeb TR, Weaver CT. 2006. Transforming growth factor-β induces development of the T(H)17 lineage. *Nature* **441:** 231–234. doi:10.1038/nature04754

Manolio TA, Collins FS, Cox NJ, Goldstein DB, Hindorff LA, Hunter DJ, McCarthy MI, Ramos EM, Cardon LR, Chakravarti A, et al. 2009. Finding the missing heritability of complex diseases. *Nature* **461:** 747–753. doi:10.1038/nature08494

Masle-Farquhar E, Jackson KJL, Peters TJ, Al-Eryani G, Singh M, Payne KJ, Rao G, Avery DT, Apps G, Kingham J, et al. 2022. STAT3 gain-of-function mutations connect leukemia with autoimmune disease by pathological NKG2D^{hi} CD8^{+} T cell dysregulation and accumulation. *Immunity* **55:** 2386–2404.e8. doi:10.1016/j.immuni.2022.11.001

Nagamine K, Peterson P, Scott HS, Kudoh J, Minoshima S, Heino M, Krohn KJ, Lalioti MD, Mullis PE, Antonarakis SE, et al. 1997. Positional cloning of the APECED gene. *Nat Genet* **17:** 393–398. doi:10.1038/ng1297-393

Nakayama M, Abiru N, Moriyama H, Babaya N, Liu E, Miao D, Yu L, Wegmann DR, Hutton JC, Elliott JF, et al. 2005. Prime role for an insulin epitope in the development of type 1 diabetes in NOD mice. *Nature* **435:** 220–223. doi:10.1038/nature03523

Nistico L, Buzzetti R, Pritchard LE, Van der Auwera B, Giovannini C, Bosi E, Larrad ME, Rios MS, Chow CC, Cockram CS, et al. 1996. The CTLA-4 gene region of chromosome 2q33 is linked to, and associated with, type 1 diabetes. Belgian Diabetes Registry. *Hum Mol Genet* **5:** 1075–1080. doi:10.1093/hmg/5.7.1075

Ogishi M, Yang R, Aytekin C, Langlais D, Bourgey M, Khan T, Ali FA, Rahman M, Delmonte OM, Chrabieh M, et al. 2021. Inherited PD-1 deficiency underlies tuberculosis and autoimmunity in a child. *Nat Med* **27:** 1646–1654. doi:10.1038/s41591-021-01388-5

Okada S, Asano T, Moriya K, Boisson-Dupuis S, Kobayashi M, Casanova JL, Puel A. 2020. Human STAT1 gain-of-function heterozygous mutations: chronic mucocutaneous candidiasis and type I interferonopathy. *J Clin Immunol* **40:** 1065–1081. doi:10.1007/s10875-020-00847-x

Orban T, Bundy B, Becker DJ, Dimeglio LA, Gitelman SE, Goland R, Gottlieb PA, Greenbaum CJ, Marks JB, Monzavi R, et al. 2014. Costimulation modulation with abatacept in patients with recent-onset type 1 diabetes: follow-up 1 year after cessation of treatment. *Diabetes Care* **37:** 1069–1075. doi:10.2337/dc13-0604

O'Shea JJ, Schwartz DM, Villarino AV, Gadina M, McInnes IB, Laurence A. 2015. The JAK-STAT pathway: impact on human disease and therapeutic intervention. *Annu Rev Med* **66:** 311–328. doi:10.1146/annurev-med-051113-024537

Pardoll DM. 2012. The blockade of immune checkpoints in cancer immunotherapy. *Nat Rev Cancer* **12:** 252–264. doi:10.1038/nrc3239

Powell BR, Buist NR, Stenzel P. 1982. An X-linked syndrome of diarrhea, polyendocrinopathy, and fatal infection in infancy. *J Pediatr* **100:** 731–737. doi:10.1016/S0022-3476(82)80573-8

Pugliese A, Zeller M, Fernandez A Jr, Zalcberg LJ, Bartlett RJ, Ricordi C, Pietropaolo M, Eisenbarth GS, Bennett ST, Patel DD. 1997. The insulin gene is transcribed in the human thymus and transcription levels correlated with allelic variation at the INS VNTR-IDDM2 susceptibility locus for type 1 diabetes. *Nat Genet* **15:** 293–297. doi:10.1038/ng0397-293

Quattrin T, Mastrandrea LD, Walker LSK. 2023. Type 1 diabetes. *Lancet* **401:** 2149–2162. doi:10.1016/S0140-6736(23)00223-4

Qureshi OS, Zheng Y, Nakamura K, Attridge K, Manzotti C, Schmidt EM, Baker J, Jeffery LE, Kaur S, Briggs Z, et al. 2011. *Trans*-endocytosis of CD80 and CD86: a molecular basis for the cell-extrinsic function of CTLA-4. *Science* **332:** 600–603. doi:10.1126/science.1202947

Robertson CC, Inshaw JRJ, Onengut-Gumuscu S, Chen WM, Santa Cruz DF, Yang H, Cutler AJ, Crouch DJM, Farber E, Bridges SL, et al. 2021. Fine-mapping, trans-ancestral and genomic analyses identify causal variants, cells, genes and drug targets for type 1 diabetes. *Nat Genet* **53:** 962–971. doi:10.1038/s41588-021-00880-5

Rosenzwajg M, Churlaud G, Mallone R, Six A, Dérian N, Chaara W, Lorenzon R, Long SA, Buckner JH, Afonso G, et al. 2015. Low-dose interleukin-2 fosters a dose-dependent regulatory T cell tuned milieu in T1D patients. *J Autoimmun* **58:** 48–58. doi:10.1016/j.jaut.2015.01.001

Rutsch N, Chamberlain CE, Dixon W, Spector L, Letourneau-Freiberg LR, Lwin WW, Philipson LH, Zarbock A, Saintus K, Wang J, et al. 2021. Diabetes with multiple autoimmune and inflammatory conditions linked to an activating SKAP2 mutation. *Diabetes Care* **44:** 1816–1825. doi:10.2337/dc20-2317

Sakaguchi S, Sakaguchi N, Asano M, Itoh M, Toda M. 1995. Immunologic self-tolerance maintained by activated T cells expressing IL-2 receptor α-chains (CD25). Breakdown of a single mechanism of self-tolerance causes various autoimmune diseases. *J Immunol* **155:** 1151–1164. doi:10.4049/jimmunol.155.3.1151

Sakaguchi S, Mikami N, Wing JB, Tanaka A, Ichiyama K, Ohkura N. 2020. Regulatory T cells and human disease. *Annu Rev Immunol* **38:** 541–566. doi:10.1146/annurev-immunol-042718-041717

Salguero MV, Arosemena M, Pollin T, Greeley SAW, Naylor RN, Letourneau-Freiberg L, Bowden TL, Wei D, Philipson LH, Lawrence JM. 2023. Monogenic forms of diabetes. In *Diabetes in America* (ed. Lawrence JM, et al.). National Institute of Diabetes and Digestive and Kidney Diseases, Bethesda, MD.

Schneider A, Rieck M, Sanda S, Pihoker C, Greenbaum C, Buckner JH. 2008. The effector T cells of diabetic subjects are resistant to regulation via $CD4^{+}FOXP3^{+}$ regulatory T cells. *J Immunol* **181:** 7350–7355. doi:10.4049/jimmunol.181.10.7350

Schreiner F, Plamper M, Dueker G, Schoenberger S, Gámez-Díaz L, Grimbacher B, Hilger AC, Gohlke B, Reutter H, Woelfle J. 2016. Infancy-onset T1DM, short stature, and severe immunodysregulation in two siblings with a homozygous LRBA mutation. *J Clin Endocrinol Metab* **101:** 898–904. doi:10.1210/jc.2015-3382

Schubert D, Bode C, Kenefeck R, Hou TZ, Wing JB, Kennedy A, Bulashevska A, Petersen BS, Schäffer AA, Grüning BA, et al. 2014. Autosomal dominant immune dysregulation syndrome in humans with CTLA4 mutations. *Nat Med* **20:** 1410–1416. doi:10.1038/nm.3746

Seidel MG, Böhm K, Dogu F, Worth A, Thrasher A, Florkin B, İkincioğullari A, Peters A, Bakhtiar S, Meeths M, et al. 2018. Treatment of severe forms of LPS-responsive beige-like anchor protein deficiency with allogeneic hematopoietic stem cell transplantation. *J Allergy Clin Immunol* **141:** 770–775.e1. doi:10.1016/j.jaci.2017.04.023

Sharfe N, Dadi HK, Shahar M, Roifman CM. 1997. Human immune disorder arising from mutation of the α chain of the interleukin-2 receptor. *Proc Natl Acad Sci* **94:** 3168–3171. doi:10.1073/pnas.94.7.3168

Shy BR, Vykunta VS, Ha A, Talbot A, Roth TL, Nguyen DN, Pfeifer WG, Chen YY, Blaeschke F, Shifrut E, et al. 2023. High-yield genome engineering in primary cells using a hybrid ssDNA repair template and small-molecule cocktails. *Nat Biotechnol* **41:** 521–531. doi:10.1038/s41587-022-01418-8

Smith JA, Yuen BTK, Purtha W, Balolong JM, Phipps JD, Crawford F, Bluestone JA, Kappler JW, Anderson MS. 2024. Aire mediates tolerance to insulin through thymic trimming of high-affinity T cell clones. *Proc Natl Acad Sci* **121:** e2320268121. doi:10.1073/pnas.2320268121

Stamatouli AM, Quandt Z, Perdigoto AL, Clark PL, Kluger H, Weiss SA, Gettinger S, Sznol M, Young A, Rushakoff R, et al. 2018. Collateral damage: insulin-dependent diabetes induced with checkpoint inhibitors. *Diabetes* **67:** 1471–1480. doi:10.2337/dbi18-0002

Taghizade N, Babayeva R, Kara A, Karakus IS, Catak MC, Bulutoglu A, Haskologlu ZS, Akay Haci I, Tunakan Dalgic C, Karabiber E, et al. 2023. Therapeutic modalities and clinical outcomes in a large cohort with LRBA deficiency and CTLA4 insufficiency. *J Allergy Clin Immunol* **152:** 1634–1645. doi:10.1016/j.jaci.2023.08.004

Tangye SG, Al-Herz W, Bousfiha A, Cunningham-Rundles C, Franco JL, Holland SM, Klein C, Morio T, Oksenhendler E, Picard C, et al. 2021. The ever-increasing array of novel inborn errors of immunity: an interim update by the IUIS Committee. *J Clin Immunol* **41:** 666–679. doi:10.1007/s10875-021-00980-1

Tesch VK, Abolhassani H, Shadur B, Zobel J, Mareika Y, Sharapova S, Karakoc-Aydiner E, Rivière JG, Garcia-Prat M, Moes N, et al. 2020. Long-term outcome of LRBA deficiency in 76 patients after various treatment modalities as evaluated by the immune deficiency and dysregulation activity (IDDA) score. *J Allergy Clin Immunol* **145:** 1452–1463. doi:10.1016/j.jaci.2019.12.896

Trotta E, Bessette PH, Silveria SL, Ely LK, Jude KM, Le DT, Holst CR, Coyle A, Potempa M, Lanier LL, et al. 2018. A human anti-IL-2 antibody that potentiates regulatory T cells by a structure-based mechanism. *Nat Med* **24:** 1005–1014. doi:10.1038/s41591-018-0070-2

Ueda H, Howson JM, Esposito L, Heward J, Snook H, Chamberlain G, Rainbow DB, Hunter KM, Smith AN, Di Genova G, et al. 2003. Association of the T-cell regulatory gene CTLA4 with susceptibility to autoimmune disease. *Nature* **423:** 506–511. doi:10.1038/nature01621

Vafiadis P, Bennett ST, Todd JA, Nadeau J, Grabs R, Goodyer CG, Wickramasinghe S, Colle E, Polychronakos C. 1997. Insulin expression in human thymus is modulated by INS VNTR alleles at the IDDM2 locus. *Nat Genet* **15:** 289–292. doi:10.1038/ng0397-289

van de Kerkhof PC, Griffiths CE, Reich K, Leonardi CL, Blauvelt A, Tsai TF, Gong Y, Huang J, Papavassilis C, Fox T. 2016. Secukinumab long-term safety experience: a pooled analysis of 10 phase II and III clinical studies in patients with moderate to severe plaque psoriasis. *J Am Acad Dermatol* **75:** 83–98.e4. doi:10.1016/j.jaad.2016.03.024

Veldhoen M, Hocking RJ, Atkins CJ, Locksley RM, Stockinger B. 2006. TGFβ in the context of an inflammatory cytokine milieu supports de novo differentiation of IL-17-producing T cells. *Immunity* **24:** 179–189. doi:10.1016/j.immuni.2006.01.001

Vibhakar R, Juan G, Traganos F, Darzynkiewicz Z, Finger LR. 1997. Activation-induced expression of human programmed death-1 gene in T-lymphocytes. *Exp Cell Res* **232:** 25–28. doi:10.1006/excr.1997.3493

Vignoli M, Ciullini Mannurita S, Fioravanti A, Tumino M, Grassi A, Guariso G, Favre C, D'Elios MM, Gambineri E. 2019. CD25 deficiency: a new conformational mutation prevents the receptor expression on cell surface. *Clin Immunol* **201:** 15–19. doi:10.1016/j.clim.2019.02.003

Villarino AV, Kanno Y, O'Shea JJ. 2017. Mechanisms and consequences of Jak-STAT signaling in the immune system. *Nat Immunol* **18:** 374–384. doi:10.1038/ni.3691

Waibel M, Wentworth JM, So M, Couper JJ, Cameron FJ, MacIsaac RJ, Atlas G, Gorelik A, Litwak S, Sanz-Villanueva L, et al. 2023. Baricitinib and β-cell function in patients with new-onset type 1 diabetes. *N Engl J Med* **389:** 2140–2150. doi:10.1056/NEJMoa2306691

Ward NC, Lui JB, Hernandez R, Yu L, Struthers M, Xie J, Santos Savio A, Dwyer CJ, Hsiung S, Yu A, et al. 2020. Persistent IL-2 receptor signaling by IL-2/CD25 fusion protein controls diabetes in NOD mice by multiple mechanisms. *Diabetes* **69:** 2400–2413. doi:10.2337/db20-0186

Warshauer JT, Bluestone JA, Anderson MS. 2020. New frontiers in the treatment of type 1 diabetes. *Cell Metab* **31:** 46–61. doi:10.1016/j.cmet.2019.11.017

Warshauer JT, Belk JA, Chan AY, Wang J, Gupta AR, Shi Q, Skartsis N, Peng Y, Phipps JD, Acenas D, et al. 2021. A human mutation in STAT3 promotes type 1 diabetes through a defect in $CD8^+$ T cell tolerance. *J Exp Med* **218:** 8. doi:10.1084/jem.20210759

Wildin RS, Ramsdell F, Peake J, Faravelli F, Casanova JL, Buist N, Levy-Lahad E, Mazzella M, Goulet O, Perroni L, et al. 2001. X-linked neonatal diabetes mellitus, enteropathy and endocrinopathy syndrome is the human equivalent of mouse scurfy. *Nat Genet* **27:** 18–20. doi:10.1038/83707

Wildin RS, Smyk-Pearson S, Filipovich AH. 2002. Clinical and molecular features of the immunodysregulation, polyendocrinopathy, enteropathy, X linked (IPEX) syndrome. *J Med Genet* **39:** 537–545. doi:10.1136/jmg.39.8.537

Wing K, Onishi Y, Prieto-Martin P, Yamaguchi T, Miyara M, Fehervari Z, Nomura T, Sakaguchi S. 2008. CTLA-4 control over $Foxp3^+$ regulatory T cell function. *Science* **322:** 271–275. doi:10.1126/science.1160062

Yu A, Snowhite I, Vendrame F, Rosenzwajg M, Klatzmann D, Pugliese A, Malek TR. 2015. Selective IL-2 responsiveness of regulatory T cells through multiple intrinsic mechanisms supports the use of low-dose IL-2 therapy in type 1 diabetes. *Diabetes* **64:** 2172–2183. doi:10.2337/db14-1322

Advancing Animal Models of Human Type 1 Diabetes

David V. Serreze, Jennifer R. Dwyer, and Jeremy J. Racine

The Jackson Laboratory, Bar Harbor, Maine 04609, USA

Correspondence: dave.serreze@jax.org

Multiple rodent models have been developed to study the basis of type 1 diabetes (T1D). However, nonobese diabetic (NOD) mice and derivative strains still provide the gold standard for dissecting the basis of the autoimmune responses underlying T1D. Here, we review the developmental origins of NOD mice, and how they and derivative strains have been used over the past several decades to dissect the genetic and immunopathogenic basis of T1D. Also discussed are ways in which the immunopathogenic basis of T1D in NOD mice and humans are similar or differ. Additionally reviewed are efforts to "humanize" NOD mice and derivative strains to provide improved models to study autoimmune responses contributing to T1D in human patients.

In most cases, type 1 diabetes (T1D) results from the ultimately T-cell-mediated autoimmune destruction of insulin-producing pancreatic β cells. Over the last several decades, multiple rodent animal models have been developed to study the pathophysiological and genetic basis of T1D development. Chief among these, and the primary focus of this review, has been the spontaneous T1D susceptible nonobese diabetic (NOD) mouse (Driver et al. 2011; Wakeland 2014). Similar to humans, T1D development in NOD mice results from complex interactions between multiple disease susceptibility genes (respectively designated *Idd* and *IDDM* genes in mice and humans) (Driver et al. 2011; Chen et al. 2018; Grant et al. 2020). The NOD mouse has been criticized for providing a limited means to identify a clinically applicable T1D intervention approach. However, the use of NOD mice indicated a murine anti-CD3 reagent mimicking clinically used teplizumab could be used to reverse recent-onset T1D (Chatenoud 2019). Treatment with the anti-CD3 teplizumab reagent has now also shown promise in human T1D patients (Chatenoud 2019; Ramos et al. 2023). Furthermore, the study of NOD mice and related strains has provided significant critical information on the shared genetic and pathophysiological basis of T1D enabling important insights into potential targets of possible future disease intervention approaches.

At this point, we will note other rodent models have also been used to study T1D development. These include BB rat-based models (Bortell and Yang 2012). Indeed, the BB-DR substrain is the only rodent model demonstrated to date to develop T1D following a viral infection, a phenomenon hypothesized by some as a disease

Cite this article as *Cold Spring Harb Perspect Med* doi: 10.1101/cshperspect.a041587

contributory factor in humans (Zipris et al. 2007). There are also more esoteric murine T1D models. One of these is a mouse model expressing in pancreatic β cells a rat insulin promoter (RIP)-driven transgene encoding the glycoprotein (GP) component of the lymphocytic choriomeningitis virus (RIP-LCMV mice). These mice develop T1D upon infection with LCMV (Van Belle et al. 2009). Another model is mice expressing an RIP-driven transgene encoding a membrane-bound form of the ovalbumin (Ova) antigen in pancreatic β cells (RIP-Ova mice). RIP-Ova mice develop T1D either upon introduction of an Ova-specific transgenic T-cell receptor (TCR), or after priming with this antigen (Wesley et al. 2010; Wang et al. 2011). Various strains of mice treated with multiple low doses of streptozotocin (MLDS) also develop T1D (Furman 2021). MLDS-induced T1D appears to entail an inflammatory component (Schott-Ohly et al. 2004; Tekula et al. 2018). However, MLDS-induced T1D is not absolutely dependent on adaptive immune responses since such treatment still elicits disease development in NOD mice made lymphocyte deficient by the introduction of the *Prkdc*^{scid} (*scid*) gene mutation (Gerling et al. 1994). Thus, while the BB rat and RIP-LCMV, RIP-Ova, and MLDS mouse models have value and use, the form of T1D developing in these rodents differs in notable ways from spontaneous disease in humans. For this reason, spontaneous T1D in NOD mice and related strains most accurately resembles that in humans, and thus have been the most widely used animal models for the study of disease immunopathogenesis. Furthermore, with many of the key genetic loci contributing to T1D being shared between mouse and human patients (Driver et al. 2011), the NOD mouse also provides a model to identify environmental factors that can impact disease development. This will be touched upon later in this review.

ORIGINS OF NOD MICE

Although the NOD strain was ultimately developed in Japan in the early 1980s, it was originally derived from "Swiss" strains (Leiter 1998). The original "Swiss" mice were outbred and imported in 1926 to the Rockefeller Institute in New York from a colony maintained in Lausanne, Switzerland. SWR/J and SJL/J became two standard strains developed at The Jackson Laboratory by inbreeding progeny of the original "Swiss" mice. In 1947, random-bred "Swiss" mice were imported to the Institute for Cancer Research in Philadelphia and became established as the outbred Ha/ICR stock. ICR mice were imported to CLEA in Japan after the Second World War where they underwent inbreeding resulting in the production of multiple derivative strains. These include the ALS and ALR strains, respectively, selected for susceptibility and resistance to the alloxan diabetogenic toxin.

NOD and other related inbred strains were derived from ICR progenitors at the Shionogi Research Laboratories in Japan by Dr. Susumu Makino (Makino et al. 1980, 1985). The original selection was for cataract development. This led to the generation of an inbred mouse strain now designated CTS that all develop cataracts. A cataract-resistant strain designated NCT was also developed. Dr. Makino wisely recognized a link between cataract and diabetes susceptibility. Thus, at the sixth generation of inbreeding (F6), he initiated the development of two additional cataract-free strains in the hope of developing a spontaneous diabetes model. At this F6 generation, Makino identified individual mice exhibiting high-fasting blood glucose levels. He then commenced selective breeding of such ICR-derived progeny exhibiting this high-fasting blood glucose phenotype. Makino also realized the need to develop a control strain, so additionally commenced selective breeding at F6 of ICR-derived progeny displaying low-fasting blood glucose levels. Serendipitously, at the F20 generation of inbreeding a female in the line originally selected for low-fasting blood glucose levels broke through into overt spontaneous T1D. The autoimmune nature of this disease was revealed by the presence of extensive leukocytic infiltration of pancreatic islets with the lesion termed "insulitis" (Makino et al. 1980, 1985). Through continued inbreeding, the progeny of this F20 diabetic female became founders for the original NOD/Shi strain. Mice within the line originally selected for high-fasting blood glucose levels never developed overt T1D, and became the inbred NON (nonobese nondiabetic) control strain. Resulting from his meticulous attention to detail, Makino's development of the NOD and NON as well as other related strains (e.g., CTS, ALS, ALR) was truly a remarkable feat.

After much international intrigue (see Leiter 1998 for details), NOD and NON breeding pairs finally arrived at the Jackson Laboratory in 1985 where they became the founders for the now widely distributed NOD/ShiLtJ and NON/ShiLtJ strains. A NOD colony earlier established by Dr. Yoko Mullen at the University of California, Los Angeles, became the origin, by way of Dr. Linda Wicker and Merck, of the also currently distributed NOD/MrkTac strain (Taconic Farms, Inc.) (Mullen 2017). The use of mouse diversity array and whole-exome capture sequencing platforms has now identified 64 single-nucleotide and two short indels distinguishing five NOD substrains held at various global locations (Simecek et al. 2015). This extent of genetic drift is comparable with similar studies carried out on C57BL6 (B6) and BALB/c substrains (Singer et al. 1993; Sittig et al. 2014).

GENETIC BASIS FOR T1D DEVELOPMENT IN NOD MICE

T1D development in humans and NOD mice is highly polygenic in nature, with over 50 loci linked to disease risk in both species (Driver et al. 2012). These are, respectively, designated as *Idd* and *IDD* genes in mice and humans. While T1D is highly polygenic in nature, particular major histocompatibility complex (MHC) and human leukocyte antigen (HLA) haplotypes are, respectively, the strongest drivers of disease development in NOD mice and human patients (Driver et al. 2011; Claessens et al. 2020; Fasolino et al. 2020; Grant et al. 2020). Within the $H2^{g7}$ MHC haplotype (designated *Idd1*) of NOD mice homozygous expression of the H2-A^{g7} coupled with an absence of H2-E class II gene products are key components of T1D development by driving pathogenic CD4 T-cell responses. The β-chain component of the H2-A^{g7} heterodimer is unique as it is characterized by histidine and serine at positions 56 and 57 in place of the normally conserved proline and aspartic acid residues (Acha-Orbea and McDevitt 1987). Transgenic analyses have shown both the histidine and serine residues at positions 56 and 57 are critical for T1D development in NOD mice (Lund et al. 1990; Miyazaki et al. 1990; Slattery et al. 1990; Stadinski et al. 2023). The conversion of aspartic acid to serine at position 57 is especially significant as non-aspartic acid residues also characterize human HLA-*DQ*β class II homologs contributing to T1D development (Todd et al. 1988). Transgenic restoration of H2-E class II expression by antigen-presenting cells (APCs) also inhibits T1D development in NOD mice (Johnson et al. 2001).

In addition to the above class II components, it is now known that while they represent common variants also characterizing some non-autoimmune prone strains, the class I molecules encoded within the $H2^{g7}$ haplotype (K^d and D^b) also exert essential diabetogenic functions in NOD mice. This was demonstrated by findings that eliminating expression of these class I molecules either through the introduction of a $\beta 2m^{null}$ mutation or their CRISPR-mediated ablation completely inhibits T1D development in NOD mice (Katz et al. 1993; Serreze et al. 1994a; Wicker et al. 1994a; Racine et al. 2018). The fact that pancreatic β cells predominantly express MHC class I molecules, probably accounts for the findings that CD8 T cells play an essential role in the initiation of T1D development in NOD mice, and also likely human patients. Indeed, an elevation in HLA class I expression by pancreatic β cells appears to be an early disease prodromal event during T1D development in humans (Richardson et al. 2016; Shapiro et al. 2021). Furthermore, T1D development in NOD mice appears to require the expression of the particular class I variants characterizing the $H2^{g7}$ MHC haplotype (Hattori et al. 1999; Pomerleau et al. 2005). NOD stocks that congenically express non-$H2^{g7}$ genes in a heterozygous state are rendered T1D resistant (Serreze et al. 2004). This indicates $H2^{g7}$ molecules not only contribute to T1D in NOD mice by activating pathogenic T cells through their antigen-presentation capabilities, but also because of their failure when in a homozygous state to mediate immune regulatory processes such as thymic negative selection normally preventing the development and/or activation of such effectors.

C57BL6 (B6), C57BL10 (B10), and NON background mice congenically carrying the NOD-derived $H2^{g7}$ MHC in a homozygous state all remain T1D free. Furthermore, the NOR strain that shares ~88% of its genome with NOD mice including the $H2^{g7}$ MHC is completely T1D resistant (Serreze et al. 1994b). Thus, the $H2^{g7}$ MHC does not independently contribute to T1D, but must do so in concert with other background genes characterizing NOD mice. Using unique breeding strategies in which the $H2^{g7}$ MHC remained fixed, and what at the time were cutting-edge, marker-identification technologies, the Todd and Wicker groups carried out backcross 1 (BC1) and F2-based segregation studies that identified multiple *Idd* genetic loci contributing to T1D development in NOD mice (Cornall et al. 1991; Todd et al. 1991; Ghosh et al. 1993). Such efforts carried out by the Todd and Wicker groups, as well as other investigators, have led to the identification of >40 non-MHC *Idd* genetic loci characterizing NOD mice (previously reviewed in Chen et al. 2018). It has also been found that genetic variation between NOD and B6 control mice results in these strains having a differing 3D chromatin architecture in thymocytes that may influence the development of autoimmunity (Fasolino et al. 2020).

While the segregation studies described above enabled the initial mapping of *Idd* loci contributing to T1D development in NOD mice, they did not allow for the identification of the actual underlying gene(s), and/or their disease-causative functions. The subsequent development of NOD stocks congenically carrying selective chromosomal segments spanning T1D resistance loci from original outcross partner strains has provided key resources to begin the identification of the actual genes controlling T1D susceptibility or resistance, and how they functionally do so. By continuous backcrossing to the NOD parental strain combined with genetic marker selection, it is possible to further truncate the size of original congenic intervals to assist in the identification and functional characterization of actual *Idd* genes. Such congenic truncation efforts have revealed that most originally identified *Idd* loci actually contain multiple genes determining T1D susceptibility. Two notable examples include the original *Idd3* locus on Chromosome (Chr.) 3 that was subsequently subdivided into the *Idd3*, *Idd10*, *Idd17*, and *Idd18* regions (Wicker et al. 1994b; Lord et al. 1995; Podolin et al. 1997), and the original *Idd5* locus on Chr. 1 that was subsequently subdivided into the *Idd5.1*, *Idd5.2*, *Idd5.3*, and *Idd5.4* regions (Cornall et al. 1991; Garchon et al. 1991; Hill et al. 2000; Hunter et al. 2007). Similarly, the original *Idd9* locus on Chr. 4 was dissected into the *Idd9.1*, *Idd9.2*, *Idd9.3*, *Idd9.4*, and *Idd9.5* subregions (Rodrigues et al. 1994; Brodnicki et al. 2000; Lyons et al. 2000; Hamilton-Williams et al. 2013).

Even with their truncations, the actual T1D controlling genes within most *Idd* locus subregions remain unknown. However, in some cases, genes likely controlling T1D within *Idd* loci have been identified (Table 1). One of these first examples was the finding that within the *Idd13* locus on Chr. 2 differing allelic variants of *β2m* contribute to T1D susceptibility or resistance. Transgenic rescue of $\beta2m^{a}$ but not $\beta2m^{b}$ expression restored T1D development in normally disease-resistant NOD.$\beta2m^{null}$ mice (Hamilton-Williams et al. 2001). This is likely due to $H2^{g7}$-encoded class I molecules taking on a different structural conformation, potentially altering their antigen-presentation patterns when dimerizing with $\beta2m^{a}$ versus $\beta2m^{b}$. A hypo-expression variant of the *Il2* gene resulting in diminished regulatory T-cell (Treg) activity was found to be a likely causal component of the NOD *Idd3* locus (Yamanouchi et al. 2007). Interestingly, a mirror image effect resulting from differing IL-2R variants has been implicated in determining T1D susceptibility in humans (Lowe et al. 2007; Todd et al. 2007). However, there has been an additional report that *Il21* gene variants may also contribute to the *Idd3* locus effect (McGuire et al. 2009). An allelic variant resulting in diminished expression of the T-cell inhibitory CTLA-4 molecule, that is also important in maintaining Treg activity, likely underlies the *Idd5.1* locus effect (Gerold et al. 2011). The *Idd10* locus effect is likely due to allelic variants of *Cd101* regulating the activity of multiple immunological cell types including Tregs (Rainbow et al. 2011; Mattner et al. 2019). By controlling the extent to which diabetogenic CD8 T cells undergo thymic deletion as well as Treg development and activity, differing expression variants of the NF-κB regulatory *Nfkbid* gene likely underlie the *Idd7* locus effect

Table 1. Identified genes likely underlying some *Idd* locus effects

Idd locus	Chromosome	Likely underlying gene	Mechanism
Idd13	2	*β2m*	Change in MHC class I conformation when dimerizing with β2m[a] (susceptibility) versus β2m[b] (resistance)
Idd3	3	*Il2*	Hypomorphic variant in NOD results in decreased Treg activity
Idd5.1	1	*Ctla4*	Hypomorphic variant in NOD results in less suppression of pathogenic T cells and diminished Treg activity
Idd10	3	*Cd101*	Unknown
Idd7	7	*Nfkbid*	NOD variant results in diminished thymic deletion of pathogenic CD8 T cells, and decreased Treg activity
Idd18.2	3	*Ptpn22*	Altering the extent of TCR signaling activity
Idd9.3	4	*Tnfrsf9*	Treg accumulation
Idd32	11	*Mtv3*	Superantigen affecting T-cell selection

(MHC) Major histocompatibility complex, (NOD) nonobese diabetic, (TCR) T-cell receptor.

on Chr. 7 (Dwyer et al. 2022). Differing expression variants of *Ptpn22* that attenuate TCR signaling are likely responsible for the *Idd18.2* locus effect (Fraser et al. 2015). Allelic variants of *PTPN22* have also been implicated in genome-wide association studies (GWAS) analyses as contributing to T1D susceptibility in humans (Armitage et al. 2021). Allelic variants of the *Tnfrsf9* gene influencing Treg accumulation have also been found to likely underlie the *Idd9.3* effect (Forsberg et al. 2019). It was recently found that the presence or absence of the endogenous *Mtv3* retrovirus is responsible for the *Idd32* locus effect (Ye et al. 2023).

Another means to assist the identification of genes underlying various *Idd* locus effects is to determine the cell types in which they manifest their activity. Means by which this can be done, and previous efforts to do so were discussed in a previous review (Chen et al. 2018). Examples include subregions of the *Idd9/11* region controlling the development of diabetogenic CD4 T cells, B lymphocytes, and Tregs. Profiling of mRNA transcripts in the appropriate cell type then enables the identification of candidate genes underlying a particular *Idd* locus effect (Chen et al. 2018). The development of CRISPR technologies now enables the engineering of identified candidate genes directly within relevant strains to test their possible diabetogenic contributions (Harrison et al. 2014).

Susceptibility or resistance variants of *Idd* genes can modulate disease development in an additive and/or epistatic fashion. An early example was combining B10-derived *Idd3* and *Idd5* congenic intervals, which conferred nearly complete T1D resistance to NOD background mice (Hill et al. 2000). It was subsequently found that it is the *Idd5.3* subregion that synergizes with *Idd3* to strongly regulate T1D susceptibility (Lin et al. 2013). Interactions between various *Idd5* subregion genes have also been identified. Interestingly, it was found that the B10-derived *Idd5.4* congenic region can actually contribute to T1D susceptibility in NOD background mice, but this effect is masked if the strong disease-protective *Idd5.1* region is also present (Hunter et al. 2007). Similar counteracting disease effects between congenic donor strain genes have been identified for the *Idd19* and *Idd6* regions on Chr. 6, the *Idd19* and *Idd20* regions also on Chr. 6, the *Idd21.1* and *Idd21.2* regions on Chr. 18, as well as the *Idd14* and *Idd31* regions on Chr. 13 (Rogner et al. 2001; Hollis-Moffatt et al. 2005; Morin et al. 2006; Wang et al. 2014).

It is clear that the actual genes contributing to T1D development in humans and NOD mice are not completely overlapping. However, it seems likely that T1D genes in humans and NOD mice function in common biochemical networks. One example noted above is the genes encoding IL-2 and its receptor, respectively, functioning in a mirroring fashion for T1D development in NOD mice and human patients. Other networks potentially influenced at differing operational points by genes contributing to T1D development on NOD mice and humans may be revealed by querying software platforms such as Ingenuity Pathway Analysis.

PATHOPHYSIOLOGY OF NOD MICE

As described above, the presence of pancreatic insulitis was the first indication that autoimmune β-cell destruction was the cause of T1D in NOD mice. In most vivariums, T1D development is more aggressive in female than male NOD mice (Leiter 1998). Insulitis development initiates at ∼4–5 weeks of age in female NOD mice. An early flow cytometry-based study evaluated the leukocytic makeup of the insulitic lesion in NOD mice at various ages (Jarpe et al. 1991). This study found the first cells infiltrating the pancreatic islets of NOD female mice were MHC class II^+ monocytes and CD8 T cells. There was a subsequent influx of CD4 T cells and B lymphocytes accompanied by a further increase in the CD8 population. Throughout the insulitis development process, the MHC class II^+ monocyte population remained fairly constant. Critically, a series of studies determined that the immune cell infiltration was in fact the cause of T1D, as adoptive transfer of splenocytes or bone marrow cells from NOD donors could recapitulate the disease in normally resistant recipients (Wicker et al. 1986, 1988; Serreze et al. 1988; LaFace and Peck 1989).

A subsequent finding that NOD-*scid* mice were completely T1D resistant indicated some or all of the lymphocyte populations in the insulitic lesion contribute to T1D development in NOD mice (Christianson et al. 1993). Adoptive transfer studies using either standard NOD-*scid* mice or a stock made MHC class I deficient by introduction of an inactivated *β2m* gene (*$β2m^{null}$*) as recipients evaluated the relative roles of CD4 and CD8 T cells from various aged NOD donors in contributing to T1D development. These studies found that a combination of both autoreactive CD4 and CD8 T cells were required to mediate most of the prodromal stages of T1D development in NOD mice (Serreze et al. 1997; DiLorenzo et al. 1998). However, only CD4 T cells from NOD donors that had already developed overt T1D could independently transfer disease to NOD-*scid.$β2m^{null}$* recipients. A recent study found that cross-presentation of β-cell autoantigens to pathogenic CD8 T cells mediated by conventional dendritic cells (cDCs) is a crucial initial step for T1D development in NOD mice (Ferris et al. 2023). It has also been reported that, at least in part, intra-islet CD4 T cells may promote T1D development in NOD mice through the activation of natural killer (NK) cells (Feuerer et al. 2009).

A critical role played by B lymphocytes for T1D development in NOD mice was provided by findings that their ablation through either a genetic approach (introducing the *$Igμ^{null}$* mutation) or antibody treatments had strong disease-protective effects (Serreze et al. 1996; Akashi et al. 1997; Noorchashm et al. 1997; Wong et al. 1998; Bouaziz et al. 2007; Hu et al. 2007; Fiorina et al. 2008; Xiu et al. 2008). Other studies found their unique ability to specifically take up β-cell autoantigens through an immunoglobulin (Ig)-mediated capture mechanism allows B lymphocytes to be the APC subtype most efficiently supporting the expansion of both diabetogenic CD4 and CD8 T cells in NOD mice (Serreze et al. 1998; Hulbert et al. 2001; Silveira et al. 2002; Mariño et al. 2012). Multiple stages of B-lymphocyte development are altered in NOD mice (Silveira et al. 2004; Acevedo-Suarez et al. 2005; Quinn et al. 2006; Mariño et al. 2008; Kendall et al. 2013), expanding the pool of antigen-specific APC capable of mediating activation of pathogenic T-cell populations. Partly based on these findings there has been significant interest in developing B-lymphocyte-targeting strategies as a possible clinically applicable T1D intervention approach.

It is currently only possible to identify humans at future T1D risk after they have already developed signs of ongoing high levels of pancreatic β-cell autoimmunity such as the presence of insulin autoantibodies (IAAs) (Bonifacio and Ziegler 2010). Thus, partly based on the animal studies described above, it was tested whether short-term treatment with the B-lymphocyte-depleting CD20-specific rituximab antibody had beneficial effects in recent-onset T1D patients (Pescovitz et al. 2009). Transient rituximab treatment allowed for early (1-year), but not long-term (2-year) preservation of C-peptide production in recent-onset T1D patients (Pescovitz et al. 2009). The lack of long-term protection may be at least partially attributable to the rebound of B lymphocytes following transient rituximab treatment. However, it has been found that B lymphocytes within the insulitic lesion of NOD mice lose cell surface CD20 expression, and thus are rendered resistant to depletion by a rituximab-like antibody (Serreze et al. 2011). Subsequent studies focused on BAFF blockade to deplete B cells in NOD mice (Zekavat et al. 2008; Mariño et al. 2014; Wang et al. 2017). This approach may in fact be more desirable than anti-CD20 treatment to attenuate diabetogenic B-lymphocyte responses (Wang et al. 2017).

Various studies in NOD mice indicate targeting of nonlymphoid cells may also provide an effective T1D intervention approach. In particular, myeloid cells including macrophages and dendritic cells (DCs) play an important role in activating diabetogenic T cells in NOD mice. This is evidenced by findings that blocking various macrophage or DC activities can inhibit T1D development in NOD mice (Hutchings et al. 1990; Nikolic et al. 2005; Saxena et al. 2007; Carrero et al. 2017; Tahvili et al. 2018; Ciecko et al. 2019). There is also evidence that developmental defects in NOD DCs limit their ability to mediate various immunological tolerance induction processes normally preventing the development or activation of autoreactive diabetogenic T-cell responses (Chilton et al. 2004; Chen et al. 2005; Huang et al. 2008; Wallet et al. 2009; Driver et al. 2010; Van Belle et al. 2010). In addition, neutrophils may also contribute to pancreatic β-cell destruction in NOD mice (Diana et al. 2013).

Thymic negative selection represents an important mechanism through which many autoreactive T cells are deleted during their early development (von Boehmer and Melchers 2010). Defects in such thymic negative selection processes reportedly contribute to the development of T1D in NOD mice and also likely humans (Kishimoto and Sprent 2001; Choisy-Rossi et al. 2004; Serreze et al. 2008). However, the activity of Tregs normally prevents the functional activation of autoreactive effector T cells that escape thymic negative selection. Defects in Treg function, and/or the ability of effector T cells to respond to their suppressive functions, appear to contribute to T1D development in both humans and NOD mice. Thus, there has been considerable interest in developing means, including IL-2-mediated expansion, through which enhancing Treg activity could provide a T1D therapeutic approach (Tang and Bluestone 2008; Bluestone et al. 2015; Perdigoto et al. 2016; Ferreira et al. 2019). Such efforts have in part been engendered by findings that IL-2 treatment can inhibit T1D development in NOD mice through the induction of Tregs (Grinberg-Bleyer et al. 2018; Nagy et al. 2021). In addition to limiting autoreactive T-cell responses, enhanced Treg activity may also inhibit T1D development by restraining pathogenic NK cells. It has also been found that numerical and functional deficiencies in invariant NK T cells (iNKT) contribute to T1D in NOD mice (Hammond et al. 2001). Treatment with the α-galactosylceramide (GalCer) iNKT superagonist reagent inhibits T1D development in NOD mice by promoting the maturation of DCs to a state capable of inducing multiple immunological tolerance mechanisms including elevating Treg activity (Chen et al. 2005). It was recently discovered that elevated expression levels of the CD226 costimulatory receptor may contribute to the diminished activity of Tregs in NOD mice (Shapiro et al. 2020; Thirawatananond et al. 2023). Diminishing CD226 expression in Tregs suppressed T1D development in NOD mice associated with increased activity of the counterreceptor TIGIT (Thirawatananond et al. 2023). Hence, developing means to diminish CD226 activity might also provide a clinically applicable T1D intervention approach.

There have been concerns that the nature of the insulitic lesion in NOD mice may not completely mimic that in human T1D patients. This is based on an examination of samples from the nPOD biorepository indicating that insulitis appears to be less severe in T1D patients than in NOD mice (Campbell-Thompson et al. 2016). A possible explanation may be that T1D develops very rapidly over a matter of weeks in NOD mice, while the disease prodromal period in humans is often years after the initial appearance of autoantibodies. Most nPOD samples are sourced from donors succumbing to a non-T1D-related death multiple years, often decades, after their initial disease diagnosis. Thus, nPOD samples likely represent a later disease phase where islet-infiltrating immune cells are not as predominant. Human pancreas samples becoming available to the scientific community at the time of initial T1D diagnosis are rare. However, Dr. Massimo Trucco (University of Pittsburgh) has provided the authors with an autopsy pancreatic micrograph from a young child who passed away within 24 hours of being diagnosed with T1D. Insulitis in this new T1D-onset patient appeared to be as severe as that in NOD mice (Fig. 1). Similar aggressive insulitis has been observed in rare samples from individuals with recent-onset T1D (Foulis 1996; Rowe et al. 2011). However, there is now a growing consensus that insulitis in patients at risk or with overt T1D can be quite heterogeneous including reaching levels similar to that in NOD mice (Atkinson and Mirmira 2023). In addition, the cellular composition of insulitic infiltrates in NOD mice and human patients also have some differences. The frequency of CD8 T cells appears to be higher in human insulitis, with B-lymphocyte levels more variable than in NOD mice (Willcox et al. 2009; Coppieters et al. 2012; Arif et al. 2014). Furthermore, it has been reported that insulitis in NOD mice is an open and dynamic process, and it is unclear to the extent to which this might also be the case in human T1D patients (Magnuson et al. 2015).

There is good concordance between the β-cell antigens targeted by T1D-causative autoreactive CD4 and CD8 T cells in human patients and NOD mice (for reviews, see Purcell et al. 2019; Amdare et al. 2021). This provides further evidence that the NOD mouse model is of value in deciphering the pathophysiological basis of T1D development in humans. To date, antigenic peptides derived from 32 different pancreatic β-cell proteins have been found to be targets of T1D contributory autoreactive CD4 and/or CD8 T cells in NOD mice or T1D patients (for review, see Amdare et al. 2021). While individual peptide sequences recognized by diabetogenic CD4 or CD8 T cells in NOD and humans can differ, in most cases they are derived from the same set of source proteins (for review, see Amdare et al. 2021). Interestingly, an increase as detected by tetramer-based flow cytometric analyses in the frequency among peripheral blood leukocytes (PBLs) of CD8 T cells recognizing the 206–214 peptide sequence derived from the β-cell antigen, islet-specific glucose-6-phosphatase catalytic subunit-related protein (originally designated IGRP, now G6pc2) marks individual NOD mice that will progress to overt T1D within 2 weeks (Trudeau et al. 2003). It is unclear whether this might also be the case in humans.

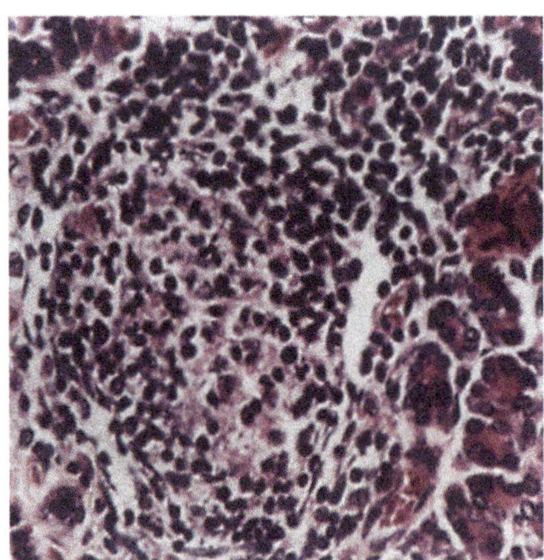
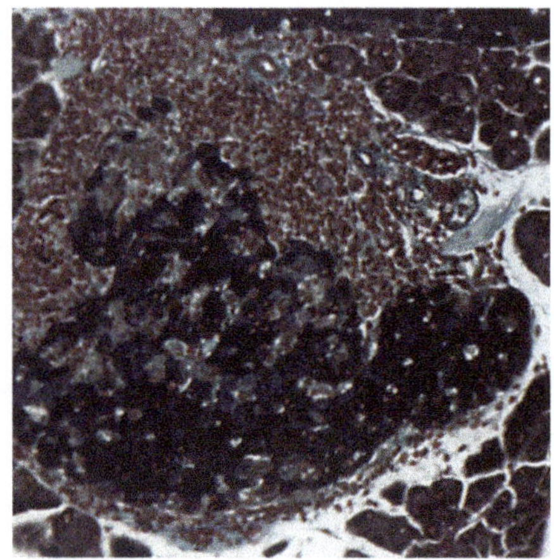

Figure 1. Representative micrograph of insulitis in an autopsy sample from a patient passing away within 24 hours of type 1 diabetes (T1D) diagnosis (*left* panel, H&E staining), and in a 12-week-old female nonobese diabetic (NOD) mouse (*right* panel, AF staining).

Multiple autoantibodies mark T1D progression in humans (So et al. 2021). IAAs usually appear before those targeting other autoantigens in humans at high future T1D risk (So et al. 2021). Insulin is also an antigenic target of autoantibodies in NOD mice (Bonifacio et al. 2001). As discussed later, B lymphocytes expressing Ig molecules recognizing peripherin are also important contributors to T1D development in NOD mice (Leeth et al. 2016).

The autoreactive T-cell responses initiating T1D development in NOD mice also appear to be primarily directed against insulin. Specifically, autoreactive CD4 T-cell responses directed against epitopes within the insulin B-chain 9–23 amino acid segment are important for T1D initiation in NOD mice. This is demonstrated by the finding of T1D resistance in "NOD B16A" mice in which their endogenous insulin 1 and 2 genes have been ablated, and replaced by a mutated proinsulin transgene with a tyrosine-to-alanine substitution at position 16 of the B-chain that allows the molecule to remain metabolically active, but not antigenic (Nakayama et al. 2005). Further support was provided by the finding that NOD mice transgenically expressing proinsulin in APC capable of inducing immunological tolerance were also rendered T1D resistant (Krishnamurthy et al. 2006). Studies by the Unanue group revealed there are two types of CD4 T cells in NOD mice recognizing insulin B-chain 9–23-derived peptides. "Type A" CD4 T cells conventionally recognize the insulin B-chain 13–21 peptide processed from the whole molecule by APC that subsequently displays the epitope bound to the sole H2-A^{g7} class II molecule encoded within the NOD *H2*^{g7} MHC haplotype that as described earlier is a primary genetic contributor to T1D in this strain (Mohan et al. 2010). "Type B" CD4 T cells respond only to a soluble insulin B12–20 peptide that cannot be processed from the whole molecule by APC (Mohan et al. 2010). Such "type B" cells escape negative selection in the thymus due to a lack of antigenic ligand expression by APC, and appear to be a major contributor to the initiation of T1D development in NOD mice, with the "type A" cells playing only a minor pathogenic role (Mohan et al. 2011). Subsequent studies found the insulin B_{12-20} peptide is directly generated in pancreatic β cells themselves from which it is secreted by a process termed "crinophagy" for subsequent direct binding to H2-A^{g7} class II molecules expressed by APC, with macrophages playing an important role for presentation to "type B" CD4 T cells (Carrero et al. 2017; Wan et al. 2018). The binding of insulin-derived peptides in alternative registers to the H2-A^{g7} class II molecule being an important component of T1D development in NOD mice has also been observed by other investigators (Crawford et al. 2011). Peptides derived from insulin or proinsulin are also the frequent targets of autoreactive T cells in human T1D patients (Nakayama et al. 2015; Purcell et al. 2019; Amdare et al. 2021). Similar to the case for NOD mice, it has been reported diabetogenic CD4 T cells from human T1D patients recognize insulin peptides bound in a particular register to disease-associated HLA class II variants (Yang et al. 2014).

A paradigm-shifting advance arising from the study of NOD mice was that some diabetogenic CD4 T cells recognize noncontiguous autoantigenic peptides (Delong et al. 2016). These include hybrid insulin peptides (HIPs), which were also found to be targeted by CD4 T cells from human T1D patients (Babon et al. 2016; Arribas-Layton et al. 2020). The HIPs identified to date have consisted of an amino acid sequence derived from insulin (this can include a portion of the normally excised C-peptide) fused to a sequence from a different β-cell secretory granule protein, or a normally noncontiguous segment of insulin itself. The first HIP was identified by the finding that the well-studied NOD-derived BDC2.5 CD4 T-cell clonotype recognizes an epitope consisting of an insulin C-peptide fragment (LQTLAL) fused to the WE14 sequence (WSMRD) derived from chromogranin-A (Delong et al. 2016). A noncontiguous antigenic peptide consisting of fused fragments from the insulin B-chain and ProSAAS has recently been shown to be targeted by BDC6.3 diabetogenic CD4 T cells from NOD mice (Wenzlau et al. 2022). Some tumor-reactive CD8 T cells were previously found to recognize noncontiguous antigenic peptides (Michaux et al. 2014; Ebstein et al. 2016). Through a process termed *cis*-peptide splicing, normally intervening amino acid sequences were removed from the β-cell protein islet amyloid polypeptide (IAPP) and receptor-type tyrosine-protein phosphatase-like N (PTPRN) resulting in the formation of noncontiguous antigenic epitopes recognized by CD8 T cells from T1D patients (Gonzalez-Duque et al. 2018; Azoury et al. 2020). There is also evidence noncontiguous autoantigenic peptides derived from the β-cell proteins secretogranin-5 (SCG5), urocortin-3, and proconvertase-2 are targeted by diabetogenic CD8 T cells in NOD mice (Azoury et al. 2020). Noncontiguous CD8 T-cell epitopes resulting from *cis*-peptide splicing are generated by proteaosome-mediated transpeptidation (Vigneron et al. 2019). The mechanism of HIP formation is less clear. However, HIPs appear to be generated in β-cell secretory granules through a transpeptidation process involving an acyl-protease intermediate (Delong et al. 2016). As noncontiguous autoantigenic epitopes are not expressed in the thymus, T cells that recognize them are not deleted during their development at this site (negative selection). Furthermore, it has been reported that Tregs in NOD mice are induced less efficiently to noncontiguous than conventional antigenic peptides (Jing et al. 2022). Both processes could represent potentially important pathogenic components of T1D development in NOD mice, and also possibly human patients.

There is also evidence autoimmune responses against neuronal antigens may be an important component of T1D pathogenesis in NOD mice as well as humans. Early support for this possibility was the finding that the neuronal protein glutamic acid decarboxylase (GAD) was a T1D-relevant autoantigen in humans (Baekkeskov et al. 1990). It was subsequently reported that the initiation of T1D development in NOD mice involved an autoimmune response against neuronal Schwann cells surrounding pancreatic islets (Winer et al. 2003). It is possible GAD-directed autoimmunity contributes to such targeting of Schwann cells. NOD mice can also develop spontaneous autoimmune encephalitis (Winer et al. 2001). The neuronal protein peripherin is also expressed in pancreatic β cells and represents the autoantigenic target of most islet-infiltrating B lymphocytes in NOD mice (Carrillo et al. 2005, 2008; Puertas et al. 2007; Garabatos et al. 2014). A NOD stock with most B lymphocytes transgenically expressing a peripherin autoreactive immunoglobulin molecule (NOD-PerIg) was found to have increased numbers of interactive cognate T cells and develop T1D at a greatly accelerated rate (Leeth et al. 2016). Autoantibodies directed against phosphorylated peripherin have also been detected in human T1D patients (Doran et al. 2016). CD4 T cells from NOD-PerIg mice were also found to have a capacity to passively transfer both peripheral and spinal nerve neuritis to NOD-*scid* recipients (Fig. 2A,B; Racine et al. 2020). If T1D onset is delayed by transient depletion of B lymphocytes, NOD-PerIg mice themselves also develop neuritis (Fig. 2C; Racine et al. 2020). These results may provide an explanation for the previous findings that there can be overlap in the autoreactive T-cell repertoires in patients with T1D or MS (Winer et al. 2001), and, unfortunately, individuals copresenting with both diseases are not rare (International Multiple Sclerosis Genetics Consortium 2009; Tettey et al. 2015).

As noted earlier, in most vivariums T1D development is more aggressive in female than male NOD mice (Leiter 1998). However, this is not universally true. For instance, in the authors' NOD colony, more than 70% of male mice can develop T1D. There is now evidence that variations in the intestinal microbiome can be an important contributor to the extent there is a gender dimorphism in T1D development in a given NOD colony. This is partly demonstrated by the finding that the gender bias in T1D development is lost in germ-free (GF) NOD mice (Yurkovetskiy et al. 2013). Several studies have found T1D can be inhibited in NOD female mice colonized by intestinal microbes from males, with the expansion of protective species under androgen control (Markle et al. 2013; Yurkovetskiy et al. 2013). Another study found male-derived T1D protective intestinal microbes elicited disease resistance through Toll receptor activity (Burrows et al. 2015). A more recent study found dietary gluten is an important factor influencing the development of intestinal microbes regulat-

 Cite this article as *Cold Spring Harb Perspect Med* doi: 10.1101/cshperspect.a041587

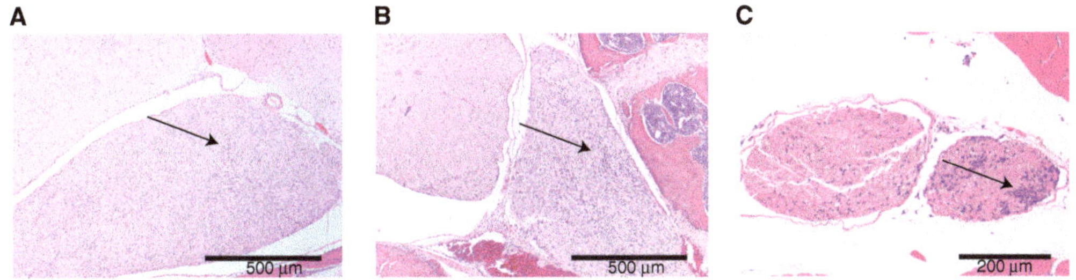

Figure 2. NOD-PerIg T cells can induce neuritis as well as type 1 diabetes (T1D). (*A*) Inflammatory damage (arrows) to peripheral sciatic nerves in NOD-*scid* recipients of NOD-PerIg T cells. (*B*) Inflammatory damage to spinal nerves in NOD-*scid* recipients of NOD-PerIg T cells. (*C*) Development of peripheral neuritis in NOD-PerIg mice in which T1D development was delayed by transient depletion of B lymphocytes by anti-CD20 treatment. (Panels reprinted, with permission, from Racine et al. 2020, originally published in *The Journal of Immunology*, © 2020, The American Association of Immunologists.)

ing T1D sensitivity (Funsten et al. 2023). The presence of segmented filamentous bacterium (SFB) has also been found to suppress T1D development in both female and male NOD mice (Kriegel et al. 2011; Fahey et al. 2017). Thus, environmental factors known to influence the varying susceptibility of common sourced NOD mice held at differing sites could include heterogeneity in the intestinal microbiome they develop. It has also been recently reported that differing immune responses to three potential species of intestinal bacteria marks those humans at T1D risk who would most benefit from the anti-CD3-mediated disease intervention approach discussed earlier (Xie et al. 2023).

HUMANIZED NOD MICE

There have been ongoing efforts to "humanize" NOD mice with the hope that experimental results obtained using these strains would have increased clinical relevance to T1D patients. To date, "humanized" mice can be placed into two major classes. One class is immunodeficient mice that can be engrafted with human cells and tissues. The other class is mice that have been genetically engineered such that various immune responses are mediated by human rather than murine molecules.

There is now a multitude of immunodeficient mouse strains that can be used as recipients for human cells and tissues (for review, see Chuprin et al. 2023). However, NOD background strains made lymphocyte deficient by the introduction of the *Prkdc*^{scid} or *Rag1*^{null} mutations, and then further engineered in various ways, represent current gold standard recipients for engrafted human cells and tissues (Chuprin et al. 2023). An important further modification of these lymphocyte-deficient NOD stocks was the introduction of an inactivated *Il2rg* (IL-2 common γ-chain receptor) gene that ablates signaling through the IL-2, IL-4, IL7, IL-9, IL-15, and IL-21 receptors (Shultz et al. 2012), resulting in what are now referred to as the NSG, NRG, and NCG strains. These combined mutations in conjunction with other NOD strain characteristics such as a lack of a central component of the complement pathway, and diminished myeloid cell phagocytic capabilities, make NSG, NRG, and NCG mice deficient in NK cells as well as lymphocytes and enable them to be efficiently engrafted with human immune cells.

NSG mice expressing transgenes encoding HLA restriction elements for human diabetogenic T cells have also been produced. These include the HLA-A2.1 class I variant characterizing many T1D patients (Valdes et al. 2005; Nejentsev et al. 2007; Noble et al. 2010; Howson et al. 2011). While not inducing overt hyperglycemia, a human HLA-A2.1-restricted IGRP-autoreactive CD8 T-cell line did adoptively transfer insulitis to such NSG-A2 mice (Unger et al. 2012). This indicated human diabetogenic T cells can be functionally activated in NSG recipients transgenically expressing appropriate HLA restriction elements.

There are some limitations to current NSG and NRG-based humanized mouse models. These include that, following their engraftment with human leukocytes or hematopoietic stem cells (HSCs), NSG and NRG recipients do not efficiently develop donor-type innate immune cells or lymphoid follicle structures (reviewed in Chuprin et al. 2023). This latter deficiency likely accounts for the finding that human B-lymphocyte engraftment and antibody production are relatively poor in NSG or NRG recipients. Multiple groups are now working on means, such as the transgenic introduction of additional hematopoietic growth factors, to overcome these current limitations of the NSG and NRG models (for review, see Chuprin et al. 2023).

As described above, other mouse models have been produced in which various immunological responses are mediated by human rather than murine molecules. Early efforts involved introducing transgenes encoding human T1D risk-associated HLA-A2.1 or B39 class I molecules into murine MHC class I–deficient NOD.$\beta 2m^{null}$ mice. These stocks were made using "HHD" transgene constructs (Pascolo et al. 1997) encoding human genomic promoter-driven HLA-A2.1 or B39-derived α1 and α2 antigen-binding domains and a covalently linked human β2m component, with the α3, transmembrane, and cytoplasmic domains of murine H2-D^b origin. Expression of either the human HLA-A2.1 or B39 class I variants was found to restore vigorous T1D development in normally completely disease-resistant NOD.$\beta 2m^{null}$ mice (Takaki et al. 2006; Schloss et al. 2018). The HLA-A2.1-expressing stock also enabled the identification of insulin and IGRP-derived antigenic peptides presented by this human class I variant to pathogenic CD8 T cells from T1D patients (Pinske et al. 2005; Ouyang et al. 2006; Mallone et al. 2007; Unger et al. 2007; Jarchum et al. 2008).

A limitation of the first-generation HLA class I transgenic NOD mice described above is the $\beta 2m^{null}$ mutation resulting in lost FcRn protein expression, a nonclassical MHC I molecule critical to serum IgG and albumin homeostasis (Chaudhury et al. 2003; Roopenian et al. 2003; Roopenian and Akilesh 2007). As a result, mice carrying a $\beta 2m^{null}$ mutation also cannot present IgG complexed antigens to T cells (Baker et al. 2014). Thus, NOD strains carrying the $\beta 2m^{null}$ mutation cannot be used to test potential antibody- or albumin delivery–based T1D interventions (Larsen et al. 2016). To overcome these limitations, CRISPR-Cas9 technologies have been used to directly ablate the classical H2-K^d and H2-D^b class I molecules normally expressed by NOD mice (resultant strain designated NOD-$cMHCI^{-/-}$) (Racine et al. 2018). As described earlier, such NOD-$cMHCI^{-/-}$ mice are completely T1D resistant. However, the introduction of the HHD-based HLA-A2.1 or B39 class I–encoding transgenes restores vigorous T1D development to NOD-$cMHCI^{-/-}$ mice (Racine et al. 2018). Thus, the availability of NOD-$cMHCI^{-/-}$ mice broadens the array of potential T1D interventions that can originally be tested in a preclinical setting.

Subsequent elimination of the H2-A^{g7} class II variant in NOD-$cMHCI^{-/-}$ mice through a CRISPR approach, resulted in a stock fully lacking expression of all classical murine MHC molecules (designated NOD-$cMHCI/II^{-/-}$) (Racine et al. 2018). Such NOD-$cMHCI/II^{-/-}$ mice serve as a platform for introducing, in a pipeline fashion, transgenes encoding any chosen combination of human HLA class I and/or II molecules. A transgene encoding the human T1D-associated DQ8 class II variant has now been introduced into NOD-$cMHCI/II^{-/-}$ mice (new strain designated NOD-$cMHCI/II^{-/-}$-DQ8) (Racine et al. 2023). Transgenes derived from T1D patients encoding disease-relevant DQ-restricted insulin autoreactive TCR molecules have also been introduced into NOD-$cMHCI/II^{-/-}$-DQ8 mice (Racine et al. 2023). One such introduced TCR, A1.9, recognizes human C-peptide$_{42-50}$ in a DQ8-restricted fashion (Pathiraja et al. 2015). Therefore, a transgene encoding human proinsulin was also introduced into NOD-$cMHCI/II^{-/-}$-DQ8-A1.9 mice (Racine et al. 2023). As shown in Figure 3, NOD-cMH$CI/II^{-/-}$-DQ8 mice generate CD4 T cells. Further, as detected by staining with a Vβ5-specific antibody, most CD4 T cells in NOD-$cMHCI/II^{-/-}$-DQ8-A1.9 mice express the transgenic human TCR (Fig. 3). Most importantly, NOD-$cMHCI/II^{-/-}$-DQ8-A1.9 mice also expressing human proinsulin develop insulitis, albeit not to a point resulting in overt hyperglycemia as this

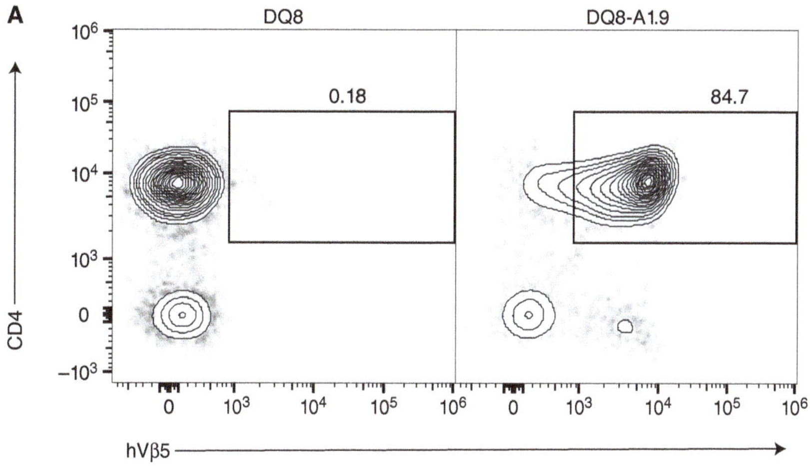

B

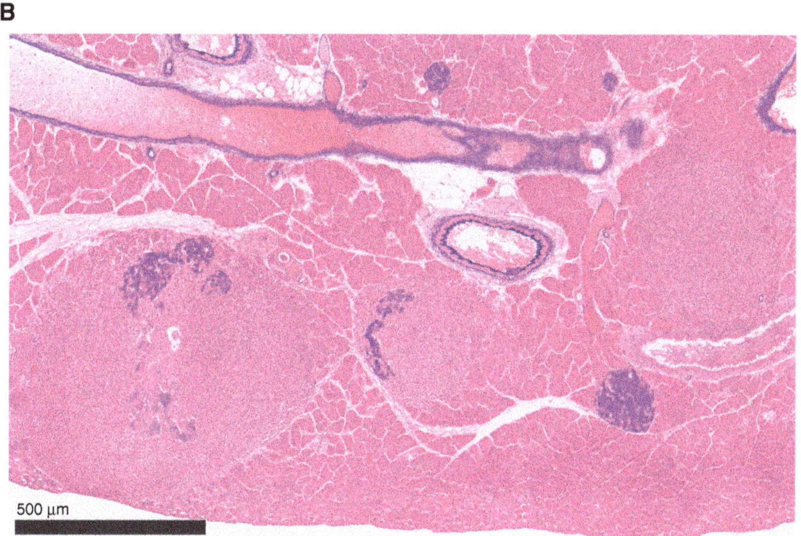

Figure 3. CD4 T cells transgenically expressing the human type 1 diabetes (T1D) patient-derived insulin-autoreactive A1.9 T-cell receptor (TCR) are functionally active in NOD-*cMHCI/II*$^{-/-}$.DQ8 mice. (*A*) CD4 T cells are generated in NOD-*cMHCI/II*$^{-/-}$.DQ8 mice (*left* panel). As assessed by positive Vβ5 staining, the human T1D patient-derived A1.9 transgenic TCR can be expressed by most CD4 T cells in NOD-*cMHCI/II*$^{-/-}$.DQ8 mice (*right* panel). (*B*) A1.9 TCR-bearing CD4 T cells in NOD-*cMHCI/II*$^{-/-}$.DQ8 background mice also coexpressing human proinsulin can mediate insulitis development.

may additionally require pathogenic class I–restricted CD8 T cells (Fig. 3). This result indicates the human A1.9 TCR-expressing CD4 T cells in NOD-*cMHCI/II*$^{-/-}$-DQ8 background mice are functionally active. Insulitis levels can be quantitatively scored in NOD background mice (Ratiu et al. 2017). Thus, such an insulitis scoring system could be used to test, in NOD-*cMHCI/II*$^{-/-}$-DQ8-A1.9 mice, the ability of potential disease intervention approaches to attenuate the activity of CD4 T cells of pathological relevance to T1D patients.

Finally, in lieu of traditional transgenic mouse models, NOD mice expressing human TCRs can be generated in a high-throughput fashion using retrogene technologies (Jing et al. 2022). Briefly, donor mice provide a bone marrow source, which is then retrovirally transformed in culture. Following transformation, bone marrow cells are used to reconstitute an immune system in irradiated recipient mice. This technology has recently been used to generate NOD.HLA-DR4^{Tg}.*H2Ab1*$^{-/-}$.*Rag1*$^{-/-}$ mice expressing GAD reactive human TCRs (Jing et al. 2022). In this model, insulitis progression required DC priming with cognate antigen, indicating peripheral tolerance mechanisms were initially keeping these human TCR–expressing T cells in check. Time will tell whether this is an antigen/epitope-specific phenomenon, or a technical hurdle that will impact all human TCR retrogenics.

To the best of our knowledge, there has been no report of human B-cell receptor (BCR) retrogenic mice. At least two separate reports have indicated that developing B cells in murine BCR retrogenic mice in vivo fail to express surface Ig molecules (French et al. 1997; Packard et al. 2016), indicating that the retrogenic approach requires modifications to study BCRs. However, the creation of functional BCR retrogenic cells in vitro can be accomplished, allowing for posttransformation transfer into recipient mice. This has been done for the diabetogenic VH125 B cell (Packard et al. 2016). Chimeric VH125 B cells (human IgG1 heavy chain) were transformed with chimeric light chains (human κ) with differing affinities toward insulin in vitro. Resulting retrogenic B cells could then be studied in vivo following transfer into recipient mice (Packard et al. 2016). While this is a step in the right direction and allows researchers and clinicians to potentially study patient-derived BCRs in vivo, technological improvements are needed to bring BCR retrogenic technology up to the levels currently available for TCR retrogenics.

CONCLUDING REMARKS

Over the previous decades, a number of animal models have been developed for the study of T1D. However, while having their limitations, NOD mice and derivative strains have provided key resources for the greatest understanding of multiple aspects of T1D development. The NOD mouse has been criticized for only providing limited insights into clinically applicable T1D interventions. In this regard, it should be noted that multiple intervention approaches reported to provide early prodromal disease-stage T1D prevention effects in NOD mice could not be replicated by independent laboratories (Grant et al. 2013). These findings indicate the NOD strain itself cannot be blamed for falsely identifying possible clinically applicable T1D interventions. As discussed earlier, such an inability to replicate some previously reported means to inhibit T1D development in NOD mice could result from differing environmental factors at varying test sites such as the makeup of the intestinal microbiome. This further stresses the need for proper experimental replication within NOD as well as relevant humanized NOD strains to potentially improve clinical translatability. Additionally, known and unknown environmental and genetic interactions, genetic drift across various colonies, and colony management specificities, can influence T1D development rates in NOD mice. This calls for a standardization in reporting of genetic (formal strain designations, substrain origin, number of generations a colony has been separated from origin source) and environmental conditions (barrier status, diet, housing, and time-of-study microbiome/pathogen screening results) that may impact intervention efficacy. Researchers are encouraged to register new alleles, strains, and phenotypes with the Mouse Genome Informatics Database (www.informatics.jax.org), which can assist in formal nomenclature assignment.

The greatest value of NOD mice has been their use in research providing a greater understanding of the pathophysiological basis of T1D. This includes the identification of largely concordant targeted β-cell autoantigens in NOD mice and T1D patients. The NOD strain has also provided insights into the identification of various immune cell populations coordinately mediating T1D, and the basis for their development and faulty regulation. Such insights include the identification of genes contributing to T1D in both NOD mice and humans. In cases where T1D genes in the two species are not identical, studies in NOD mice have been useful in identifying common potentially targetable biochemical networks in which they may operate. The increasing use of various "humanized" NOD mouse models should further enhance the identification of potential targets for possible future

 Cite this article as *Cold Spring Harb Perspect Med* doi: 10.1101/cshperspect.a041587

clinically applicable disease intervention approaches. In conclusion, the areas of increased understanding of the pathophysiological basis of T1D enabled by NOD mouse studies continue to provide great value to the biomedical research community.

REFERENCES

Acevedo-Suarez CA, Hulbert C, Woodward EJ, Thomas JW. 2005. Uncoupling of anergy from developmental arrest in anti-insulin B cells supports the development of autoimmune diabetes. *J Immunol* **174:** 827–833. doi:10.4049/jimmunol.174.2.827

Acha-Orbea H, McDevitt HO. 1987. The first external domain of the nonobese diabetic mouse class II I-Aβ chain is unique. *Proc Natl Acad Sci* **84:** 2435–2439. doi:10.1073/pnas.84.8.2435

Akashi T, Nagafuchi S, Anzai K, Kondo S, Kitamura D, Wakana S, Ono J, Kikuchi M, Niho Y, Watanabe T. 1997. Direct evidence for the contribution of B cells to the progression of insulitis and the development of diabetes in non-obese diabetic mice. *Int Immunol* **9:** 1159–1164. doi:10.1093/intimm/9.8.1159

Amdare N, Purcell AW, DiLorenzo TP. 2021. Noncontiguous T cell epitopes in autoimmune diabetes: from mice to men and back again. *J Biol Chem* **297:** 100827. doi:10.1016/j.jbc.2021.100827

Arif S, Leete P, Nguyen V, Marks K, Nor NM, Estorninho M, Kronenberg-Versteeg D, Bingley PJ, Todd JA, Guy C, et al. 2014. Blood and islet phenotypes indicate immunological heterogeneity in type 1 diabetes. *Diabetes* **63:** 3835–3845. doi:10.2337/db14-0365

Armitage LH, Wallet MA, Mathews CE. 2021. Influence of PTPN22 allotypes on innate and adaptive immune function in health and disease. *Front Immunol* **12:** 636618. doi:10.3389/fimmu.2021.636618

Arribas-Layton D, Guyer P, Delong T, Dang M, Chow IT, Speake C, Greenbaum CJ, Kwok WW, Baker RL, Haskins K, et al. 2020. Hybrid insulin peptides are recognized by human T cells in the context of DRB1*04:01. *Diabetes* **69:** 1492–1502. doi:10.2337/db19-0620

Atkinson MA, Mirmira RG. 2023. The pathogenic "symphony" in type 1 diabetes: a disorder of the immune system, β cells, and exocrine pancreas. *Cell Metab* **35:** 1500–1518. doi:10.1016/j.cmet.2023.06.018

Azoury ME, Tarayrah M, Afonso G, Pais A, Colli ML, Maillard C, Lavaud C, Alexandre-Heymann L, Gonzalez-Duque S, Verdier Y, et al. 2020. Peptides derived from insulin granule proteins are targeted by $CD8^+$ T cells across MHC class I restrictions in humans and NOD mice. *Diabetes* **69:** 2678–2690. doi:10.2337/db20-0013

Babon JA, DeNicola ME, Blodgett DM, Crèvecoeur I, Buttrick TS, Maehr R, Bottino R, Naji A, Kaddis J, Elyaman W, et al. 2016. Analysis of self-antigen specificity of islet-infiltrating T cells from human donors with type 1 diabetes. *Nat Med* **22:** 1482–1487. doi:10.1038/nm.4203

Baekkeskov S, Aanstoot HJ, Christgau S, Reetz A, Solimena M, Cascalho M, Folli F, Richter-Olesen H, De Camilli P. 1990. Identification of the 64K autoantigen in insulin-dependent diabetes as the GABA-synthesizing enzyme glutamic acid decarboxylase. *Nature* **347:** 151–156. doi:10.1038/347151a0

Baker K, Rath T, Pyzik M, Blumberg RS. 2014. The role of FcRn in antigen presentation. *Front Immunol* **5:** 408. doi:10.3389/fimmu.2014.00408

Bluestone JA, Buckner JH, Fitch M, Gitelman SE, Gupta S, Hellerstein MK, Herold KC, Lares A, Lee MR, Li K, et al. 2015. Type 1 diabetes immunotherapy using polyclonal regulatory T cells. *Sci Transl Med* **7:** a189. doi:10.1126/scitranslmed.aad4134

Bonifacio E, Ziegler AG. 2010. Advances in the prediction and natural history of type 1 diabetes. *Endocrinol Metab Clin North Am* **39:** 513–525. doi:10.1016/j.ecl.2010.05.007

Bonifacio E, Atkinson MA, Eisenbarth GS, Serreze DV, Kay TW, Lee-Chan E, Singh B. 2001. International workshop on lessons from animal models for human type 1 diabetes: identification of insulin but not glutamic acid decarboxylase or IA-2 as specific autoantigens of humoral autoimmunity in nonobese diabetic mice. *Diabetes* **50:** 2451–2458. doi:10.2337/diabetes.50.11.2451

Bortell R, Yang C. 2012. The BB rat as a model of human type 1 diabetes. *Methods Mol Biol* **933:** 31–44. doi:10.1007/978-1-62703-068-7_3

Bouazi JD, Yanaba K, Venturi GM, Wang Y, Tisch RM, Poe JC, Tedder TF. 2007. Therapeutic B cell depletion impairs adaptive and autoreactive $CD4^+$ T cell activation in mice. *Proc Natl Acad Sci* **104:** 20878–20883. doi:10.1073/pnas.0709205105

Brodnicki TC, McClive P, Couper S, Morahan G. 2000. Localization of Idd11 using NOD congenic mouse strains: elimination of Slc9a1 as a candidate gene. *Immunogenetics* **51:** 37–41. doi:10.1007/s002510050006

Burrows MP, Volchkov P, Kobayashi KS, Chervonsky AV. 2015. Microbiota regulates type 1 diabetes through Toll-like receptors. *Proc Natl Acad Sci* **112:** 9973–9977. doi:10.1073/pnas.1508740112

Campbell-Thompson M, Fu A, Kaddis JS, Wasserfall C, Schatz DA, Pugliese A, Atkinson MA. 2016. Insulitis and β-cell mass in the natural history of type 1 diabetes. *Diabetes* **65:** 719–731. doi:10.2337/db15-0779

Carrero JA, McCarthy DP, Ferris ST, Wan X, Hu H, Zinselmeyer BH, Vomund AN, Unanue ER. 2017. Resident macrophages of pancreatic islets have a seminal role in the initiation of autoimmune diabetes of NOD mice. *Proc Natl Acad Sci* **114:** E10418–E10427. doi:10.1073/pnas.1713543114

Carrillo J, Puertas MC, Alba A, Ampudia RM, Pastor X, Planas R, Riutort N, Alonso N, Pujol-Borrell R, Santamaria P, et al. 2005. Islet-infiltrating B-cells in nonobese diabetic mice predominantly target nervous system elements. *Diabetes* **54:** 69–77. doi:10.2337/diabetes.54.1.69

Carrillo J, Puertas MC, Planas R, Pastor X, Alba A, Stratmann T, Pujol-Borrell R, Ampudia RM, Vives-Pi M, Verdaguer J. 2008. Anti-peripherin B lymphocytes are positively selected during diabetogenesis. *Mol Immunol* **45:** 3152–3162. doi:10.1016/j.molimm.2008.03.003

Chatenoud L. 2019. A future for CD3 antibodies in immunotherapy of type 1 diabetes. *Diabetologia* **62:** 578–581. doi:10.1007/s00125-018-4808-7

Chaudhury C, Mehnaz S, Robinson JM, Hayton WL, Pearl DK, Roopenian DC, Anderson CL. 2003. The major histocompatibility complex-related Fc receptor for IgG (FcRn) binds albumin and prolongs its lifespan. *J Exp Med* **197:** 315–322. doi:10.1084/jem.20021829

Chen YG, Choisy-Rossi CM, Holl TM, Chapman HD, Besra GS, Porcelli SA, Shaffer DJ, Roopenian D, Wilson SB, Serreze DV. 2005. Activated NKT cells inhibit autoimmune diabetes through tolerogenic recruitment of dendritic cells to pancreatic lymph nodes. *J Immunol* **174:** 1196–1204. doi:10.4049/jimmunol.174.3.1196

Chen YG, Mathews CE, Driver JP. 2018. The role of NOD mice in type 1 diabetes research: lessons from the past and recommendations for the future. *Front Endocrinol (Lausanne)* **9:** 51. doi:10.3389/fendo.2018.00051

Chilton PM, Rezzoug F, Fugier-Vivier I, Weeter LA, Xu H, Huang Y, Ray MB, Ildstad ST. 2004. Flt3-ligand treatment prevents diabetes in NOD mice. *Diabetes* **53:** 1995–2002. doi:10.2337/diabetes.53.8.1995

Choisy-Rossi CM, Holl TM, Pierce MA, Chapman HD, Serreze DV. 2004. Enhanced pathogenicity of diabetogenic T cells escaping a non-MHC gene-controlled near death experience. *J Immunol* **173:** 3791–3800. doi:10.4049/jimmunol.173.6.3791

Christianson SW, Shultz LD, Leiter EH. 1993. Adoptive transfer of diabetes into immunodeficient NOD-*scid/scid* mice: relative contributions of CD4$^+$ and CD8$^+$ T lymphocytes from diabetic versus prediabetic NOD. NON-*Thy* 1^a donors. *Diabetes* **42:** 44–55. doi:10.2337/diab.42.1.44

Chuprin J, Buettner H, Seedhom MO, Greiner DL, Keck JG, Ishikawa F, Shultz LD, Brehm MA. 2023. Humanized mouse models for immuno-oncology research. *Nat Rev Clin Oncol* **20:** 192–206. doi:10.1038/s41571-022-00721-2

Ciecko AE, Foda B, Barr JY, Ramanathan S, Atkinson MA, Serreze DV, Geurts AM, Lieberman SM, Chen YG. 2019. Interleukin-27 is essential for type 1 diabetes development and Sjögren syndrome-like inflammation. *Cell Rep* **29:** 3073–3086.e5. doi:10.1016/j.celrep.2019.11.010

Claessens LA, Wesselius J, van Lummel M, Laban S, Mulder F, Mul D, Nikolic T, Aanstoot HJ, Koeleman BPC, Roep BO. 2020. Clinical and genetic correlates of islet-autoimmune signatures in juvenile-onset type 1 diabetes. *Diabetologia* **63:** 351–361. doi:10.1007/s00125-019-05032-3

Coppieters KT, Dotta F, Amirian N, Campbell PD, Kay TW, Atkinson MA, Roep BO, von Herrath MG. 2012. Demonstration of islet-autoreactive CD8 T cells in insulitic lesions from recent onset and long-term type 1 diabetes patients. *J Exp Med* **209:** 51–60. doi:10.1084/jem.20111187

Cornall RJ, Prins JB, Todd J, Pressey A, DeLarto N, Wicker L, Peterson L. 1991. Type 1 diabetes in mice is linked to the interleukin-1 receptor and Lsh/Ity/Bcg genes on chromosome 1. *Nature* **353:** 262–265. doi:10.1038/353262a0

Crawford F, Stadinski B, Jin N, Michels A, Nakayama M, Pratt P, Marrack P, Eisenbarth G, Kappler JW. 2011. Specificity and detection of insulin-reactive CD4$^+$ T cells in type 1 diabetes in the nonobese diabetic (NOD) mouse. *Proc Natl Acad Sci* **108:** 16729–16734. doi:10.1073/pnas.1113954108

Delong T, Wiles TA, Baker RL, Bradley B, Barbour G, Reisdorph R, Armstrong M, Powell RL, Reisdorph N, Kumar N, et al. 2016. Pathogenic CD4 T cells in type 1 diabetes recognize epitopes formed by peptide fusion. *Science* **351:** 711–714. doi:10.1126/science.aad2791

Diana J, Simoni Y, Furio L, Beaudoin L, Agerberth B, Barrat F, Lehuen A. 2013. Crosstalk between neutrophils, B-1a cells and plasmacytoid dendritic cells initiates autoimmune diabetes. *Nat Med* **19:** 65–73. doi:10.1038/nm.3042

DiLorenzo TP, Graser RT, Ono T, Christianson GJ, Chapman HD, Roopenian DC, Nathenson SG, Serreze DV. 1998. Major histocompatibility complex class I–restricted T cells are required for all but the end stages of diabetes development in nonobese diabetic mice and use a prevalent T cell receptor α chain gene rearrangement. *Proc Natl Acad Sci* **95:** 12538–12543. doi:10.1073/pnas.95.21.12538

Doran TM, Morimoto J, Simanski S, Koesema EJ, Clark LF, Pels K, Stoops SL, Pugliese A, Skyler JS, Kodadek T. 2016. Discovery of phosphorylated peripherin as a major humoral autoantigen in type 1 diabetes mellitus. *Cell Chem Biol* **23:** 618–628. doi:10.1016/j.chembiol.2016.04.006

Driver JP, Scheuplein F, Chen YG, Grier AE, Wilson SB, Serreze DV. 2010. Invariant natural killer T-cell control of type 1 diabetes: a dendritic cell genetic decision of a silver bullet or Russian roulette. *Diabetes* **59:** 423–432. doi:10.2337/db09-1116

Driver JP, Serreze DV, Chen YG. 2011. Mouse models for the study of autoimmune type 1 diabetes: a NOD to similarities and differences to human disease. *Semin Immunopathol* **33:** 67–87. doi:10.1007/s00281-010-0204-1

Driver JP, Chen YG, Mathews CE. 2012. Comparative genetics: synergizing human and NOD mouse studies for identifying genetic causation of type 1 diabetes. *Rev Diabet Stud* **9:** 169–187. doi:10.1900/RDS.2012.9.169

Dwyer JR, Racine JJ, Chapman HD, Quinlan A, Presa M, Stafford GA, Schmitz I, Serreze DV. 2022. Nfkbid overexpression in nonobese diabetic mice elicits complete type 1 diabetes resistance in part associated with enhanced thymic deletion of pathogenic CD8 T cells and increased numbers and activity of regulatory T cells. *J Immunol* **209:** 227–237. doi:10.4049/jimmunol.2100558

Ebstein F, Textoris-Taube K, Keller C, Golnik R, Vigneron N, Van den Eynde BJ, Schuler-Thurner B, Schadendorf D, Lorenz FK, Uckert W, et al. 2016. Proteasomes generate spliced epitopes by two different mechanisms and as efficiently as non-spliced epitopes. *Sci Rep* **6:** 24032. doi:10.1038/srep24032

Fahey JR, Lyons BL, Olekszak HL, Mourino AJ, Ratiu JJ, Racine JJ, Chapman HD, Serreze DV, Baker DL, Hendrix NK. 2017. Antibiotic-associated manipulation of the gut microbiota and phenotypic restoration in NOD mice. *Comp Med* **67:** 335–343.

Fasolino M, Goldman N, Wang W, Cattau B, Zhou Y, Petrovic J, Link VM, Cote A, Chandra A, Silverman M, et al. 2020. Genetic variation in type 1 diabetes reconfigures the 3D chromatin organization of T cells and alters gene expression. *Immunity* **52:** 257–274.e11. doi:10.1016/j.immuni.2020.01.003

Ferreira LMR, Muller YD, Bluestone JA, Tang Q. 2019. Next-generation regulatory T cell therapy. *Nat Rev Drug Discov* **18:** 749–769. doi:10.1038/s41573-019-0041-4

Ferris ST, Liu T, Chen J, Ohara RA, Ou F, Wu R, Kim S, Murphy TL, Murphy KM. 2023. WDFY4 deficiency in NOD mice ameliorates autoimmune diabetes and insulitis. *Proc Natl Acad Sci* **120:** e2219956120. doi:10.1073/pnas.2219956120

Feuerer M, Shen Y, Littman DR, Benoist C, Mathis D. 2009. How punctual ablation of regulatory T cells unleashes an autoimmune lesion within the pancreatic islets. *Immunity* **31:** 654–664. doi:10.1016/j.immuni.2009.08.023

Fiorina P, Vergani A, Dada S, Jurewicz M, Wong M, Law K, Wu E, Tian Z, Abdi R, Guleria I, et al. 2008. Targeting CD22 reprograms B-cells and reverses autoimmune diabetes. *Diabetes* **57:** 3013–3024. doi:10.2337/db08-0420

Forsberg MH, Foda B, Serreze DV, Chen YG. 2019. Combined congenic mapping and nuclease-based gene targeting for studying allele-specific effects of Tnfrsf9 within the Idd9.3 autoimmune diabetes locus. *Sci Rep* **9:** 4316. doi:10.1038/s41598-019-40898-8

Foulis AK. 1996. The pathology of the endocrine pancreas in type 1 (insulin-dependent) diabetes mellitus. *APMIS* **104:** 161–167. doi:10.1111/j.1699-0463.1996.tb00702.x

Fraser HI, Howlett S, Clark J, Rainbow DB, Stanford SM, Wu DJ, Hsieh YW, Maine CJ, Christensen M, Kuchroo V, et al. 2015. *Ptpn22* and *Cd2* variations are associated with altered protein expression and susceptibility to type 1 diabetes in nonobese diabetic mice. *J Immunol* **195:** 4841–4852. doi:10.4049/jimmunol.1402654

French MB, Allison J, Cram DS, Thomas HE, Dempsey-Collier M, Silva A, Georgiou HM, Kay TW, Harrison LC, Lew AM. 1997. Transgenic expression of mouse proinsulin II prevents diabetes in non-obese diabetic mice. *Diabetes* **46:** 34–39. doi:10.2337/diab.46.1.34

Funsten MC, Yurkovetskiy LA, Kuznetsov A, Reiman D, Hansen CHF, Senter KI, Lee J, Ratiu J, Dahal-Koirala S, Antonopoulos DA, et al. 2023. Microbiota-dependent proteolysis of gluten subverts diet-mediated protection against type 1 diabetes. *Cell Host Microbe* **31:** 213–227.e9. doi:10.1016/j.chom.2022.12.009

Furman BL. 2021. Streptozotocin-induced diabetic models in mice and rats. *Curr Protoc* **1:** e78. doi:10.1002/0471141755.ph0547s70

Garabatos N, Alvarez R, Carrillo J, Carrascal J, Izquierdo C, Chapman HD, Presa M, Mora C, Serreze DV, Verdaguer J, et al. 2014. In vivo detection of peripherin-specific autoreactive B cells during type 1 diabetes pathogenesis. *J Immunol* **192:** 3080–3090. doi:10.4049/jimmunol.1301053

Garchon HJ, Bendossa P, Eloy L, Bach JF. 1991. Identification and mapping to chromosome 1 of a susceptibility locus for periinsulitis in non-obese diabetic mice. *Nature* **353:** 260–262. doi:10.1038/353260a0

Gerling IC, Friedman H, Greiner DL, Shultz LD, Leiter EH. 1994. Multiple low-dose streptozocin-induced diabetes in NOD-*scid/scid* mice in the absence of functional lymphocytes. *Diabetes* **43:** 433–440. doi:10.2337/diab.43.3.433

Gerold KD, Zheng P, Rainbow DB, Zernecke A, Wicker LS, Kissler S. 2011. The soluble CTLA-4 splice variant protects from type 1 diabetes and potentiates regulatory T-cell function. *Diabetes* **60:** 1955–1963. doi:10.2337/db11-0130

Ghosh S, Palmer SM, Rodrigues NR, Cordell HJ, Hearne CM, Cornall RJ, Prins JB, McShane P, Lathrop GM, Peterson LB, et al. 1993. Polygenic control of autoimmune diabetes in nonobese diabetic mice. *Nat Genet* **4:** 404–409. doi:10.1038/ng0893-404

Gonzalez-Duque S, Azoury ME, Colli ML, Afonso G, Turatsinze JV, Nigi L, Lalanne AI, Sebastiani G, Carre A, Pinto S, et al. 2018. Conventional and neo-antigenic peptides presented by β cells are targeted by circulating naïve CD8$^+$ T cells in type 1 diabetic and healthy donors. *Cell Metab* **28:** 946–960.e6. doi:10.1016/j.cmet.2018.07.007

Grant CW, Moran-Paul CM, Duclos SK, Guberski DL, Arreaza-Rubin G, Spain LM. 2013. Testing agents for prevention or reversal of type 1 diabetes in rodents. *PLoS ONE* **8:** e72989. doi:10.1371/journal.pone.0072989

Grant SFA, Wells AD, Rich SS. 2020. Next steps in the identification of gene targets for type 1 diabetes. *Diabetologia* **63:** 2260–2269. doi:10.1007/s00125-020-05248-8

Grinberg-Bleyer Y, Caron R, Seeley JJ, De Silva NS, Schindler CW, Hayden MS, Klein U, Ghosh S. 2018. The alternative NF-κB pathway in regulatory T cell homeostasis and suppressive function. *J Immunol* **200:** 2362–2371. doi:10.4049/jimmunol.1800042

Hamilton-Williams EE, Serreze DV, Charlton B, Johnson EA, Marron MP, Müllbacher A, Slattery RM. 2001. Transgenic rescue implicates β_2-microglobulin as a diabetes susceptibility gene in nonobese diabetic (NOD) mice. *Proc Natl Acad Sci* **98:** 11533–11538. doi:10.1073/pnas.191383798

Hamilton-Williams EE, Rainbow DB, Cheung J, Christensen M, Lyons PA, Peterson LB, Steward CA, Sherman LA, Wicker LS. 2013. Fine mapping of type 1 diabetes regions Idd9.1 and Idd9.2 reveals genetic complexity. *Mamm Genome* **24:** 358–375. doi:10.1007/s00335-013-9466-y

Hammond KJ, Pellicci DG, Poulton LD, Naidenko OV, Scalzo AA, Baxter AG, Godfrey DI. 2001. CD1d-restricted NKT cells: an interstrain comparison. *J Immunol* **167:** 1164–1173. doi:10.4049/jimmunol.167.3.1164

Harrison MM, Jenkins BV, O'Connor-Giles KM, Wildonger J. 2014. A CRISPR view of development. *Genes Dev* **28:** 1859–1872. doi:10.1101/gad.248252.114

Hattori M, Yamato E, Itoh N, Senpuku H, Fujisawa T, Yoshino M, Fukuda M, Matsumoto E, Toyonaga T, Nakagawa I, et al. 1999. Homologous recombination of the MHC class I K region defines new MHC-linked diabetogenic susceptibility gene(s) in nonobese diabetic mice. *J Immunol* **163:** 1721–1724. doi:10.4049/jimmunol.163.4.1721

Hill NJ, Lyons PA, Armitage N, Todd JA, Wicker LS, Peterson LB. 2000. The NOD *Idd5* locus controls insulitis and diabetes and overlaps the orthologous CTLA4/IDDM12 and NRAMP1 loci in humans. *Diabetes* **49:** 1744–1747. doi:10.2337/diabetes.49.10.1744

Hollis-Moffatt JE, Hook SM, Merriman TR. 2005. Colocalization of mouse autoimmune diabetes loci *Idd21.1* and *Idd21.2* with *IDDM6* (human) and *Iddm3* (rat). *Diabetes* **54:** 2820–2825. doi:10.2337/diabetes.54.9.2820

Howson JM, Stevens H, Smyth DJ, Walker NM, Chandler KA, Bingley PJ, Todd JA. 2011. Evidence that HLA class I and II associations with type 1 diabetes, autoantibodies to GAD and autoantibodies to IA-2, are distinct. *Diabetes* **60:** 2635–2644. doi:10.2337/db11-0131

Hu CY, Rodriguez-Pinto D, Du W, Ahuja A, Henegariu O, Wong FS, Shlomchik MJ, Wen L. 2007. Treatment with CD20-specific antibody prevents and reverses autoimmune diabetes in mice. *J Clin Invest* **117:** 3857–3867. doi:10.1172/JCI32405

Huang Y, Fugier-Vivier IJ, Miller T, Elliott MJ, Xu H, Bozulic LD, Chilton PM, Ildstad ST. 2008. Plasmacytoid precursor dendritic cells from NOD mice exhibit impaired function:

are they a component of diabetes pathogenesis? *Diabetes* **57:** 2360–2370. doi:10.2337/db08-0356

Hulbert C, Riseili B, Rojas M, Thomas JW. 2001. B cell specificity contributes to the outcome of diabetes in nonobese diabetic mice. *J Immunol* **167:** 5535–5538. doi:10.4049/jimmunol.167.10.5535

Hunter K, Rainbow D, Plagnol V, Todd JA, Peterson LB, Wicker LS. 2007. Interactions between *Idd5.1/Ctla4* and other type 1 diabetes genes. *J Immunol* **179:** 8341–8349. doi:10.4049/jimmunol.179.12.8341

Hutchings P, Rosen H, O'Reilly L, Gordon S, Cooke A. 1990. Transfer of diabetes in mice prevented by blockade of adhesion-promoting receptor on macrophages. *Nature* **348:** 639–642. doi:10.1038/348639a0

International Multiple Sclerosis Genetics Consortium (IMS GC). 2009. The expanding genetic overlap between multiple sclerosis and type I diabetes. *Genes Immun* **10:** 11–14. doi:10.1038/gene.2008.83

Jarchum I, Nichol L, Trucco M, Santamaria P, DiLorenzo TP. 2008. Identification of novel IGRP epitopes targeted in type 1 diabetes patients. *Clin Immunol* **127:** 359–365. doi:10.1016/j.clim.2008.01.015

Jarpe A, Hickman M, Anderson J, Winter W, Peck A. 1991. Flow cytometric enumeration of mononuclear cell populations infiltrating the islets of Langerhan in prediabetic NOD mice: development of a model of autoimmune insulitis for type I diabetes. *Reg Immunol* **3:** 305–317.

Jing Y, Kong Y, McGinty J, Blahnik-Fagan G, Lee T, Orozco-Figueroa S, Bettini ML, James EA, Bettini M. 2022. T-cell receptor/HLA humanized mice reveal reduced tolerance and increased immunogenicity of posttranslationally modified GAD65 epitope. *Diabetes* **71:** 1012–1022. doi:10.2337/db21-0993

Johnson EA, Silveira P, Chapman HD, Leiter EH, Serreze DV. 2001. Inhibition of autoimmune diabetes in nonobese diabetic mice by transgenic restoration of H2-E MHC class II expression: additive, but unequal, involvement of multiple APC subtypes. *J Immunol* **167:** 2404–2410. doi:10.4049/jimmunol.167.4.2404

Katz J, Benoist C, Mathis D. 1993. Major histocompatibility complex class I molecules are required for the development of insulitis in non-obese diabetic mice. *Eur J Immunol* **23:** 3358–3360. doi:10.1002/eji.1830231244

Kendall PL, Case JB, Sullivan AM, Holderness JS, Wells KS, Liu E, Thomas JW. 2013. Tolerant anti-insulin B cells are effective APCs. *J Immunol* **190:** 2519–2526. doi:10.4049/jimmunol.1202104

Kishimoto H, Sprent J. 2001. A defect in central tolerance in NOD mice. *Nat Immunol* **2:** 1025–1031. doi:10.1038/ni726

Kriegel MA, Sefik E, Hill JA, Wu HJ, Benoist C, Mathis D. 2011. Naturally transmitted segmented filamentous bacteria segregate with diabetes protection in nonobese diabetic mice. *Proc Natl Acad Sci* **108:** 11548–11553. doi:10.1073/pnas.1108924108

Krishnamurthy B, Dudek N, McKenzie MD, Purcell AW, Brooks AG, Gellert S, Colman PG, Harrison LC, Lew AM, Thomas HE, et al. 2006. Responses against islet antigens in NOD mice are prevented by tolerance to proinsulin but not IGRP. *J Clin Invest* **116:** 3258–3265. doi:10.1172/JCI29602

LaFace DW, Peck AB. 1989. Reciprocal allogeneic bone marrow transplantation between NOD mice and diabetes-nonsusceptible mice associated with transfer and prevention of autoimmune diabetes. *Diabetes* **38:** 894–901. doi:10.2337/diab.38.7.894

Larsen MT, Kuhlmann M, Hvam ML, Howard KA. 2016. Albumin-based drug delivery: harnessing nature to cure disease. *Mol Cell Ther* **4:** 3. doi:10.1186/s40591-016-0048-8

Leeth CM, Racine J, Chapman HD, Arpa B, Carrillo J, Carrascal J, Wang Q, Ratiu J, Egia-Mendikute L, Rosell-Mases E, et al. 2016. B-lymphocytes expressing an immunoglobulin specificity recognizing the pancreatic β-cell autoantigen peripherin are potent contributors to type 1 diabetes development in NOD mice. *Diabetes* **65:** 1977–1987. doi:10.2337/db15-1606

Leiter EH. 1998. NOD mice and related strains: origins, husbandry, and biology introduction. In *NOD mice and related strains: research applications in diabetes, AIDS, cancer and other diseases* (ed. Leiter E, Atkinson M), pp. 1–36. RG Landis, Austin, TX.

Lin X, Hamilton-Williams EE, Rainbow DB, Hunter KM, Dai YD, Cheung J, Peterson LB, Wicker LS, Sherman LA. 2013. Genetic interactions among *Idd3*, *Idd5.1*, *Idd5.2*, and *Idd5.3* protective loci in the nonobese diabetic mouse model of type 1 diabetes. *J Immunol* **190:** 3109–3120. doi:10.4049/jimmunol.1203422

Lord CJ, Denny P, Hill NJ, Lyons PA, Peterson LB, Podolin PL, Renjilian RJ, Wicker LS, Todd JA. 1995. Mapping the diabetes polygene Idd3 on mouse chromosome 3 by use of novel congenic strains. *Autoimmunity* **6:** 563–570. doi:10.1007/BF00352359

Lowe CE, Cooper JD, Brusko T, Walker NM, Smyth DJ, Bailey R, Bourget K, Plagnol V, Field S, Atkinson M, et al. 2007. Large-scale genetic fine mapping and genotype-phenotype associations implicate polymorphism in the IL2RA region in type 1 diabetes. *Nat Genet* **39:** 1074–1082. doi:10.1038/ng2102

Lund T, O'Reilly L, Hutchings P, Kanagawa O, Simpson E, Gravely R, Chandler P, Dyson J, Picard JK, Edwards A, et al. 1990. Prevention of insulin-dependent diabetes mellitus in non-obese diabetic mice by transgenes encoding modified I-A β-chain or normal I-E α-chain. *Nature* **345:** 727–729. doi:10.1038/345727a0

Lyons PA, Hancock WW, Denny P, Lord CJ, Hill NJ, Armitage N, Siegmund T, Todd JA, Phillipps MS, Hess JF, et al. 2000. The NOD *Idd9* genetic interval influences the pathogenicity of insulitis and contains molecular variants of *Cd30*, *Tnfr2*, and *Cd137*. *Immunity* **13:** 107–115. doi:10.1016/s1074-7613(00)00012-1

Magnuson AM, Thurber GM, Kohler RH, Weissleder R, Mathis D, Benoist C. 2015. Population dynamics of islet-infiltrating cells in autoimmune diabetes. *Proc Natl Acad Sci* **112:** 1511–1516. doi:10.1073/pnas.1423769112

Makino S, Kunimoto K, Muraoka Y, Mizushima Y, Katagiri K, Tochino Y. 1980. Breeding of a non-obese, diabetic strain of mice. *Exp Anim* **29:** 1–13. doi:10.1538/expanim1978.29.1_1

Makino S, Hayashi Y, Muraoka Y, Tochino Y. 1985. Establishment of the nonobese-diabetic (NOD) mouse. In *Current topics in clinical and experimental aspects of diabetes mellitus* (ed. Sakamoto N, Min HK, Baba S), pp. 25–32. Elsevier, Amsterdam.

Mallone R, Martinuzzi E, Blancou P, Novelli G, Afonzo G, Dolz M, Bruno G, Chaillous L, Chatenoud L, Bach JM, et al. 2007. $CD8^+$ T cell responses identify β-cell autoimmunity in human type 1 diabetes. *Diabetes* **56:** 613–621. doi:10.2337/db06-1419

Mariño E, Batten M, Groom J, Walters S, Liuwantara D, Mackay F, Grey ST. 2008. Marginal-zone B-cells of non-obese diabetic mice expand with diabetes onset, invade the pancreatic lymph nodes, and present autoantigen to diabetogenic T-cells. *Diabetes* **57:** 395–404. doi:10.2337/db07-0589

Mariño E, Tan B, Binge L, Mackay CR, Grey ST. 2012. B-cell cross-presentation of autologous antigen precipitates diabetes. *Diabetes* **61:** 2893–2905. doi:10.2337/db12-0006

Mariño E, Walters SN, Villanueva JE, Richards JL, Mackay CR, Grey ST. 2014. BAFF regulates activation of self-reactive T cells through B-cell dependent mechanisms and mediates protection in NOD mice. *Eur J Immunol* **44:** 983–993. doi:10.1002/eji.201344186

Markle JG, Frank DN, Mortin-Toth S, Robertson CE, Feazel LM, Rolle-Kampczyk U, von Bergen M, McCoy KD, Macpherson AJ, Danska JS. 2013. Sex differences in the gut microbiome drive hormone-dependent regulation of autoimmunity. *Science* **339:** 1084–1088. doi:10.1126/science.1233521

Mattner J, Mohammed JP, Fusakio ME, Giessler C, Hackstein CP, Opoka R, Wrage M, Schey R, Clark J, Fraser HI, et al. 2019. Genetic and functional data identifying Cd101 as a type 1 diabetes (T1D) susceptibility gene in nonobese diabetic (NOD) mice. *PLoS Genet* **15:** e1008178. doi:10.1371/journal.pgen.1008178

McGuire HM, Vogelzang A, Hill N, Flodström-Tullberg M, Sprent J, King C. 2009. Loss of parity between IL-2 and IL-21 in the NOD Idd3 locus. *Proc Natl Acad Sci* **106:** 19438–19443. doi:10.1073/pnas.0903561106

Michaux A, Larrieu P, Stroobant V, Fonteneau JF, Jotereau F, Van den Eynde BJ, Moreau-Aubry A, Vigneron N. 2014. A spliced antigenic peptide comprising a single spliced amino acid is produced in the proteasome by reverse splicing of a longer peptide fragment followed by trimming. *J Immunol* **192:** 1962–1971. doi:10.4049/jimmunol.1302032

Miyazaki T, Uno M, Uehira M, Kikutani H, Kishimoto T, Kimoto M, Nishimoto H, Miyazaki J, Yamamura K. 1990. Direct evidence for the contribution of the unique $I\text{-}A^{nod}$ to the development of insulitis in non-obese diabetic mice. *Nature* **345:** 722–724. doi:10.1038/345722a0

Mohan JF, Levisetti MG, Calderon B, Herzog JW, Petzold SJ, Unanue ER. 2010. Unique autoreactive T cells recognize insulin peptides generated within the islets of Langerhans in autoimmune diabetes. *Nat Immunol* **11:** 350–354. doi:10.1038/ni.1850

Mohan JF, Petzold SJ, Unanue ER. 2011. Register shifting of an insulin peptide-MHC complex allows diabetogenic T cells to escape thymic deletion. *J Exp Med* **208:** 2375–2383. doi:10.1084/jem.20111502

Morin J, Boitard C, Vallois D, Avner P, Rogner UC. 2006. Mapping of the murine type 1 diabetes locus Idd20 by genetic interaction. *Mamm Genome* **17:** 1105–1112. doi:10.1007/s00335-006-0076-9

Mullen Y. 2017. Development of the nonobese diabetic mouse and contribution of animal models for understanding type 1 diabetes. *Pancreas* **46:** 455–466. doi:10.1097/MPA.0000000000000828

Nagy N, Kaber G, Kratochvil MJ, Kuipers HF, Ruppert SM, Yadava K, Yang J, Heilshorn SC, Long SA, Pugliese A, et al. 2021. Weekly injection of IL-2 using an injectable hydrogel reduces autoimmune diabetes incidence in NOD mice. *Diabetologia* **64:** 152–158. doi:10.1007/s00125-020-05314-1

Nakayama T, Abiru N, Moriyama H, Babaya N, Liu E, Miao D, Yu L, Wegmann DR, Hutton JC, Elliott JF, et al. 2005. Prime role for an insulin epitope in the development of type 1 diabetes in NOD mice. *Nature* **435:** 220–223. doi:10.1038/nature03523

Nakayama M, McDaniel K, Fitzgerald-Miller L, Kiekhaefer C, Snell-Bergeon JK, Davidson HW, Rewers M, Yu L, Gottlieb P, Kappler JW, et al. 2015. Regulatory vs. inflammatory cytokine T-cell responses to mutated insulin peptides in healthy and type 1 diabetic subjects. *Proc Natl Acad Sci* **112:** 4429–4434. doi:10.1073/pnas.1502967112

Nejentsev S, Howson JMM, Walker NM, Szeszko J, Field SF, Stevens HE, Reynolds P, Hardy M, King E, Masters J, et al. 2007. Localization of type 1 diabetes susceptibility to the MHC class I genes *HLA-B* and *HLA-A*. *Nature* **450:** 887–892. doi:10.1038/nature06406

Nikolic T, Geutskens SB, van Rooijen N, Drexhage HA, Leenen PJ. 2005. Dendritic cells and macrophages are essential for the retention of lymphocytes in (peri)-insulitis of the nonobese diabetic mouse: a phagocyte depletion study. *Lab Invest* **85:** 487–501. doi:10.1038/labinvest.3700238

Noble JA, Valdes AM, Varney MD, Carlson JA, Moonsamy P, Fear AL, Lane JA, Lavant E, Rappner R, Louey A, et al. 2010. HLA class I and genetic susceptibility to type 1 diabetes: results from the Type 1 Diabetes Genetics Consortium. *Diabetes* **59:** 2972–2979. doi:10.2337/db10-0699

Noorchashm H, Noorchashm N, Kern J, Rostami SY, Barker CF, Naji A. 1997. B-cells are required for the initiation of insulitis and sialitis in nonobese diabetic mice. *Diabetes* **46:** 941–946. doi:10.2337/diab.46.6.941

Ouyang Q, Standifer NE, Qin H, Gottlieb PA, Verchere CB, Nepom GT, Tan R, Panagiotopoulos C. 2006. Recognition of HLA-class I–restricted β-cell epitopes in type 1 diabetes. *Diabetes* **55:** 3068–3074. doi:10.2337/db06-0065

Packard TA, Smith MJ, Conrad FJ, Johnson SA, Getahun A, Lindsay RS, Hinman RM, Friedman RS, Thomas JW, Cambier JC. 2016. B cell receptor affinity for insulin dictates autoantigen acquisition and B cell functionality in autoimmune diabetes. *J Clin Med* **5:** 98. doi:10.3390/jcm5110098

Pascolo S, Bervas N, Ure JM, Smith AG, Lemonnier FA, Pérarnau B. 1997. HLA-A2.1-restricted education and cytolytic activity of $CD8^+$ T lymphocytes from β2 microglobulin (β2m) HLA-A2.1 monochain transgenic $H\text{-}2D^b$ β2m double knockout mice. *J Exp Med* **185:** 2043–2051. doi:10.1084/jem.185.12.2043

Pathiraja V, Kuehlich JP, Campbell PD, Krishnamurthy B, Loudovaris T, Coates PT, Brodnicki TC, O'Connell PJ, Kedzierska K, Rodda C, et al. 2015. Proinsulin-specific, HLA-DQ8, and HLA-DQ8-transdimer-restricted $CD4^+$ T cells infiltrate islets in type 1 diabetes. *Diabetes* **64:** 172–182. doi:10.2337/db14-0858

Perdigoto AL, Chatenoud L, Bluestone JA, Herold KC. 2016. Inducing and administering Tregs to treat human disease. *Front Immunol* **6:** 654. doi:10.3389/fimmu.2015.00654

Pescovitz MD, Greenbaum CJ, Krause-Steinrauf H, Becker DJ, Gitelman SE, Goland R, Gottlieb PA, Marks JB, McGee PF, Moran AM, et al. 2009. Rituximab, B-lymphocyte depletion, and preservation of β-cell function. *N Engl J Med* **361:** 2143–2152. doi:10.1056/NEJMoa0904452

Pinske GGM, Tysma OHM, Bergen CAM, Kester MGD, Ossendorp F, van Veelen PA, Keymeulen B, Pipeleers D, Drijfhout JW, Roep BO. 2005. Autoreactive CD8 T cells associated with β cell destruction in type 1 diabetes. *Proc Natl Acad Sci* **102:** 18425–18430. doi:10.1073/pnas.0508621102

Podolin PL, Denny P, Lord CJ, Hill NJ, Todd JA, Peterson LB, Wicker LS, Lyons PA. 1997. Congenic mapping of the insulin-dependent diabetes (*Idd*) gene, *Idd10*, localizes two genes mediating the *Idd10* effect and eliminates the candidate *Fcgr1*. *J Immunol* **159:** 1835–1843. doi:10.4049/jimmunol.159.4.1835

Pomerleau DP, Bagley RJ, Serreze DV, Mathews CE, Leiter EH. 2005. Major histocompatibility complex-linked diabetes susceptibility in NOD mice: subcongenic analysis localizes a component of *Idd16* at the *H2-D* end of the diabetogenic $H2^{g7}$ complex. *Diabetes* **54:** 1603–1606. doi:10.2337/diabetes.54.5.1603

Puertas MC, Carrillo J, Pastor X, Ampudia RM, Planas R, Alba A, Bruno R, Pujol-Borrell R, Estanyol JM, Vives-Pi M, et al. 2007. Peripherin is a relevant neuroendocrine autoantigen recognized by islet-infiltrating B lymphocytes. *J Immunol* **178:** 6533–6539. doi:10.4049/jimmunol.178.10.6533

Purcell AW, Sechi S, DiLorenzo TP. 2019. The evolving landscape of autoantigen discovery and characterization in type 1 diabetes. *Diabetes* **68:** 879–886. doi:10.2337/dbi18-0066

Quinn WJ III, Noorchashm N, Crowley JE, Reed AJ, Noorchashm H, Naji A, Cancro MP. 2006. Cutting edge: impaired transitional B cell production and selection in the nonobese diabetic mouse. *J Immunol* **176:** 7159–7164. doi:10.4049/jimmunol.176.12.7159

Racine JJ, Stewart I, Ratiu J, Christianson G, Lowell E, Helm K, Allocco J, Maser RS, Chen YG, Lutz CM, et al. 2018. Improved murine MHC-deficient HLA transgenic NOD mouse models for type 1 diabetes therapy development. *Diabetes* **67:** 923–935. doi:10.2337/db17-1467

Racine JJ, Chapman HD, Doty R, Cairns BM, Hines TJ, Tadenev ALD, Anderson LC, Green T, Dyer ME, Wotton JM, et al. 2020. T cells from NOD-*Perig* mice target both pancreatic and neuronal tissue. *J Immunol* **205:** 2026–2038. doi:10.4049/jimmunol.2000114

Racine JJ, Misherghi A, Dwyer JR, Maser R, Forte E, Bedard O, Sattler S, Pugliese A, Landry L, Elso C, et al. 2023. HLA-DQ8 supports development of insulitis mediated by insulin-reactive human TCR-transgenic T cells in nonobese diabetic mice. *J Immunol* **211:** 1792–1805. doi:10.4049/jimmunol.2300303

Rainbow DB, Moule C, Fraser HI, Clark J, Howlett SK, Burren O, Christensen M, Moody V, Steward CA, Mohammed JP, et al. 2011. Evidence that *Cd101* is an autoimmune diabetes gene in nonobese diabetic mice. *J Immunol* **187:** 325–336. doi:10.4049/jimmunol.1003523

Ramos EL, Dayan CM, Chatenoud L, Sumnik Z, Simmons KM, Szypowska A, Gitelman SE, Knecht LA, Niemoeller E, Tian W, et al. 2023. Teplizumab and β-cell function in newly diagnosed type 1 diabetes. *N Engl J Med* **389:** 2151–2161. doi:10.1056/NEJMoa2308743

Ratiu JJ, Racine JJ, Hasham MG, Wang Q, Branca JA, Chapman HD, Zhu J, Donghia N, Philip V, Schott WH, et al. 2017. Genetic and small molecule disruption of the AID/RAD51 axis similarly protects nonobese diabetic mice from type 1 diabetes through expansion of regulatory B lymphocytes. *J Immunol* **198:** 4255–4267. doi:10.4049/jimmunol.1700024

Richardson SJ, Rodriguez-Calvo T, Gerling IC, Mathews CE, Kaddis JS, Russell MA, Zeissler M, Leete P, Krogvold L, Dahl-Jørgensen K, et al. 2016. Islet cell hyperexpression of HLA class I antigens: a defining feature in type 1 diabetes. *Diabetologia* **59:** 2448–2458. doi:10.1007/s00125-016-4067-4

Rodrigues NR, Cornall RJ, Chandler P, Simpson E, Wicker LS, Peterson LB, Todd JA. 1994. Mapping of an insulin-dependent diabetes locus, Idd9, in NOD mice to chromosome 4. *Mamm Genome* **5:** 167–170. doi:10.1007/BF00352349

Rogner UC, Boitard C, Morin J, Melanitou E, Avner P. 2001. Three loci on mouse chromosome 6 influence onset and final incidence of type I diabetes in NOD.C3H congenic strains. *Genomics* **74:** 163–171. doi:10.1006/geno.2001.6508

Roopenian DC, Akilesh S. 2007. FcRn: the neonatal Fc receptor comes of age. *Nat Rev Immunol* **7:** 715–725. doi:10.1038/nri2155

Roopenian DC, Christianson GJ, Sproule TJ, Brown AC, Akilesh S, Jung N, Petkova S, Avanessian L, Choi EY, Shaffer DJ, et al. 2003. The MHC class I-like IgG receptor controls perinatal IgG transport, IgG homeostasis, and fate of IgG-Fc-coupled drugs. *J Immunol* **170:** 3528–3533. doi:10.4049/jimmunol.170.7.3528

Rowe PA, Campbell-Thompson ML, Schatz DA, Atkinson MA. 2011. The pancreas in human type 1 diabetes. *Semin Immunopathol* **33:** 29–43. doi:10.1007/s00281-010-0208-x

Saxena V, Ondr JK, Magnusen AF, Munn DH, Katz JD. 2007. The countervailing actions of myeloid and plasmacytoid dendritic cells control autoimmune diabetes in the nonobese diabetic mouse. *J Immunol* **179:** 5041–5053. doi:10.4049/jimmunol.179.8.5041

Schloss J, Ali R, Racine JJ, Chapman HD, Serreze DV, DiLorenzo TP. 2018. HLA-B*39:06 efficiently mediates type 1 diabetes in a mouse model incorporating reduced thymic insulin expression. *J Immunol* **200:** 3353–3363. doi:10.4049/jimmunol.1701652

Schott-Ohly P, Lgssiar A, Partke HJ, Hassan M, Friesen N, Gleichmann H. 2004. Prevention of spontaneous and experimentally induced diabetes in mice with zinc sulfate-enriched drinking water is associated with activation and reduction of NF-κB and AP-1 in islets, respectively. *Exp Biol Med (Maywood)* **229:** 1177–1185. doi:10.1177/153537020422901113

Serreze DV, Leiter EH, Worthen SM, Shultz LD. 1988. NOD marrow stem cells adoptively transfer diabetes to resistant (NOD × NON)F1 mice. *Diabetes* **37:** 252–255. doi:10.2337/diab.37.2.252

Serreze DV, Leiter EH, Christianson GJ, Greiner D, Roopenian DC. 1994a. MHC class I deficient NOD-*B2m*^{null} mice are diabetes and insulitis resistant. *Diabetes* **43:** 505–509. doi:10.2337/diab.43.3.505

Serreze DV, Prochazka M, Reifsnyder PC, Bridgett M, Leiter EH. 1994b. Use of recombinant congenic and congenic strains of NOD mice to identify a new insulin-dependent diabetes resistance gene. *J Exp Med* **180:** 1553–1558. doi:10.1084/jem.180.4.1553

Serreze DV, Chapman HD, Varnum DS, Hanson MS, Reifsnyder PC, Richard SD, Fleming SA, Leiter EH, Shultz LD. 1996. B lymphocytes are essential for the initiation of T cell-mediated autoimmune diabetes: analysis of a new "speed congenic" stock of NOD.Igμ null mice. *J Exp Med* **184:** 2049–2053. doi:10.1084/jem.184.5.2049

Serreze DV, Chapman HD, Varnum DS, Gerling I, Leiter EH, Shultz LD. 1997. Initiation of autoimmune diabetes in NOD/Lt mice is MHC class I-dependent. *J Immunol* **158:** 3978–3986. doi:10.4049/jimmunol.158.8.3978

Serreze DV, Fleming SA, Chapman HD, Richard SD, Leiter EH, Tisch RM. 1998. B lymphocytes are critical antigen-presenting cells for the initiation of T cell-mediated autoimmune diabetes in nonobese diabetic mice. *J Immunol* **161:** 3912–3918. doi:10.4049/jimmunol.161.8.3912

Serreze DV, Holl TM, Marron MP, Graser RT, Johnson EA, Choisy-Rossi C, Slattery RM, Lieberman SM, DiLorenzo TP. 2004. MHC class II molecules play a role in the selection of autoreactive class I-restricted CD8 T cells that are essential contributors to type 1 diabetes development in nonobese diabetic mice. *J Immunol* **172:** 871–879. doi:10.4049/jimmunol.172.2.871

Serreze DV, Choisy-Rossi CM, Grier A, Holl TM, Chapman HD, Gahagan JR, Osborne MA, Zhang W, King BL, Brown A, et al. 2008. Through regulation of TCR expression levels, an *Idd7* region gene(s) interactively contributes to the impaired thymic deletion of autoreactive diabetogenic CD8$^+$ T cells in nonobese diabetic mice. *J Immunol* **180:** 3250–3259. doi:10.4049/jimmunol.180.5.3250

Serreze DV, Chapman HD, Niens M, Dunn R, Kehry MR, Driver JP, Haller MJ, Wasserfall C, Atkinson M. 2011. Loss of intra-islet CD20 expression may complicate efficacy of B-cell-directed type 1 diabetes therapies. *Diabetes* **60:** 2914–2921. doi:10.2337/db11-0705

Shapiro MR, Yeh WI, Longfield JR, Gallagher J, Infante CM, Wellford S, Posgai AL, Atkinson MA, Campbell-Thompson M, Lieberman SM, et al. 2020. CD226 deletion reduces type 1 diabetes in the NOD mouse by impairing thymocyte development and peripheral T cell activation. *Front Immunol* **11:** 2180. doi:10.3389/fimmu.2020.02180

Shapiro MR, Thirawatananond P, Peters L, Sharp RC, Ogundare S, Posgai AL, Perry DJ, Brusko TM. 2021. De-coding genetic risk variants in type 1 diabetes. *Immunol Cell Biol* **99:** 496–508. doi:10.1111/imcb.12438

Shultz LD, Brehm MA, Bavari S, Greiner DL. 2012. Humanized mice as a preclinical tool for infectious disease and biomedical research. *Ann NY Acad Sci* **1245:** 50–54. doi:10.1111/j.1749-6632.2011.06310.x

Silveira P, Johnson EA, Chapman HD, Tisch RM, Serreze DV. 2002. The preferential ability of B lymphocytes to act as diabetogenic APC in NOD mice depends on expression of self-antigen-specific immunoglobulin receptors. *Eur J Immunol* **32:** 3657–3666. doi:10.1002/1521-4141(200212)32:12<3657::AID-IMMU3657>3.0.CO;2-E

Silveira PA, Dombrowsky J, Johnson E, Chapman HD, Nemazee D, Serreze DV. 2004. B cell selection defects underlie the development of diabetogenic APCs in nonobese diabetic mice. *J Immunol* **172:** 5086–5094. doi:10.4049/jimmunol.172.8.5086

Simecek P, Churchill GA, Yang H, Rowe LB, Herberg L, Serreze DV, Leiter EH. 2015. Genetic analysis of substrain divergence in non-obese diabetic (NOD) mice. *G3 (Bethesda)* **5:** 771–775. doi:10.1534/g3.115.017046

Singer SM, Tisch R, Yang XD, McDevitt HO. 1993. An Ab^d transgene prevents diabetes in nonobese diabetic mice by inducing regulatory T cells. *Proc Natl Acad Sci* **90:** 9566–9570. doi:10.1073/pnas.90.20.9566

Sittig LJ, Jeong C, Tixier E, Davis J, Barrios-Camacho CM, Palmer AA. 2014. Phenotypic instability between the near isogenic substrains BALB/cJ and BALB/cByJ. *Mamm Genome* **25:** 564–572. doi:10.1007/s00335-014-9531-1

Slattery RM, Kjer-Nielsen L, Allison J, Charlton B, Mandel T, Miller JFAP. 1990. Prevention of diabetes in non-obese diabetic I-A^k transgenic mice. *Nature* **345:** 724–726. doi:10.1038/345724a0

So M, Speake C, Steck AK, Lundgren M, Colman PG, Palmer JP, Herold KC, Greenbaum CJ. 2021. Advances in type 1 diabetes prediction using islet autoantibodies: beyond a simple count. *Endocr Rev* **42:** 584–604. doi:10.1210/endrev/bnab013

Stadinski BD, Cleveland SB, Brehm MA, Greiner DL, Huseby PG, Huseby ES. 2023. I-A^{g7} β56/57 polymorphisms regulate non-cognate negative selection to CD4$^+$ T cell orchestrators of type 1 diabetes. *Nat Immunol* **24:** 652–663. doi:10.1038/s41590-023-01441-0

Tahvili S, Törngren M, Holmberg D, Leanderson T, Ivars F. 2018. Paquinimod prevents development of diabetes in the non-obese diabetic (NOD) mouse. *PLoS ONE* **13:** e0196598. doi:10.1371/journal.pone.0196598

Takaki T, Marron MP, Mathews CE, Guttman ST, Bottino R, Trucco M, DiLorenzo TP, Serreze DV. 2006. HLA-A*0201-restricted T cells from humanized NOD mice recognize autoantigens of potential clinical relevance to type 1 diabetes. *J Immunol* **176:** 3257–3265. doi:10.4049/jimmunol.176.5.3257

Tang Q, Bluestone JA. 2008. The Foxp3$^+$ regulatory T cell: a jack of all trades, master of regulation. *Nat Immunol* **9:** 239–244. doi:10.1038/ni1572

Tekula S, Khurana A, Anchi P, Godugu C. 2018. Withaferin-A attenuates multiple low doses of Streptozotocin (MLD-STZ) induced type 1 diabetes. *Biomed Pharmacother* **106:** 1428–1440. doi:10.1016/j.biopha.2018.07.090

Tettey P, Simpson S Jr, Taylor BV, van der Mei IA. 2015. The co-occurrence of multiple sclerosis and type 1 diabetes: shared aetiologic features and clinical implication for MS aetiology. *J Neurol Sci* **348:** 126–131. doi:10.1016/j.jns.2014.11.019

Thirawatananond P, Brown ME, Sachs LK, Arnoletti JM, Yeh WI, Posgai AL, Shapiro MR, Chen YG, Brusko TM. 2023. Treg-specific CD226 deletion reduces diabetes incidence in NOD mice by improving regulatory T-cell stability. *Diabetes* **72:** 1629–1640. doi:10.2337/db23-0307

Todd JA, Acha-Orbea H, Bell JI, Chao N, Fronek Z, Jacob CO, McDermott M, Sinha AA, Timmerman L, Steinman L, et al. 1988. A molecular basis for MHC class II-associated autoimmunity. *Science* **240:** 1003–1009. doi:10.1126/science.3368786

Todd JA, Aitman TJ, Cornall RJ, Ghosh S, Hall JRS, Hearne CM, Knight AM, Love JM, McAleer MA, Prins JB, et al. 1991. Genetic analysis of autoimmune type 1 diabetes mellitus in mice. *Nature* **351:** 542–547. doi:10.1038/351542a0

Todd JA, Walker NM, Cooper JD, Smyth DJ, Downes K, Plagnol V, Bailey R, Nejentsev S, Field SF, Payne F, et al. 2007. Robust associations of four new chromosome regions from genome-wide analyses of type 1 diabetes. *Nat Genet* **39:** 857–864. doi:10.1038/ng2068

Trudeau JD, Kelly-Smith C, Verchere CB, Elliott JF, Dutz JP, Finegood DT, Santamaria P, Tan R. 2003. Prediction of spontaneous autoimmune diabetes in NOD mice by quantification of autoreactive T cells in blood. *J Clin Invest* **111:** 217–223. doi:10.1172/JCI16409

Unger WW, Pinkse GG, Mulder-van der Kracht S, van der Slik AR, Kester MG, Ossendorp F, Drijfhout JW, Serreze DV, Roep BO. 2007. Human clonal CD8 autoreactivity to an IGRP islet epitope shared between mice and men. *Ann NY Acad Sci* **1103:** 192–195. doi:10.1196/annals.1394.024

Unger WW, Pearson T, Abreu JR, Laban S, van der Slik AR, der Kracht SM, Kester MG, Serreze DV, Shultz LD, Griffioen M, et al. 2012. Islet-specific CTL cloned from a type 1 diabetes patient cause β-cell destruction after engraftment into HLA-A2 transgenic NOD/scid/IL2RG null mice. *PLoS ONE* **7:** e49213. doi:10.1371/journal.pone.0049213

Valdes AM, Erlich HA, Noble JA. 2005. Human leukocyte antigen class I B and C loci contribute to type 1 diabetes (T1D) susceptibility and age at T1D onset. *Hum Immunol* **66:** 301–313. doi:10.1016/j.humimm.2004.12.001

Van Belle TL, Taylor P, von Herrath MG. 2009. Mouse models for type 1 diabetes. *Drug Discov Today Dis Models* **6:** 41–45. doi:10.1016/j.ddmod.2009.03.008

Van Belle TL, Juntti T, Liao J, von Herrath MG. 2010. Pre-existing autoimmunity determines type 1 diabetes outcome after Flt3-ligand treatment. *J Autoimmun* **34:** 445–452. doi:10.1016/j.jaut.2009.11.010

Vigneron N, Stroobant V, Ferrari V, Abi Habib J, Van den Eynde BJ. 2019. Production of spliced peptides by the proteasome. *Mol Immunol* **113:** 93–102. doi:10.1016/j.molimm.2018.03.030

von Boehmer H, Melchers F. 2010. Checkpoints in lymphocyte development and autoimmune disease. *Nat Immunol* **11:** 14–20. doi:10.1038/ni.1794

Wakeland EK. 2014. Hunting autoimmune disease genes in NOD: early steps on a long road to somewhere important (hopefully). *J Immunol* **193:** 3–6. doi:10.4049/jimmunol.1401200

Wallet MA, Flores RR, Wang Y, Yi Z, Kroger CJ, Mathews CE, Earp HS, Matsushima G, Wang B, Tisch R. 2009. MerTK regulates thymic selection of autoreactive T cells. *Proc Natl Acad Sci* **106:** 4810–4815. doi:10.1073/pnas.0900683106

Wan X, Zinselmeyer BH, Zakharov PN, Vomund AN, Taniguchi R, Santambrogio L, Anderson MS, Lichti CF, Unanue ER. 2018. Pancreatic islets communicate with lymphoid tissues via exocytosis of insulin peptides. *Nature* **560:** 107–111. doi:10.1038/s41586-018-0341-6

Wang CJ, Schmidt EM, Attridge K, Kenefeck R, Wardzinski L, Chamberlain JL, Soulier A, Clough LE, Manzotti CN, Narendran P, et al. 2011. Immune regulation by CTLA-4-relevance to autoimmune diabetes in a transgenic mouse model. *Diabetes Metab Res Rev* **27:** 946–950. doi:10.1002/dmrr.1277

Wang N, Elso CM, Mackin L, Mannering SI, Strugnell RA, Wijburg OL, Brodnicki TC. 2014. Congenic mice reveal genetic epistasis and overlapping disease loci for autoimmune diabetes and listeriosis. *Immunogenetics* **66:** 501–506. doi:10.1007/s00251-014-0782-5

Wang Q, Racine JJ, Ratiu JJ, Wang S, Ettinger R, Wasserfall C, Atkinson MA, Serreze DV. 2017. Transient BAFF blockade inhibits type 1 diabetes development in nonobese diabetic mice by enriching immunoregulatory B lymphocytes sensitive to deletion by anti-CD20 cotherapy. *J Immunol* **199:** 3757–3770. doi:10.4049/jimmunol.1700822

Wenzlau JM, DiLisio JE, Barbour G, Dang M, Hohenstein AC, Nakayama M, Delong T, Baker RL, Haskins K. 2022. Insulin B-chain hybrid peptides are agonists for T cells reactive to insulin B:9-23 in autoimmune diabetes. *Front Immunol* **13:** 926650. doi:10.3389/fimmu.2022.926650

Wesley JD, Sather BD, Perdue NR, Ziegler SF, Campbell DJ. 2010. Cellular requirements for diabetes induction in DO11.10xRIPmOVA mice. *J Immunol* **185:** 4760–4768. doi:10.4049/jimmunol.1000820

Wicker LS, Miller BJ, Mullen Y. 1986. Transfer of autoimmune diabetes mellitus with T cells from nonobese diabetic mice. *Transplant Proc* **XVIII:** 809–811.

Wicker LS, Miller BJ, Chai A, Terada M, Mullen Y. 1988. Expression of genetically determined diabetes and insulitis in the nonobese diabetic (NOD) mouse at the level of bone marrow-derived cells. Transfer of diabetes and insulitis to nondiabetic (NOD × B10)F1 mice with bone marrow cells from NOD mice. *J Exp Med* **167:** 1801–1810. doi:10.1084/jem.167.6.1801

Wicker LS, Leiter EH, Todd JA, Renjilian RJ, Peterson E, Fischer PA, Podolin PL, Zijlstra M, Jaenisch R, Peterson LB. 1994a. β2-Microglobulin-deficient NOD mice do not develop insulitis or diabetes. *Diabetes* **43:** 500–504. doi:10.2337/diab.43.3.500

Wicker LS, Todd JA, Prins JB, Podolin PL, Renjilian RJ, Peterson LB. 1994b. Resistance alleles at two non-major histocompatibility complex-linked insulin-dependent diabetes loci on chromosome 3, *Idd3* and *Idd10*, protect nonobese diabetic mice from diabetes. *J Exp Med* **180:** 1705–1713. doi:10.1084/jem.180.5.1705

Willcox A, Richardson SJ, Bone AJ, Foulis AK, Morgan NG. 2009. Analysis of islet inflammation in human type 1 diabetes. *Clin Exp Immunol* **155:** 173–181. doi:10.1111/j.1365-2249.2008.03860.x

Winer S, Astsaturov I, Cheung R, Gunaratnam L, Kubiak V, Cortez MA, Moscarello M, O'Connor PW, McKerlie C, Becker DJ, et al. 2001. Type I diabetes and multiple sclerosis patients target islet plus central nervous system autoantigens; nonimmunized nonobese diabetic mice can develop autoimmune encephalitis. *J Immunol* **166:** 2831–2841. doi:10.4049/jimmunol.166.4.2831

Winer S, Tsui H, Lau A, Li X, Cheung RK, Sampson A, Afifiyan F, Elford A, Jackowski G, Becker DJ, et al. 2003. Autoimmune islet destruction in spontaneous type 1 diabetes is not β-cell exclusive. *Nat Med* **9:** 198–205. doi:10.1038/nm818

Wong FS, Visintin I, Wen L, Granata J, Flavell R, Janeway CA. 1998. The role of lymphocyte subsets in accelerated diabetes in nonobese diabetic-rat insulin promoter-B7-1 (NOD-RIP-B7-1) mice. *J Exp Med* **187:** 1985–1993. doi:10.1084/jem.187.12.1985

Xie QY, Oh S, Wong A, Yau C, Herold KC, Danska JS. 2023. Immune responses to gut bacteria associated with time to diagnosis and clinical response to T cell-directed therapy for type 1 diabetes prevention. *Sci Transl Med* **15:** eadh0353. doi:10.1126/scitranslmed.adh0353

Xiu Y, Wong CP, Bouaziz JD, Hamaguchi Y, Wang Y, Pop SM, Tisch RM, Tedder TF. 2008. B lymphocyte depletion by CD20 monoclonal antibody prevents diabetes in nonobese diabetic mice despite isotype-specific differences in FcγR effector functions. *J Immunol* **180:** 2863–2875. doi:10.4049/jimmunol.180.5.2863

Yamanouchi J, Rainbow D, Serra P, Howlett S, Hunter K, Garner VE, Gonzalez-Munoz A, Clark J, Veijola R, Cubbon R, et al. 2007. Interleukin-2 gene variation impairs regulatory T cell function and causes autoimmunity. *Nat Genet* **39:** 329–337. doi:10.1038/ng1958

Yang J, Chow IT, Sosinowski T, Torres-Chinn N, Greenbaum CJ, James EA, Kappler JW, Davidson HW, Kwok WW. 2014. Autoreactive T cells specific for insulin B:11-23 recognize a low-affinity peptide register in human subjects with autoimmune diabetes. *Proc Natl Acad Sci* **111:** 14840–14845. doi:10.1073/pnas.1416864111

Ye C, Clements SA, Gu W, Geurts AM, Mathews CE, Serreze DV, Chen YG, Driver JP. 2023. Deletion of $V\beta3^{+}CD4^{+}$ T cells by endogenous mouse mammary tumor virus 3 prevents type 1 diabetes induction by autoreactive $CD8^{+}$ T cells. *Proc Natl Acad Sci* **120:** e2312039120. doi:10.1073/pnas.2312039120

Yurkovetskiy L, Burrows M, Khan AA, Graham L, Volchkov P, Becker L, Antonopoulos D, Umesaki Y, Chervonsky AV. 2013. Gender bias in autoimmunity is influenced by microbiota. *Immunity* **39:** 400–412. doi:10.1016/j.immuni.2013.08.013

Zekavat G, Rostami SY, Badkerhanian A, Parsons RF, Koeberlein B, Yu M, Ward CD, Migone TS, Yu L, Eisenbarth GS, et al. 2008. In vivo BLyS/BAFF neutralization ameliorates islet-directed autoimmunity in nonobese diabetic mice. *J Immunol* **181:** 8133–8144. doi:10.4049/jimmunol.181.11.8133

Zipris D, Lien E, Nair A, Xie JX, Greiner DL, Mordes JP, Rossini AA. 2007. TLR9-signaling pathways are involved in Kilham rat virus-induced autoimmune diabetes in the biobreeding diabetes-resistant rat. *J Immunol* **178:** 693–701. doi:10.4049/jimmunol.178.2.693

Cross Talk between β Cells and Immune Cells: What We Know, What We Think We Know, and What We Should Learn

Fatoumata Samassa,[1] Capucine Holtzmann,[1,2] and Roberto Mallone[1,3,4]

[1]Université Paris Cité, Institut Cochin, CNRS, INSERM, Cochin-Port-Royal, Bâtiment Cassini - 123, F-75014 Paris, France

[2]Ecole Normale Supérieure, F-69342 Lyon, France

[3]Assistance Publique Hôpitaux de Paris, Service de Diabétologie et Immunologie Clinique, Cochin Hospital, F-75014 Paris, France

[4]Indiana Biosciences Research Institute, Indianapolis, Indiana 46202, USA

Correspondence: roberto.mallone@inserm.fr

Type 1 diabetes (T1D) is a disease whose pathogenesis is driven by both immune dysregulation and β-cell dysfunction. While the specialized structure and function of β cells make them vulnerable to autoimmunity, several surface receptor/ligand pairs underlie the cross talk engaged with T lymphocytes and other immune subsets. The expression of these ligands on β cells is coordinately up-regulated by the exposure to interferons, notably the type I interferons that represent the signature cytokines since the early preclinical stages of T1D. Yet, their interaction with receptors expressed on T lymphocytes can favor either β-cell vulnerability or protection. Despite several knowledge gaps, this novel holistic view of autoimmunity that incorporates both immune and β-cell-derived pathogenic drivers is starting to translate into novel therapeutic strategies aimed at decreasing vulnerability and/or increasing these protective mechanisms. This review summarizes the current knowledge in this evolving field, the assumptions that are often taken for granted but lack formal evidence, and the blind spots in this landscape that may hide further therapeutic opportunities.

It is now widely recognized that type 1 diabetes (T1D) is a disease not only of autoimmunity, but also of β cells themselves (Mallone and Eizirik 2020; Carré et al. 2021). Moreover, work by us (Culina et al. 2018; Gonzalez-Duque et al. 2018; Azoury et al. 2020) and others (Wiedeman et al. 2020; Guyer et al. 2022) have highlighted the existence of a universal state of "benign" islet autoimmunity. This benign state is characterized by the presence of circulating islet-reactive $CD8^+$ and $CD4^+$ T cells in the blood of all individuals, irrespective of T1D status. These T cells display a largely naive-like phenotype and, upon in vitro differentiation, can give rise to cytotoxic $CD8^+$ T cells with a β-cell-lytic potency that is similar for T1D and healthy donors. $CD8^+$ T cells with the

Cite this article as *Cold Spring Harb Perspect Med* doi: 10.1101/cshperspect.a041604

same antigen reactivity are, however, found enriched in the pancreas of T1D donors, suggesting their preferential recruitment to the target organ in the disease setting. Simply said, we are all autoimmune, and the next question opened by this novel paradigm is to understand why we are not all diabetic. The mechanisms driving benign autoimmunity toward a progressive state are likely diverse, but a key role may be played by β cells and by their cross talk with pathogenic T cells. We will here review current knowledge in support of this possibility, highlight areas of uncertainty for future work, and discuss the implications for β-cell-protective therapies that are starting to offer novel treatment options.

THE BIOLOGY OF β CELLS MAKES THEM SUSCEPTIBLE TO AUTOIMMUNITY

Some specific anatomical and functional features of β cells render them ideal autoimmune targets (Mallone and Eizirik 2020). These features are shared by most endocrine cells and may explain why endocrinopathies rank high in the list of autoimmune diseases, in terms of prevalence and of breadth of organs involved.

First, β cells have very high biosynthetic rates for insulin, which need to constantly adapt to glycemic levels (e.g., increasing by more than 10-fold and to ~50% of total protein production at high glucose concentrations) (Schuit et al. 1988). This requirement imposes a high basal state of endoplasmic reticulum (ER) stress, which is usually maintained at physiological levels by the unfolded protein response but can be readily decompensated by additional stressors. This may also favor the role of insulin as a central autoantigen of T1D, as its high and modulable rates of biosynthesis favor mistranscription and mistranslation events that generate unstable byproducts. Such byproducts are a major source of antigenic peptide presentation via their degradation by the proteasome (Carré and Mallone 2021). The same may apply to the signature autoimmune target proteins of other endocrine cells (e.g., thyroglobulin in thyrocytes).

Second, β cells are endowed with a rich vascularization through which they secrete insulin in the bloodstream. This rich vascularization may also ease the egress of antigen-presenting cells phagocyting β-cell products toward pancreatic lymph nodes for the initial T-cell priming, and the subsequent homing of primed T cells to the islets.

Third, the release of insulin and its antigenic byproducts in the bloodstream and their uptake by distant antigen-presenting cells may further favor this initial T-cell priming (Wan et al. 2018; Unanue and Wan 2019). The same principle may apply to other granule proteins (e.g., secretogranin-5, urocortin-3, and proconvertase-2) (Gonzalez-Duque et al. 2018; Azoury et al. 2020), which are secreted with insulin and undergo the same intermediate processing in the ER and granules to generate their bioactive products (Carré and Mallone 2021). While these granule proteins are also expressed by α cells (see below), $CD8^+$ T cells recognizing them are as diabetogenic as those recognizing insulin upon transfer in immunodeficient NOD/*scid* mice (Azoury et al. 2020).

Collectively, these features make β cells alluring targets for autoimmunity.

WHY ONLY β CELLS AND NOT α CELLS?

Alpha cells and glucagon share many of the above features with β cells and insulin, yet they are not targeted by autoimmunity in T1D or any other autoimmune disease. This puzzling phenomenon has been recently reviewed (Eizirik et al. 2023). While no satisfactory explanation can be provided to date, two observations may offer hypotheses for future investigation. First, our recent immunopeptidomics work to identify the antigenic peptides displayed by HLA class I molecules (Carré et al. 2023) revealed that the top-ranking source protein for HLA-bound peptides retrieved from primary human islets is glucagon rather than insulin, suggesting that α cells can efficiently present peptides for T-cell recognition. Second, glucagon-reactive $CD8^+$ T cells are not present in the insulitis infiltrates (Anderson et al. 2021), suggesting that this exposure of HLA-bound glucagon peptides does not lead to efficient T-cell priming and/or homing to the islets.

Different hypotheses may explain these observations. One hypothesis points to the context of insulin versus glucagon release, as insulin is released together with high Zn^{2+} concentrations, which might provide an adjuvant-like signal favoring immunogenic T-cell responses upon uptake by antigen-presenting cells (Haase et al. 2008; Yu et al. 2011). Moreover, while the secretion of proinsulin (and its byproducts) is a well-established marker of β-cell stress that may favor T-cell priming at a distance, it is not known whether the same applies to proglucagon for α cells, which are less amenable to such stress. The leader sequence of insulin is also a rich epitope hotspot (Kronenberg-Versteeg et al. 2018), while that of glucagon seems less favorable in terms of HLA-binding motifs (Carré et al. 2023). Of further note, it is unknown whether neoantigens generated either at the pretranslational level (i.e., mRNA open reading frame and splice variants) or posttranslationally (i.e., biochemical modifications, hybrid glucagon peptides) can be generated by α cells.

A second hypothesis is that, contrary to insulin, the expression of glucagon-related peptides is not mainly restricted to α cells, and their expression in enteroendocrine L cells in the tolerogenic gut microenvironment may impose a physiological state of peripheral immune tolerance to glucagon. Moreover, central tolerance to glucagon may also be at play, as the *GCG* gene is expressed in mature human thymic medullary epithelial cells at higher levels than *INS* (median ± SD RPKM 8.9 ± 1.2 vs. 1.2 ± 0.9), according to published data sets (Carter et al. 2022).

A third hypothesis is that the presentation of glucagon and other α-cell antigens may not lead to autoimmunity because of an intrinsic resistance of α cells.

RECEPTOR/LIGAND PAIRS FAVORING THE T-CELL/β-CELL CROSS TALK

One major driver for the transition from benign to pathological islet autoimmunity may be the loss of immune ignorance toward β cells. Under physiological conditions, the visibility of β cells to $CD8^+$ T cells is limited, due to a weak expression of HLA class I molecules. While this is a common theme in multiple tissues, work by Moon and colleagues (2015) aligns with our description of a benign state of islet autoimmunity hardwired in the immune system, due to a marginal thymic deletion process (Culina et al. 2018). These authors highlighted how steady-state tolerance to β-cell antigens does not rely on T-cell deletion, but rather on immune ignorance.

Another common theme in several autoimmune diseases is the presence of an early type I interferon (IFN) signature (Szymczak et al. 2021). Type I IFNs (mainly IFN-α and IFN-β) are also the earliest cytokine signatures observed in individuals at risk for T1D (Ferreira et al. 2014; Kallionpää et al. 2014).

Surface HLA Class I

One of the main outcomes of this IFN exposure is the up-regulation of surface HLA class I molecules, resulting in an increased presentation of antigenic peptides (Gonzalez-Duque et al. 2018). This presentation is increased in terms of both peptide quantity and breadth and includes posttranslationally modified peptides presented only under IFN-stimulated conditions (Carré et al. 2023).

HLA class I up-regulation may thus break immune ignorance and lead to autoimmune priming. Our recent work (Carré et al. 2023) revealed another unexpected twist that may contribute to this loss of ignorance. While the resting β-cell peptidome was dominated by the presentation of HLA-A-restricted peptides, IFN-α skewed HLA class I up-regulation toward HLA-B allotypes, translating into a major increase in HLA-B-restricted peptides with different binding motifs and into an increased activation of HLA-B-restricted versus HLA-A-restricted $CD8^+$ T cells. We further observed that the long-described histopathological hallmark of HLA class I hyperexpression in the islets of T1D patients (Richardson et al. 2016) preferentially involves HLA-B, and that islet-infiltrating $CD8^+$ T cells from T1D donors can recognize HLA-B-restricted granule peptides. Thus, the inflammatory milieu of insulitis may skew the autoimmune response toward different epitopes presented by HLA-B, hence recruiting a distinct T-cell repertoire that remains largely unexplored and may be relevant to T1D pathogenesis. Indeed, very few HLA-B-restricted epitopes have been identified to date, as most studies have focused on the most prevalent HLA-A2 allotype (James et al. 2020). Although remaining unnoticed, this preferential HLA-B up-regulation can also be found in several previous publications comparing islets exposed or not to IFNs or retrieved from T1D versus nondiabetic organ donors (Russell et al. 2019; Chandra et al. 2022; Giusti et al. 2022; Szymczak et al. 2022; Elgamal et al. 2023), as well as tumor cells exposed to IFNs (Javitt et al. 2019). This finding is also relevant in view of the notions that HLA-B*39:06 is the strongest T1D-predisposing HLA class I allele (Nejentsev et al. 2007), and that HLA-B but not HLA-A matching improves both kidney and islet allograft survival (Thorogood et al. 1990; Lemos et al. 2023). This novel paradigm of preferential HLA-B up-regulation may also apply to other autoimmune and antitumor responses featuring type I IFN signatures.

Extracellular HLA Class I Forms

While HLA class I is typically retained on the cell surface for antigen presentation, extracellular forms also exist, either contained in extracellular vesicles (~44 kD) or as soluble isoforms (~34 kD) generated by metalloprotease cleavage (Demaria et al. 1999; Haynes et al. 2002) or by alternative mRNA splicing lacking exon 5 (~39 kD) (Krangel 1986). However, most studies do not provide a clear distinction between these different pathways. While this shedding process is physiological (Ritz et al. 2017), it is up-regulated in several autoimmune (Adamashvili et al. 1995, 2003) and cancer settings (Campoli and Ferrone 2008). While extracellular HLA class I molecules carry bound peptides (Ritz et al. 2017), it is unknown how this peptidome compares to that of surface HLA class I. Interestingly, however, HLA-B allotypes have also been found enriched in extracellular vesicles, along with their peptide ligands (Bauzá-Martinez et al. 2021). Similarly, soluble HLA class I has been reported to activate $CD8^+$ T cells through peptide transfer to surface HLA class I (Allard et al. 2014) or to induce their apoptosis (Zavazava and Krönke 1996; Puppo et al. 2000; Contini et al. 2003). Interestingly, the T1D susceptibility allele HLA-A24, which is associated with a rapid β-cell decline (Nakanishi et al. 1993), has been reported to yield higher levels of serum extracellular HLA class I (Zavazava et al. 1990; Adamashvili et al. 1996). It has also been reported that the decline of extracellular HLA is synchronous to that of β-cell function in T1D patients, and faster in HLA-$A24^+$ patients (Nakanishi et al. 1997). Extracellular HLA class I levels were abnormally elevated in T1D patients and in their nondiabetic relatives compared to controls and correlated with the presence of an HLA-A24 haplotype (Adamashvili et al. 1997). Whether soluble HLA class I molecules are also released by β cells is under investigation.

RECEPTOR/LIGAND PAIRS THAT MAY INHIBIT THE T-CELL/β-CELL CROSS TALK

While the role of HLA class I up-regulation in sensitizing β cells for autoimmune T-cell recognition and subsequent destruction is now well established, less is known about inhibitory pathways that may protect β cells, or at least attempt to do so. The pathways discussed below are not meant to provide a comprehensive list—many others are likely to exist but are either poorly documented in β cells or awaiting to be discovered. The same applies to receptor/ligand pairs favoring the T-cell/β-cell cross talk, and to the same or other inhibitory ligands acting in *trans* (e.g., expressed on antigen-presenting cells). A role for intracellular factors (e.g., the DNA methylation enzyme TET2 favoring β-cell killing) (Rui et al. 2021) and soluble mediators (e.g., protective growth/differentiation factor GDF15) (Nakayasu et al. 2020) expressed by β cells has also been documented, but is not discussed here.

PD-1/PD-L1

The most studied receptor/ligand pair involves PD-1, expressed on activated $CD8^+$ T cells and remaining high on exhausted T cells; and PD-L1, which is expressed on β cells and only marginally on α cells (Colli et al. 2018; Osum et al. 2018). Soluble PD-L1 isoforms generated by mRNA alternative splicing have also been described in cancer cells (Wang et al. 2021), but not in β cells. The up-regulation of both molecules is an inte-

 Cite this article as *Cold Spring Harb Perspect Med* doi: 10.1101/cshperspect.a041604

gral part of the T-cell/β-cell cross talk, as PD-L1 levels on β cells correlate with the extent of T-cell infiltration and likely reflect its up-regulation by IFN-γ produced by activated T cells, which concomitantly up-regulate PD-1. The PD-L1 pathway is critical in the maintenance of tolerance in NOD mice. It is regulated, at least in part, by 12/15-lipoxygenase (Piñeros et al. 2022), and restored following antigen-specific or anti-CD3 therapy (Fife et al. 2006). However, whether PD-L1 expression in β cells is a critical part of this mechanism is uncertain. In principle, PD-1 engagement by its ligands PD-L1 and, to a lesser extent, PD-L2, would be expected to inhibit the cytotoxic activity of $CD8^+$ T cells against β cells. However, direct evidence is lacking. In cancer patients, clinical antitumor responses to therapeutic PD-1 blockade correlate with tumor PD-L1 expression and $CD8^+$ T-cell infiltration (Herbst et al. 2014; Tumeh et al. 2014). While this has led to the speculation that PD-L1 may shield tumor cells from T-cell lysis, PD-L1 expression by other cells (e.g., myeloid cells) in the tumor microenvironment is also critical (Herbst et al. 2014). Indeed, it has been shown that the relative contributions of PD-L1 on tumor and nontumor cells are context-dependent (Juneja et al. 2017). The expression of PD-1 by stem-like $CD8^+$ T cells in draining lymph nodes, both in cancer patients and in the pancreatic lymph nodes of NOD mice (Gearty et al. 2022), may also represent a key operational site for this protective pathway (Samassa and Mallone 2022). This is in line with the notion that therapeutic PD-1 blockade in cancer patients also targets $PD\text{-}1^+$ stem-like $CD8^+$ T cells rather than their terminally differentiated/exhausted counterparts infiltrating the tumor (Im et al. 2016).

HLA-E

HLA-E is a nonclassical, nearly monomorphic HLA class I molecule, with only two dominant alleles described (HLA-E*01:01 and HLA-E*01:03) and a murine ortholog called Qa-1. Soluble HLA-E isoforms, mostly generated by cleavage of the cell surface isoforms by metalloproteases, have also been described in endothelial cells (Coupel et al. 2007), but not in β cells. Under physiological conditions, it presents a specific set of nonamer peptides derived from the leader sequence of HLA-A, -B, -C, and -G molecules (Braud et al. 1997). Under cell stress and infection conditions, this peptide repertoire extends to homologous peptides derived from stress (e.g., heat shock protein 60; HSP60) and microbial proteins (e.g., CMV UL40) (van Hall et al. 2010). Its interactions with NKG2/CD94 innate receptors on natural killer (NK) cells and a subset of $CD8^+$ T cells have been extensively studied (Gunturi et al. 2004), with a predominant inhibitory effect mediated by a higher affinity binding to the inhibitory NKG2A compared to the activating NKG2C isoform (Valés-Gómez et al. 1999).

Later studies documented the recognition of peptide/HLA-E complexes by α/β T-cell receptors (TCRs) expressed on $CD8^+$ T cells (Pietra et al. 2001, 2023; García et al. 2002). In murine models, the peptide presented drives the ensuing response of Qa-1-restricted $CD8^+$ T cells toward different outcomes. When pathogen-derived peptides are recognized, Qa-1-restricted $CD8^+$ T cells acquire cytotoxic properties. In contrast, self-derived peptides are recognized by a regulatory subset of Qa-1-restricted $CD8^+$ T cells with immunosuppressive properties (Kim and Cantor 2011; Kim et al. 2011). These regulatory $CD8^+$ T cells selectively eliminate activated, but not naive, $CD4^+$ T cells through recognition of peptide/Qa-1 complexes expressed by these cells and up-regulated upon activation, preventing experimental autoimmune encephalomyelitis (Jiang et al. 1998; Hu et al. 2004) and diabetes (Panoutsakopoulou et al. 2004). These immunosuppressive properties are dependent on the recognition of peptide/Qa-1 complexes by α/β TCRs rather than by the CD94/NKG2A receptors also expressed by these regulatory $CD8^+$ T cells. Indeed, C57BL/6 mice carrying a Qa-1 mutation disrupting CD8 coreceptor binding but preserving the CD94/NKG2A interaction develop antinuclear autoantibodies and a lupus-like syndrome due to a dysregulated activity of $Qa\text{-}1^{high}$ follicular T helper cells (Kim et al. 2011). Similarly, HLA-E-restricted regulatory $CD8^+$ T cells have been described in humans. In recent-onset T1D, this regulatory subset displays decreased suppression of autoreactive CD4$^+$ T cells in vitro, which can be restored by stimulation with dendritic cells loaded with an HLA-E-binding HSP60 leader sequence peptide (Jiang et al. 2010).

HLA-E overexpression is well-documented in cancer cells, but its potential role in immune escape is not settled. In renal cell carcinoma, HLA-E expression did not correlate with poor prognosis or with the extent of T-cell infiltration, but was inversely correlated with CD56$^+$ infiltration, possibly indicative of NK-cell inhibition (Seliger et al. 2016). In colorectal cancer, HLA-E expression was instead correlated with an unfavorable prognosis and with a higher CD8$^+$ infiltration (Bossard et al. 2012). A negative correlation with CD57$^+$ infiltration and in vitro inhibition of NK cytotoxicity has also been reported (Levy et al. 2008).

In T1D, residual insulin-containing islets of diabetic donors feature a hyperexpression of HLA-E, which is higher in α than in β cells (Lundberg et al. 2016; Colli et al. 2020). As for the well-documented hyperexpression of classical HLA class I molecules, this is instead not observed in insulin-deficient islets (i.e., lacking residual β cells). While histopathological and gene expression studies on pancreas tissues are very limited, functional studies are lacking altogether. Although it is postulated that this HLA-E hyperexpression may represent a defense mechanism for β cells, this hypothesis has not been formally tested outside the setting of alloimmune islet rejection (Parent et al. 2021). Our recent immunopeptidomics analysis of HLA-bound peptides presented by β cells (Carré et al. 2023) has also provided information about the peptides predicted to be HLA-E-restricted. Several potential ligands derived from β-cell-enriched proteins were identified, which may offer a starting point for more in-depth functional studies of HLA-E-restricted CD8$^+$ T cells that may be relevant to T1D pathogenesis.

Collectively, this literature from the cancer and autoimmunity fields exemplifies the debate surrounding the potential role of HLA-E in protecting target cells, including pancreatic β cells, and the uncertainty surrounding the relative role of NK versus T cells and of the CD94/NKG2A versus TCR recognition pathways.

Other Nonclassical HLA Class I Molecules

Two other nonclassical HLA class I molecules, namely, HLA-F (Richardson et al. 2016; Russell et al. 2019) and HLA-G (Cirulli et al. 2006), have also been found to be hyperexpressed in the islets of T1D donors, both at the RNA and protein level (Wyatt et al. 2019). They share with HLA-E a limited polymorphism and the same pattern of expression in the pancreas, namely, their localization in both β and α cells and their dependency on the presence of residual β cells, as they are only found (hyper)expressed in insulin-containing islets. Interestingly, while the usual expression of HLA-F and HLA-G is mostly cytoplasmic, surface expression is also observed in pancreatic endocrine cells (Cirulli et al. 2006; Richardson et al. 2016). Similar to HLA-E, a protective role has been postulated based on their reported inhibition of the activation of NK and other immune cells: through inhibitory immunoglobulin (Ig)-like transcript (ILT)2 and ILT4 receptors (Allan et al. 2002), killer Ig-like receptors (KIRs) (Goodridge et al. 2013), and leukocyte Ig-like receptor (LIR)1 (Dulberger et al. 2017) for HLA-F, and through ILT2/ILT4 (Allan et al. 2002), KIRs and CD160 (Wyatt et al. 2019) for HLA-G. Also in this case, however, this possibility has not been formally tested in the T1D setting. The receptor/ligand pairs that may favor β-cell vulnerability versus protection are summarized in Figure 1.

THERAPEUTIC HARNESSING OF β-CELL PROTECTION

The increased appreciation of a β-cell component in the pathogenesis of T1D (Mallone et al. 2022) has prompted the development of novel therapeutic strategies with agents that may decrease β-cell vulnerability. While such agents may eventually find their place for both T1D prevention at preclinical stages 1–2 and intervention at clinical stage 3, they have so far been tested only at stage 3.

Verapamil

One promising β-cell-protective agent is verapamil, a calcium channel blocker that inhibits thioredoxin-interacting protein (TXNIP, a media-

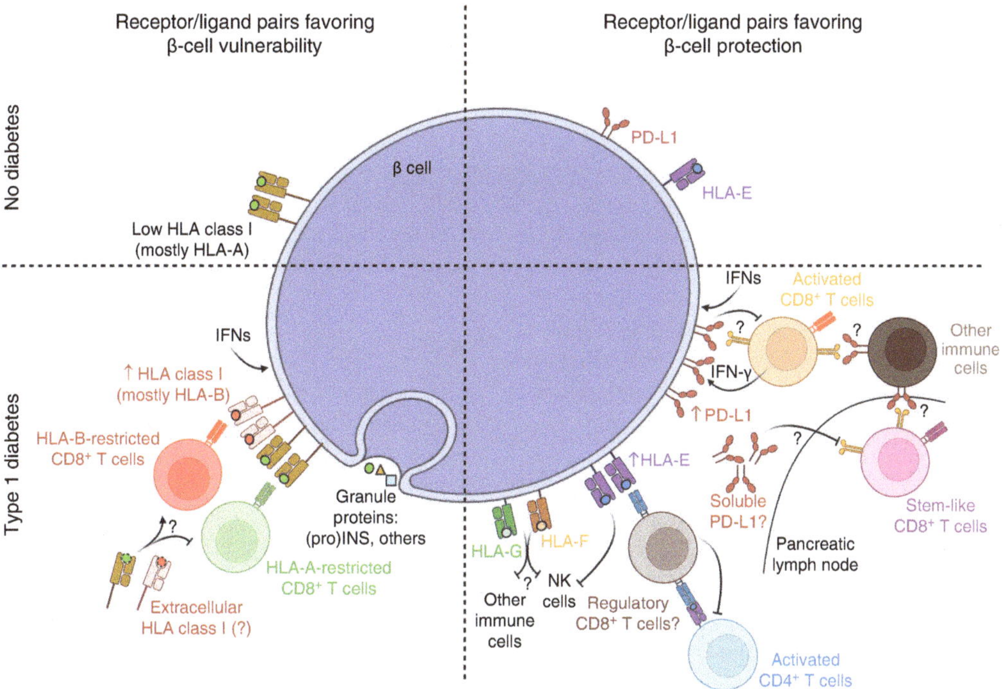

Figure 1. Receptor/ligand pairs that may favor β-cell vulnerability versus protection. See text for details. (Figure generated with BioRender, https://biorender.com.)

tor of oxidative stress). The C-peptide preservation reported in a pilot phase 2 trial (Ovalle et al. 2018) was recently confirmed in the larger CLVer trial on children and adolescents with new-onset T1D, who showed a 30% higher C-peptide level at 1 year when treated with verapamil compared to placebo, without significant side effects (Forlenza et al. 2023). The VER-A-T1D phase 2 trial (NCT04545151) is testing this treatment in adults. Further studies are needed to determine the optimal duration of treatment, with follow-up studies suggesting that the benefit is lost after drug discontinuation (Xu et al. 2022). Moreover, TXNIP is the most up-regulated gene in human islets exposed to high glucose (Shalev et al. 2002), and it induces β-cell apoptosis, acting in synergy with glucotoxicity (Chen et al. 2008). As such, verapamil treatment may also be relevant for type 2 diabetes (Wang et al. 2022). It is currently unknown whether it may also protect β cells from T-cell-mediated lysis, but the fact that glucotoxicity can sensitize β cells for killing by $CD8^+$ T cells recognizing the key T-cell epitope preproinsulin 15–24 (Skowera et al. 2008) suggests that this may be the case. Moreover, ancillary mechanistic studies documented a decreased expression of HLA-A/B/C, HLA-G, and HLA-DPA1/DRA in verapamil-treated human islets, and identified chromogranin A as a novel candidate circulating biomarker of β-cell stress inversely correlated with C-peptide levels (Xu et al. 2022). Clinical trials to test more potent TXNIP inhibitors that may improve clinical benefits are under consideration (Thielen et al. 2020).

Imatinib

Although C-peptide preservation was not maintained after treatment discontinuation, encouraging results were also obtained with the tyrosine kinase inhibitor imatinib, which has been shown to reduce insulin resistance and ER stress and to improve β-cell survival in the presence of various stressors, including autoimmunity (Gitelman et al. 2021). The safety profile was less favorable for this drug, with 38% of treated patients requiring a temporary dose reduction and 13% discontinuing treatment altogether due to side effects. Treatment in combination with other agents may allow lower dosing regimens.

Combination Therapies

Combination therapies with immunomodulatory and β-cell-protective agents are widely advocated to achieve synergistic effects by targeting distinct yet connected pathogenic mechanisms. This is similar and somehow specular to what has been obtained in the oncology field by combining immunotherapeutic agents to potentiate immune responses against tumor cells, and chemotherapeutic agents to decrease tumor burden and enhance its vulnerability. A first trial of this kind combining an anti-IL-21 blocking antibody with the GLP-1 receptor agonist liraglutide achieved superior C-peptide preservation at 1 year compared to placebo (von Herrath et al. 2021). Importantly, this benefit was lower than with either agent alone, suggesting the relevance of such combination strategies.

IFN Signaling Inhibitors

Another approach to achieve synergistic effects is to use agents, such as inhibitors of IFN signaling, that can block these critical signaling pathways in β cells in addition to blunting T-cell activation. One first promising example is provided by the BANDIT trial, which tested the oral drug baricitinib, a JAK1/2 inhibitor, in new-onset T1D children and adults (Waibel et al. 2023). No decline in C peptide was observed during the 48 weeks of treatment as compared to that of the placebo arm (48% comparative median increase for baricitinib vs. placebo), with nonsignificant yet reduced insulin doses and HbA1c levels. Adverse events were similar in the two treatment arms, with no serious adverse events. While loss of efficacy is to be expected after treatment discontinuation based on the experience with other autoimmune conditions, this favorable safety profile makes continuous treatment feasible. Besides their blunting of IFN signaling in β cells, JAK1/2 inhibitors have pleiotropic effects that may contribute to this clinical benefit, including reduced IFN-γ production and islet homing of T cells (through down-regulation of CXCL10 release by β cells and of adhesion molecules on islet endothelium) and inhibition of other IFN-γ-mediated effects on different immune subsets.

Trials with other IFN signaling inhibitors are underway (e.g., using abrocitinib [JAK1]/ritlecitinib [JAK3]) (NCT05743244), with several other molecules available for consideration (Chaimowitz et al. 2020; Russell et al. 2023).

Outlook

It is important to note that IFNs up-regulate the expression of both activatory (HLA class I, most notably HLA-B) and inhibitory surface ligands (PD-L1, HLA-E, HLA-F, and HLA-G). Indeed, a recent study (Chandra et al. 2022) showed that a TYK2 inhibitor (which inhibits IFN-α signaling) only partially protected IFN-α-sensitized β cells from T-cell-mediated lysis. This was likely due to the fact that the treatment inhibited the up-regulation of HLA class I, but also that of PD-L1. Thus, the ideal therapeutic agent should be able to dissociate these two effects by decreasing the expression of HLA class I and increasing that of potentially protective ligands. The group of R. Scharfmann recently reported that tryptophan is one such prototype β-cell-protective agent, as it was capable of up-regulating PD-L1 expression, alone or in combination with IFN-γ, and to inhibit the IFN-γ-induced up-regulation of HLA class I and of the T-cell homing chemokine CXCL10 (Rachdi et al. 2023). The group of D. Eizirik also observed that silencing STAT2 prevents IFN-α-induced HLA class I but not PD-L1 up-regulation (Marroqui et al. 2017; Colli et al. 2018). Dissociating these two opposing modulatory effects may thus prove feasible in the future. Of further note, all the candidate β-cell-protective agents trialed to date are already on the market for treating other conditions, and their repurposing for T1D may accelerate clinical approval. The therapeutic targets and agents discussed above are summarized in Figure 2.

CONCLUDING REMARKS

Beta cells are active players in the pathogenesis of T1D and are earning a well-deserved attention to

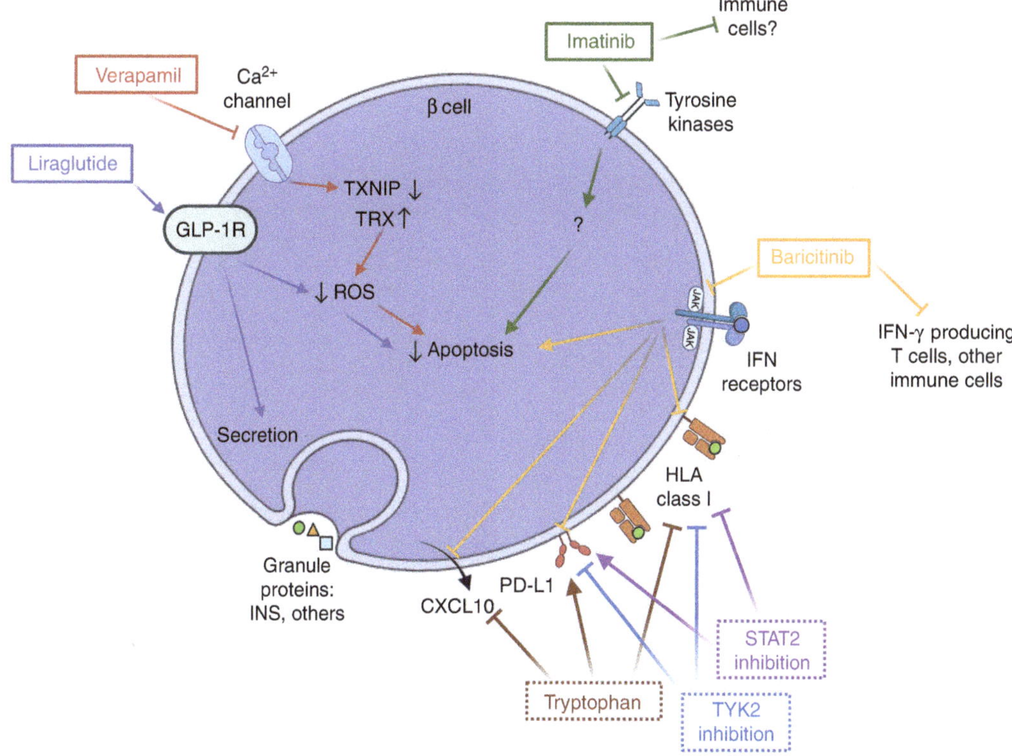

Figure 2. Therapeutic targets and agents to harness β-cell protection. Targets and agents with dashed contours have not been tested in clinical trials to date. See text for details. (Figure generated with BioRender, https://biorender.com.)

advance our understanding of disease mechanisms and to develop novel treatment strategies complementary to immunotherapies. The available literature highlights how this field of investigation is still in its infancy in terms of mechanistic insights, and that some components of the β-cell cross talk with immune cells are sometimes given as granted without formal proof. The first success stories of clinical trials with β-cell-protective agents encourage the scientific community to pursue this promising avenue, and to keep an open mindset to spot the next opportunities for progress.

ACKNOWLEDGMENTS

The work on this topic in the laboratory of R. Mallone is supported by Agence Nationale de la Recherche (ANR-19-CE15-0014-01), an EFSD Young Investigator Research Award to F. Samassa, and the Innovative Medicines Initiative 2 Joint Undertaking under grant agreements 945268 (INNODIA HARVEST), which receive support from the EU Horizon 2020 program, JDRF, and The Leona M. and Harry B. Helmsley Charitable Trust.

REFERENCES

Adamashvili IM, McDonald JC, Fraser PA, Milford EL, Pressly TA, Gelder FB. 1995. Soluble class I HLA antigens in patients with rheumatoid arthritis and their families. *J Rheumatol* **22:** 1025–1031.

Adamashvili IM, Fraser PA, McDonald JC. 1996. Association of serum concentrations of soluble class I HLA with HLA allotypes. *Transplantation* **61:** 984–987. doi:10.1097/00007890-199603270-00028

Adamashvili I, McVie R, Gelder F, Gautreaux M, Jaramillo J, Roggero T, McDonald J. 1997. Soluble HLA class I antigens in patients with type I diabetes and their family members.

Hum Immunol **55:** 176–183. doi:10.1016/s0198-8859(97)00096-7

Adamashvili I, Wolf R, Aultman D, Milford EL, Jaffe S, Hall V, Pressly T, Minagar A, Kelley R. 2003. Soluble HLA-I (s-HLA-I) synthesis in systemic lupus erythematosus. *Rheumatol Int* **23:** 294–300. doi:10.1007/s00296-003-0306-3

Allan DSJ, Lepin EJM, Braud VM, O'Callaghan CA, McMichael AJ. 2002. Tetrameric complexes of HLA-E, HLA-F, and HLA-G. *J Immunol Methods* **268:** 43–50. doi:10.1016/s0022-1759(02)00199-0

Allard M, Oger R, Benlalam H, Florenceau L, Echasserieau K, Bernardeau K, Labarrière N, Lang F, Gervois N. 2014. Soluble HLA-I/peptide monomers mediate antigen-specific CD8 T cell activation through passive peptide exchange with cell-bound HLA-I molecules. *J Immunol* **192:** 5090–5097. doi:10.4049/jimmunol.1303226

Anderson AM, Landry LG, Alkanani AA, Pyle L, Powers AC, Atkinson MA, Mathews CE, Roep BO, Michels AW, Nakayama M. 2021. Human islet T cells are highly reactive to preproinsulin in type 1 diabetes. *Proc Natl Acad Sci* **118:** e2107208118. doi:10.1073/pnas.2107208118

Azoury ME, Tarayrah M, Afonso G, Pais A, Colli ML, Maillard C, Lavaud C, Alexandre-Heymann L, Gonzalez-Duque S, Verdier Y, et al. 2020. Peptides derived from insulin granule proteins are targeted by CD8$^+$ T cells across MHC class I restrictions in humans and NOD mice. *Diabetes* **69:** 2678–2690. doi:10.2337/db20-0013

Bauzá-Martinez J, Heck AJR, Wu W. 2021. HLA-B and cysteinylated ligands distinguish the antigen presentation landscape of extracellular vesicles. *Commun Biol* **4:** 825. doi:10.1038/s42003-021-02364-y

Bossard C, Bézieau S, Matysiak-Budnik T, Volteau C, Laboisse CL, Jotereau F, Mosnier JF. 2012. HLA-E/β2 microglobulin overexpression in colorectal cancer is associated with recruitment of inhibitory immune cells and tumor progression. *Int J Cancer* **131:** 855–863. doi:10.1002/ijc.26453

Braud V, Jones EY, McMichael A. 1997. The human major histocompatibility complex class Ib molecule HLA-E binds signal sequence-derived peptides with primary anchor residues at positions 2 and 9. *Eur J Immunol* **27:** 1164–1169. doi:10.1002/eji.1830270517

Campoli M, Ferrone S. 2008. Tumor escape mechanisms: potential role of soluble HLA antigens and NK cells activating ligands. *Tissue Antigens* **72:** 321–334. doi:10.1111/j.1399-0039.2008.01106.x

Carré A, Mallone R. 2021. Making insulin and staying out of autoimmune trouble: the β-cell conundrum. *Front Immunol* **12:** 639682. doi:10.3389/fimmu.2021.639682

Carré A, Richardson SJ, Larger E, Mallone R. 2021. Presumption of guilt for T cells in type 1 diabetes: lead culprits or partners in crime depending on age of onset? *Diabetologia* **64:** 15–25. doi:10.1007/s00125-020-05298-y

Carré A, Zhou Z, Perez-Hernandez J, Samassa F, Lekka C, Manganaro A, Oshima M, Liao H, Parker R, Nicastri A, et al. 2023. Interferon-α promotes neo-antigen formation and preferential HLA-B-restricted antigen presentation in pancreatic β-cells. bioRxiv doi:10.1101/2023.1109.1115.557918

Carter JA, Stromich L, Peacey M, Chapin SR, Velten L, Steinmetz LM, Brors B, Pinto S, Meyer HV. 2022. Transcriptomic diversity in human medullary thymic epithelial cells. *Nat Commun* **13:** 4296. doi:10.1038/s41467-022-31750-1

Chaimowitz NS, Ebenezer SJ, Hanson IC, Anderson M, Forbes LR. 2020. STAT1 gain of function, type 1 diabetes, and reversal with JAK inhibition. *N Engl J Med* **383:** 1494–1496. doi:10.1056/NEJMc2022226

Chandra V, Ibrahim H, Halliez C, Prasad RB, Vecchio F, Dwivedi OP, Kvist J, Balboa D, Saarimäki-Vire J, Montaser H, et al. 2022. The type 1 diabetes gene TYK2 regulates β-cell development and its responses to interferon-α. *Nat Commun* **13:** 6363. doi:10.1038/s41467-022-34069-z

Chen J, Saxena G, Mungrue IN, Lusis AJ, Shalev A. 2008. Thioredoxin-interacting protein: a critical link between glucose toxicity and β-cell apoptosis. *Diabetes* **57:** 938–944. doi:10.2337/db07-0715

Cirulli V, Zalatan J, McMaster M, Prinsen R, Salomon DR, Ricordi C, Torbett BE, Meda P, Crisa L. 2006. The class I HLA repertoire of pancreatic islets comprises the nonclassical class Ib antigen HLA-G. *Diabetes* **55:** 1214–1222. doi:10.2337/db05-0731

Colli ML, Hill JLE, Marroquí L, Chaffey J, Dos Santos RS, Leete P, Coomans de Brachène A, Paula FMM, Op de Beeck A, Castela A, et al. 2018. PDL1 is expressed in the islets of people with type 1 diabetes and is up-regulated by interferons-α and-γ via IRF1 induction. *EBioMedicine* **36:** 367–375. doi:10.1016/j.ebiom.2018.09.040

Colli ML, Ramos-Rodríguez M, Nakayasu ES, Alvelos MI, Lopes M, Hill JLE, Turatsinze JV, Coomans de Brachène A, Russell MA, Raurell-Vila H, et al. 2020. An integrated multi-omics approach identifies the landscape of interferon-α-mediated responses of human pancreatic β cells. *Nat Commun* **11:** 2584. doi:10.1038/s41467-020-16327-0

Contini P, Ghio M, Poggi A, Filaci G, Indiveri F, Ferrone S, Puppo F. 2003. Soluble HLA-A,-B,-C and -G molecules induce apoptosis in T and NK CD8$^+$ cells and inhibit cytotoxic T cell activity through CD8 ligation. *Eur J Immunol* **33:** 125–134. doi:10.1002/immu.200390015

Coupel S, Moreau A, Hamidou M, Horejsi V, Soulillou JP, Charreau B. 2007. Expression and release of soluble HLA-E is an immunoregulatory feature of endothelial cell activation. *Blood* **109:** 2806–2814. doi:10.1182/blood-2006-06-030213

Culina S, Lalanne AI, Afonso G, Cerosaletti K, Pinto S, Sebastiani G, Kuranda K, Nigi L, Eugster A, Østerbye T, et al. 2018. Islet-reactive CD8$^+$ T cell frequencies in the pancreas, but not in blood, distinguish type 1 diabetic patients from healthy donors. *Sci Immunol* **3:** eaao4013. doi:10.1126/sciimmunol.aao4013

Demaria S, DeVito-Haynes LD, Salter RD, Burlingham WJ, Bushkin Y. 1999. Peptide-conformed β2m-free class I heavy chains are intermediates in generation of soluble HLA by the membrane-bound metalloproteinase. *Hum Immunol* **60:** 1216–1226. doi:10.1016/s0198-8859(99)00113-5

Dulberger CL, McMurtrey CP, Hölzemer A, Neu KE, Liu V, Steinbach AM, Garcia-Beltran WF, Sulak M, Jabri B, Lynch VJ, et al. 2017. Human leukocyte antigen f presents peptides and regulates immunity through interactions with NK cell receptors. *Immunity* **46:** 1018–1029.e7. doi:10.1016/j.immuni.2017.06.002

Eizirik DL, Szymczak F, Mallone R. 2023. Why does the immune system destroy pancreatic β-cells but not α-cells in type 1 diabetes? *Nat Rev Endocrinol* **19:** 425–434. doi:10.1038/s41574-023-00826-3

Elgamal RM, Kudtarkar P, Melton RL, Mummey HM, Benaglio P, Okino ML, Gaulton KJ. 2023. An integrated map of cell type-specific gene expression in pancreatic islets. *Diabetes* **72:** 1719–1728. doi:10.2337/db23-0130

Ferreira RC, Guo H, Coulson RM, Smyth DJ, Pekalski ML, Burren OS, Cutler AJ, Doecke JD, Flint S, McKinney EF, et al. 2014. A type I interferon transcriptional signature precedes autoimmunity in children genetically at risk for type 1 diabetes. *Diabetes* **63:** 2538–2550. doi:10.2337/db13-1777

Fife BT, Guleria I, Gubbels BM, Eagar TN, Tang Q, Bour-Jordan H, Yagita H, Azuma M, Sayegh MH, Bluestone JA. 2006. Insulin-induced remission in new-onset NOD mice is maintained by the PD-1-PD-L1 pathway. *J Exp Med* **203:** 2737–2747. doi:10.1084/jem.20061577

Forlenza GP, McVean J, Beck RW, Bauza C, Bailey R, Buckingham B, DiMeglio LA, Sherr JL, Clements M, Neyman A, et al. 2023. Effect of verapamil on pancreatic β cell function in newly diagnosed pediatric type 1 diabetes: a randomized clinical trial. *JAMA* **329:** 990–999. doi:10.1001/jama.2023.2064

García P, Llano M, de Heredia AB, Willberg CB, Caparrós E, Aparicio P, Braud VM, López-Botet M. 2002. Human T cell receptor-mediated recognition of HLA-E. *Eur J Immunol* **32:** 936–944. doi:10.1002/1521-4141(200204)32:4<936::AID-IMMU936>3.0.CO;2-M

Gearty SV, Dündar F, Zumbo P, Espinosa-Carrasco G, Shakiba M, Sanchez-Rivera FJ, Socci ND, Trivedi P, Lowe SW, Lauer P, et al. 2022. An autoimmune stem-like CD8 T cell population drives type 1 diabetes. *Nature* **602:** 156–161. doi:10.1038/s41586-021-04248-x

Gitelman SE, Bundy BN, Ferrannini E, Lim N, Blanchfield JL, DiMeglio LA, Felner EI, Gaglia JL, Gottlieb PA, Long SA, et al. 2021. Imatinib therapy for patients with recent-onset type 1 diabetes: a multicentre, randomised, double-blind, placebo-controlled, phase 2 trial. *Lancet Diabetes Endocrinol* **9:** 502–514. doi:10.1016/S2213-8587(21)00139-X

Giusti L, Tesi M, Ciregia F, Marselli L, Zallocco L, Suleiman M, De Luca C, Del Guerra S, Zuccarini M, Trerotola M, et al. 2022. The protective action of metformin against pro-inflammatory cytokine-induced human islet cell damage and the mechanisms involved. *Cells* **11:** 2465. doi:10.3390/cells11152465

Gonzalez-Duque S, Azoury ME, Colli ML, Afonso G, Turatsinze JV, Nigi L, Lalanne AI, Sebastiani G, Carré A, Pinto S, et al. 2018. Conventional and neo-antigenic peptides presented by β cells are targeted by circulating naïve $CD8^+$ T cells in type 1 diabetic and healthy donors. *Cell Metab* **28:** 946–960.e6. doi:10.1016/j.cmet.2018.07.007

Goodridge JP, Burian A, Lee N, Geraghty DE. 2013. HLA-F and MHC class I open conformers are ligands for NK cell Ig-like receptors. *J Immunol* **191:** 3553–3562. doi:10.4049/jimmunol.1300081

Gunturi A, Berg RE, Forman J. 2004. The role of CD94/NKG2 in innate and adaptive immunity. *Immunol Res* **30:** 29–34. doi:10.1385/IR:30:1:029

Guyer P, Arribas-Layton D, Manganaro A, Speake C, Lord S, Eizirik DL, Kent SC, Mallone R, James EA. 2022. Recognition of mRNA splice variant and secretory granule epitopes by $CD4^+$ T cells in type 1 diabetes. *Diabetes* **72:** 85–96. doi:10.2337/db22-0191

Haase H, Ober-Blöbaum JL, Engelhardt G, Hebel S, Heit A, Heine H, Rink L. 2008. Zinc signals are essential for lipopolysaccharide-induced signal transduction in monocytes. *J Immunol* **181:** 6491–6502. doi:10.4049/jimmunol.181.9.6491

Haynes LD, Bushkin Y, Love RB, Burlingham WJ. 2002. Interferon-γ drives the metalloproteinase-dependent cleavage of HLA class I soluble forms from primary human bronchial epithelial cells. *Hum Immunol* **63:** 893–901. doi:10.1016/s0198-8859(02)00461-5

Herbst RS, Soria JC, Kowanetz M, Fine GD, Hamid O, Gordon MS, Sosman JA, McDermott DF, Powderly JD, Gettinger SN, et al. 2014. Predictive correlates of response to the anti-PD-L1 antibody MPDL3280A in cancer patients. *Nature* **515:** 563–567. doi:10.1038/nature14011

Hu D, Ikizawa K, Lu L, Sanchirico ME, Shinohara ML, Cantor H. 2004. Analysis of regulatory CD8 T cells in Qa-1-deficient mice. *Nat Immunol* **5:** 516–523. doi:10.1038/ni1063

Im SJ, Hashimoto M, Gerner MY, Lee J, Kissick HT, Burger MC, Shan Q, Hale JS, Lee J, Nasti TH, et al. 2016. Defining $CD8^+$ T cells that provide the proliferative burst after PD-1 therapy. *Nature* **537:** 417–421. doi:10.1038/nature19330

James EA, Mallone R, Kent SC, DiLorenzo TP. 2020. T-cell epitopes and neo-epitopes in type 1 diabetes: a comprehensive update and reappraisal. *Diabetes* **69:** 1311–1335. doi:10.2337/dbi19-0022

Javitt A, Barnea E, Kramer MP, Wolf-Levy H, Levin Y, Admon A, Merbl Y. 2019. Pro-inflammatory cytokines alter the immunopeptidome landscape by modulation of HLA-B expression. *Front Immunol* **10:** 141. doi:10.3389/fimmu.2019.00141

Jiang H, Kashleva H, Xu LX, Forman J, Flaherty L, Pernis B, Braunstein NS, Chess L. 1998. T cell vaccination induces T cell receptor Vβ-specific Qa-1-restricted regulatory $CD8^+$ T cells. *Proc Natl Acad Sci* **95:** 4533–4537. doi:10.1073/pnas.95.8.4533

Jiang H, Canfield SM, Gallagher MP, Jiang HH, Jiang Y, Zheng Z, Chess L. 2010. HLA-E-restricted regulatory $CD8^+$ T cells are involved in development and control of human autoimmune type 1 diabetes. *J Clin Invest* **120:** 3641–3650. doi:10.1172/JCI43522

Juneja VR, McGuire KA, Manguso RT, LaFleur MW, Collins N, Haining WN, Freeman GJ, Sharpe AH. 2017. PD-L1 on tumor cells is sufficient for immune evasion in immunogenic tumors and inhibits CD8 T cell cytotoxicity. *J Exp Med* **214:** 895–904. doi:10.1084/jem.20160801

Kallionpää H, Elo LL, Laajala E, Mykkänen J, Ricaño-Ponce I, Vaarma M, Laajala TD, Hyöty H, Ilonen J, Veijola R, et al. 2014. Innate immune activity is detected prior to seroconversion in children with HLA-conferred type 1 diabetes susceptibility. *Diabetes* **63:** 2402–2414. doi:10.2337/db13-1775

Kim HJ, Cantor H. 2011. Regulation of self-tolerance by Qa-1-restricted $CD8^+$ regulatory T cells. *Semin Immunol* **23:** 446–452. doi:10.1016/j.smim.2011.06.001

Kim HJ, Wang X, Radfar S, Sproule TJ, Roopenian DC, Cantor H. 2011. $CD8^+$ T regulatory cells express the Ly49 class I MHC receptor and are defective in autoimmune prone B6-Yaa mice. *Proc Natl Acad Sci* **108:** 2010–2015. doi:10.1073/pnas.1018974108

Krangel MS. 1986. Secretion of HLA-A and -B antigens via an alternative RNA splicing pathway. *J Exp Med* **163:** 1173–1190. doi:10.1084/jem.163.5.1173

Kronenberg-Versteeg D, Eichmann M, Russell MA, de Ru A, Hehn B, Yusuf N, van Veelen PA, Richardson SJ, Morgan NG, Lemberg MK, et al. 2018. Molecular pathways for immune recognition of preproinsulin signal peptide in type 1 diabetes. *Diabetes* **67:** 687–696. doi:10.2337/db17-0021

Legoux FP, Lim JB, Cauley AW, Dikiy S, Ertelt J, Mariani TJ, Sparwasser T, Way SS, Moon JJ. 2015. CD4$^+$ T cell tolerance to tissue-restricted self antigens is mediated by antigen-specific regulatory T cells rather than deletion. *Immunity* **43:** 896–908. doi:10.1016/j.immuni.2015.10.011

Lemos JRN, Baidal DA, Poggioli R, Fuenmayor V, Chavez C, Alvarez A, Ricordi C, Alejandro R. 2023. HLA-B matching prolongs allograft survival in islet cell transplantation. *Cell Transplant* **32:** 9636897231166529. doi:10.1177/0963 6897231166529

Levy EM, Bianchini M, Von Euw EM, Barrio MM, Bravo AI, Furman D, Domenichini E, Macagno C, Pinsky V, Zucchini C, et al. 2008. Human leukocyte antigen-E protein is overexpressed in primary human colorectal cancer. *Int J Oncol* **32:** 633–641.

Lundberg M, Krogvold L, Kuric E, Dahl-Jørgensen K, Skog O. 2016. Expression of interferon-stimulated genes in insulitic pancreatic islets of patients recently diagnosed with type 1 diabetes. *Diabetes* **65:** 3104–3110. doi:10.2337/db16-0616

Mallone R, Eizirik DL. 2020. Presumption of innocence for β cells: why are they vulnerable autoimmune targets in type 1 diabetes? *Diabetologia* **63:** 1999–2006. doi:10.1007/s001 25-020-05176-7

Mallone R, Halliez C, Rui J, Herold KC. 2022. The β-cell in type 1 diabetes pathogenesis: a victim of circumstances or an instigator of tragic events? *Diabetes* **71:** 1603–1610. doi:10.2337/dbi21-0036

Marroqui L, Dos Santos RS, Op de Beeck A, Coomans de Brachène A, Marselli L, Marchetti P, Eizirik DL. 2017. Interferon-α mediates human β cell HLA class I overexpression, endoplasmic reticulum stress and apoptosis, three hallmarks of early human type 1 diabetes. *Diabetologia* **60:** 656–667. doi:10.1007/s00125-016-4201-3

Nakanishi K, Kobayashi T, Murase T, Nakatsuji T, Inoko H, Tsuji K, Kosaka K. 1993. Association of HLA-A24 with complete β-cell destruction in IDDM. *Diabetes* **42:** 1086–1093. doi:10.2337/diab.42.7.1086

Nakanishi K, Kobayashi T, Komatsu Y, Kogawa N, Hagihara M, Tsuji K. 1997. Synchronous decline of serum-soluble HLA class I antigen and β-cell function in insulin-dependent diabetes mellitus. *Clin Immunol Immunopathol* **85:** 246–252. doi:10.1006/clin.1997.4456

Nakayasu ES, Syed F, Tersey SA, Gritsenko MA, Mitchell HD, Chan CY, Dirice E, Turatsinze JV, Cui Y, Kulkarni RN, et al. 2020. Comprehensive proteomics analysis of stressed human islets identifies GDF15 as a target for type 1 diabetes intervention. *Cell Metab* **31:** 363–374.e6. doi:10.1016/j.cmet.2019.12.005

Nejentsev S, Howson JM, Walker NM, Szeszko J, Field SF, Stevens HE, Reynolds P, Hardy M, King E, Masters J, et al. 2007. Localization of type 1 diabetes susceptibility to the MHC class I genes HLA-B and HLA-A. *Nature* **450:** 887–892. doi:10.1038/nature06406

Osum KC, Burrack AL, Martinov T, Sahli NL, Mitchell JS, Tucker CG, Pauken KE, Papas K, Appakalai B, Spanier JA, et al. 2018. Interferon-γ drives programmed death-ligand 1 expression on islet β cells to limit T cell function during autoimmune diabetes. *Sci Rep* **8:** 8295. doi:10.1038/s41598-018-26471-9

Ovalle F, Grimes T, Xu G, Patel AJ, Grayson TB, Thielen LA, Li P, Shalev A. 2018. Verapamil and β cell function in adults with recent-onset type 1 diabetes. *Nat Med* **24:** 1108–1112. doi:10.1038/s41591-018-0089-4

Panoutsakopoulou V, Huster KM, McCarty N, Feinberg E, Wang R, Wucherpfennig KW, Cantor H. 2004. Suppression of autoimmune disease after vaccination with autoreactive T cells that express Qa-1 peptide complexes. *J Clin Invest* **113:** 1218–1224. doi:10.1172/JCI20772

Parent AV, Faleo G, Chavez J, Saxton M, Berrios DI, Kerper NR, Tang Q, Hebrok M. 2021. Selective deletion of human leukocyte antigens protects stem cell-derived islets from immune rejection. *Cell Rep* **36:** 109538. doi:10.1016/j.celrep.2021.109538

Pietra G, Romagnani C, Falco M, Vitale M, Castriconi R, Pende D, Millo E, Anfossi S, Biassoni R, Moretta L, et al. 2001. The analysis of the natural killer-like activity of human cytolytic T lymphocytes revealed HLA-E as a novel target for TCR α/β-mediated recognition. *Eur J Immunol* **31:** 3687–3693. doi:10.1002/1521-4141(200112)31:12<3687::aid-immu3687>3.0.co;2-c

Pietra G, Romagnani C, Mazzarino P, Falco M, Millo E, Moretta A, Moretta L, Mingari MC. 2003. HLA-E-restricted recognition of cytomegalovirus-derived peptides by human CD8$^+$ cytolytic T lymphocytes. *Proc Natl Acad Sci* **100:** 10896–10901. doi:10.1073/pnas.1834449100

Piñeros AR, Kulkarni A, Gao H, Orr KS, Glenn L, Huang F, Liu Y, Gannon M, Syed F, Wu W, et al. 2022. Proinflammatory signaling in islet β cells propagates invasion of pathogenic immune cells in autoimmune diabetes. *Cell Rep* **39:** 111011. doi:10.1016/j.celrep.2022.111011

Puppo F, Contini P, Ghio M, Brenci S, Scudeletti M, Filaci G, Ferrone S, Indiveri F. 2000. Soluble human MHC class I molecules induce soluble Fas ligand secretion and trigger apoptosis in activated CD8$^+$ Fas (CD95)$^+$ T lymphocytes. *Int Immunol* **12:** 195–203. doi:10.1093/intimm/12.2.195

Rachdi L, Zhou Z, Berthault C, Lourenço C, Fouque A, Domet T, Armanet M, You S, Peakman M, Mallone R, et al. 2023. Tryptophan metabolism promotes immune evasion in human pancreatic β cells. *EBioMedicine* **95:** 104740. doi:10.1016/j.ebiom.2023.104740

Richardson SJ, Rodriguez-Calvo T, Gerling IC, Mathews CE, Kaddis JS, Russell MA, Zeissler M, Leete P, Krogvold L, Dahl-Jørgensen K, et al. 2016. Islet cell hyperexpression of HLA class I antigens: a defining feature in type 1 diabetes. *Diabetologia* **59:** 2448–2458. doi:10.1007/s00125-016-4067-4

Ritz D, Gloger A, Neri D, Fugmann T. 2017. Purification of soluble HLA class I complexes from human serum or plasma deliver high quality immuno peptidomes required for biomarker discovery. *Proteomics* **17:** 10.1002/pmic.201600364 doi:10.1002/pmic.201600364

Rui J, Deng S, Perdigoto AL, Ponath G, Kursawe R, Lawlor N, Sumida T, Levine-Ritterman M, Stitzel ML, Pitt D, et al.

2021. Tet2 controls the responses of β cells to inflammation in autoimmune diabetes. *Nat Commun* **12:** 5074. doi:10.1038/s41467-021-25367-z

Russell MA, Redick SD, Blodgett DM, Richardson SJ, Leete P, Krogvold L, Dahl-Jørgensen K, Bottino R, Brissova M, Spaeth JM, et al. 2019. HLA class II antigen processing and presentation pathway components demonstrated by transcriptome and protein analyses of islet β-cells from donors with type 1 diabetes. *Diabetes* **68:** 988–1001. doi:10.2337/db18-0686

Russell MA, Richardson SJ, Morgan NG. 2023. The role of the interferon/JAK-STAT axis in driving islet HLA-I hyperexpression in type 1 diabetes. *Front Endocrinol* **14:** 1270325. doi:10.3389/fendo.2023.1270325

Samassa F, Mallone R. 2022. Self-antigens, benign autoimmunity and type 1 diabetes: a β-cell and T-cell perspective. *Curr Opin Endocrinol Diabetes Obes* **29:** 370–378. doi:10.1097/MED.0000000000000735

Schuit FC, In't Veld PA, Pipeleers DG. 1988. Glucose stimulates proinsulin biosynthesis by a dose-dependent recruitment of pancreatic β cells. *Proc Natl Acad Sci* **85:** 3865–3869. doi:10.1073/pnas.85.11.3865

Seliger B, Jasinski-Bergner S, Quandt D, Stoehr C, Bukur J, Wach S, Legal W, Taubert H, Wullich B, Hartmann A. 2016. HLA-E expression and its clinical relevance in human renal cell carcinoma. *Oncotarget* **7:** 67360–67372. doi:10.18632/oncotarget.11744

Shalev A, Pise-Masison CA, Radonovich M, Hoffmann SC, Hirshberg B, Brady JN, Harlan DM. 2002. Oligonucleotide microarray analysis of intact human pancreatic islets: identification of glucose-responsive genes and a highly regulated TGFβ signaling pathway. *Endocrinology* **143:** 3695–3698. doi:10.1210/en.2002-220564

Skowera A, Ellis RJ, Varela-Calviño R, Arif S, Huang GC, Van-Krinks C, Zaremba A, Rackham C, Allen JS, Tree TI, et al. 2008. CTLs are targeted to kill β cells in patients with type 1 diabetes through recognition of a glucose-regulated preproinsulin epitope. *J Clin Invest* **118:** 3390–3402. doi:10.1172/JCI35449

Szymczak F, Colli ML, Mamula MJ, Evans-Molina C, Eizirik DL. 2021. Gene expression signatures of target tissues in type 1 diabetes, lupus erythematosus, multiple sclerosis, and rheumatoid arthritis. *Sci Adv* **7:** eabd7600. doi:10.1126/sciadv.abd7600

Szymczak F, Alvelos MI, Marín-Cañas S, Castela Â, Demine S, Colli ML, Op de Beeck A, Thomaidou S, Marselli L, Zaldumbide A, et al. 2022. Transcription and splicing regulation by NLRC5 shape the interferon response in human pancreatic β cells. *Sci Adv* **8:** eabn5732. doi:10.1126/sciadv.abn5732

Thielen LA, Chen J, Jing G, Moukha-Chafiq O, Xu G, Jo S, Grayson TB, Lu B, Li P, Augelli-Szafran CE, et al. 2020. Identification of an anti-diabetic, orally available small molecule that regulates TXNIP expression and glucagon action. *Cell Metab* **32:** 353–365.e8. doi:10.1016/j.cmet.2020.07.002

Thorogood J, Persijn GG, Schreuder GM, D'Amaro J, Zantvoort FA, van Houwelingen JC, van Rood JJ. 1990. The effect of HLA matching on kidney graft survival in separate posttransplantation intervals. *Transplantation* **50:** 146–149. doi:10.1097/00007890-199007000-00027

Tumeh PC, Harview CL, Yearley JH, Shintaku IP, Taylor EJ, Robert L, Chmielowski B, Spasic M, Henry G, Ciobanu V, et al. 2014. PD-1 blockade induces responses by inhibiting adaptive immune resistance. *Nature* **515:** 568–571. doi:10.1038/nature13954

Unanue ER, Wan X. 2019. The immunoreactive platform of the pancreatic islets influences the development of autoreactivity. *Diabetes* **68:** 1544–1551. doi:10.2337/dbi18-0048

Valés-Gómez M, Reyburn HT, Erskine RA, López-Botet M, Strominger JL. 1999. Kinetics and peptide dependency of the binding of the inhibitory NK receptor CD94/NKG2-A and the activating receptor CD94/NKG2-C to HLA-E. *EMBO J* **18:** 4250–4260. doi:10.1093/emboj/18.15.4250

van Hall T, Oliveira CC, Joosten SA, Ottenhoff THM. 2010. The other Janus face of Qa-1 and HLA-E: diverse peptide repertoires in times of stress. *Microbes Infect* **12:** 910–918. doi:10.1016/j.micinf.2010.07.011

von Herrath M, Bain SC, Bode B, Clausen JO, Coppieters K, Gaysina L, Gumprecht J, Hansen TK, Mathieu C, Morales C, et al. 2021. Anti-interleukin-21 antibody and liraglutide for the preservation of β-cell function in adults with recent-onset type 1 diabetes: a randomised, double-blind, placebo-controlled, phase 2 trial. *Lancet Diabetes Endocrinol* **9:** 212–224. doi:10.1016/S2213-8587(21)00019-X

Waibel M, Wentworth JM, So M, Couper JJ, Cameron FJ, MacIsaac RJ, Atlas G, Gorelik A, Litwak S, Sanz-Villanueva L, et al. 2023. Baricitinib and β-cell function in patients with new-onset type 1 diabetes. *N Engl J Med* **389:** 2140–2150. doi:10.1056/NEJMoa2306691

Wan X, Zinselmeyer BH, Zakharov PN, Vomund AN, Taniguchi R, Santambrogio L, Anderson MS, Lichti CF, Unanue ER. 2018. Pancreatic islets communicate with lymphoid tissues via exocytosis of insulin peptides. *Nature* **560:** 107–111. doi:10.1038/s41586-018-0341-6

Wang C, Weng M, Xia S, Zhang M, Chen C, Tang J, Huang D, Yu H, Sun W, Zhang H, et al. 2021. Distinct roles of programmed death ligand 1 alternative splicing isoforms in colorectal cancer. *Cancer Sci* **112:** 178–193. doi:10.1111/cas.14690

Wang CY, Huang KC, Lu CW, Chu CH, Huang CN, Chen HS, Lee IT, Chen JF, Chen CC, Chen CS, et al. 2022. A randomized controlled trial of R-form verapamil added to ongoing metformin therapy in patients with type 2 diabetes. *J Clin Endocrinol Metab* **107:** e4063–e4071. doi:10.1210/clinem/dgac436

Wiedeman AE, Muir VS, Rosasco MG, DeBerg HA, Presnell S, Haas B, Dufort MJ, Speake C, Greenbaum CJ, Serti E, et al. 2020. Autoreactive CD8$^+$ T cell exhaustion distinguishes subjects with slow type 1 diabetes progression. *J Clin Invest* **130:** 480–490. doi:10.1172/JCI126595

Wyatt RC, Lanzoni G, Russell MA, Gerling I, Richardson SJ. 2019. What the HLA-I!—classical and non-classical HLA class I and their potential roles in type 1 diabetes. *Curr Diab Rep* **19:** 159. doi:10.1007/s11892-019-1245-z

Xu G, Grimes TD, Grayson TB, Chen J, Thielen LA, Tse HM, Li P, Kanke M, Lin TT, Schepmoes AA, et al. 2022. Exploratory study reveals far reaching systemic and cellular effects of verapamil treatment in subjects with type 1 diabetes. *Nat Commun* **13:** 1159. doi:10.1038/s41467-022-28826-3

Yu M, Lee WW, Tomar D, Pryshchep S, Czesnikiewicz-Guzik M, Lamar DL, Li G, Singh K, Tian L, Weyand CM, et al. 2011. Regulation of T cell receptor signaling by activation-induced zinc influx. *J Exp Med* **208:** 775–785. doi:10.1084/jem.20100031

Zavazava N, Krönke M. 1996. Soluble HLA class I molecules induce apoptosis in alloreactive cytotoxic T lymphocytes. *Nat Med* **2:** 1005–1010. doi:10.1038/nm0996-1005

Zavazava N, Westphal E, Muller-Ruchholtz W. 1990. Characterization of soluble HLA molecules in sweat and quantitative HLA differences in serum of healthy individuals. *J Immunogenet* **17:** 387–394. doi:10.1111/j.1744-313x.1990.tb00890.x

Inflammatory β-Cell Stress and Immune Surveillance in Type 1 Diabetes

Anil Bhushan[1] and Peter J. Thompson[2,3]

[1]Diabetes Center, University of California San Francisco, San Francisco, California 94143, USA

[2]Diabetes Envisioned and Accomplished in Manitoba (DREAM), Children's Hospital Research Institute of Manitoba, Winnipeg, Manitoba R3E 3P4, Canada

[3]Department of Physiology and Pathophysiology, Rady Faculty of Health Sciences, University of Manitoba, Winnipeg, Manitoba R3E 0W2, Canada

Correspondence: peter.thompson@umanitoba.ca

Recent years have seen increased recognition for the role of β-cell stress as a contributing factor to the autoimmune destruction process that ultimately results in symptomatic type 1 diabetes (T1D). Preclinical studies have discovered a variety of stress responses in the β-cell that occur at presymptomatic stages and contribute to disease progression, but unifying explanations of how these mechanisms operate to promote disease progression remain incomplete. We propose that stressed β-cells transition into β-cells expressing inflammatory molecules that provoke an immune response to restore homeostasis by coordinating islet repair and the removal of stressed cells. However, when immune surveillance fails, stressed β-cells accumulate and contribute to autoimmunity. Therapies directed toward stressed β-cells to either curb their inflammatory signaling or to eliminate them (essentially doing the job of the failed immune surveillance) are moving from animal models into the clinic with promising initial results, although the understanding of how the immune response is coordinated by stressed β-cells is not clear. In this article, we discuss β-cell stress responses implicated in T1D pathogenesis based on evidence from humans and highlight existing knowledge gaps in their mechanisms. Future work in this field is poised to target T1D by simultaneously targeting stressed β-cells and the failed immune response to halt the progression of autoimmunity and prevent β-cell destruction.

Autoimmunity has been axiomatic to type 1 diabetes (T1D) pathology since its immune basis was first demonstrated (Gale 2001). Stemming from discoveries made in the 1970s that showed the presence of serum autoantibodies with reactivity to islet/β-cell antigens in insulin-dependent diabetes donors (Bottazzo et al. 1974; MacCuish et al. 1974), the etiological basis for what was then referred to as "juvenile-onset diabetes," was distinguished from what is now called type 2 diabetes (T2D) and increasingly regarded as an autoimmune disease (Craighead 1978). Viewing T1D as an autoimmune disease has been the foundational paradigm driving the decades-long development and clinical testing of immunotherapies (Bluestone et al. 2021), and has recently led to

Cite this article as *Cold Spring Harb Perspect Med* doi: 10.1101/cshperspect.a041605

the first Food and Drug Administration (FDA)-approved intervention capable of delaying symptomatic T1D, the anti-CD3 monoclonal antibody therapy teplizumab (Herold et al. 2019).

However, autoimmunity in T1D occurs in the context of the pancreas and is driven by interactions between the immune system and dysfunctional β-cells, a concept that has now become generally accepted, as reviewed elsewhere (Carré et al. 2021; Roep et al. 2021; Mallone et al. 2022). This has led to a shift in viewing T1D as strictly an immune disease, to now appreciating T1D as a disease of the immune system and dysfunctional cells of the pancreas. Recent findings have overturned or challenged previous assumptions about T1D including (1) observations demonstrating residual β-cells in the majority of long-standing T1D donors (Oram et al. 2019); (2) genome-wide association studies (GWAS) that have demonstrated many T1D-associated risk polymorphisms in genes expressed in islets/β-cells (Størling and Pociot 2017); (3) evidence for substantial differences islet and immune pathology in T1D donors based on age at symptomatic disease onset (Leete et al. 2020); and (4) a clearer clinical picture of the natural history of T1D (Insel et al. 2015) with strong evidence for islet and β-cell dysfunction in early presymptomatic stages (Brissova et al. 2018; Evans-Molina et al. 2018; Doliba et al. 2022; Warncke et al. 2022). For example, in our previous work studying β-cell dysfunction, our view of T1D evolved as a result of the identification of a novel population of stressed β-cells that displayed a senescent-like phenotype accompanied by an inflammatory profile in both nonobese diabetic (NOD) mice and human T1D donor pancreatic samples (Thompson et al. 2019b). Notably, β-cells expressing senescence markers also accumulate in mouse models of T2D (Aguayo-Mazzucato et al. 2019) as well as in a mouse model of maturity-onset diabetes of the young (MODY) in a sex-specific manner (Walker et al. 2021). Together these studies have implicated β-cell senescence as a novel pathological mechanism of β-cell dysfunction not only in T1D but also T2D and monogenic diabetes (Cha et al. 2023).

Building upon these advances, our ability to study the role of islet/β-cell stress in T1D has grown exponentially with the advent of single-cell technologies (Carrano et al. 2017). These technologies have led to major high-throughput imaging studies (Damond et al. 2019; Wang et al. 2019) and single-cell multiomic studies (Chiou et al. 2021a,b; Benaglio et al. 2022; Fasolino et al. 2022; Elgamal et al. 2023) that have furnished insights into cell-type-specific gene regulatory networks, epigenetic mechanisms, functions of risk-associated GWAS polymorphisms and other molecular changes in islet cells during the progression of the disease at the single-cell scale. Importantly, these discoveries have been made by investigators working in large research consortia on behalf of the diabetes research community, where data have been made publicly available in user-friendly interfaces (Kaestner et al. 2019; Kudtarkar et al. 2023), facilitating access for the rest of the field. In a relatively short time, as compared with the decades of study on immunotherapies, a growing focus on the β-cell stress in T1D has already resulted in clinical translation of non-immune-based interventions to allay the decline in β-cell mass and function, postdiagnosis (Brawerman and Thompson 2020).

A wide variety of β-cell stress responses and phenotypes have been reported in T1D and extensively reviewed elsewhere (Roep et al. 2021; Vived et al. 2023). These include the type I interferon (IFN) response (Marroqui et al. 2021), the unfolded protein response (UPR) (Sahin et al. 2021), stress response senescence (Thompson and Bhushan 2022), proinsulin processing defects (Sims et al. 2020), altered β-cell identity (Moin and Butler 2019), defective autophagy (Muralidharan et al. 2021), and polyamine biosynthesis (Sims et al. 2023). In this article, we focus our discussion on the UPR and senescence and highlight studies where they have been shown to be involved or play a role in T1D, with an emphasis on evidence from studies using human donor specimens and recent clinical trials. Major gaps in knowledge remain regarding how these β-stress responses arise and interrelate with one another during disease progression. We advance the hypothesis that inflammatory signaling is a common feature between UPR and senescence, providing an explanation as to how they both can accelerate disease progression and interact with the immune system. UPR and senescence are stressed states in which β-cells acquire inflammatory secretomes, which could provoke immune surveillance leading to either restoration of islet homeostasis if appropriately and efficiently resolved, or acceleration of T1D pathology if surveillance fails. Ultimately understanding how stressed β-cells in the pancreas interact with an immune response that results in β-cell destruction in T1D needs to be investigated to develop therapies that are disease-specific and provide a durable response.

WHY THE β-CELL?

It has been known for many years that of all the endocrine islet cells, β-cells are the most vulnerable to both intrinsic sources of stress (such as from glucose metabolism, reactive oxygen species, insulin synthesis, and protein folding) and extrinsic sources of stress (such as nutrient excess, inflammatory mediators, and viral infections). The origins of this β-cell fragility may lie in their developmental history and the requirement of β-cell replication in the postnatal period for expansion. β-cell maturation in which β-cells acquire the ability to precisely sense glucose and secrete insulin occurs after the expansion phase and is accompanied by turning off a number of housekeeping metabolic genes referred to as β-cell "disallowed" genes (Rutter et al. 2020). These special features of β-cells are also modified by polymorphisms in genes expressed in β-cells. After the HLA class II locus, the *INS* gene is the next-highest risk-conferring locus for T1D development, followed by a number of other β-cell-expressed genes (Pociot 2017). Regardless of the reasons why β-cells are more prone to stress and ultimately become the targets of autoimmunity in T1D, it is now appreciated that stressed β-cells are a promising target of disease-modifying therapy in T1D.

β-CELL UPR

As a professional secretory cell, β-cells experience constant endoplasmic reticulum (ER) stress due to the high rates of synthesis and processing of insulin and use the UPR to mitigate this stress. The UPR is an essential and ubiquitous cellular response to protein folding and synthesis sensed in the ER and consisting of three main branches in mammals (Fig. 1A; Sahin et al. 2021). Upon sensing ER stress, membrane-bound adaptor proteins, IRE1α, PERK, and ATF6 become activated and trigger downstream changes aimed at balancing cell stress mitigation and restoration of homeostasis with apoptosis (Fig. 1A; Ghosh et al. 2019). In β-cells, these adaptive changes include transcriptional activation of UPR target genes by cleaved ATF6 and spliced XBP1 (XBP1s), changes in redox balance, global suppression of mRNA translation by eIF2α, among others (Fig. 1A). If mitigation measures fail, the adaptive UPR shifts toward a terminal response in a mechanism dependent on TXNIP (Lerner et al. 2012; Oslowski et al. 2012).

Cellular stress impacts protein folding, thus the UPR is also well situated to sense danger in the form of aberrantly produced or misfolded proteins and contribute to immune responses. One way in which the UPR tunes immune responses is through the modulation of cytokine production (Logue et al. 2018; Smith 2018). These cytokines are soluble secreted proteins of the interleukins, IFNs, and tumor necrosis factor (TNF) family members among other secreted factors. The UPR influences cytokine production on multiple levels, from stimulation of pattern recognition receptors (PRRs) to modulation of inflammatory signaling pathways, and the regulation of cytokine transcription factors (Smith 2018). UPR can enhance PRRs that could potentially cause increased cytokine production in the absence of infection leading to inflammatory conditions in β-cells, such as Janus kinase/signal transducer and activator of transcription (JAK/STAT) signaling. In the β-cells, the triggering of the JAK/STAT pathway, such as downstream from type I IFN signaling (Fig. 1B) or in response to other cytokines results in phosphorylation of the STAT family of proteins, which together with IRF transcription factors activates expression of interferon-stimulated genes (ISGs) (Fig. 1B). Notably, the JAK/STAT pathway in β-cells leads to up-regulation of HLA class I expression, persistent ER stress, and chemokine production (Marroqui et al. 2021). Chemokines including

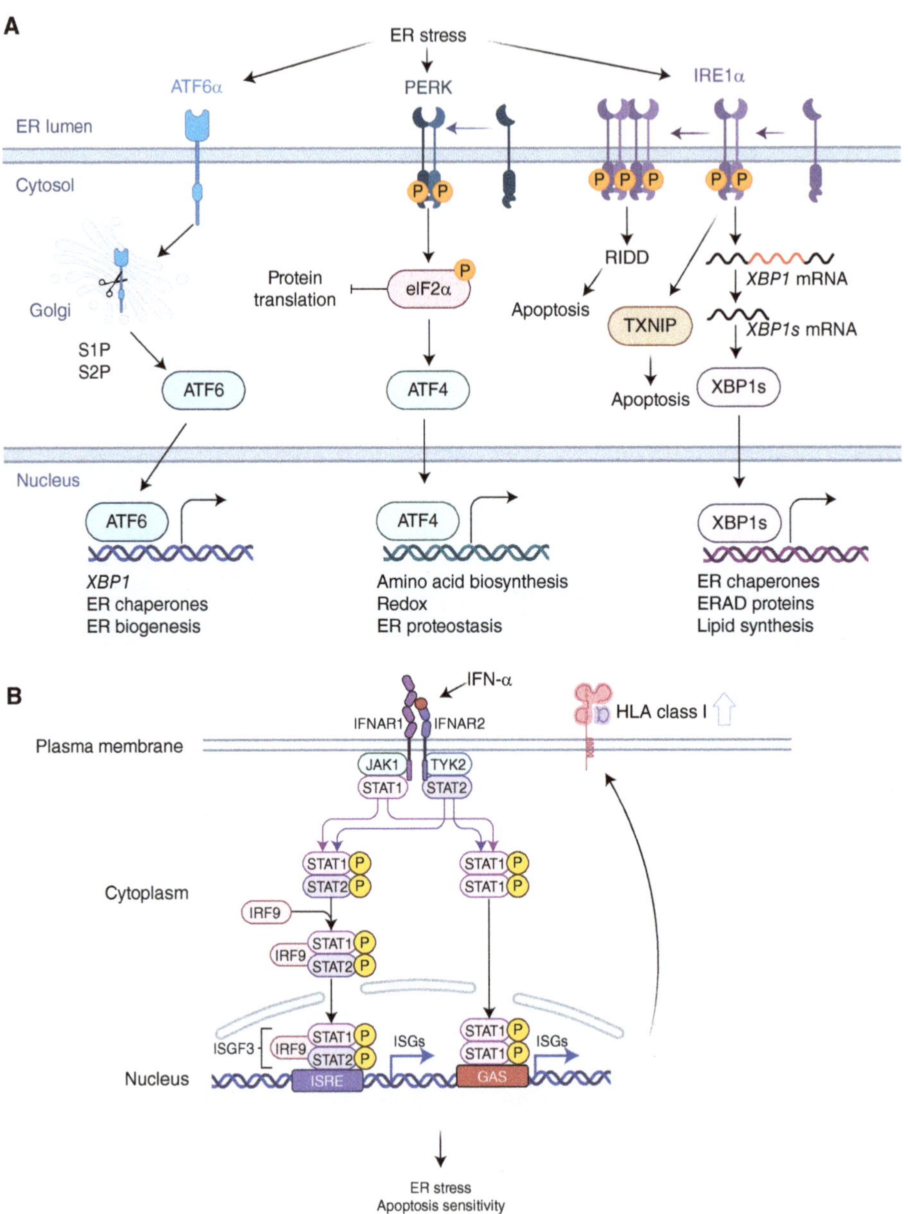

Figure 1. Overview of human β-cell unfolded protein response (UPR) and interferon (IFN)-mediated Janus kinase/signal transducer and activator of transcription (JAK/STAT) signaling. (*A*) UPR is activated in response to unfolded proteins in the lumen of the endoplasmic reticulum (ER), and resulting in ER stress leading to IRE1α, PERK, or ATF6 activation. IRE1α RNAse and kinase activities lead to regulated IRE1 dependent decay (RIDD) and XBP1 mRNA splicing. RIDD is capable of promoting apoptosis in the absence of resolution of ER stress. Spliced XBP1 (XBP1s) is a transcription factor that activates UPR genes downstream from IRE1 signaling to promote adaptive responses, such as ER-associated degradation (ERAD). Chronic stress leads to hyperactivation of IRE1α, up-regulation of TXNIP expression, and apoptosis. PERK phosphorylates eIF2a to shut down translation and can also activate a transcriptional response involving ATF4. ATF6 is cleaved in the Golgi and translocates to the nucleus where it regulates UPR genes to promote adaptive responses. (The figure is based on data from Sahin et al. 2021 and was created with BioRender, biorender.com.) (*B*) IFN signaling is activated upon IFNα/β binding to the receptor IFNAR triggering activation of JAK/STAT signaling and interferon stimulated gene (ISG) activation from phospho-STAT1/2 and IRF9 transcription factors. This leads to chemokine production (CXCL9, CXCL10), ER stress, and up-regulation of HLA class I. IFN signaling further sensitizes β-cells to UPR-mediated apoptosis due to chronic ER stress. (Figure generated with BioRender, biorender.com.)

Cite this article as *Cold Spring Harb Perspect Med* doi: 10.1101/cshperspect.a041605

CXCL10 and CXCL9 can promote the recruitment of T cells to islets (Christen and Kimmel 2020), consistent with a potential mechanism of immune surveillance. ER stress resulting from JAK/STAT signaling (Fig. 1B) could also elicit a feedforward loop exacerbating UPR (Fig. 1A), which links the type I IFN response with UPR in β-cells (Marroqui et al. 2021). A recent phase II clinical trial using JAK/STAT pathway inhibitor baricitinib in stage 3 new-onset T1D patients showed a beneficial effect in reducing the decline in residual β-cell function (Waibel et al. 2023), supporting the role of this stress pathway as an effective drug target in T1D.

Our understanding of the role of β-cell UPR in T1D is largely derived from studies in mouse models and rodent β-cell lines. Early work showed that markers of UPR precede insulitis and hyperglycemia in NOD mice (Tersey et al. 2012) and later work demonstrated that small molecule inhibition of IRE1α protects against spontaneous diabetes development and can even reverse new-onset hyperglycemia in NOD mice (Morita et al. 2017). Similarly, the bile acid tauroursodeoxycholic acid (TUDCA), which promotes protein folding and stability, can reduce the incidence of diabetes in NOD mice and in a virally induced T-cell-mediated model of diabetes (Engin et al. 2013). Notably, the protective effect of TUDCA required ATF6; mice with *Atf6α* knockout in β-cells were not protected in this model (Engin et al. 2013). Genetic evidence from β-cell-specific *Ire1α* and *Atf6α* knockout NOD mice has revealed previously unanticipated complexity in the UPR. Despite putative adaptive mechanisms, deletion of either of these UPR sensors in NOD mice leads to short-term negative consequences for β-cell differentiation and stress, but at later stages becomes protective and leads to a reduced incidence of disease in NOD mice (Lee et al. 2020, 2023). While the IRE1 and ATF6 branches are involved in T1D, mutation of PERK is known to lead to neonatal diabetes (Cnop et al. 2017), highlighting an essential role for β-cell survival and function distinct from the other two branches. In contrast with studies over the past 10 years in mouse models, comparatively less is understood about UPR mechanisms in human β-cells in T1D. Some evidence suggests that UPR is diminished in residual β-cells in T1D donors (Marhfour et al. 2012; Engin et al. 2013), but a comprehensive analysis of UPR branches and downstream markers across the natural history of T1D in humans has not been performed. Nevertheless, clinical trials using UPR modulating agents have strongly supported the role of this stress response in promoting β-cell loss during new-onset/stage 3 T1D, as will be discussed in detail below.

β-CELL SENESCENCE

A subpopulation of β-cells undergo a stress response that results in senescence during T1D (Fig. 2). Cellular senescence is the consequence of a stress response that can occur at any time but is more prone to occur during aging, leading to a permanent cell cycle and growth arrest and the development of several hallmark features (Di Micco et al. 2021). Features shared by most senescent cell types include up-regulation of cyclin-dependent kinase inhibitors, a DNA damage response, up-regulation of prosurvival signaling pathways, elevation of lysosomal β-galactosidase (termed senescence-associated-β-galactosidase [SA-βgal]) and secretion of a unique collection of cytokines, chemokines, proteases, shed receptors and growth factors, microRNAs, and extracellular vesicles termed senescence-associated secretory phenotype (SASP) (Di Micco et al. 2021). SASP generates an immune response (Marin et al. 2023) and elicits immune surveillance in other tissues to promote senescent cell clearance (Xue et al. 2007; Kang et al. 2011; Tasdemir et al. 2016). Senescent β-cells that arise during T1D in NOD mice and humans were shown to exhibit most of the same features of senescence in other cell types (Fig. 2; Cha et al. 2023). Senescent β-cells in NOD mice accumulate during the late prediabetic stage at ~14–16 weeks of age before the onset of hyperglycemia and are defined by elevated p21 expression, $p16^{Ink4a}$, a prosurvival phenotype mediated by up-regulation of Bcl-2, a DNA damage response indicated by Ser139-phosphorylated histone H2A.X (γ-H2A.X), high SA-βgal activity, and a SASP (Cha et al. 2023). As these cells are resistant

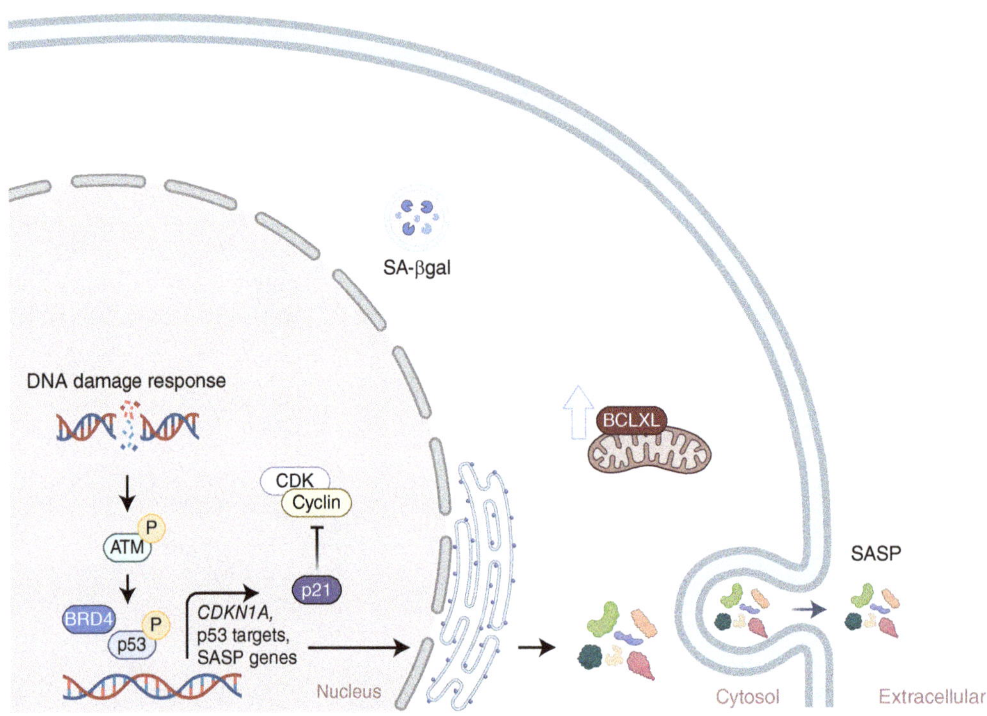

Figure 2. Overview of human β-cell senescence. The specific stress triggers that cause DNA damage leading to β-cell senescence during type 1 diabetes (T1D) are not known; however, direct DNA damage is sufficient to elicit downstream senescence phenotypes. DNA damage provokes a DNA damage response involving autophosphorylation of sensor kinase ATM at Ser1981, which phosphorylates and activates p53. p53 drives a transcriptional program involving *CDKN1A* (encoding p21), senescence-associated secretory phenotype (SASP) genes and other p53 target genes. Senescence/SASP gene activation also involves bromodomain and extraterminal domain (BET) proteins such as BRD4. Up-regulation of p21 suppresses cyclin-dependent kinase/cyclin complexes (CDK/cyclin) in the nucleus. Senescent β-cells also up-regulate senescence-associated β-galactosidase (SA-βgal) activity in the lysosome and increase expression of antiapoptotic gene *BCL2L1* (and potential up-regulation of protein BCL-XL). Expression of SASP genes leads to the secretion of SASP factors including GDF15, IGFBP4, CXCL1, and IL-8. (Figure generated with BioRender, biorender.com.)

to apoptosis due to the up-regulation of Bcl-2, they are particularly sensitive to Bcl-2 inhibitors, which exploit this sensitivity to trigger apoptosis. This family of drugs is known as senolytic compounds as they preferentially eliminate senescent cells (Kirkland and Tchkonia 2020). Senolytic treatment of NOD mice at late prediabetic stages eliminated senescent β-cells, preserved healthy β-cell mass, and maintained glucose control without an apparent effect on the immune system (Thompson et al. 2019b). A major caveat is that Bcl-2 inhibitors eliminated all senescent cells, not just senescent β-cells. However, the lesson from these studies is that elimination of senescent cells reduced immune infiltration and β-cell destruction. Indeed we also found that suppression of the SASP with a bromodomain and extraterminal domain (BET) domain family inhibitor iBET-762, slowed disease progression in NOD mice (Thompson et al. 2019a), consistent with earlier work using an older generation BET protein inhibitor iBET-151 (Fu et al. 2014). We postulated an endogenous mechanism of immune surveillance normally restrains senescent β-cell accumulation in NOD mice, but failed during disease progression, which led us to identify cell surface receptors up-regulated on senescent β-cells to identify immune targets. Indeed, senescent β-cells were found to up-regulate MHC class I and adaptor molecule *β-2-microglobulin* by single-cell RNA-seq analysis (Thompson et al. 2019b), suggesting an altered dialogue with the immune system. In additional studies, we found that other senescent cell types up-regulated an MHC class I–like molecule CD1d, which presents lipid antigens to invariant natural killer T (iNKT) cells, leading us to explore the role of iNKT cells in the immune surveillance of senescent cells in adipose tissue and lung (Arora et al. 2021). Thus, a unifying feature of our previous work in this field was that stressed cells (in this case senescent) have altered interactions with the immune system and escape from surveillance, promoting their accumulation, which accelerates disease progression.

In contrast with studies in NOD mice, considerably less is known about senescence in human β-cells during T1D. In human pancreas studies on a small cohort of donors ($n = 6$ per group), recent-onset T1D (0–6 yr) and AA+ donors (1–3 autoantibodies) had higher frequencies of β-cells expressing p21 but not p16^{INK4A}, and higher frequencies of β-cells with elevated SA-βgal activity and SASP factors IL-6 and SERPINE1 (Thompson et al. 2019b). Markers of the p21 senescence program are also apparent in residual β-cells in T1D donors as assessed by single-cell RNA-seq data analysis (Lee et al. 2023). While it is not known what stressor(s) causes β-cells to activate a senescence response in during the natural history of T1D, similar phenotypes can be evoked in human islet β-cells or EndoC-βH5 human fetal-derived β-cells in culture upon exposure to chemically induced sublethal DNA double-strand break damage (Brawerman et al. 2022b). Senescence phenotypes induced by DNA damage in human β-cell models include stable activation of the ATM-p53-p21 pathway, a p53-driven and BET protein-dependent transcriptional program, up-regulation and secretion of SASP factors, and up-regulation of *BCL2L1* mRNA levels, encoding BCL-XL (Fig. 3; Thompson et al. 2019a; Brawerman et al. 2022b). In contrast with other cell types, p16^{INK4a} mRNA or protein is not up-regulated during the senescence response to DNA damage in human islet or EndoC cells (Fig. 3; Thompson et al. 2019a,b; Brawerman et al. 2022b), suggesting p21 plays a more dominant role. In further support of the idea that unrepaired DNA damage elicits senescence, a higher frequency of human β-cells had markers of DNA damage and repair in recently diagnosed stage 3 T1D donors as compared with control normoglycemic donors, which correlated with degree of islet insulitis (Horwitz et al. 2018). Whatever the mechanisms that trigger senescence in β-cells, this stress response is apparently unique to β-cells during T1D, since α-cells do not show the same signatures of senescence in NOD mice or T1D donor pancreas (Brawerman et al. 2022a). Although there is ample evidence to support the involvement of β-cell senescence in T1D in humans, our current knowledge of this response still has major gaps and is not yet sufficient to justify clinical trials of senescence-targeted agents in new-onset T1D patients, as has been done for agents targeting UPR. Future work to elucidate the mechanisms that drive senescence in β-cells during T1D, its impacts of insulin secretion and immune signaling, and the development of agents with appropriate specificity to target β-cell senescence pathways will be required to move this field forward into a clinical setting.

INTERACTIONS BETWEEN β-CELL STRESS RESPONSES IN T1D

A critical element that is often overlooked in the discussion of β-cell stress pathways is the heterogeneity among stress responses and how they relate to one another. While the field has come to recognize that heterogeneity exists on multiple levels among β-cells within an islet and between islets (Miranda et al. 2021), it is less appreciated that stress responses in β-cells do not occur in isolation of each other and that different stress responses may be occurring in β-cells that reside in the same islet during T1D, a feature that may correspond to clinical heterogeneity in the disease (Thompson et al. 2023). The best example of this is the way in which proinflammatory cytokine stress leads to apoptosis in some islet β-cells, but some cells survive this stress and remain alive (Stancill et al. 2021). Similarly, the induction of a generally sublethal stress of chemical DNA dou-

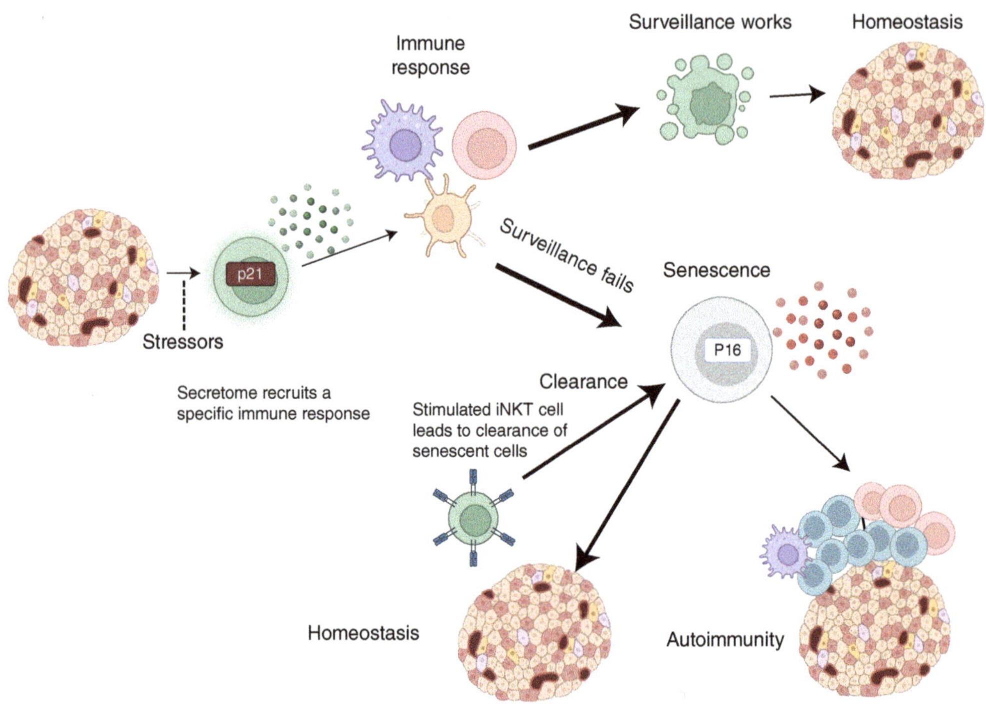

Figure 3. Mechanism of immune surveillance of stressed β-cells in type 1 diabetes (T1D). We hypothesize that p21 expression drives an early surveillance secretome from β-cells, activating resident immune cells to remove these stressed β-cells and restore homeostasis. However, if this response fails, β-cells progress to late-stage senescence (elevated $p16^{Ink4a}$) and senescence-associated secretory phenotype (SASP) accumulate, a process that accelerates autoimmunity and T1D progression. Activation of invariant natural killer T (iNKT) cells with α-galactosylceramide leads to a systemic surveillance response that may clear senescent β-cells from islets. (Figure generated with BioRender, biorender.com.)

ble-strand break damage in human islets nevertheless leads some β-cells to activate senescence while others undergo apoptosis (Brawerman et al. 2022a). Thus, exposure to the same stressor can lead to different outcomes for different β-cells within a population. Moreover, within each of the stress responses outlined above, there are some common molecular underpinnings. For instance, the type I IFN response involves ER stress signaling through the PERK and IRE1α branches as a result of chemokine production (Marroqui et al. 2021), providing a clear link between the IFN pathway and UPR. Late-stage senescence can also lead to a type I IFN response in some cell types (De Cecco et al. 2019). Similarly, while DNA damage is a potent inducer of senescence in β-cells (Brawerman et al. 2022b), it can also elicit UPR activation in other cell types (Dufey et al. 2020). Disruption of one stress response may trigger another as was shown in a recent study in which it was found that deletion of UPR mediator *Atf6α* in β-cells leads to an early senescence program that is ultimately protective against spontaneous diabetes development in NOD mice (Lee et al. 2023). Major knowledge gaps remain in understanding the interrelationships between β-cell stress phenotypes, and investigating this heterogeneity is likely to be a fruitful area of investigation in T1D for many years to come.

CLINICAL TRANSLATION OF AGENTS TARGETING β STRESS IN T1D

In just the past 6 years, there have been four published placebo-controlled, adequately powered

 Cite this article as *Cold Spring Harb Perspect Med* doi: 10.1101/cshperspect.a041605

multisite clinical trials using agents that act on β-cell stress in T1D (Ovalle et al. 2018; Gitelman et al. 2021; Forlenza et al. 2023; Waibel et al. 2023). All tested agents were administered orally alongside normal insulin regimens and were used within 30–100 days after clinical disease diagnosis at stage 3 symptomatic T1D, as it is well known that residual β-cell function continues to decline for up to 5 years after diagnosis (Oram et al. 2019), and passing the hurdle of efficacy at the diagnosis stage is an important milestone to support additional trials at earlier disease stages (as was done with teplizumab). Even though agents mitigating β-cell stress are most likely to show the best efficacy during presymptomatic T1D stages where there are more β-cells left, these recent trials have paved the way for further work and provided important insights, translating preclinical studies from the NOD model to humans. The main takeaway from these studies is that it is possible to target stressed β-cells directly to slow the decline in functional β-cell mass after clinical diagnosis of T1D. On the other hand, excitement from these early trials is tempered by issues with dose-related side effects, the need for continual administration, and the unclear long-term effects on the health of pediatric populations most likely to benefit from these agents.

CLINICAL TRANSLATION OF UPR AGENTS

Agents that shift the UPR fate decision toward adaptation and survival and away from terminal UPR and apoptosis have been tested in randomized double-blind phase II placebo-controlled clinical trials at stage 3 symptomatic diabetes onset. These agents include the inhibitor TXNIP verapamil (NCT02372253 and NCT04233034) (Ovalle et al. 2018; Forlenza et al. 2023) and the IRE1α modulator imatinib (NCT01781975) (Gitelman et al. 2021). One clinical trial is still ongoing for the use of the bile acid derivative TUDCA (NCT02218619), previously shown to delay diabetes in NOD mice (Engin et al. 2013).

In the first clinical trial targeting β-cell stress in T1D, verapamil, an FDA-approved calcium channel blocker and vasodilator initially used in the 1960s for treating heart disease (Arefanian et al. 2023), was tested in a small trial where adult T1D patients (ages 18–45) within 100 days of diagnosis received 400 mg/day oral dose of verapamil (n = 11) or a placebo (n = 13) for 12 months (Ovalle et al. 2018). Measures of stimulated C-peptide levels and changes (mixed meal test), insulin use, glucose monitor time in range, and HbA1c were monitored at 3, 6, and 12 months. Notably, patients who received verapamil showed better outcomes across these measurements as compared with placebo and there were no substantial differences in adverse outcomes or measures of blood pressure (Ovalle et al. 2018). Following this trial, a larger pediatric trial was recently conducted using verapamil (n = 47 initial analysis) or placebo (n = 38 initial analysis) on patients ages 7–17 (Forlenza et al. 2023). This trial used a dose-escalation protocol where subjects were progressively stratified, moving from 60–120 mg/day up to 240–360 mg/day, as tolerated by the end of the trial. Once again, this trial observed a benefit of oral daily verapamil treatment over 52 weeks, with improvements to C-peptide, HbA1c, lower use of insulin, and better glycemic control in verapamil-treated patients as compared with placebo controls (Forlenza et al. 2023). However, there were more adverse events noted in the verapamil-treated cohort as compared with the control, including nausea/vomiting, headache, constipation, and electrocardiogram abnormalities (Forlenza et al. 2023). As this trial was done with pediatric patients where the effects of continual dosing (up to 1 yr) with verapamil have not been determined, long-term safety concerns have been raised (Hsu et al. 2023). In addition, verapamil has a wide variety of effects that go beyond only its effects on TXNIP expression (Xu et al. 2022) and how these may be altered in a pediatric population remains to be determined. Also, the effect of verapamil is rapidly reversible with discontinuation of use (Xu et al. 2022), indicating it has only a temporal and acutely stabilizing effect on β-cell function.

The tyrosine kinase ABL inhibitor imatinib was tested in a phase II randomized double-blind placebo-controlled trial on newly diagnosed (<100 d) adult T1D patients (Gitelman et al. 2021). Imatinib has been widely used in the treatment of leukemia, where it preferentially triggers apoptosis in cells overexpressing ABL due to gene translocation and fusion (Welsh 2022). Earlier work indicated that imatinib (also known as Gleevec), inhibits the interaction of ABL with IRE1α leading to a shift in UPR toward an adaptive response and reversing established insulitis and diabetes in the NOD mouse model (Morita et al. 2017). Although the effect of imatinib was suggested to be directly on β-cell UPR, it was later shown that the effect on T1D reversal in NOD mice required B cells, where the drug was found to improve reactive oxygen species levels in B cells, which helped β-cells recover from hyperglycemic stress (Wilson et al. 2019). In the trial, adult patients received 400 mg of the drug ($n = 45$) or placebo ($n = 22$) orally each day for 26 weeks, followed by assessment of β-cell function, glycemic control, and insulin use up to 24 months from protocol start (Gitelman et al. 2021). The study found a significant preservation of β-cell function effective within the first 3–6 months (in imatinib-treated subjects while taking the drug), but the effect was not sustained longer after cessation of imatinib (Gitelman et al. 2021). Unfortunately, there were a large number and wide range of adverse events in the imatinib group (172 events) as compared with the placebo (28 events), including infections, and endocrine, nervous, psychiatric, respiratory, and most commonly gastrointestinal symptoms (Gitelman et al. 2021), suggesting dosing needs to be carefully titrated and monitored. This concern is especially important in light of observations that the dose at which imatinib has protective effects on β-cells (micromolar range) is orders of magnitude higher than the dose at which it is selective for ABL inhibition (nanomolar range) (Welsh 2022), and thus high dosing is likely to lead to off-target effects and toxicity.

CLINICAL TRANSLATION OF SENESCENCE-TARGETED AGENTS

Senescence-targeted therapies have not yet been tested in clinical trials for T1D. However, approaches to target senescence in other diseases use one of two different modalities: senolytics and senomorphics. Senolytics target key prosurvival signaling pathways in senescent cells and tip the apoptosis-survival balance toward apoptosis preferentially in senescent cells (Chaib et al. 2022). Senomorphics modify the senescent cell phenotype in a beneficial way, most commonly by inhibiting or suppressing the inflammatory component of SASP to neutralize its deleterious effects on the tissue microenvironment (Huang et al. 2022). Evidence-based trials in T1D using senescence-targeting agents would require (1) knowledge of the specific prosurvival signaling or SASP regulation in human β-cells to target with these agents, and (2) noninvasive biomarker(s) to measure the burden of senescent β-cells and efficacy of the senescence-targeted therapy in patients in the clinic. Previous work showed that senescent β-cells in NOD mice use up-regulation of Bcl-2 protein levels as a druggable mechanism to resist apoptosis (Thompson et al. 2019b), and senescent human β-cells arising in aged human donor islets can be depleted with the BCL-2 family inhibitor ABT-263 (Aguayo-Mazzucato et al. 2019). Whether this occurs in senescent β-cells in T1D donors has not been established and thus the mechanisms of the prosurvival signaling in senescent human β-cells in T1D remain to be determined. The mechanism of SASP in senescent β-cells in NOD mice and a DNA damage–induced human islet senescence model involves BET protein-mediated transcriptional activation (Thompson et al. 2019a), which is amenable to targeting using small molecule BET inhibitors that block BET protein binding to chromatin. BET inhibitors have been clinically tested in patients with solid malignancies involving BRD4-driven transcriptional programs and have shown promise (Piha-Paul et al. 2020). However, since BET proteins are ubiquitously expressed, these inhibitors would most likely have many adverse off-target effects in other tissues if used for T1D patients. In addition, no biomarkers are yet available to monitor senescent β-cell burden. Nevertheless, clinical translation of senescence-targeted approaches for treating T1D is on the horizon and the benefits and drawbacks of targeting senescence with pharmacological agents must be carefully considered.

While senolytics are very effective in eliminating all the negative effects of senescent cells, recent work suggests that there are beneficial aspects of some types of senescent cells, particularly those expressing high levels of p16^{INK4A} (Grosse et al. 2020). Therefore, caution is warranted with senolytic agents that act by nonspecifically removing any kind of senescent cell. An additional consideration is achieving the optimal dose, because senolytics act on ubiquitous targets senescent cells are sensitized to these agents but normal cells can also be affected (Chaib et al. 2022). Since senolytics trigger apoptosis of the senescent cell population, the question is raised of how this would impact overall functional β-cell mass and disease progression at different stages of T1D. Senolytic agents would likely be most effective at early stages (stages 1 and 2) and would not be very effective after onset of stage 3 clinical disease because there are already so few remaining β-cells in most patients. On the other hand, senomorphic agents could preserve β-cell function by mitigating the negative impacts of inflammatory SASP factors. As a disadvantage, senomorphic agents do not specifically act on senescent cells; they act on a variety of ubiquitous cell signaling pathways, leading to problematic off-target effects.

A third approach to target senescent cells that has recently emerged is the use of activating the immune system to clear senescent cells (Prata et al. 2018). Chimeric antigen receptor (CAR) T cells specific to senescence-associated antigens, activation of iNKT cells, and programmed cell death 1 ligand 1 (PDL1) blockade have all been used in mouse models as a way to harness the immune system to eliminate pathologic senescent cells during aging and in various diseases involving liver, adipose, and lung (Amor et al. 2020; Arora et al. 2021; Wang et al. 2022). In terms of clinical trials for targeting senescence in other diseases, promising results have been obtained from small early phases I and II clinical trials using senolytic therapies. The senolytic combination of dasatinib and quercetin (D+Q) has shown positive outcomes with minimal adverse effects in age-related diseases, including idiopathic pulmonary fibrosis, diabetic kidney disease, and Alzheimer's disease (Hickson et al. 2019; Justice et al. 2019; Gonzales et al. 2023). Therefore, the road to using these senescence-targeted agents in T1D will be informed by ongoing and completed clinical trials in other fields.

IMMUNE SURVEILLANCE OF STRESSED β-CELLS

How can different stress responses such as UPR and senescence aggravate disease progression? Secretion of inflammatory factors, leading to an immune surveillance response aimed at restoring homeostasis, which eventually fails, is a unifying mechanism to explain how different stress responses like UPR and senescence could promote T1D progression. We propose that UPR stressed or senescent β-cells accumulate because of a failure of immune surveillance, a notion supported by studies in other tissues during aging and cancer (Fig. 3; Ovadya et al. 2018; Yousefzadeh et al. 2021). Chemokine production from UPR stressed β-cells (Fig. 1A,B) or SASP from senescent β-cells (Fig. 2) could trigger immune surveillance, but failure of surveillance would favor their accumulation, ultimately promoting T1D (Fig. 3). Accordingly, agents that shift UPR toward an adaptive response (Engin et al. 2013) block JAK/STAT signaling (Li and McDevitt 2011), remove senescent cells (Thompson et al. 2019b), or inhibit SASP (Thompson et al. 2019a) all significantly delay T1D onset in NOD mice. Although it remains to be determined how senescent β-cells interact with the islet-resident immune compartment, recently published data indicate that senescent cells in adipose and lung interact with the innate immune compartment with clearance mechanisms attributable to iNKT cells (Arora et al. 2021). iNKT cells function as an endogenous immune surveillance mechanism that normally recognizes pathological senescent cells and initiates their removal to maintain tissue homeostasis. iNKT cells, unlike other T cells, are activated by lipid antigens bound to CD1d, an MHC class I–related molecule (Godfrey et al. 2010). CD1d, typically expressed by antigen-presenting cells, showed elevated expression in senescent preadipocytes and lung fibroblasts compared to control/nonsenescent cells (Arora et al. 2021), suggesting a link between senescence and iNKT regulation. Earlier work has established a link between iNKTs and T1D. iNKT cell frequencies in circulation are reduced in NOD mice and T1D patients (Poulton et al. 2001; Kis et al. 2007; Roman-Gonzalez et al. 2009; Beristain-Covarrubias et al. 2015) as well as during aging (Jing et al. 2007). Stimulating iNKT cells with α-galactosylceramide, a synthetic ligand for CD1d, was sufficient to prevent diabetes in NOD mice (Hong et al. 2001; Sharif et al. 2001). Thus, it is plausible that iNKT activation could promote immune surveillance and clearance of senescent β-cells in the context of T1D (Fig. 3). The observation that lipid antigens presented by dendritic cells lead to stimulation contrasts with lipid antigens presented by B cells that result in iNKT cell anergy (Parekh et al. 2005) and suggests that it is possible senescent cells that up-regulate CD1d could induce iNKT cell anergy. However, this anergy can be overcome by direct stimulation of iNKT cells with α-galactosylceramide resulting in clearance to senescent cells in different tissues (Arora et al. 2021).

UPR and senescence both result in β-cells acquiring a secretory profile that likely generates different immune responses. Recent work suggests that in response to cellular stress, macrophages are recruited to allow repair but in the absence of repair, immune surveillance mediated by T lymphocytes removes the damaged cells (Sturmlechner et al. 2021). We propose that early p21 expression likewise initially drives immune surveillance of β-cells by islet-resident immune cells (Fig. 3). However, when immune surveillance fails, β-cells acquire a late senescent fate leading to accumulation (Fig. 3). In this scenario, the same stressed β-cell could move from ER stress as an early response to senescence as a late response as it evades immune clearance.

CONCLUDING REMARKS

Our knowledge of the mechanisms of β-cell stress pathways, and how they interrelate and influence T1D pathology is still in its infancy as compared with the decades of effort invested in studying the immune system. As it is increasingly being recognized that stressed islets/β-cells play an important role in the immune response in T1D, future efforts to decipher stress response pathways in islet cells and how they may be targeted therapeutically remain a promising endeavor for the field. Defective immune surveillance of stressed inflammatory β-cells early in the disease is a unifying concept to explain how diverse mechanisms such as UPR and senescence can both promote T1D progression. The first clinical trials using agents targeting β-cell UPR in new-onset T1D patients have taught us lessons that will pave the way for applying these and other interventions at earlier disease stages where there are more functional β-cells and hence more potential for beneficial clinical impact. Designing immunotherapies that take islet cell stress into account and are tailored to the individual at early disease stages may well be the next frontier in personalized medicine for T1D.

ACKNOWLEDGMENTS

We apologize to our colleagues whose work could not be cited due to space limitations. The laboratory of P.J.T. is supported by grants from the Canadian Institutes of Health Research (PJT-479641, TDP-485691, and TDP-485915), the Juvenile Diabetes Research Foundation (4-SRA-2023-1182-S-N and 4-SRA-2023-1384-S-N), a new investigator operating grant from Research Manitoba (5351), an operating grant from the Health Sciences Centre Foundation Winnipeg, and an End Diabetes 2022 Award from Diabetes Canada (OG-3-22-5694-PT). The laboratory of A.B. is supported by the JDRF Center of Excellence Grant and NIH R01DK121794.

REFERENCES

Aguayo-Mazzucato C, Andle J, Lee TB, Midha A, Talemal L, Chipashvili V, Hollister-Lock J, van Deursen J, Weir G, Bonner-Weir S. 2019. Acceleration of β cell aging determines diabetes and senolysis improves disease outcomes. *Cell Metab* **30:** 129–142.e4. doi:10.1016/j.cmet.2019.05.006

Amor C, Feucht J, Leibold J, Ho YJ, Zhu C, Alonso-Curbelo D, Mansilla-Soto J, Boyer JA, Li X, Giavridis T, et al. 2020. Senolytic CAR T cells reverse senescence-associated pathologies. *Nature* **583:** 127–132. doi:10.1038/s41586-020-2403-9

Arefanian H, Koti L, Sindhu S, Ahmad R, Al Madhoun A, Al-Mulla F. 2023. Verapamil chronicles: advances from cardiovascular to pancreatic β-cell protection. *Front Pharmacol* **14:** 1–10. doi:10.3389/fphar.2023.1322148

Arora S, Thompson PJ, Wang Y, Bhattacharyya A, Apostolopoulou H, Hatano R, Naikawadi RP, Shah A, Wolters PJ, Koliwad SK, et al. 2021. Invariant natural killer T cells coordinate clearance of senescent cells. *Med* **2:** 938–950.e8. doi:10.1016/j.medj.2021.04.014

Benaglio P, Zhu H, Okino ML, Yan J, Elgamal R, Nariai N, Beebe E, Korgaonkar K, Qiu Y, Donovan MKR, et al. 2022.

Type 1 diabetes risk genes mediate pancreatic β cell survival in response to proinflammatory cytokines. *Cell Genom* **2:** 100214. doi:10.1016/j.xgen.2022.100214

Beristain-Covarrubias N, Canche-pool E, Gomez-diaz R, Sanchez-torres LE, Ortiz-Navarrete V. 2015. Reduced iNKT cells numbers in type 1 diabetes patients and their first-degree relatives. *Immun Inflamm Dis* **3:** 411–419. doi:10.1002/iid3.79

Bluestone JA, Buckner JH, Herold KC. 2021. Immunotherapy: building a bridge to a cure for type 1 diabetes. *Science* **373:** 510–516. doi:10.1126/science.abh1654

Bottazzo GF, Florin-Christensen A, Doniach D. 1974. Islet-cell antibodies in diabetes mellitus with autoimmune polyendocrine deficiencies. *Lancet* **304:** 1279–1283. doi: 10.1016/s0140-6736(74)90140-8

Brawerman G, Thompson PJ. 2020. β Cell therapies for preventing type 1 diabetes: from bench to bedside. *Biomolecules* **10:** 1681. doi:10.3390/biom10121681

Brawerman G, Ntranos V, Thompson PJ. 2022a. α Cell dysfunction in type 1 diabetes is independent of a senescence program. *Front Endocrinol* **13:** 932516. doi:10.3389/fendo.2022.932516

Brawerman G, Pipella J, Thompson PJ. 2022b. DNA damage to β cells in culture recapitulates features of senescent β cells that accumulate in type 1 diabetes. *Mol Metab* **62:** 101524. doi:10.1016/j.molmet.2022.101524

Brissova M, Haliyur R, Saunders D, Shrestha S, Dai C, Blodgett DM, Bottino R, Campbell-Thompson M, Aramandla R, Poffenberger G, et al. 2018. α Cell function and gene expression are compromised in type 1 diabetes. *Cell Rep* **22:** 2667–2676. doi:10.1016/j.celrep.2018.02.032

Carrano AC, Mulas F, Zeng C, Sander M. 2017. Interrogating islets in health and disease with single-cell technologies. *Mol Metab* **6:** 991–1001. doi:10.1016/j.molmet.2017.04.012

Carré A, Richardson SJ, Larger E, Mallone R. 2021. Presumption of guilt for T cells in type 1 diabetes: lead culprits or partners in crime depending on age of onset? *Diabetologia* **64:** 15–25. doi:10.1007/s00125-020-05298-y

Cha J, Aguayo-Mazzucato C, Thompson PJ. 2023. Pancreatic β-cell senescence in diabetes: mechanisms, markers and therapies. *Front Endocrinol (Lausanne)* **14:** 1212716. doi:10.3389/fendo.2023.1212716

Chaib S, Tchkonia T, Kirkland JL. 2022. Cellular senescence and senolytics: the path to the clinic. *Nat Med* **28:** 1556–1568. doi:10.1038/s41591-022-01923-y

Chiou J, Geusz RJ, Okino ML, Han JY, Miller M, Melton R, Beebe E, Benaglio P, Huang S, Korgaonkar K, et al. 2021a. Interpreting type 1 diabetes risk with genetics and single-cell epigenomics. *Nature* **594:** 398–402. doi:10.1038/s41586-021-03552-w

Chiou J, Zeng C, Cheng Z, Han JY, Schlichting M, Miller M, Mendez R, Huang S, Wang J, Sui Y, et al. 2021b. Single-cell chromatin accessibility identifies pancreatic islet cell type- and state-specific regulatory programs of diabetes risk. *Nat Genet* **53:** 455–466. doi:10.1038/s41588-021-00823-0

Christen U, Kimmel R. 2020. Chemokines as drivers of the autoimmune destruction in type 1 diabetes: opportunity for therapeutic intervention in consideration of an optimal treatment schedule. *Front Endocrinol (Lausanne)* **11:** 1–12. doi:10.3389/fendo.2020.591083

Cnop M, Toivonen S, Igoillo-Esteve M, Salpea P. 2017. Endoplasmic reticulum stress and eIF2α phosphorylation: the Achilles heel of pancreatic β cells. *Mol Metab* **6:** 1024–1039. doi:10.1016/j.molmet.2017.06.001

Craighead JE. 1978. Current views on the etiology of insulin-dependent diabetes mellitus. *N Engl J Med* **299:** 1439–1445. doi:10.1056/NEJM197812282992605

Damond N, Engler S, Zanotelli VRT, Schapiro D, Wasserfall CH, Kusmartseva I, Nick HS, Thorel F, Herrera PL, Atkinson MA, et al. 2019. A map of human type 1 diabetes progression by imaging mass cytometry. *Cell Metab* **29:** 755–768.e5. doi:10.1016/j.cmet.2018.11.014

De Cecco M, Ito T, Petrashen AP, Elias AE, Skvir NJ, Criscione SW, Caligiana A, Brocculi G, Adney EM, Boeke JD, et al. 2019. L1 drives IFN in senescent cells and promotes age-associated inflammation. *Nature* **566:** 73–78. doi:10.1038/s41586-018-0784-9

Di Micco R, Krizhanovsky V, Baker D, d'Adda di Fagagna F. 2021. Cellular senescence in ageing: from mechanisms to therapeutic opportunities. *Nat Rev Mol Cell Biol* **22:** 75–95. doi:10.1038/s41580-020-00314-w

Doliba NM, Rozo AV, Roman J, Qin W, Traum D, Gao L, Liu J, Manduchi E, Liu C, Golson ML, et al. 2022. α Cell dysfunction in islets from nondiabetic, glutamic acid decarboxylase autoantibody–positive individuals. *J Clin Invest* **132:** e156243. doi:10.1172/JCI156243

Dufey E, Bravo-San Pedro JM, Eggers C, González-Quiroz M, Urra H, Sagredo AI, Sepulveda D, Pihán P, Carreras-Sureda A, Hazari Y, et al. 2020. Genotoxic stress triggers the activation of IRE1α-dependent RNA decay to modulate the DNA damage response. *Nat Commun* **11:** 1–13. doi:10.1038/s41467-020-15694-y

Elgamal RM, Kudtarkar P, Melton RL, Mummey HM, Benaglio P, Okino ML, Gaulton KJ. 2023. An integrated map of cell type-specific gene expression in pancreatic islets. *Diabetes* **72:** 1719–1728. doi:10.2337/db23-0130

Engin F, Yermalovich A, Nguyen T, Hummasti S, Fu W, Eizirik DL, Mathis D, Hotamisligil GS. 2013. Restoration of the unfolded protein response in pancreatic β cells protects mice against type 1 diabetes. *Sci Transl Med* **5:** 211ra156. doi:10.1126/scitranslmed.3006534

Evans-Molina C, Sims EK, Dimeglio LA, Ismail HM, Steck AK, Palmer JP, Krischer JP, Geyer S, Xu P, Sosenko JM. 2018. β Cell dysfunction exists for more than 5 years prior to type 1 diabetes diagnosis. *JCI Insight* **3:** e120877. doi:10.1172/jci

Fasolino M, Schwartz GW, Patil AR, Mongia A, Golson ML, Wang YJ, Morgan A, Liu C, Schug J, Liu J, et al. 2022. Single-cell multi-omics analysis of human pancreatic islets reveals novel cellular states in type 1 diabetes. *Nat Metab* **4:** 284–299. doi:10.1038/s42255-022-00531-x

Forlenza GP, McVean J, Beck RW, Bauza C, Bailey R, Buckingham B, Dimeglio LA, Sherr JL, Clements M, Neyman A, et al. 2023. Effect of verapamil on pancreatic β cell function in newly diagnosed pediatric type 1 diabetes: a randomized clinical trial. *J Am Med Assoc* **329:** 990–999. doi:10.1001/jama.2023.2064

Fu W, Farache J, Clardy SM, Hattori K, Mander P, Lee K, Rioja I, Weissleder R, Prinjha RK, Benoist C, et al. 2014. Epigenetic modulation of type-1 diabetes via a dual effect on pancreatic macrophages and β cells. *eLife* **3:** e04631. doi:10.7554/eLife.04631

Gale EAM. 2001. The discovery of type 1 diabetes. *Diabetes* **50:** 217–226. doi:10.2337/diabetes.50.2.217

Ghosh R, Colon-Negron K, Papa FR. 2019. Endoplasmic reticulum stress, degeneration of pancreatic islet β-cells, and therapeutic modulation of the unfolded protein response in diabetes. *Mol Metab* **27:** S60–S68. doi:10.1016/j.molmet.2019.06.012

Gitelman SE, Bundy BN, Ferrannini E, Lim N, Blanchfield JL, DiMeglio LA, Felner EI, Gaglia JL, Gottlieb PA, Long SA, et al. 2021. Imatinib therapy for patients with recent-onset type 1 diabetes: a multicentre, randomised, double-blind, placebo-controlled, phase 2 trial. *Lancet Diabetes Endocrinol* **9:** 502–514. doi:10.1016/S2213-8587(21)00139-X

Godfrey DI, Stankovic S, Baxter AG. 2010. Raising the NKT cell family. *Nat Immunol* **11:** 197–206. doi:10.1038/ni.1841

Gonzales MM, Garbarino VR, Kautz TF, Palavicini JP, Lopez-Cruzan M, Dehkordi SK, Mathews JJ, Zare H, Xu P, Zhang B, et al. 2023. Senolytic therapy in mild Alzheimer's disease: a phase 1 feasibility trial. *Nat Med* **29:** 2481–2488. doi:10.1038/s41591-023-02543-w

Grosse L, Wagner N, Emelyanov A, Molina C, Lacas-Gervais S, Wagner KD, Bulavin DV. 2020. Defined p16High senescent cell types are indispensable for mouse healthspan. *Cell Metab* **32:** 87–99.e6. doi:10.1016/j.cmet.2020.05.002

Herold KC, Bundy BN, Alice Long S, Bluestone JA, DiMeglio LA, Dufort MJ, Gitelman SE, Gottlieb PA, Krischer JP, Linsley PS, et al. 2019. An anti-CD3 antibody, teplizumab, in relatives at risk for type 1 diabetes. *N Engl J Med* **381:** 603–613. doi:10.1056/NEJMoa1902226

Hickson LTJ, Langhi Prata LGP, Bobart SA, Evans TK, Giorgadze N, Hashmi SK, Herrmann SM, Jensen MD, Jia Q, Jordan KL, et al. 2019. Senolytics decrease senescent cells in humans: preliminary report from a clinical trial of Dasatinib plus Quercetin in individuals with diabetic kidney disease. *EBioMedicine* **47:** 446–456. doi:10.1016/j.ebiom.2019.08.069

Hong S, Wilson MT, Serizawa I, Wu L, Singh N, Naidenko OV, Miura T, Haba T, Scherer DC, Wei J, et al. 2001. The natural killer T-cell ligand α-galactosylceramide prevents autoimmune diabetes in non-obese diabetic mice. *Nat Med* **7:** 1052–1056. doi:10.1038/nm0901-1052

Horwitz E, Krogvold L, Zhitomirsky S, Swisa A, Fischman M, Lax T, Dahan T, Hurvitz N, Weinberg-Corem N, Klochendler A, et al. 2018. β-Cell DNA damage response promotes islet inflammation in type 1 diabetes. *Diabetes* **67:** 2305–2311. doi:10.2337/db17-1006

Hsu NC, Tsai HB, Hsu CH. 2023. Verapamil and pancreatic β cell function in pediatric type 1 diabetes. *J Am Med Assoc* **330:** 380. doi:10.1001/jama.2023.9110

Huang W, Hickson LTJ, Eirin A, Kirkland JL, Lerman LO. 2022. Cellular senescence: the good, the bad and the unknown. *Nat Rev Nephrol* **18:** 611–627. doi:10.1038/s41581-022-00601-z

Insel RA, Dunne JL, Atkinson MA, Chiang JL, Dabelea D, Gottlieb PA, Greenbaum CJ, Herold KC, Krischer JP, Lernmark A, et al. 2015. Staging presymptomatic type 1 diabetes: a scientific statement of JDRF, the Endocrine Society, and the American Diabetes Association. *Diabetes Care* **38:** 1964–1974. doi:10.2337/dc15-1419

Jing Y, Gravenstein S, Rao Chaganty N, Chen N, Lyerly KH, Joyce S, Deng Y. 2007. Aging is associated with a rapid decline in frequency, alterations in subset composition, and enhanced Th2 response in CD1d-restricted NKT cells from human peripheral blood. *Exp Gerontol* **42:** 719–732. doi:10.1016/j.exger.2007.01.009

Justice JN, Nambiar AM, Tchkonia T, LeBrasseur NK, Pascual R, Hashmi SK, Prata L, Masternak MM, Kritchevsky SB, Musi N, et al. 2019. Senolytics in idiopathic pulmonary fibrosis: results from a first-in-human, open-label, pilot study. *EBioMedicine* **40:** 554–563. doi:10.1016/j.ebiom.2018.12.052

Kaestner KH, Powers AC, Naji A, Atkinson MA. 2019. NIH initiative to improve understanding of the pancreas, islet, and autoimmunity in type 1 diabetes: the Human Pancreas Analysis Program (HPAP). *Diabetes* **68:** 1394–1402. doi:10.2337/db19-0058

Kang TW, Yevsa T, Woller N, Hoenicke L, Wuestefeld T, Dauch D, Hohmeyer A, Gereke M, Rudalska R, Potapova A, et al. 2011. Senescence surveillance of pre-malignant hepatocytes limits liver cancer development. *Nature* **479:** 547–551. doi:10.1038/nature10599

Kirkland JL, Tchkonia T. 2020. Senolytic drugs: from discovery to translation. *J Intern Med* **288:** 518–536. doi:10.1111/joim.13141

Kis J, Engelmann P, Farkas K, Richman G, Eck S, Lolley J, Jalahej H, Borowiec M, Kent SC, Treszl A, et al. 2007. Reduced $CD4^+$ subset and Th1 bias of the human iNKT cells in type 1 diabetes mellitus. *J Leukoc Biol* **81:** 654–662. doi:10.1189/jlb.1106654

Kudtarkar P, Costanzo MC, Sun Y, Jang D, Koesterer R, Mychaleckyj JC, Nayak U, Onengut-Gumuscu S, Rich SS, Flannick JA, et al. 2023. Leveraging type 1 diabetes human genetic and genomic data in the T1D knowledge portal. *PLoS Biol* **21:** e3002233. doi:10.1371/journal.pbio.3002233

Lee H, Lee YS, Harenda Q, Pietrzak S, Oktay HZ, Schreiber S, Liao Y, Sonthalia S, Ciecko AE, Chen YG, et al. 2020. β Cell dedifferentiation induced by IRE1α deletion prevents type 1 diabetes. *Cell Metab* **31:** 822–836.e5. doi:10.1016/j.cmet.2020.03.002

Lee H, Sahin GS, Chen C, Hatzoglou M, Sonthalia S, Cañas SM, Oktay HZ, Duckworth AT, Brawerman G, Thompson PJ, Hatzoglou M, et al. 2023. Stress-induced β cell early senescence confers protection against type 1 diabetes. *Cell Metab* 2200–2215.e9. doi:10.1016/j.cmet.2023.10.014

Leete P, Oram RA, McDonald TJ, Shields BM, Ziller C, Roep BO, Tree TI, Patel K, Hammersley S, Bolt R, et al. 2020. Studies of insulin and proinsulin in pancreas and serum support the existence of aetiopathological endotypes of type 1 diabetes associated with age at diagnosis. *Diabetologia* **63:** 1258–1267. doi:10.1007/s00125-020-05115-6

Lerner AG, Upton JP, Praveen PVK, Ghosh R, Nakagawa Y, Igbaria A, Shen S, Nguyen V, Backes BJ, Heiman M, et al. 2012. IRE1α induces thioredoxin-interacting protein to activate the NLRP3 inflammasome and promote programmed cell death under irremediable ER stress. *Cell Metab* **16:** 250–264. doi:10.1016/j.cmet.2012.07.007

Li Q, McDevitt HO. 2011. The role of interferon α in initiation of type I diabetes in the NOD mouse. *Clin Immunol* **140:** 3–7. doi:10.1016/j.clim.2011.04.010

Logue SE, McGrath EP, Cleary P, Greene S, Mnich K, Almanza A, Chevet E, Dwyer RM, Oommen A, Legembre P, et al. 2018. Inhibition of IRE1 RNase activity modulates the tumor cell secretome and enhances response to chemotherapy. *Nat Commun* **9:** 3267. doi:10.1038/s41467-018-05763-8

MacCuish AC, Irvine WJ, Barnes EW, Duncan LJ. 1974. Antibodies to pancreatic islet cells in insulin-dependent diabetics with coexistent autoimmune disease. *Lancet* **304:** 1529–1531. doi:10.1016/s0140-6736(74)90281-5

Mallone R, Halliez C, Rui J, Herold KC. 2022. The β-cell in type 1 diabetes pathogenesis: a victim of circumstances or an instigator of tragic events? *Diabetes* **71:** 1603–1610. doi:10.2337/dbi21-0036

Marhfour I, Lopez XM, Lefkaditis D, Salmon I, Allagnat F, Richardson SJ, Morgan NG, Eizirik DL. 2012. Expression of endoplasmic reticulum stress markers in the islets of patients with type 1 diabetes. *Diabetologia* **55:** 2417–2420. doi:10.1007/s00125-012-2604-3

Marin I, Boix O, Garcia-Garijo A, Sirois I, Caballe A, Zarzuela E, Ruano I, Attolini CS-O, Prats N, López-Domínguez JA, et al. 2023. Cellular senescence is immunogenic and promotes antitumor immunity. *Cancer Discov* **13:** 410–431. doi:10.1158/2159-8290.CD-22-0523

Marroqui L, Perez-Serna AA, Babiloni-Chust I, Dos Santos RS. 2021. Type I interferons as key players in pancreatic β-cell dysfunction in type 1 diabetes. *Int Rev Cell Mol Biol* **359:** 1–80. doi:10.1016/bs.ircmb.2021.02.011

Miranda MA, Macias-Velasco JF, Lawson HA. 2021. Pancreatic β-cell heterogeneity in health and diabetes: classes, sources, and subtypes. *Am J Physiol Endocrinol Metab* **320:** E716–E731. doi:10.1152/ajpendo.00649.2020

Moin ASM, Butler AE. 2019. Alterations in β cell identity in type 1 and type 2 diabetes. *Curr Diab Rep* **19:** 83. doi:10.1007/s11892-019-1194-6

Morita S, Villalta SA, Feldman HC, Register AC, Rosenthal W, Hoffmann-Petersen IT, Mehdizadeh M, Ghosh R, Wang L, Colon-Negron K, et al. 2017. Targeting ABL-IRE1α signaling spares ER-stressed pancreatic β cells to reverse autoimmune diabetes. *Cell Metab* **25:** 883–897.e8. doi:10.1016/j.cmet.2017.03.018

Muralidharan C, Conteh AM, Marasco MR, Crowder JJ, Kuipers J, de Boer P, Giepmans BNG, Linnemann AK. 2021. Pancreatic β cell autophagy is impaired in type 1 diabetes. *Diabetologia* **64:** 865–877. doi:10.1007/s00125-021-05387-6

Oram RA, Sims EK, Evans-Molina C. 2019. β Cells in type 1 diabetes: mass and function; sleeping or dead? *Diabetologia* **62:** 567–577. doi:10.1007/s00125-019-4822-4

Oslowski CM, Hara T, O'Sullivan-Murphy B, Kanekura K, Lu S, Hara M, Ishigaki S, Zhu LJ, Hayashi E, Hui ST, et al. 2012. Thioredoxin-interacting protein mediates ER stress-induced β cell death through initiation of the inflammasome. *Cell Metab* **16:** 265–273. doi:10.1016/j.cmet.2012.07.005

Ovadya Y, Landsberger T, Leins H, Vadai E, Gal H, Biran A, Yosef R, Sagiv A, Agrawal A, Shapira A, et al. 2018. Impaired immune surveillance accelerates accumulation of senescent cells and aging. *Nat Commun* **9:** 5435. doi:10.1038/s41467-018-07825-3

Ovalle F, Grimes T, Xu G, Patel AJ, Grayson TB, Thielen LA, Li P, Shalev A. 2018. Verapamil and β cell function in adults with recent-onset type 1 diabetes. *Nat Med* **24:** 1108–1112. doi:10.1038/s41591-018-0089-4

Parekh VV, Wilson MT, Olivares-Villagómez D, Singh AK, Wu L, Wang CR, Joyce S, Van Kaer L. 2005. Glycolipid antigen induces long-term natural killer T cell anergy in mice. *J Clin Invest* **115:** 2572–2583. doi:10.1172/JCI24762

Piha-Paul SA, Hann CL, French CA, Cousin S, Braña I, Cassier PA, Moreno V, de Bono JS, Harward SD, Ferron-Brady G, et al. 2020. Phase 1 study of Molibresib (GSK525762), a bromodomain and extra-terminal domain protein inhibitor, in NUT carcinoma and other solid tumors. *JNCI Cancer Spectr* **4:** 1–9.

Pociot F. 2017. Type 1 diabetes genome-wide association studies: not to be lost in translation. *Clin Transl Immunol* **6:** e162–e167. doi:10.1038/cti.2017.51

Poulton LD, Smyth MJ, Hawke CG, Silveira P, Shepherd D, Naidenko OV, Godfrey DI, Baxter AG. 2001. Cytometric and functional analyses of NK and NKT cell deficiencies in NOD mice. *Int Immunol* **13:** 887–896. doi:10.1093/intimm/13.7.887

Prata LGPL, Ovsyannikova IG, Tchkonia T, Kirkland JL. 2018. Senescent cell clearance by the immune system: emerging therapeutic opportunities. *Semin Immunol* **40:** 101275. doi:10.1016/j.smim.2019.04.003

Roep BO, Thomaidou S, van Tienhoven R, Zaldumbide A. 2021. Type 1 diabetes mellitus as a disease of the β-cell (do not blame the immune system?). *Nat Rev Endocrinol* **17:** 150–161. doi:10.1038/s41574-020-00443-4

Roman-Gonzalez A, Moreno ME, Alfaro JM, Uribe F, Latorre-Sierra G, Rugeles MT, Montoya CJ. 2009. Frequency and function of circulating invariant NKT cells in autoimmune diabetes mellitus and thyroid diseases in Colombian patients. *Hum Immunol* **70:** 262–268. doi:10.1016/j.humimm.2009.01.012

Rutter GA, Georgiadou E, Martinez-Sanchez A, Pullen TJ. 2020. Metabolic and functional specialisations of the pancreatic β cell: gene disallowance, mitochondrial metabolism and intercellular connectivity. *Diabetologia* **63:** 1990–1998. doi:10.1007/s00125-020-05205-5

Sahin GS, Lee H, Engin F. 2021. An accomplice more than a mere victim: the impact of β-cell ER stress on type 1 diabetes pathogenesis. *Mol Metab* **54:** 101365. doi:10.1016/j.molmet.2021.101365

Sharif S, Arreaza GA, Zucker P, Mi QS, Sondhi J, Naidenko OV, Kronenberg M, Koezuka Y, Delovitch TL, Gombert JM, et al. 2001. Activation of natural killer T cells by α-galactosylceramide treatment prevents the onset and recurrence of autoimmune type 1 diabetes. *Nat Med* **7:** 1057–1062. doi:10.1038/nm0901-1057

Sims EK, Mirmira RG, Evans-Molina C. 2020. The role of β-cell dysfunction in early type 1 diabetes. *Curr Opin Endocrinol Diabetes Obes* **27:** 215–224. doi:10.1097/MED.0000000000000548

Sims EK, Kulkarni A, Hull A, Woerner SE, Cabrera S, Mastrandrea LD, Hammoud B, Sarkar S, Nakayasu ES, Mastracci TL, et al. 2023. Inhibition of polyamine biosynthesis preserves β cell function in type 1 diabetes. *Cell Rep Med* **4:** 101261. doi:10.1016/j.xcrm.2023.101261

Smith JA. 2018. Regulation of cytokine production by the unfolded protein response; implications for infection and autoimmunity. *Front Immunol* **9:** 1–21. doi:10.3389/fimmu.2018.00422

Stancill JS, Kasmani MY, Khatun A, Cui W, Corbett JA. 2021. Cytokine and nitric oxide-dependent gene regulation in islet endocrine and nonendocrine cells. *Function (Oxf)* **3:** zqab063. doi:10.1093/function/zqab063

Størling J, Pociot F. 2017. Type 1 diabetes candidate genes linked to pancreatic islet cell inflammation and β-cell apoptosis. *Genes (Basel)* **8:** 72. doi:10.3390/genes8020072

Sturmlechner I, Zhang C, Sine CC, van Deursen EJJ, Jeganathan KB, Hamada N, Grasic J, Friedman D, Stutchman JT, Can I, et al. 2021. P21 produces a bioactive secretome that places stressed cells under immunosurveillance. *Science* **374:** eabb3420. doi:10.1126/science.abb3420

Tasdemir N, Banito A, Roe JS, Alonso-Curbelo D, Camiolo M, Tschaharganeh DF, Huang CH, Aksoy O, Bolden JE, Chen CC, et al. 2016. BRD4 connects enhancer remodeling to senescence immune surveillance. *Cancer Discov* **6:** 612–629. doi:10.1158/2159-8290.CD-16-0217

Tersey SA, Nishiki Y, Templin AT, Cabrera SM, Stull ND, Colvin SC, Evans-Molina C, Rickus JL, Maier B, Mirmira RG. 2012. Islet β-cell endoplasmic reticulum stress precedes the onset of type 1 diabetes in the nonobese diabetic mouse model. *Diabetes* **61:** 818–827. doi:10.2337/db11-1293

Thompson PJ, Bhushan A. 2022. Diabetes: senescence in type 1 diabetes. In *Cellular senescence in disease* (ed. Serrano M, Muñoz-Espín D), pp. 269–288. Academic, London.

Thompson PJ, Shah A, Apostolopolou H, Bhushan A. 2019a. BET proteins are required for transcriptional activation of the senescent islet cell secretome in type 1 diabetes. *Int J Mol Sci* **20:** 4776. doi:10.3390/ijms20194776

Thompson PJ, Shah A, Ntranos V, Van Gool F, Atkinson M, Bhushan A. 2019b. Targeted elimination of senescent β cells prevents type 1 diabetes. *Cell Metab* **29:** 1045–1060.e10. doi:10.1016/j.cmet.2019.01.021

Thompson PJ, Pipella J, Rutter GA, Gaisano HY, Santamaria P. 2023. Islet autoimmunity in human type 1 diabetes: initiation and progression from the perspective of the β cell. *Diabetologia* **66:** 1971–1982. doi:10.1007/s00125-023-05970-z

Vived C, Lee-Papastavros A, Aparecida da Silva Pereira J, Yi P, MacDonald TL. 2023. β Cell stress and endocrine function during T1D: what's next to discover? *Endocrinology* **165:** 1–12. doi:10.1210/endocr/bqad162

Waibel M, Wentworth JM, So M, Ph D, Couper JJ, Cameron FJ, Gorelik A, Sc M, Litwak S, Ph D, et al. 2023. Baricitinib and β-cell function in patients with new-onset type 1 diabetes. *N Engl J Med* **389:** 2140–2150. doi:10.1056/NEJMoa2306691

Walker EM, Cha J, Tong X, Guo M, Liu JH, Yu S, Iacovazzo D, Mauvais-Jarvis F, Flanagan SE, Korbonits M, et al. 2021. Sex-biased islet β cell dysfunction is caused by the MODY MAFA S64F variant by inducing premature aging and senescence in males. *Cell Rep* **37:** 109813. doi:10.1016/j.celrep.2021.109813

Wang YJ, Traum D, Schug J, Gao L, Liu C, Atkinson MA, Powers AC, Feldman MD, Naji A, Chang KM, et al. 2019. Multiplexed in situ imaging mass cytometry analysis of the human endocrine pancreas and immune system in type 1 diabetes. *Cell Metab* **29:** 769–783.e4. doi:10.1016/j.cmet.2019.01.003

Wang TW, Johmura Y, Suzuki N, Omori S, Migita T, Yamaguchi K, Hatakeyama S, Yamazaki S, Shimizu E, Imoto S, et al. 2022. Blocking PD-L1–PD-1 improves senescence surveillance and ageing phenotypes. *Nature* **611:** 358–364. doi:10.1038/s41586-022-05388-4

Warncke K, Weiss A, Achenbach P, Von Dem Berge T, Berner R, Casteels K, Groele L, Hatzikotoulas K, Hommel A, Kordonouri O, et al. 2022. Elevations in blood glucose before and after the appearance of islet autoantibodies in children. *J Clin Invest* **132:** e162123. doi:10.1172/JCI162123

Welsh N. 2022. Are off-target effects of imatinib the key to improving β-cell function in diabetes? *Ups J Med Sci* doi:10.48101/ujms.v127.8841

Wilson CS, Spaeth JM, Karp J, Stocks BT, Hoopes EM, Stein RW, Moore DJ. 2019. B lymphocytes protect islet β cells in diabetes-prone NOD mice treated with imatinib. *JCI Insight* **5:** e125317. doi:10.1172/jci.insight.125317

Xu G, Grimes TD, Grayson TB, Chen J, Thielen LA, Tse HM, Li P, Kanke M, Lin TT, Schepmoes AA, et al. 2022. Exploratory study reveals far reaching systemic and cellular effects of verapamil treatment in subjects with type 1 diabetes. *Nat Commun* **13:** 1159. doi:10.1038/s41467-022-28826-3

Xue W, Zender L, Miething C, Dickins RA, Hernando E, Krizhanovsky V, Cordon-Cardo C, Lowe SW. 2007. Senescence and tumour clearance is triggered by p53 restoration in murine liver carcinomas. *Nature* **445:** 656–660. doi:10.1038/nature05529

Yousefzadeh MJ, Flores RR, Zhu Y, Schmiechen ZC, Brooks RW, Trussoni CE, Cui Y, Angelini L, Lee KA, McGowan SJ, et al. 2021. An aged immune system drives senescence and ageing of solid organs. *Nature* **594:** 100–105. doi:10.1038/s41586-021-03547-7

The Chicken or the Egg Dilemma: Understanding the Interplay between the Immune System and the β Cell in Type 1 Diabetes

Maria Skjøtt Hansen,[1] Pravil Pokharel,[2] Jon Piganelli,[2] and Lori Sussel[1]

[1]Barbara Davis Center for Diabetes, University of Colorado Anschutz Medical Campus, Aurora, Colorado 80045, USA

[2]Division of Endocrinology Diabetes and Metabolism, Indiana University School of Medicine, Indianapolis, Indiana 46202, USA

Correspondence: lori.sussel@cuanschutz.edu

In this review, we explore the complex interplay between the immune system and pancreatic β cells in the context of type 1 diabetes (T1D). While T1D is predominantly considered a T-cell-mediated autoimmune disease, the inability of human leukocyte antigen (HLA)-risk alleles alone to explain disease development suggests a role for β cells in initiating and/or propagating disease. This review delves into the vulnerability of β cells, emphasizing their susceptibility to endoplasmic reticulum (ER) stress and protein modifications, which may give rise to neoantigens. Additionally, we discuss the role of viral infections as contributors to T1D onset, and of genetic factors with dual impacts on the immune system and β cells. A greater understanding of the interplay between environmental triggers, autoimmunity, and the β cell will not only lead to insight as to why the islet β cells are specifically targeted by the immune system in T1D but may also reveal potential novel therapeutic interventions.

Type 1 diabetes (T1D) is an autoimmune disease that develops when the immune system erroneously attacks and destroys the insulin-producing β cells in the pancreas. It is widely accepted that T1D is a T-cell-mediated autoimmune disorder, with the highest genetic risk factor being specific human leukocyte antigen (HLA) alleles. However, it has become increasingly appreciated that the pathogenesis of T1D involves both the immune system and the targeted β cell (Mallone and Eizirik 2020; Roep et al. 2021). One of the main arguments for the involvement of the β cell is the inability of the HLA risk alleles to fully explain disease risk (Noble and Erlich 2012). The genes located in the HLA class II region on chromosome 6p21 have the strongest association with predisposition to and protection against T1D development. The HLA DR3–DQ2 or DR4–DQ8 haplotypes confer the highest risk of disease development and are found in ~90% of patients with T1D (Rønningen et al. 1991). However, the same haplotypes are represented in ~40% of the general population, meaning that the vast ma-

Cite this article as *Cold Spring Harb Perspect Med* doi: 10.1101/cshperspect.a041591

jority of individuals with the high-risk HLA haplotype never develop T1D (Field 2002). Thus, the HLA genes alone do not explain disease development. Additionally, autoreactive $CD8^+$ T cells, the final mediators of β-cell destruction, circulate at similar levels in healthy individuals as compared to patients with T1D. However, patients with T1D present with infiltrating autoreactive $CD4^+$ and $CD8^+$ T cells in the islet, suggesting that local factors within the pancreas are promoting homing of the T cells to the β cells. Therefore, although autoimmunity is the primary cause of T1D, it is likely that the islet β cells also play a major role in the development of disease.

Presuming that the β cell is partially responsible for the autoimmune attack, the next question is whether it plays a role in disease initiation and/or in disease propagation. While the pathogenesis of T1D has been studied for decades, the etiology of the disease remains poorly understood. Furthermore, much less is known about the initial series of events that take place before the appearance of the first islet autoantibody. In this work, we discuss features of β cells and the immune system that potentially set up a "perfect storm" to trigger T1D (Fig. 1).

β-CELL RISK GENES

While a defective immune system is inevitably the central driver of autoimmunity, it remains unclear why the β cell becomes the primary and only target in T1D. Recent genome-wide association studies (GWASs) have suggested that although the most significant genetic predisposition to T1D is conferred by the HLA complex, many single-nucleotide polymorphisms (SNPs) in non-HLA loci also contribute to the disease (Fløyel et al. 2015). Furthermore, there is emerging research to suggest that β cells may be genetically predisposed to increased stress in individuals with T1D, as several genes in T1D susceptibility loci are involved in the regulation of islet inflammation and β-cell apoptosis, including *PTPN2*, *BACH2*, and *IFIH1/MDA5*, among others.

PTPN2 (Protein Tyrosine Phosphatase, Nonreceptor Type 2) is a gene that encodes a protein called T-cell protein tyrosine phosphatase (TCPTP). This protein plays a key role in the regulation of immune responses by modulating the activity of certain signaling pathways in immune cells, including T cells. Mutations in the *PTPN2* gene have been associated with several autoimmune diseases, including T1D. It has also been demonstrated that the *PTPN2* risk variant rs1893217 causes a decrease in *PTPN2* expression and contributes to the sensitivity of β cells to immune- or virus-mediated apoptosis (Moore et al. 2009). The risk variant also reduces IL-2 receptor signaling, which decreases $FOXP3^+$ Tregs in patients with T1D, thus dysregulating Treg function (Bettini and Bettini 2021). While an important role for PTPN2 in regulating immune system function has been established, it is still unclear why or how the pancreatic β cells are specifically targeted. One indication that PTPN2 may have functions outside of T cells was from studies in mice that have shown that global deletion of *Ptpn2* leads to rampant autoimmunity, whereas T-cell-specific inactivation of *Ptpn2* causes less severe autoimmune phenotypes. Interestingly, PTPN2 is also highly expressed in β cells and the knockdown of *PTPN2* in human β-cell lines sensitized β cells to cytotoxicity (Roca-Rivada et al. 2023). Furthermore, mouse islets carrying a β-cell deletion of Ptpn2 displayed impaired glucose-stimulated insulin secretion and reduced glucose-induced metabolic flux in response to cytokine treatment, suggesting β cells lacking Ptpn2 were inherently more susceptible to inflammatory stress due to maladaptive metabolic fitness (Roca-Rivada et al. 2023; Kim et al. 2024). These findings suggest that PTPN2 is important for both modulating T-cell activity and β-cell function/survival, and defects in both the immune system and the β cell will result in exacerbated β-cell destruction in the context of an autoimmune environment.

IFIH1 (Interferon Induced with Helicase C Domain 1), also known as *MDA5* (Melanoma Differentiation-Associated Protein 5), is a gene that encodes a protein involved in the innate immune system. *IFIH1/MDA5* plays a crucial role in detecting viral RNA, particularly double-stranded RNA (dsRNA), which is a common molecular pattern associated with viral in-

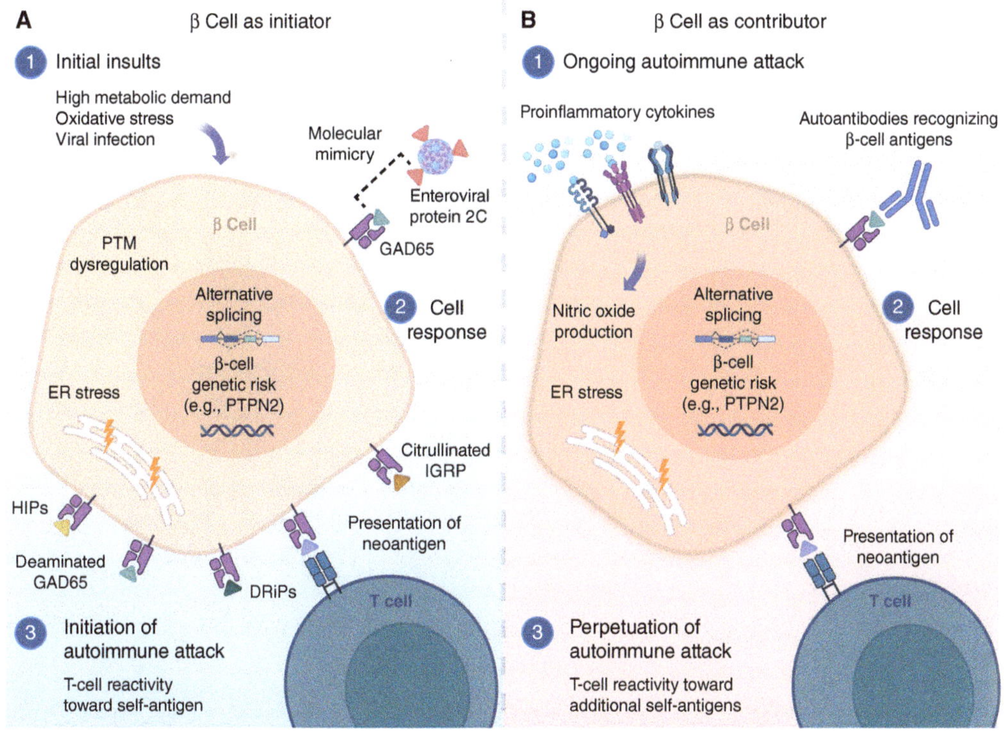

Figure 1. The β cell as initiator versus contributor of the autoimmune attack. The β cell potentially plays a role as both an initiator and a contributor to the autoimmune attack in type 1 diabetes (T1D). (*A*) External factors such as high metabolic demand, oxidative stress, or viral infection, may serve as the initial insult on the β cell, resulting in β-cell stress. Increased endoplasmic reticulum (ER) stress can trigger the dysregulation of posttranslational modifications (PTMs) and/or alternative splicing events, which can result in the formation of neoantigens. These neoantigens, such as citrullinated peptides, hybrid peptides, or defective ribosomal products, are then presented on the cell surface to be recognized as "foreign" by an autoreactive T cell. In addition, viral infections could potentially cause the T-cell-targeting of β cells through molecular mimicry between viral and β-cell proteins, or through inflammation-driven bystander activation of preexisting autoreactive T cells. In each scenario, an individual must also possess a genetic susceptibility that causes faulty central and peripheral tolerance, leading to the generation of autoreactive T cells. (*B*) Once an autoimmune attack has been initiated, the presence of proinflammatory cytokines as well as β-cell-specific autoantibodies can perpetuate the β-cell destruction. Increased local inflammation can lead to increased ER stress, alternative splicing, and nitric oxide production, exacerbating neoantigen generation and presentation. In both the initiation and perpetuation of an autoimmune attack, β-cell risk genes can heighten the susceptibility of β cells to stress responses and amplify their immunogenicity.

fections, including coxsackievirus B (CVB). When IFIH1/MDA5 recognizes viral RNA, it triggers a signaling pathway that leads to the production of type I interferons and other inflammatory cytokines, an environment that can place the β cell at risk (Blum and Tse 2020). GWASs have shown a strong association between *IFIH1/MDA5* variants and T1D. More recently, Knebel et al. (2024) identified a direct role for sensing dsRNA within β cells for the development of T1D. In this study, disruption of the RNA editing enzyme ADAR (adenosine deaminases acting on RNA) in β cells resulted in a robust IFIH1/MDA5-dependent interferon response, in addition to islet inflammation and β-cell failure and destruction. Furthermore, the interferon response was enhanced in conditions of elevated glucose, suggesting that a combination of increased β-cell exertion and islet inflammation led to β-cell failure.

BACH2 (BTB and CNC Homology 1, Basic Leucine Zipper Transcription Factor 2) encodes a transcription factor that has been characterized to play a crucial role in the development and function of immune cells (Cooper et al. 2008; Kometani et al. 2013; Roychoudhuri et al. 2013). Dysregulation of the *BACH2* gene has been associated with autoimmune diseases, including T1D, primarily due to its functions in the immune system. However, the Eizirik laboratory has demonstrated that BACH2 is also expressed in human and rodent islets and its expression is modulated by proinflammatory cytokines (Marroquí et al. 2014). Furthermore, inhibition of BACH2 in β cells aggravated cytokine-induced β-cell death, again demonstrating the existence of a complex relationship between the β cell and the immune system.

These are just a few examples of how an underlying genetic defect compromises β-cell function. Interestingly, in most cases, a single genetic defect affects both the immune system and the β cell, which could provide some insight as to why a global defect in the immune system specifically targets the pancreatic β cells.

Is the β Cell an Easy Target?

Although certain polymorphisms in β-cell genes are linked to an increased risk of disease due to heightened susceptibility, this alone does not fully account for the remarkable specificity of the autoimmune attack on β cells. While α cells are dysfunctional in T1D, they neither provoke an immune response nor face destruction. This difference in immunogenicity has been attributed to variations in the expression of antiapoptotic genes, proapoptotic genes, as well as endoplasmic reticulum (ER) stress-related genes (Eizirik et al. 2023). This raises the question of whether the β cell is inherently more immunogenic, especially under certain conditions. Indeed, it has been proposed that the inherent secretory function of the β cell makes it highly vulnerable to an immune attack (Piganelli et al. 2021; Sahin et al. 2021). The β cell produces almost one million molecules of pre-proinsulin per minute under stimulated conditions, putting a tremendous burden on the ER for proper protein folding, trafficking, and secretion (Scheuner and Kaufman 2008; Sahin et al. 2021). The ER ensures that only properly folded and assembled proteins are transported to their final destinations, while misfolded or damaged proteins are retained and degraded by the ER-associated degradation (ERAD) pathway (Hwang and Qi 2018).

Several lines of evidence suggest that ER stress may contribute to β-cell dysfunction and death in T1D (Fig. 2). First, β cells have a highly developed and active ER, due to their high demand for insulin synthesis and secretion (Araki et al. 2003). Therefore, they are particularly vulnerable to ER stress caused by a variety of factors, such as genetic mutations, environmental toxins, hypoxia, hypoglycemia, and inflammatory cytokines. Second, ER stress can activate inflammatory pathways, such as nuclear factor κB (NF-κB), which can exacerbate the autoimmune attack on β cells by increasing the expression of proinflammatory genes and antigen presentation molecules (Babon et al. 2016; Marré et al. 2018). Analogously, ER stress can lead to increased IL-1β production and secretion through induction of the unfolded protein response (UPR) mediator thioredoxin-interacting protein (TXNIP) (Maedler et al. 2002; Lerner et al. 2012; Oslowski et al. 2012). Third, ER stress can impair insulin biosynthesis and secretion, leading to glucose intolerance and hyperglycemia, which can further aggravate ER stress and create a vicious cycle. Fourth, ER stress can induce apoptosis of β cells through a variety of mechanisms, such as activation of caspases, induction of proapoptotic genes, and release of calcium from the ER (Ron 2002; Marré et al. 2015).

Several studies have demonstrated the presence of ER stress markers in β cells of animal models and human patients with T1D. For example, Harding and Ron (2002) described a role for ER stress in rare forms of clinical and experimental diabetes caused by mutations affecting the ER stress–activated pancreatic ER kinase (PERK) and its downstream effector, the translation initiation complex eukaryotic initiation

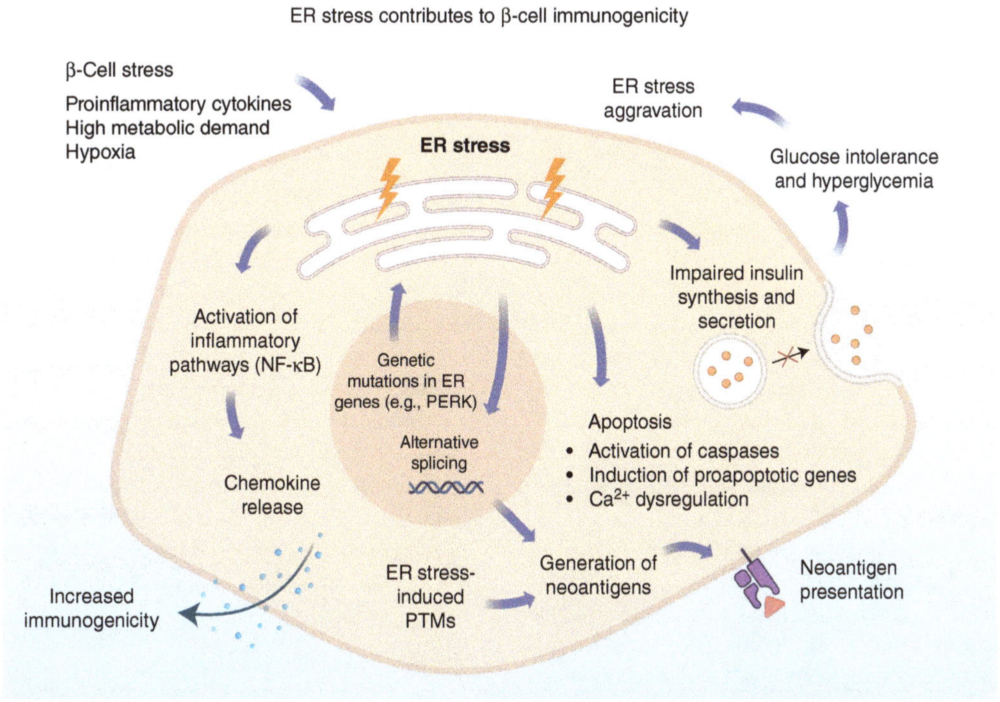

Figure 2. Endoplasmic reticulum (ER) stress as a contributor of β-cell immunogenicity. The high secretory demand of β cells causes them to be inherently susceptible to ER stress. β-Cell ER stress can activate inflammatory pathways, increasing the expression of proinflammatory genes and human leukocyte antigen (HLA) molecules, as well as increasing chemokine release. Additionally, ER stress can impair insulin production and secretion, causing glucose intolerance and hyperglycemia, further exacerbating the stress response. Through activation of caspases, ER calcium release, and induction of proapoptotic genes, ER stress can induce apoptosis. ER stress may also result in dysregulation of alternative splicing events, as well as posttranslational modifications (PTMs), causing the formation of neoantigens. Finally, genetic predisposition may render some individuals more susceptible to ER stress, increasing the likelihood of triggering an autoimmune response. Overall, ER stress is likely a major contributor to the autoimmune response in type 1 diabetes (T1D), through the exacerbation of stress, inflammation, and immunogenicity.

factor 2 (eIF2). They also suggested that ER stress may play a role in more common forms of diabetes. *Perk* KO mice have been found to develop irreversible abnormalities soon after birth, such as high blood sugar levels, low insulin levels, and impaired β-cell function, resulting from their inability to maintain the integrity of the ER (Harding et al. 2001). Similarly, polymorphisms in the Tyrosine kinase 2 (TYK2) gene have been associated with protection against T1D. TYK2 and JAK1 are activated by IFN-α, and through activation of a variety of downstream pathways, JAK1/TYK2 kinases cause inflammation, ER stress, and overexpression of HLA class I. SNPs in TYK2 that decrease its activity are associated with protection against T1D as well as other autoimmune diseases, suggesting a genetic basis for these stress/inflammatory pathways (Coomans de Brachène et al. 2020; Pellenz et al. 2021). Tersey's group (2012) also showed that islet β cells from prediabetic nonobese diabetic (NOD) mice, a widely used model of T1D, displayed increased expression of ER stress markers, morphological alterations in ER structure, and activation of NF-κB target genes. Furthermore, they found that exposure of MIN6 cells, a mouse insulinoma cell line, to a mixture of proinflammatory cytokines caused ER stress and translational blockade. Additionally, it has been proposed that ER stress may be involved in β-cell death that is induced by nitric oxide, an effector molecule implicated in T1D pathogenesis (Oyadomari et al. 2001). The connection between T1D and ER stress is further highlighted by the observation that administering taurourso deoxycholic acid (TUDCA), a chemical ER stress reliever, during the prediabetic phase substantially reduces the incidence of diabetes in T1D mouse models (Engin et al. 2013). Supporting this concept, islets from alloxan-induced diabetes-resistant (ALR/LT) mice, with genomes 70% similar to NOD mice but resistant to autoimmune destruction, demonstrate increased expression of ER stress–response molecules, including heat shock proteins, glucose-regulated protein 94 (GRP94), GRP78, protein disulfide isomerase, and calreticulin (Yang et al. 2008). These studies and many others implicate β-cell ER stress as a major contributor to the autoimmune response in T1D (reviewed extensively in Marré et al. 2015; Brozzi and Eizirik 2016; Sahin et al. 2021).

NEOANTIGEN FORMATION

The specificity of the autoimmune attack toward β cells in T1D is likely attributed to the presentation of epitopes unique to β cells. However, the identification and characterization of neoepitopes in T1D is a challenging task, as they may be rare, heterogeneous, and/or dynamic events. Moreover, the mechanisms by which neoepitopes are generated and presented to T cells are not fully understood. Advances in mass spectrometry, peptide synthesis, and T-cell assays have enabled the discovery and validation of several neoepitopes in T1D (James et al. 2018), and the expanding catalog of neoepitopes holds promise for shedding new light on the etiology and progression of the disease, as well as new opportunities for diagnosis and intervention.

While there is substantial evidence supporting the role of β-cell ER stress contributing to β-cell dysfunction and/or death in response to T1D, the role of ER stress in disease initiation is less clear. One potential mechanism has been suggested by the observation that ER stress can lead to the formation of posttranslational modifications (PTMs) of multiple β-cell proteins. This idea is supported by the identification of PTM of proteins such as insulin, chromogranin A, and glutamic acid decarboxylase 65 (GAD65) (Sherr et al. 2008), known autoantigens that contribute to the development of autoimmunity directed against the β cell. Furthermore, PTMs that arise as a consequence of ER stress or inflammation are unlikely to be well represented in the thymus, indicating that PTMs represent a likely means of undermining self-tolerance, thereby becoming preferential T-cell targets (James et al. 2018). In the context of a genetic predisposition to autoimmunity, such as the prodiabetes HLA alleles, the presentation of these modified neoantigens could trigger autoreactive T cells and initiate pathological processes.

HYBRID INSULIN PEPTIDES

One relatively new and notable example of PTMs in T1D is hybrid insulin peptides (HIPs). These peptides are formed through a process of transpeptidation that results in the covalent fusion between the carboxy-terminal carboxylic acid group of insulin C-peptide fragments with amino-terminal amine groups of other peptides, such as chromogranin A (Delong et al. 2012) or secretogranin II (Herold et al. 2021). HIPs are recognized by $CD4^+$ T cells in both mouse models and human patients with T1D (Delong et al. 2016). Additional studies found that proinsulin C-peptide fragments linked to islet amyloid polypeptide IAPP1, IAPP2, neuropeptide-Y, or insulin A chain were recognized by $CD4^+$ T cells from the pancreatic islets (Babon et al. 2016). Hybrid peptides were also detected in a human β-cell line by using HLA-peptidomics and found to elicit responses from $CD8^+$ T cells in the blood and pancreas of T1D patients (Azoury et al. 2020). There is growing evidence for the existence of these HIPs, and their formation would explain how endogenous β-cell proteins can become autoantigens that are perceived as "foreign" to the immune system.

 Cite this article as *Cold Spring Harb Perspect Med* doi: 10.1101/cshperspect.a041591

DEAMIDATED GAD65

Deamidated forms of GAD65, another major autoantigen in T1D have also been described. The deamidation reaction converts glutamine residues into glutamic acid, altering the structure and immunogenicity of the expressed peptide (McGinty et al. 2014). Deamidated GAD65 has been shown to be recognized by both $CD4^+$ and $CD8^+$ T cells in T1D (Marré et al. 2015).

CITRULLINATED PEPTIDES

Citrullination is another PTM in β cells that is linked to T1D. Citrullination converts arginine residues to citrulline, which can affect the binding and recognition of the peptide by HLA molecules and T cells (Yang et al. 2021). Citrullinated islet-specific glucose-6-phosphatase catalytic subunit-related protein (IGRP) has been characterized as an autoantigen in T1D and is recognized by $CD8^+$ T cells (Lieberman et al. 2003). Autoantibodies, circulating $CD4^+$ T cells, and islet-infiltrating $CD4^+$ T cells have been found to react against citrullinated GRP78 epitopes in individuals with T1D (Buitinga et al. 2018). In addition, circulating $CD4^+$ T cells reactive against citrullinated GAD65 and citrullinated IAPP have been detected in people with T1D (Babon et al. 2016). Furthermore, glucokinase, the primary glucose sensor and regulator of glucose homeostasis, is recognized by circulating $CD4^+$ T cells when citrullinated. Interestingly, glucokinase citrullination has been found to impair islet responses to glucose and overall glucose homeostasis, establishing a direct link between PTMs and β-cell function (Yang et al. 2022).

DEFECTIVE RIBOSOMAL PRODUCTS

Another type of modified protein that has been proposed to escape thymic education and peripheral tolerance is defective ribosomal products (DRiPs). DRiPs arise from the translation of untranslated regions (UTRs), ribosomal frameshifting, or alternative translation initiation. In tumor cells, the DRiPS generates a unique class of tumor-associated antigens selectively expressed by malignant cells. Analogously, Roep and his group discovered an alternative open reading frame within human insulin mRNA, that encoded a peptide much more immunogenic than the peptide encoded by the standard reading frame (Kracht et al. 2017). They also found that cytotoxic T cells directed against this peptide were present in the circulation of individuals diagnosed with T1D (Kracht et al. 2017). This peptide, which they referred to as an INS-DRiP, is an out-of-frame translation product, likely formed as a result of leaky ribosome scanning for translation initiation at a downstream start codon. Translation initiation at position 341 in the insulin mRNA generates an alternative polypeptide in a +2 reading frame that does not share any sequence identity with the canonical insulin product (Kracht et al. 2017). This study reveals another source of potential self-epitopes and implicates a primary role for the β cell in triggering autoimmunity in T1D.

NEOANTIGENS FORMED BY ALTERNATIVE SPLICING

Splicing is a normal cellular process in which precursor mRNAs (pre-mRNA) are converted into mature mRNAs by the removal of introns and joining of exons. Alternative splicing results in the joining of exons in different combinations, or the inclusion of introns, to form different protein isoforms. It has been estimated that ~95% of human genes undergo alternative splicing, generating on average four isoforms per gene (Baralle and Giudice 2017). Protein isoforms formed by alternative splicing often possess different binding affinities and functional capabilities, allowing cells to fine-tune their transcriptome and generate proteome diversity to gain functional specialization. RNA-binding proteins (RBPs) regulate splicing by binding to *cis*-regulatory sequence elements in the pre-mRNA and enhancing or suppressing spliceosome recruitment to splice sites (Horn et al. 2023). Several studies using immortalized β-cell lines and in rat primary β cells have shown that cytokine treatment and other stressors cause both aberrant splicing and dysregulation of RBPs (Ortis et al. 2010; Jeffery et al. 2019). Furthermore, in islets from donors with type 2 diabetes (T2D), 26% of alternative splicing events were found to be dysregulated compared to control islets (Jeffery et al. 2019). Alternative splicing alterations can be caused by defects in *cis*-regulatory elements, such as mutations or SNPs in splicing enhancers or silencers, or by defects in splicing factors (Juan-Mateu et al. 2016). In one example, decreased expression of GLIS3, a gene implicated in both T1D and T2D, results in aberrant splicing of the proapoptotic BH3-only gene *BIM*, causing increased β-cell apoptosis both before and after cytokine exposure (Nogueira et al. 2013). This effect is mediated by the splicing factor SRSF6/SRp55, which functions downstream from GLIS3. In addition to *BIM*, SRSF6 also regulates splicing of *LMO7*, another gene significantly associated with T1D. SRSF6 knockdown in EndoC-βH1 cells mimics the *LMO7* splicing effects seen when treating the cells with proinflammatory cytokines (Alvelos et al. 2021). These data reveal a new layer of potential risk mechanisms that are invisible at the transcript expression level but potent when looking at splice variants and the resulting protein isoforms.

The implication that alternative splicing can lead to the formation of protein isoforms with different protein-binding capacities, poses an important question in the field of autoimmune diseases: Can alternative splicing also lead to the generation of neoantigens? While the premise for neoantigens formed by alternative splicing is strong, only a few groups have been able to show that alternative splicing in the β cell leads to the presentation of more immunogenic peptides. Using a combination of peptidomics and transcriptomics, Mallone and his group identified several potentially novel β-cell neoantigens derived from splice variants. The majority of these peptides presented on β-cell HLA class I were splice isoforms of secretory granule proteins, such as CHGA, UCN3, and IAPP. Recognition of the peptides by circulating $CD8^+$ T cells from HLA-$A2^+$ healthy donors confirmed their capability to elicit an immune response (Gonzalez-Duque et al. 2018). Alternative splicing and differential expression of isoforms of the islet autoantigen G6PC2 (formerly known as IGRP) between pancreas and thymus in human donors has been proposed to contribute to the generation of autoreactive T cells. $CD8^+$ T cells recognizing G6PC2 isoforms exclusive to pancreatic islets could be detected at higher levels than isoforms present in both the pancreas and thymus, possibly due to failure of thymic negative selection. Interestingly, the autoreactive T cells were present in T1D subjects and healthy controls at similar levels, showing that the presence of autoreactive $CD8^+$ T cells alone is not sufficient to cause T1D (de Jong et al. 2013).

THE CHICKEN OR THE EGG?

It is crucial to note that while the generation of neoepitopes in β cells may initiate or perpetuate autoimmunity in T1D, evidence suggests that β cells do not spontaneously "poke" or provoke the immune system without provocation. It is believed that the initial triggers of autoimmunity likely arise from environmental factors, such as chemical exposures and other stressors that inflict damage that leads to neoepitope formation in one or more of the mechanisms described above (Richardson et al. 2016). However, the up-regulation of HLA and the subsequent presentation of neoantigens in β cells, while potentially perpetuating insulitis, is a natural stress response aimed at displaying abnormal proteins for immune clearance (Coppieters et al. 2012). In most situations, β cells are attempting to restore homeostasis, not incite attack; however, in the context of genetically susceptible HLA haplotypes and immune regulators, the interplay between β-cell abnormalities and an abnormal immune response converge to initiate and/or perpetuate autoimmunity (Noble et al. 2002). But exactly how vulnerable are the β cells in individuals without T1D? Does everyone have β cells capable of rapid and remarkably abundant protein synthesis at any given moment, but with the accompanying drawback that β cells are constantly sitting on the edge of immune destruction? Or is the high susceptibility of the β cells to destruction a trait specific to patients with T1D? It is possible that HIPs and DRiPs commonly occur in nondiabetic individuals with no repercussions, but are abnormally revealed and/or up-regulated in conditions where the β cells are ultimately targeted for destruction. Currently, the technologies to detect these neopeptides are not sensitive enough to answer this question. However, we do know that increased β-cell workload, as seen in conditions like T2D, gestational diabetes, or obesity, does not necessarily lead to T1D. Despite being pushed to their limits, and likely experiencing ER stress, β cells in these conditions remain intact. This suggests that β-cell stress alone is inadequate for triggering disease onset, indicating there may be an underlying genetic predisposition intrinsic to β cells in T1D individuals. On the other hand, directly interfering with the immune system, such as administering immune checkpoint inhibitors such as PD-1 inhibitors, can result in fulminant T1D, albeit in a small fraction of treated patients (Ikegami et al. 2016; Baden et al. 2018). Overall, the specific extent of the intrinsic immune system and β-cell dysfunctions needed for disease onset remains subject to the ongoing debate, although it is likely to require a combination of defects in both systems.

THE ROLE OF VIRAL INFECTION

Viral infections have long been suggested to be potential β-cell-related triggers for the development of T1D, although—as with many aspects of T1D—the exact relationship between a viral infection and T1D is complex and not fully understood. Several mechanisms through which a viral infection can contribute to T1D, include β-cell stress, virus-induced inflammation surrounding the β cell, and molecular mimicry of endogenous β-cell proteins. A β-cell stress mechanism stems from the idea that viral infections can interfere with protein translation or degrade ER proteins and induce ER stress (Atkinson et al. 1994). As discussed above, β cells are inordinately sensitive to ER stress, and this could catalyze detrimental cellular responses that could trigger or exacerbate an immune response.

In addition, there is evidence that viral infections induce an inflammatory response that may trigger an autoimmune reaction against pancreatic β cells. β cells can be directly exposed to viral infection as they express specific coxsackievirus and adenovirus receptors. Epidemiological and clinical studies strongly support the involvement of enteroviruses, in particular CVB, in the pathogenesis of T1D (Hober and Sauter 2010; Yeung et al. 2011; Allen et al. 2018; Ilonen et al. 2019). However, the pathological mechanisms that trigger the initiation or progression of CVB-induced autoimmunity against islet antigens in T1D are not yet fully elucidated. One theory is bystander activation of preexisting autoreactive T cells through the initiation of inflammation (Isaacs et al. 2021). For example, a viral infection could trigger heterologous T cells to mount an inflammatory attack that spills over onto β cells. The inflammation then causes tissue damage, which releases sequestered islet antigens. Antigen-presenting cells then pick up these autoantigens and display them to autoreactive T cells, inciting the cells to turn their fire onto the β cells. The escape of autoreactive T cells into the periphery is the linchpin; an individual would also have to have a genetic susceptibility that causes faulty central and peripheral tolerance to allow for the escape of and propagation of the autoreactive T cells to target β cells. While viral infection is in fact higher in children diagnosed with T1D compared to siblings or age-matched controls, infection is relatively common in all three groups. In a study from the United Kingdom, evidence of enteroviral RNA sequences was found in 27% of children with T1D, compared to 4.9% in age-matched controls (Nairn et al. 1999). In a study from Sweden, enterovirus was found in 50% of children with T1D, in 26% of their siblings, and in none of the control subjects (Yin et al. 2002). A caveat of this particular study was the low sample size (24 children with T1D). In another study, 46% of newly diagnosed children with T1D showed the presence of antibodies to the CVB compared to 34% of their siblings (Frisk et al. 1992).

Alternatively, it has been suggested that CVB infection promotes T1D by initially infecting macrophages, rather than the β cells directly, and the subsequent presentation of islet antigens by the infected macrophages activates autoreactive T cells to attack the β cells (Horwitz et al. 2004). The key event would be when inflammation leads to the uptake and display of β-cell antigens. If this antigen presentation occurs on a small scale, β-cell loss remains limited; however, if the inflammation becomes chronic, self-reactive T cells would become activated to β-cell antigens leading to a break in tolerance to self-tissue and, ultimately T-cell-mediated β-cell death.

There is also evidence that some viral proteins resemble proteins found in pancreatic β cells, leading to a cross-reaction by the immune system. For example, studies have shown that epitopes from CVB share structural similarities with epitopes from β cells to activate autoreactive T cells that can cross-react with β cells and contribute to their destruction (Coppieters et al. 2012). In the case of IA-2, the dominant epitope has been shown to elicit T-cell responses in relatives of patients with T1D (Honeyman et al. 1998). This suggests that the epitope may be involved in the early stages of the disease process. The fact that the epitope shares sequence similarity with proteins from viruses and bacteria suggests that these pathogens may trigger the development of autoimmunity to IA-2. The shared sequence similarity between two other IA-2 epitopes and amino acid sequences in milk, wheat, and bean proteins is also intriguing. This suggests that exposure to these common dietary proteins may also contribute to the development of autoimmunity to IA-2 (Honeyman et al. 1998). For instance, cross-reactivity between epitopes present in CVB and GAD65 has been documented (Atkinson et al. 1994). Molecular mimicry between the enteroviral protein 2C and GAD65 has also been implicated as a possible autoimmunity-triggering mechanism, since 2C and GAD65 share a common amino acid sequence called PEVRE (Hober and Sauter 2010).

Overall, while a single viral species may not be a risk factor for developing T1D, viral infections may be instrumental in initiating autoimmune diabetes in a subset of cases. It is very likely some or all of the mechanisms described above are at play, depending on the individual. A key scenario in this progression focuses on the normal immune response in clearing an infectious agent from infected tissue, such as the pancreas. Virally infected host cells respond by releasing signals, which mobilize immune cells to the site to subvert the infection, ultimately clearing the pathogen at which point tissue gradually returns to a state of normalcy as inflammation subsides, and repair processes predominate. But some individuals develop chronic infections because their immune systems are unable to eradicate the pathogen, or their immune cells become depleted after prolonged contact with the virus. In the context of a chronic infection, the immune system's ability to distinguish between self and nonself can become compromised. This again suggests a complex interplay between the targeted β cell and a dysfunctional immune system—with both contributing to the development of autoimmunity.

Moreover, it has been suggested that a lower expression of genes associated with viral recognition and innate immune response in β cells, as compared to α cells, contributes to their inadequate resistance against coxsackievirus infection (Eizirik et al. 2023). For example, the T1D risk gene *IFH1* encodes a helicase involved in the recognition of viral dsRNA and is much higher expressed in α cells compared to β cells. This aligns with the observation that α cells clear viruses more effectively than β cells (Marroqui et al. 2015), and perhaps partially explains why α cells are not targeted for destruction in T1D. Intriguingly, in a phase 2 trial involving children and adolescents with newly diagnosed T1D, a combination therapy with two antiviral drugs, pleconaril and ribavirin, resulted in higher endogenous insulin production than placebo after 12 months (Krogvold et al. 2023). This prolongation of the honeymoon phase upon treatment with antiviral drugs suggests that enteroviral infection likely plays a role in the autoimmune destruction process, and that eliminating the virus may decelerate—though not entirely halt—β-cell destruction.

Finally, infection with the SARS-CoV-2 virus has been associated with an increased incidence of T1D, although with inconsistent results. Large studies conducted in Finland, Scotland, Romania, and Germany revealed a heightened incidence of T1D during the pan-

 Cite this article as *Cold Spring Harb Perspect Med* doi: 10.1101/cshperspect.a041591

demic (Vlad et al. 2021; Kamrath et al. 2022; Salmi et al. 2022; McKeigue et al. 2023). However, studies using the same data sources as the German study, albeit with a shorter observation period, indicated no rise in T1D during the COVID-19 pandemic compared to previous years (Tittel et al. 2020). A nationwide study in Denmark also reported an increased incidence of T1D, yet no link was established between T1D development, and a positive SARS-CoV-2 test (Zareini et al. 2023). Finally, a study that simultaneously screened for the presence of islet autoantibodies and SARS-CoV-2 antibodies in Colorado, United States, and Bavaria, Germany, found no association between SARS-CoV-2 infection and autoimmune signatures related to the development of T1D (Rewers et al. 2022). Ultimately, the link between SARS-CoV-2 infection and T1D incidence remains unclear, with conflicting findings across studies. Further research will be needed to determine whether there is a causative link between SARS-CoV-2 infection and T1D.

SUMMARY

Understanding the intricate sequence of events that contribute to the development of T1D will be instrumental in our ability to develop long-term therapies. With the advent of single-cell technologies, there is a growing appreciation for a heterogeneous immune response within islets of individuals with T1D, including specific T-cell populations, as well as B cells and macrophages. Similarly, there is heterogeneity within the β-cell population. Ultimately, it will be important to parse out the relative roles of the immune system and the β cells that set in motion an immune response that ultimately breaks self-tolerance and leads to β-cell destruction. By unraveling the mysteries surrounding the interplay of autoimmunity, environmental triggers (i.e., stressors, viruses), and dysfunctional β-cell responses, we pave the way for interventions that target the root cause of the disease.

ACKNOWLEDGMENTS

We thank members of the Sussel and Piganelli Laboratories for discussions about the content of the review and members of the Sussel Laboratory for their critical reading of the manuscript. Funding for the authors includes support from the Diabetes Research Connection (M.S.H.), R01 DK082590, R01 DK118155, U01 DK127505, P30 DK057516 (L.S.), and R01 DK132583 (J.P.).

REFERENCES

Allen DW, Kim KW, Rawlinson WD, Craig ME. 2018. Maternal virus infections in pregnancy and type 1 diabetes in their offspring: systematic review and meta-analysis of observational studies. *Rev Med Virol* **28:** e1974. doi:10.1002/rmv.1974

Alvelos MI, et al. 2021. The RNA-binding profile of the splicing factor SRSF6 in immortalized human pancreatic β-cells. *Life Sci Alliance* **4**. doi:10.26508/lsa.202000825

Araki E, Oyadomari S, Mori M. 2003. Impact of endoplasmic reticulum stress pathway on pancreatic β-cells and diabetes mellitus. *Exp Biol Med* **228:** 1213–1217. doi:10.1177/153537020322801018

Atkinson MA, et al. 1994. Cellular immunity to a determinant common to glutamate decarboxylase and coxsackie virus in insulin-dependent diabetes. *J Clin Invest* **94:** 2125–2129.

Azoury ME, Tarayrah M, Afonso G, Pais A, Colli ML, Maillard C, Lavaud C, Alexandre-Heymann L, Gonzalez-Duque S, Verdier Y, et al. 2020. Peptides derived from insulin granule proteins are targeted by $CD8^+$ T cells across MHC class I restrictions in humans and NOD mice. *Diabetes* **69:** 2678–2690. doi:10.2337/db20-0013

Babon JA, DeNicola ME, Blodgett DM, Crèvecoeur I, Buttrick TS, Maehr R, Bottino R, Naji A, Kaddis J, Elyaman W, et al. 2016. Analysis of self-antigen specificity of islet-infiltrating T cells from human donors with type 1 diabetes. *Nat Med* **22:** 1482–1487. doi:10.1038/nm.4203

Baden MY, Imagawa A, Abiru N, Awata T, Ikegami H, Uchigata Y, Oikawa Y, Osawa H, Kajio H, Kawasaki E, et al. 2018. Characteristics and clinical course of type 1 diabetes mellitus related to anti-programmed cell death-1 therapy. *Diabetol Int* **10:** 58–66. doi:10.1007/s13340-018-0362-2

Baralle FE, Giudice J. 2017. Alternative splicing as a regulator of development and tissue identity. *Nat Rev: Molec Cell Biol* **18:** 437–451. doi:10.1038/nrm.2017.27

Bettini M, Bettini ML. 2021. Function, failure, and the future potential of Tregs in type 1 diabetes. *Diabetes* **70:** 1211–1219. doi:10.2337/dbi18-0058

Brozzi F, Eizirik DL. 2016. ER stress and the decline and fall of pancreatic β cells in type 1 diabetes. *Ups J Med Sci* **121:** 133–139. doi:10.3109/03009734.2015.1135217

Buitinga M, Callebaut A, Marques Câmara Sodré F, Crèvecoeur I, Blahnik-Fagan G, Yang ML, Bugliani M, Arribas-Layton D, Marré M, Cook DP, et al. 2018. Inflammation-induced citrullinated glucose-regulated protein 78 elicits immune responses in human type 1 diabetes. *Diabetes* **67:** 2337–2348. doi:10.2337/db18-0295

Coomans de Brachène A, Castela A, Op de Beeck A, Mirmira RG, Marselli L, Marchetti P, Masse C, Miao W, Leit S,

Evans-Molina C, et al. 2020. Preclinical evaluation of tyrosine kinase 2 inhibitors for human β-cell protection in type 1 diabetes. *Diabetes Obes Metab* **22:** 1827–1836. doi:10.1111/dom.14104

Cooper JD, Smyth DJ, Smiles AM, Plagnol V, Walker NM, Allen JE, Downes K, Barrett JC, Healy BC, Mychaleckyj JC, et al. 2008. Meta-analysis of genome-wide association study data identifies additional type 1 diabetes risk loci. *Nat Genet* **40:** 1399–1401. doi:10.1038/ng.249

Coppieters KT, Boettler T, von Herrath M. 2012. Virus infections in type 1 diabetes. *Cold Spring Harb Perspect Med* **2:** a007682. doi:10.1101/cshperspect.a007682

de Jong VM, Abreu JR, Verrijn Stuart AA, van der Slik AR, Verhaeghen K, Engelse MA, Blom B, Staal FJ, Gorus FK, Roep BO. 2013. Alternative splicing and differential expression of the islet autoantigen IGRP between pancreas and thymus contributes to immunogenicity of pancreatic islets but not diabetogenicity in humans. *Diabetologia* **56:** 2651–2658. doi:10.1007/s00125-013-3034-6

Delong T, Baker RL, He J, Barbour G, Bradley B, Haskins K. 2012. Diabetogenic T-cell clones recognize an altered peptide of chromogranin A. *Diabetes* **61:** 3239–3246. doi:10.2337/db12-0112

Delong T, Wiles TA, Baker RL, Bradley B, Barbour G, Reisdorph R, Armstrong M, Powell RL, Reisdorph N, Kumar N, et al. 2016. Pathogenic CD4 T cells in type 1 diabetes recognize epitopes formed by peptide fusion. *Science* **351:** 711–714. doi:10.1126/science.aad2791

Eizirik DL, Szymczak F, Mallone R. 2023. Why does the immune system destroy pancreatic β-cells but not α-cells in type 1 diabetes? *Nat Rev Endocrinol* **19:** 425–434. doi:10.1038/s41574-023-00826-3

Engin F, et al. 2013. Restoration of the unfolded protein response in pancreatic β cells protects mice against type 1 diabetes. *Sci Trans Med* **5:** 211ra156. doi:10.1126/scitranslmed.3006534

Field LL. 2002. Genetic linkage and association studies of type I diabetes: challenges and rewards. *Diabetologia* **45:** 21–35. doi:10.1007/s125-002-8241-7

Fløyel T, Kaur S, Pociot F. 2015. Genes affecting β-cell function in type 1 diabetes. *Curr Diab Rep* **15:** 97. doi:10.1007/s11892-015-0655-9

Frisk G, Friman G, Tuvemo T, Fohlman J, Diderholm H. 1992. Coxsackie B virus IgM in children at onset of type 1 (insulin-dependent) diabetes mellitus: evidence for IgM induction by a recent or current infection. *Diabetologia* **35:** 249–253. doi:10.1007/BF00400925

Gonzalez-Duque S, Azoury ME, Colli ML, Afonso G, Turatsinze JV, Nigi L, Lalanne AI, Sebastiani G, Carré A, Pinto S, et al. 2018. Conventional and neo-antigenic peptides presented by β cells are targeted by circulating naive $CD8^+$ T cells in type 1 diabetic and healthy donors. *Cell Metab* **28:** 946–960.e6. doi:10.1016/j.cmet.2018.07.007

Harding HP, Ron D. 2002. Endoplasmic reticulum stress and the development of diabetes: a review. *Diabetes* **51:** S455–S461. doi:10.2337/diabetes.51.2007.s455

Harding HP, Zeng H, Zhang Y, Jungries R, Chung P, Plesken H, Sabatini DD, Ron D. 2001. Diabetes mellitus and exocrine pancreatic dysfunction in perk$^{-/-}$ mice reveals a role for translational control in secretory cell survival. *Mol Cell* **7:** 1153–1163. doi:10.1016/s1097-2765(01)00264-7

Herold Z, Doleschall M, Somogyi A. 2021. Role and function of granin proteins in diabetes mellitus. *World J Diabetes* **12:** 1081–1092. doi:10.4239/wjd.v12.i7.1081

Hober D, Sauter P. 2010. Pathogenesis of type 1 diabetes mellitus: interplay between enterovirus and host. *Nat Rev Endocrinol* **6:** 279–289. doi:10.1038/nrendo.2010.27

Honeyman MC, Stone NL, Harrison LC. 1998. T-cell epitopes in type 1 diabetes autoantigen tyrosine phosphatase IA-2: potential for mimicry with rotavirus and other environmental agents. *Molec Med* **4:** 231–239.

Horn T, et al. 2023. Position-dependent effects of RNA-binding proteins in the context of co-transcriptional splicing. *NPJ Syst Biol Appl* **9:** 1–22. doi:10.1038/s41540-022-00264-3

Horwitz MS, Ilic A, Fine C, Balasa B, Sarvetnick N. 2004. Coxsackieviral-mediated diabetes: induction requires antigen-presenting cells and is accompanied by phagocytosis of β cells. *Clin Immunol* **110:** 134–144. doi:10.1016/j.clim.2003.09.014

Hwang J, Qi L. 2018. Quality control in the endoplasmic reticulum: crosstalk between ERAD and UPR pathways. *Trends Biochem Sci* **43:** 593–605. doi:10.1016/j.tibs.2018.06.005

Ikegami H, Kawabata Y, Noso S. 2016. Immune checkpoint therapy and type 1 diabetes. *Diabetol Int* **7:** 221–227. doi:10.1007/s13340-016-0276-9

Ilonen J, Lempainen J, Veijola R. 2019. The heterogeneous pathogenesis of type 1 diabetes mellitus. *Nat Rev Endocrinol* **15:** 635–650. doi:10.1038/s41574-019-0254-y

Isaacs SR, Foskett DB, Maxwell AJ, Ward EJ, Faulkner CL, Luo JYX, Rawlinson WD, Craig ME, Kim KW. 2021. Viruses and type 1 diabetes: from enteroviruses to the virome. *Microorganisms* **9:** 1519. doi:10.3390/microorganisms9071519

James EA, Pietropaolo M, Mamula MJ. 2018. Immune recognition of β-cells: neoepitopes as key players in the loss of tolerance. *Diabetes* **67:** 1035–1042. doi:10.2337/dbi17-0030

Jeffery N, et al. 2019. Cellular stressors may alter islet hormone cell proportions by moderation of alternative splicing patterns. *Hum Molec Genet* **28:** 2763–2774. doi:10.1093/hmg/ddz094

Juan-Mateu J, Villate O, Eizirik DL. 2016. Mechanisms in endocrinology: alternative splicing: the new frontier in diabetes research. *Eur J Endocrinol* **174:** R225–R238. doi:10.1530/EJE-15-0916

Kamrath C, Rosenbauer J, Eckert AJ, Siedler K, Bartelt H, Klose D, Sindichakis M, Herrlinger S, Lahn V, Holl RW. 2022. Incidence of type 1 diabetes in children and adolescents during the COVID-19 pandemic in Germany: results from the DPV registry. *Diabetes Care* **45:** 1762–1771. doi:10.2337/dc21-0969

Kim YK, Kim YR, Wells KL, Sarbaugh D, Guney M, Tsai CF, Zee T, Karsenty G, Nakayasu ES, Sussel L. 2024. PTPN2 regulates metabolic flux to affect β cell susceptibility to inflammatory stress. *Diabetes* **73:** 434–447. doi:10.2337/db23-0355

Knebel UE, Peleg S, Dai C, Cohen-Fultheim R, Jonsson S, Poznyak K, Israeli M, Zamashanski L, Glaser B, Levanon EY, et al. 2024. Disrupted RNA editing in β cells mimics early-stage type 1 diabetes. *Cell Metab* **36:** 48–61.e6. doi:10.1016/j.cmet.2023.11.011

Kometani K, Nakagawa R, Shinnakasu R, Kaji T, Rybouchkin A, Moriyama S, Furukawa K, Koseki H, Takemori T, Kurosaki T. 2013. Repression of the transcription factor Bach2 contributes to predisposition of IgG1 memory B cells toward plasma cell differentiation. *Immunity* **39:** 136–147. doi:10.1016/j.immuni.2013.06.011

Kracht MJ, van Lummel M, Nikolic T, Joosten AM, Laban S, van der Slik AR, van Veelen PA, Carlotti F, de Koning EJ, Hoeben RC, et al. 2017. Autoimmunity against a defective ribosomal insulin gene product in type 1 diabetes. *Nat Med* **23:** 501–507. doi:10.1038/nm.4289

Krogvold L, Mynarek IM, Ponzi E, Mørk FB, Hessel TW, Roald T, Lindblom N, Westman J, Barker P, Hyöty H, et al. 2023. Pleconaril and ribavirin in new-onset type 1 diabetes: a phase 2 randomized trial. *Nat Med* **29:** 2902–2908. doi:10.1038/s41591-023-02576-1

Lerner AG, Upton JP, Praveen PV, Ghosh R, Nakagawa Y, Igbaria A, Shen S, Nguyen V, Backes BJ, Heiman M, et al. 2012. IRE1α induces thioredoxin-interacting protein to activate the NLRP3 inflammasome and promote programmed cell death under irremediable ER stress. *Cell Metab* **16:** 250–264. doi:10.1016/j.cmet.2012.07.007

Lieberman SM, Evans AM, Han B, Takaki T, Vinnitskaya Y, Caldwell JA, Serreze DV, Shabanowitz J, Hunt DF, Nathenson SG, et al. 2003. Identification of the β cell antigen targeted by a prevalent population of pathogenic $CD8^+$ T cells in autoimmune diabetes. *Proc Natl Acad Sci* **100:** 8384–8388. doi:10.1073/pnas.0932778100

Maedler K, Sergeev P, Ris F, Oberholzer J, Joller-Jemelka HI, Spinas GA, Kaiser N, Halban PA, Donath MY. 2002. Glucose-induced β cell production of IL-1β contributes to glucotoxicity in human pancreatic islets. *J Clin Invest* **110:** 851–860. doi:10.1172/JCI15318

Mallone R, Eizirik DL. 2020. Presumption of innocence for β cells: why are they vulnerable autoimmune targets in type 1 diabetes? *Diabetologia* **63:** 1999–2006. doi:10.1007/s00125-020-05176-7

Marré ML, James EA, Piganelli JD. 2015. B cell ER stress and the implications for immunogenicity in type 1 diabetes. *Front Cell Dev Biol* **3:** 67. doi:10.3389/fcell.2015.00067

Marré ML, McGinty JW, Chow I-T, DeNicola ME, Beck NW, Kent SC, Powers AC, Bottino R, Harlan DM, Greenbaum CJ, et al. 2018. Modifying enzymes are elicited by ER stress, generating epitopes that are selectively recognized by $CD4^+$ T cells in patients with type 1 diabetes. *Diabetes* **67:** 1356–1368. doi:10.2337/db17-1166

Marroquí L, Santin I, Dos Santos RS, Marselli L, Marchetti P, Eizirik DL. 2014. *BACH2*, a candidate risk gene for type 1 diabetes, regulates apoptosis in pancreatic β-cells via JNK1 modulation and crosstalk with the candidate gene *PTPN2*. *Diabetes* **63:** 2516–2527. doi:10.2337/db13-1443

Marroqui L, Lopes M, dos Santos RS, Grieco FA, Roivainen M, Richardson SJ, Morgan NG, Op de Beeck A, Eizirik DL. 2015. Differential cell autonomous responses determine the outcome of coxsackievirus infections in murine pancreatic α and β cells. *eLife* **4:** e06990. doi:10.7554/eLife.06990

McGinty JW, Chow IT, Greenbaum C, Odegard J, Kwok WW, James EA. 2014. Recognition of posttranslationally modified GAD65 epitopes in subjects with type 1 diabetes. *Diabetes* **63:** 3033–3040. doi:10.2337/db13-1952

McKeigue PM, McGurnaghan S, Blackbourn L, Bath LE, McAllister DA, Caparrotta TM, Wild SH, Wood SN, Stockton D, Colhoun HM. 2023. Relation of incident type 1 diabetes to recent COVID-19 infection: cohort study using e-health record linkage in Scotland. *Diabetes Care* **46:** 921–928. doi:10.2337/dc22-0385

Moore F, Colli ML, Cnop M, Esteve MI, Cardozo AK, Cunha DA, Bugliani M, Marchetti P, Eizirik DL. 2009. PTPN2, a candidate gene for type 1 diabetes, modulates interferon-γ-induced pancreatic β-cell apoptosis. *Diabetes* **58:** 1283–1291. doi:10.2337/db08-1510

Nairn C, Galbraith DN, Taylor KW, Clements GB. 1999. Enterovirus variants in the serum of children at the onset of type 1 diabetes mellitus. *Diabet Med* **16:** 509–513. doi:10.1046/j.1464-5491.1999.00098.x

Noble JA, Valdes AM, Bugawan TL, Apple RJ, Thomson G, Erlich HA. 2002. The HLA class I A locus affects susceptibility to type 1 diabetes. *Hum Immunol* **63:** 657–664. doi:10.1016/s0198-8859(02)00421-4

Noble JA, Erlich HA. 2012. Genetics of type 1 diabetes. *Cold Spring Harb Perspect Med* **2:** a007732. doi:10.1101/cshperspect.a007732

Nogueira TC, Paula FM, Villate O, Colli ML, Moura RF, Cunha DA, Marselli L, Marchetti P, Cnop M, Julier C, Eizirik DL. 2013. GLIS3, a susceptibility gene for type 1 and type 2 diabetes, modulates pancreatic β cell apoptosis via regulation of a splice variant of the BH3-only protein Bim. *PLoS Genet* **9:** e1003532. doi:10.1371/journal.pgen.1003532

Ortis F, Naamane N, Flamez D, Ladriere L, Moor F, Cunha DA, Colli ML, Thykjaer T, Thorsen K, Orntoft TF, Eizirik DL. 2010. Cytokines interleukin-1β and tumor necrosis factor-α regulate different transcriptional and alternative splicing networks in primary β-cells. *Diabetes* **59:** 358–374. doi:10.2337/db09-1159

Oslowski CM, Hara T, O'Sullivan-Murphy B, Kanekura K, Lu S, Hara M, Ishigaki S, Zhu LJ, Hayashi E, Hui ST, et al. 2012. Thioredoxin-interacting protein mediates ER stress-induced β cell death through initiation of the inflammasome. *Cell Metab* **16:** 265–273. doi:10.1016/j.cmet.2012.07.005

Oyadomari S, Takeda K, Takiguchi M, Gotoh T, Matsumoto M, Wada I, Akira S, Araki E, Mori M. 2001. Nitric oxide-induced apoptosis in pancreatic β cells is mediated by the endoplasmic reticulum stress pathway. *Proc Natl Acad Sci* **98:** 10845–10850. doi:10.1073/pnas.191207498

Pellenz FM, Dieter C, Lemos NE, Bauer AC, Souza BM, Crispim D. 2021. Association of TYK2 polymorphisms with autoimmune diseases: a comprehensive and updated systematic review with meta-analysis. *Genet Mol Biol* **44:** e20200425. doi:10.1590/1678-4685-GMB-2020-0425

Piganelli JD, Mamula MJ, James EA. 2021. The role of β cell stress and neo-epitopes in the immunopathology of type 1 diabetes. *Front Endocrinol* **11:** 624590. doi:10.3389/fendo.2020.624590

Rewers M, Bonifacio E, Ewald D, Geno Rasmussen C, Jia X, Pyle L, Ziegler AG, ASK Study Group and Fr1da Study Group. 2022. SARS-CoV-2 infections and presymptomatic type 1 diabetes autoimmunity in children and adolescents from Colorado, USA, and Bavaria, Germany. *J Am Med Assoc* **328:** 1252–1255. doi:10.1001/jama.2022.14092

Richardson SJ, Rodriguez-Calvo T, Gerling IC, Mathews CE, Kaddis JS, Russell MA, Zeissler M, Leete P, Krogvold L, Dahl-Jorgensen K, et al. 2016. Islet cell hyperexpression of HLA class I antigens: a defining feature in type 1 diabetes. *Diabetologia* **59:** 2448–2458. doi:10.1007/s00125-016-4067-4

Roca-Rivada A, Marín-Cañas S, Colli ML, Vinci C, Sawatani T, Marselli L, Cnop M, Marchetti P, Eizirik DL. 2023. Inhibition of the type 1 diabetes candidate gene PTPN2 aggravates TNF-α-induced human β cell dysfunction and death. *Diabetologia* **66:** 1544–1556. doi:10.1007/s00125-023-05908-5

Roep BO, Thomaidou S, van Tienhoven R, Zaldumbide A. 2021. Type 1 diabetes mellitus as a disease of the β-cell (do not blame the immune system?). *Nat Rev Endocrinol* **17:** 150–161. doi:10.1038/s41574-020-00443-4

Ron D. 2002. Translational control in the endoplasmic reticulum stress response. *J Clin Invest* **110:** 1383–1388. doi:10.1172/JCI16784

Roychoudhuri R, Hirahara K, Mousavi K, Clever D, Klebanoff CA, Bonelli M, Sciumè G, Zare H, Vahedi G, Dema B, et al. 2013. BACH2 represses effector programs to stabilize T(reg)-mediated immune homeostasis. *Nature* **498:** 506–510. doi:10.1038/nature12199

Rønningen KS, Spurkland A, Iwe T, Vartdal F, Thorsby E. 1991. Distribution of HLA-DRB1, -DQA1 and -DQB1 alleles and DQA1-DQB1 genotypes among Norwegian patients with insulin-dependent diabetes mellitus. *Tissue Antigens* **37:** 105–111. doi:10.1111/j.1399-0039.1991.tb01854.x

Sahin GS, Lee H, Engin F. 2021. An accomplice more than a mere victim: the impact of β-cell ER stress on type 1 diabetes pathogenesis. *Mol Metab* **54:** 101365. doi:10.1016/j.molmet.2021.101365

Salmi H, Heinonen S, Hästbacka J, Lääperi M, Rautiainen P, Miettinen PJ, Vapalahti O, Hepojoki J, Knip M. 2022. New-onset type 1 diabetes in Finnish children during the COVID-19 pandemic. *Arc Dis Childhood* **107:** 180–185. doi:10.1136/archdischild-2020-321220

Scheuner D, Kaufman RJ. 2008. The unfolded protein response: a pathway that links insulin demand with β-cell failure and diabetes. *Endocr Rev* **29:** 317–333. doi:10.1210/er.2007-0039

Sherr J, Sosenko J, Skyler JS, Herold KC. 2008. Prevention of type 1 diabetes: the time has come. *Nat Clin Pract Endocrinol Metab* **4:** 334–343. doi:10.1038/ncpendmet0832

Tittel SR, Rosenbauer J, Kamrath C, Ziegler J, Reschke F, Hammersen J, Mönkemöller K, Pappa A, Kapellen T, Holl RW, et al. 2020. Did the COVID-19 lockdown affect the incidence of pediatric type 1 diabetes in Germany? *Diabetes Care* **43:** e172–e173. doi:10.2337/dc20-1633

Vlad A, Serban V, Timar R, Sima A, Botea V, Albai O, Timar B, Vlad M. 2021. Increased incidence of type 1 diabetes during the COVID-19 pandemic in Romanian children. *Medicina (Kaunas)* **57:** 973. doi:10.3390/medicina57090973

Yang P, Li M, Guo D, Gong F, Adam B-L, Atkinson MA, Wang C-Y. 2008. Comparative analysis of the islet proteome between NOD/Lt and ALR/Lt mice. *Ann NY Acad Sci* **1150:** 68–71. doi:10.1196/annals.1447.002

Yang ML, Sodré FMC, Mamula MJ, Overbergh L. 2021. Citrullination and PAD enzyme biology in type 1 diabetes—regulators of inflammation, autoimmunity, and pathology. *Front Immunol* **12:** 678953. doi:10.3389/fimmu.2021.678953

Yang ML, Horstman S, Gee R, Guyer P, Lam TT, Kanyo J, Perdigoto AL, Speake C, Greenbaum CJ, Callebaut A, et al. 2022. Citrullination of glucokinase is linked to autoimmune diabetes. *Nat Commun* **13:** 1870. doi:10.1038/s41467-022-29512-0

Yeung WCG, Rawlinson WD, Craig ME. 2011. Enterovirus infection and type 1 diabetes mellitus: systematic review and meta-analysis of observational molecular studies. *Br Med J* **342:** d35. doi:10.1136/bmj.d35

Yin H, Berg AK, Tuvemo T, Frisk G. 2002. Enterovirus RNA is found in peripheral blood mononuclear cells in a majority of type 1 diabetic children at onset. *Diabetes* **51:** 1964–1971. doi:10.2337/diabetes.51.6.1964

Zareini B, Sørensen KK, Eiken PA, Fischer TK, Kristensen PL, Lendorf ME, Pedersen-Bjergaard U, Torp-Pedersen C, Nolsoe RLM. 2023. Association of COVID-19 and development of type 1 diabetes: a Danish nationwide register study. *Diabetes Care* **46:** 1477–1482. doi:10.2337/dc23-0428

The Human Pancreas in Type 1 Diabetes: Lessons Learned from the Network of Pancreatic Organ Donors with Diabetes

Irina Kusmartseva,[1] Amanda Posgai,[1] Mingder Yang,[1] Richard Oram,[2] Mark Atkinson,[1] Alberto Pugliese,[3] and Carmella Evans-Molina[4]

[1]Department of Pathology, Immunology, and Laboratory Medicine, College of Medicine, University of Florida, Gainesville, Florida 32610, USA

[2]Clinical and Biomedical Sciences, Faculty of Health and Life Sciences, University of Exeter, Exeter EX1 2LU, United Kingdom

[3]Department of Diabetes Immunology, Arthur Riggs Diabetes and Metabolism Research Institute, City of Hope, Duarte, California 91010, USA

[4]Center for Diabetes and Metabolic Diseases, Indiana University School of Medicine, Indianapolis, Indiana 46202, USA

Correspondence: cevansmo@iupui.edu

The Network for Pancreatic Organ Donors with Diabetes (nPOD) has helped shape the contemporary understanding of type 1 diabetes (T1D) pathogenesis in humans through the procurement, distribution to scientists, and collaborative study of human pancreata and disease-related tissues from organ donors with T1D and islet autoantibody positivity. Since its inception in 2007, nPOD has collected tissues from 600 donors, and these resources have been distributed across 22 countries to more than 290 projects, resulting in nearly 350 publications. Research projects supported by nPOD span the breadth of diabetes research, including studies on T1D immunology and β-cell biology, and have uniquely unveiled abnormalities in other pancreatic cell types. In this article, we will detail the history and programmatic features of nPOD, as well as highlight key scientific findings from nPOD studies. We will present our view for the future of nPOD and discuss how the success of the program has established a precedent whereby knowledge gaps in biomedical research can be addressed through the study of human tissues.

The Network for Pancreatic Organ Donors with Diabetes (nPOD) program was formed in 2007. nPOD's mission, throughout 17 years of continuous operation, is to improve our collective knowledge of human type 1 diabetes (T1D) pathogenesis through the procurement, distribution to scientists, and collaborative study of human pancreata and disease-related tissues from organ donors with T1D and islet autoantibody (AAb) positivity. Since its genesis, nPOD has collected

Cite this article as *Cold Spring Harb Perspect Med* doi: 10.1101/cshperspect.a041588

organs, tissues, DNA, and RNA from more than 600 donors, and these resources have been distributed across 22 countries to nearly 300 projects in both academic and industry settings, resulting in almost 350 publications (www.jdrfnpod.org/publications/npod-publications). Furthermore, nPOD has helped facilitate the development of a robust and collaborative community of T1D investigators that incorporates multiple disciplines. In parallel, nPOD has served as a model system for other organ donor-based research programs developed in the diabetes research community and beyond (HuBMAP Consortium 2019; Kaestner et al. 2019; Shapira et al. 2022), thus establishing a precedent whereby knowledge voids related to disease pathogenesis in humans are addressed through the study of organ donor tissues. The goal of this paper is to highlight the history and unique programmatic features of nPOD and to summarize key scientific findings from the nPOD program that have enhanced our understanding of T1D pathogenesis, including immune, endocrine, and exocrine contributions to disease.

HISTORY OF THE GENESIS OF NPOD

Historically, studies of serum and peripheral blood have predominated human T1D research, largely because investigations of pancreatic tissues have been limited by the difficulty of obtaining suitable samples. Commonly, human pancreatic specimens were from retrospective collection of tissues obtained at autopsy from individuals who died at or near the time of symptomatic diabetes onset (Gepts 1965; Foulis et al. 1986). While pragmatic, this approach to obtaining pancreas tissue has several significant limitations, including poor tissue quality, limited quantity, and restrictive sample format. In addition, lack of lymphoid tissue availability, limited knowledge of clinical histories, and minimal capability to perform modern assessments of β-cell function, immune cell profiling, and metabolic control significantly hampered information that could be gleaned from studies on these otherwise highly valuable pancreata.

In 2006, in response to a request by Dr. George Eisenbarth, the Juvenile Diabetes Research Foundation (JDRF) formed a task force to design a system that would provide investigators with access to transplant-quality pancreata obtained from organ donors with T1D and at increased risk for T1D. The concept that T1D research would be advanced by the availability of these human pancreata was not a significant controversy; however, the task force faced many hurdles. Concerns existed over financial, logistical, practical, and ethical limitations and whether these limitations could be overcome to expand such a program across the country. Following 6 months of in-depth analysis by a committee comprised of T1D researchers, JDRF staff, JDRF lay review committee members, Organ Procurement Organization (OPO) administrators, and tissue procurement officers, nPOD was conceptualized and initiated (Campbell-Thompson et al. 2012a; Pugliese et al. 2014; Kaddis et al. 2015).

OVERVIEW OF THE nPOD PROGRAM AND BIOREPOSITORY

The structure of nPOD includes three main components: (1) the Administrative Coordinating Center, (2) the Organ Processing and Pathology Core (OPPC), and (3) the Immunology Core (Fig. 1). The Administrative Coordinating Center has well-established partnerships with all 56 OPOs across the United States, enabling nPOD to obtain transplant-quality tissues (Fig. 1). Upon acceptance of a donor offer, organs are processed within 24 hours of procurement at the OPPC at the University of Florida (UF) Diabetes Institute according to established standard operating procedures (SOPs) (Fig. 2; Campbell-Thompson et al. 2012b,c). Every donor pancreas is evaluated using histology and immunohistochemistry to provide baseline characterization of tissue quality, pancreatic islet morphology, and detection of insulitis according to standard criteria (Campbell-Thompson et al. 2013). The images of stained slides and de-identified donor information are shared via the nPOD Online Pathology System and nPOD Data Portal (npod.org/for-investigators/data-portal). The Immunology Core works alongside the OPPC to apply state-of-the-art technologies to define immune correlates of disease and to generate single cell data

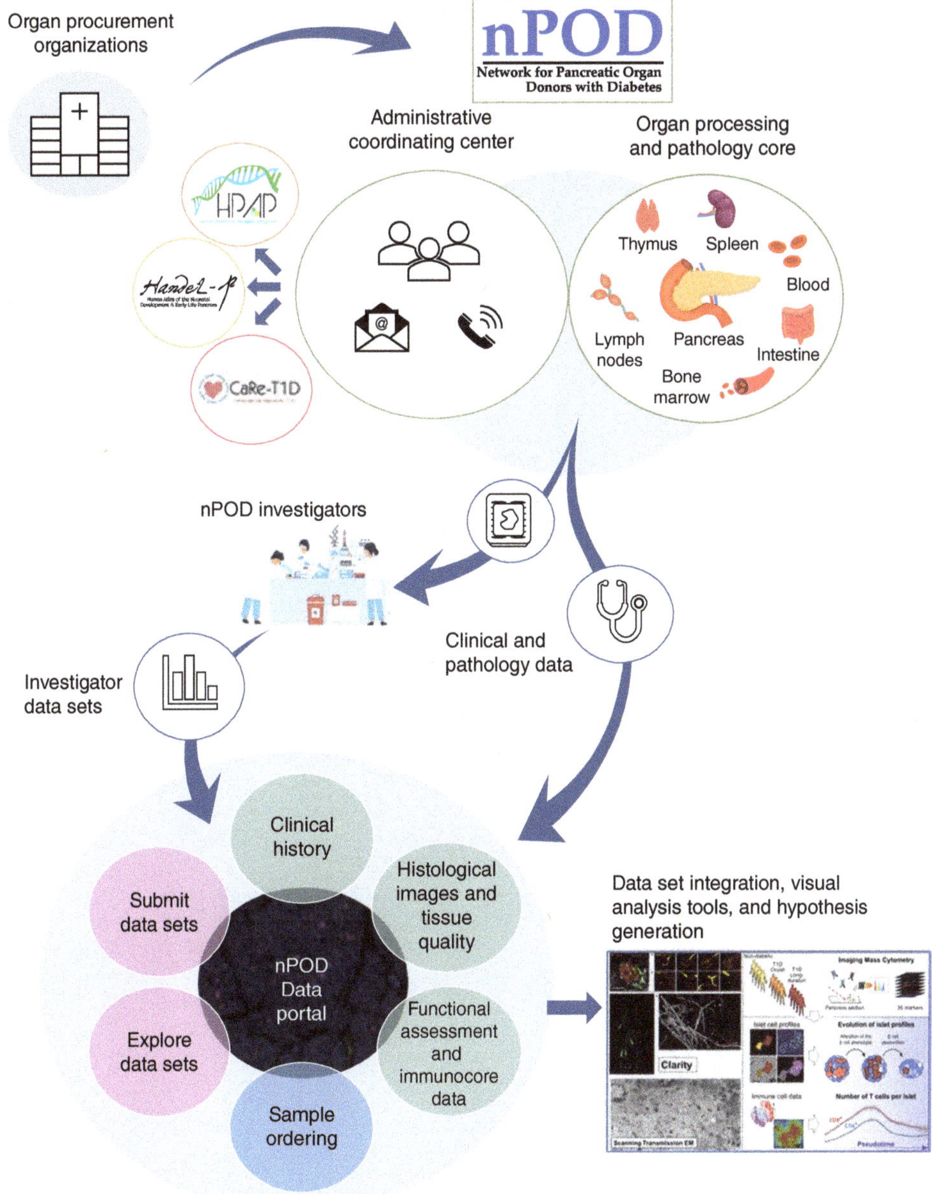

Figure 1. Network for Pancreatic Organ donors with Diabetes (nPOD) organizational structure. Organizational flow chart of nPOD operations.

(Fuhrman et al. 2015; Haller et al. 2016; Seay et al. 2016, 2017; Chen et al. 2017; Driver et al. 2017; Newby et al. 2017; Sebastiani et al. 2017; Yeh et al. 2017; Ahmed et al. 2019; Khosravi-Maharlooei et al. 2019; Peters et al. 2019; Shapiro et al. 2019, 2020a,b; Beam et al. 2020; Dean et al. 2020; Motwani et al. 2020) to support high-level bioinformatic and machine learning analyses. The standardized assessments performed by the OPPC and Immunology Core ensure that each donated organ undergoes rigorous phenotyping and analysis to provide baseline categorization,

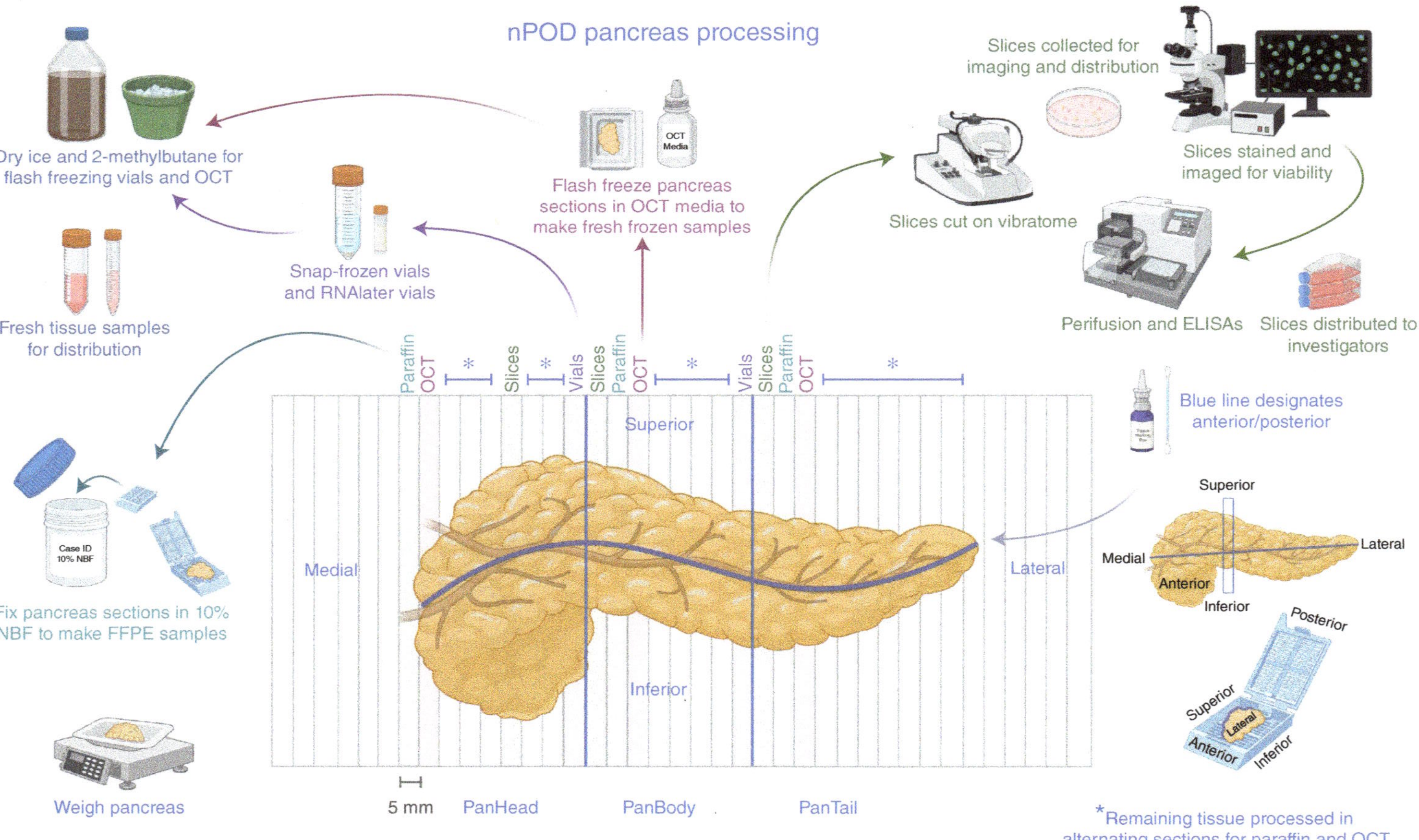

Figure 2. Pancreas processing schematic. Pancreas processing is guided by a set of rigorous standard operating procedures for each organ brought into the program.

thus ensuring that repetitive experiments do not need to be performed by investigators receiving downstream tissues. The current status of the nPOD biorepository is summarized in Figure 3.

SCIENTIFIC IMPACT OF THE nPOD PROGRAM

The nPOD program has helped shape the contemporary understanding of human T1D by providing multiple investigators with access to pancreas and lymphoid tissues, and by promoting collaborative and coordinated analyses of tissues collected under rigorous conditions with extensive baseline phenotyping. Importantly, nPOD has leveraged tissue collection from donors with T1D at different disease stages, including the preclinical stages (defined by the presence of islet AAb in donors without T1D), the peridiagnostic period, established disease extending for many years after diagnosis, and rare transplant recipients who developed recurrence of T1D despite immunosuppression (Fig. 3). While nPOD studies can only be cross sectional, the availability of specimens from various disease stages increases our understanding of the natural history of disease development, which has critical implications for the design of clinical trials and intervention studies. Finally, nPOD studies have led to critical validation of earlier findings from peripheral blood of living individuals and have generated novel discoveries that are only possible given access to human tissues and state-of-the-art methodologies (Fig. 4).

In the sections below, we summarize how analysis of nPOD tissue has advanced our understanding of human T1D. We summarize new opportunities for genotype–phenotype association studies, and we discuss challenges and surprises encountered during the construction of this unique human organ donor research program. Finally, we end with a vision for coordinated investigation of several future opportunities and key questions (Table 1).

T1D IMMUNOLOGY

T1D is primarily considered a T-cell-mediated autoimmune disease. However, many key questions remain regarding the timing and contribution of insulitis to human T1D, the sequence and composition of islet-infiltrating immune cells, and the repertoire of antigens and epitopes recognized by these immune cells. One of the motivating factors for the formation of nPOD was the need to test the hypothesis that AAb positivity would be associated with the presence of insulitis in the pancreas (Insel et al. 2015). By examining donors at different disease stages, a recent analysis of nPOD donors illustrated that the propor-

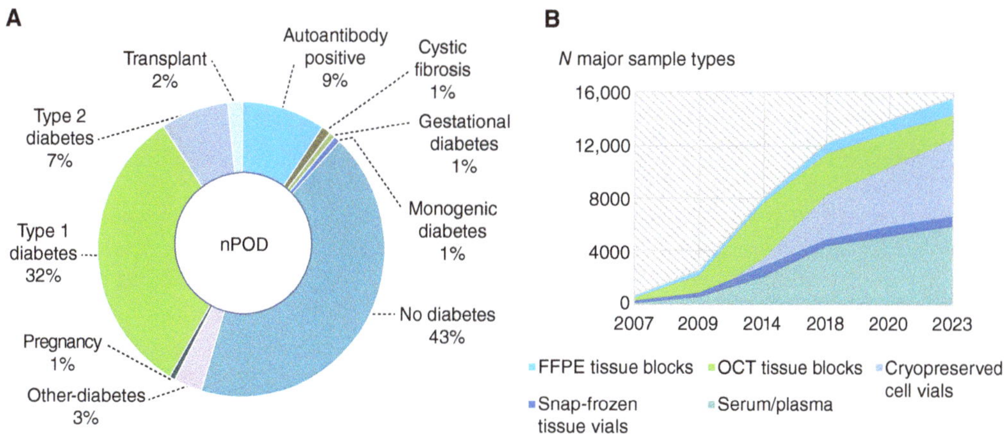

Figure 3. Overview of the Network for Pancreatic Organ donors with Diabetes (nPOD) biorepository. (*A*) The distribution of donor diagnoses within the nPOD biorepository. (*B*) The cumulative acquisition of tissues brought into the biorepository.

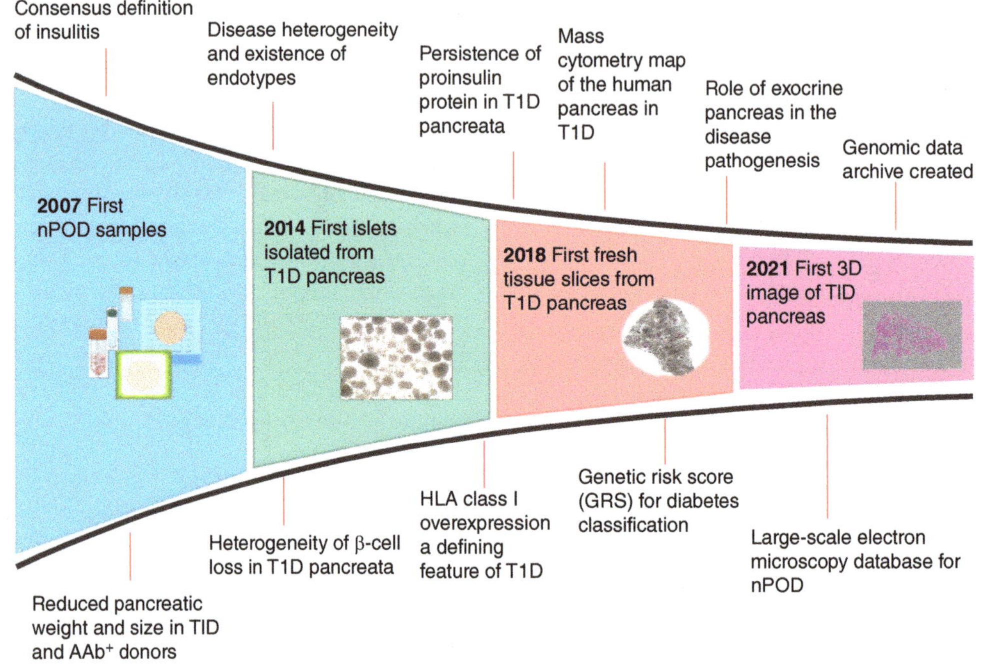

Figure 4. Timeline of Network for Pancreatic Organ donors with Diabetes (nPOD) program evolution including key programmatic advancements and scientific discoveries.

tion of infiltrated islets and the density of infiltrating T cells evolves during disease progression, with infiltration becoming apparent in double AAb–positive pre-T1D donors (Apaolaza et al. 2023). However, insulitis and β-cell loss are rarely found in donors with AAb positivity, especially those with a single AAb. In those that had insulitis, the immune cell infiltration was typically mild, restricted to a small number of islets, and associated with limited evidence of β-cell loss, suggesting that the mere presence of AAb may not be a reflection of ongoing islet destruction. This finding needs to be considered in clinical trials, as certain therapies may not be ideal at this stage of disease, at least in the absence of signs of metabolic abnormalities that could indicate β-cell loss and dysfunction. However, as described elsewhere in this article, several studies by nPOD investigators have demonstrated pancreatic alterations among AAb-positive donors, even those with a single AAb. Thus, it appears that abnormalities in β cells, α cells, and even exocrine cells may be present in earlier disease stages (Fig. 5), with active autoimmune destruction of islets becoming prominent closer to diagnosis. This concept is also supported by longitudinal studies of at-risk relatives of individuals with T1D (Bogun et al. 2020).

The examination of nPOD donors has allowed for advanced and accurate characterization, assessment, and quantification of pancreas pathology at multiple disease stages. nPOD investigators have developed a consensus definition of insulitis (Campbell-Thompson et al. 2013), which is now used by most research studies, thus providing more uniformity in interpretation. Critically, new reagents to detect autoreactive T cells have led to the demonstration that T cells with reactivity against islet antigens are found in insulitis lesions, which is a fundamental validation of the T-cell-driven nature of T1D. Moreover, it appears that the diversity of the immune response increases over time, suggesting epitope spreading (Coppieters et al. 2012). Different patterns of insulitis have been reported based on the relative proportions of B and T cells,

Table 1. Key questions and future opportunities

Key Question 1	What are the key differences in disease phenotype and pathogenesis when stage 3 T1D is diagnosed in children versus adults?
Key Question 2	How do changes in prohormone processing and posttranslational antigenic processing defects contribute to T1D development?
Key Question 3	What is the role of the exocrine pancreas in T1D development?
Key Question 4	How can nPOD most effectively facilitate translational studies to advance immunotherapies (e.g., CAR-Treg), β-cell surrogate therapies, or other therapies for T1D? How can nPOD leverage live tissue platforms to test candidate therapeutics? How can nPOD activities be better integrated with new clinical trial results? In turn, how can clinical trial results inform nPOD priorities and activities?
Key Question 5	Which β or islet cell–specific targets will be most useful for a variety of studies, including imaging, small molecule delivery, and immune targeting efforts (e.g., CAR-Treg, therapeutic antibodies)?
Key Question 6	How might nPOD studies better guide clinical trials seeking to understand diversity (e.g., ancestry/race, age, social determinants of health), polygenic disease risk, and therapeutic targets for T1D prevention and reversal?

(T1D) Type 1 diabetes, (nPOD) Network for Pancreatic Organ Donors with Diabetes.

supporting the concept of disease endotypes that may be related to some extent to age (Arif et al. 2014; Battaglia et al. 2020; Leete et al. 2020).

Recent studies have relied on advanced methodologies, including mass cytometry, to analyze the cellular composition of islet cell infiltrates and determine the phenotype of immune cells both in the islets and in the exocrine compartment, leading to a better understanding of cellular networks and interactions (Damond et al. 2019; Wang et al. 2019). Using islets and pancreatic lymph nodes, nPOD researchers have identified and characterized key features of islet-infiltrating T and B cells (Smith et al. 2015; Babon et al. 2016; Michels et al. 2017; Anderson et al. 2021; Stensland et al. 2023), leading to the confirmation of previously known epitopes and the discovery of novel T- and B-cell reactivities, including those reacting against native epitopes, neoepitopes, and epitopes resulting from alternatively spliced variants (Guyer et al. 2023). For example, Babon et al. (2016) recovered and characterized islet-infiltrating T cells from nine donors between 6 and 30 years of age with 2–20 years since T1D diagnosis (Babon et al. 2016). The study assessed a comprehensive set of antigen specificities and represents one of the most expansive analyses of islet-infiltrating T cells in T1D donors, with more than 250 T-cell lines or clones obtained. Among those characterized, many T cells reacted against known autoantigens, including neoepitopes (McGinty et al. 2015; Delong et al. 2016), and functional analyses revealed proinflammatory profiles typical of effector phenotypes. This systematic evaluation demonstrated the existence of a broad repertoire of T-cell responses, likely resulting from heterogeneity in HLA restriction, environmental factors, and disease stage. Considering the wide range of disease duration among the donors examined, the demonstration of autoreactive islet-infiltrating T cells ex vivo is consistent with the expanded pathology assessment of insulitis in nPOD donors. Together, these findings suggest that islet autoimmunity is chronic and continues for years after diagnosis.

The ability to study islet-infiltrating immune cells from disease-relevant human tissues has also allowed for the creation of multiple new tools for the assessment of autoimmunity in T1D. These advancements include the assembly of databases inclusive of T-cell receptor (TCR) and B-cell receptor (BCR) data (Seay et al. 2016; Linsley et al. 2023) and the engineering of T cells that express T1D-associated TCRs (Michels et al. 2017), which can be used in a variety of experimental studies. Additionally, TCRs can be exploited for therapeutic application, for example, by expressing known T1D-associated clones on transduced regulatory T cells (Treg) or chimeric antigen receptor (CAR)-Treg cells (Yang et al. 2022; Hunt et al. 2023; Obarorakpor et al. 2023;

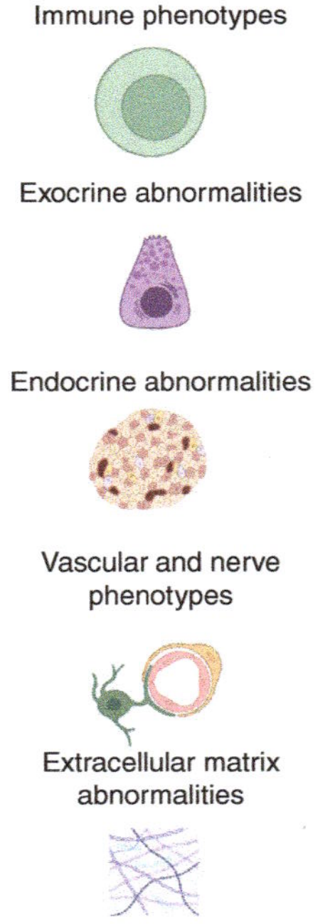

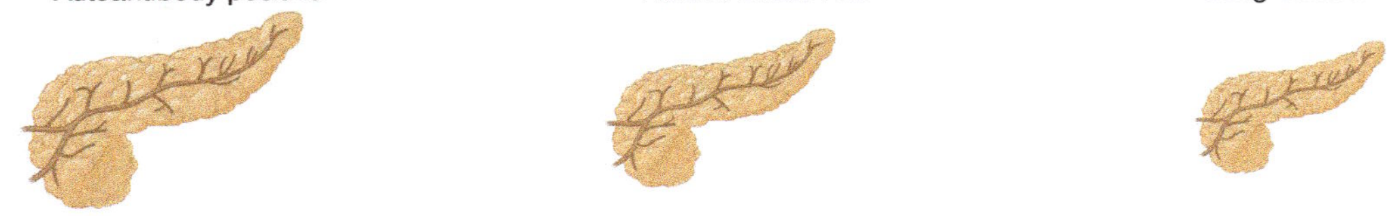

	Autoantibody positive	Recent-onset T1D	Long-duration T1D
	Pancreas size ↓	Pancreas size ↓↓	Pancreas size ↓↓↓
Immune phenotypes	Insulitis is mild and restricted to a small number of islets	Insulitis is commonly observed	Insulitis frequency declines with diabetes duration and affects ICIs
Exocrine abnormalities	HLA class I overexpression is lobular and present in ICIs	HLA class I overexpression is lobular and present in ICIs	HLA class I overexpression is lobular and present in ICIs
	Very low HLA class II expression	HLA class II present in a subset of ICIs	HLA class II present in a subset of ICIs
	No reduction in acinar cells size and number	Reduced acinar cell size and increased acinar number	Reduced acinar cell size and number
Endocrine abnormalities	β-Cell mass relatively preserved	β-Cell mass reductions are heterogeneous at time of stage 3 onset (60%–95%)	β-Cell mass reduced 88%–95%
	Proinsulin$^+$ area and PI/I ratio increased	PI/I ratio increased	Proinsulin persistence in some β cells even in the context of negative C-peptide
	α-Cell dysfunction described in GAD$^+$ donors; mass unchanged	α-Cell dysfunction; mass unchanged	α-Cell dysfunction; mass unchanged
Vascular and nerve phenotypes	Islet axon numbers were significantly lower in AAb-positive donors compared to T1D individuals, exocrine axon density was unaltered	Islet axon numbers were significantly lower in AAb-positive donors compared to T1D individuals, exocrine axon density was unaltered	TH axons found in close approximation to islet α cells in T1D individuals with long-standing diabetes
	Impaired islet pericyte and capillary responses to vasoactive stimuli	Islet vessels with smaller diameter and higher density compared to control donors	Islet vessels with smaller diameter and higher density compared to control donors
Extracellular matrix abnormalities	Increased hyaluronan (HA) deposition that was colocalized with insulitis	HA is significantly increased both within and around the islet	HA is significantly increased both within and around the islet

Figure 5. The human pancreas in type 1 diabetes (T1D) exhibits abnormalities in multiple cellular compartments. Overview of immune, exocrine, endocrine, vascular, nerve, and extracellular matrix abnormalities in the human pancreas from autoantibody (AAb)-positive donors, donors with recent-onset T1D, and long-duration T1D. (PI/I) Proinsulin/insulin, (ICI) insulin-containing islets, (GAD) glutamic acid decarboxylase, (HA) hyaluronan, (AAb$^+$) autoantibody positive.

Shapiro et al. 2023; Spanier et al. 2023). Michels et al. (2017) analyzed islet-infiltrating T cells from nPOD donors, focusing on proinsulin-specific CD4$^+$ T cells. The sequencing of islet-infiltrating TCRs revealed diverse repertoires, yet there was evidence of clonal expansion and many TCR sequences were detected in multiple islets. Seay et al. (2016) studied the pancreas, pancreatic lymph nodes, spleen, irrelevant lymph nodes, and peripheral blood from 18 nPOD donors diagnosed with T1D 4–32 years before death. Consistent with the data of Michels et al. (2017) on the same donors, this study showed initial evidence for the existence of "public" TCRs that are shared among patients. Additional evidence for public TCRs derives from the observation that reoccurrence of T1D in the transplanted pancreas was associated with the reappearance of TCR sequences of GAD65 autoreactive CD4$^+$ T cells (Vendrame et al. 2010), and this overlapped with sequences from a large number of the nPOD T1D donors studied by Seay et al. (2016).

Additional studies have helped define critical pathological abnormalities in the immunopathogenesis of T1D. For example, nPOD collaborative studies have validated two important features that were initially considered controversial: the hyperexpression of HLA class I molecules in islets (Richardson et al. 2016) and the aberrant expression of HLA class II molecules (Russell et al. 2019; Quesada-Masachs et al. 2022) on a subset of β cells. Both phenomena are now characterized in much greater depth, quantified, and the hyperexpression of the class I HLA molecule can now be considered a bona fide therapeutic target, potentially amenable to manipulation using JAK or TYK2 inhibition (Coomans de Brachène et al. 2018, 2020; Chandra et al. 2022; Waibel et al. 2023). nPOD studies have led also to the identification of key components of the extracellular matrix (ECM) that are important in immunopathogenesis, including the formation of tertiary lymphoid organs in the pancreas of individuals with T1D (Korpos et al. 2021). Finally, the recent implementation of the pancreas slice platform by nPOD has allowed for examination of functional interactions between immune cells and islet cells in living tissue (Panzer et al. 2020; Huber et al. 2021). This platform could also be used as a tool to model islet autoimmunity and examine therapeutic responses in human tissues.

THE ENDOCRINE PANCREAS IN T1D

A Role for the β Cell in T1D Pathophysiology

Historically, the vast abundance of research on T1D pathogenesis has been directed at improving our understanding of the autoimmune features underlying this disease, with much less emphasis placed on the contributory role(s) of pancreatic islets and β cells (Atkinson and Mirmira 2023). The collaborative nature of the nPOD community, access to human tissues, and the development of programs like the National Institutes of Health (NIH) Human Islet Research Network (HIRN) are helping reshape historical views surrounding the role of the β cell in T1D pathophysiology (Fig. 5). Notably, nPOD-supported studies have provided unique insight into the trajectory of β-cell loss in early stage disease and the extent of β-cell destruction at stage 3 T1D onset. It is now well-appreciated that β-cell mass is markedly heterogeneous in normal populations, with nearly a fourfold variation in β-cell mass among nondiabetic donors (Olehnik et al. 2017). An inherent limitation of all postmortem pancreas studies is that the data represent a series of cross-sectional observations, and it is impossible to know where a particular donor falls within this continuum of starting β-cell mass. Notwithstanding this limitation, a key finding from the analysis of nPOD tissues is that the extent of β-cell destruction at stage 3 T1D onset is heterogeneous and incomplete, ranging from 60% to 95% loss (Damond et al. 2019; Atkinson and Mirmira 2023). The extent of β-cell loss at diagnosis may not match the severity of clinical presentation, and in some organ donors, modest reductions in β-cell mass have been associated with death from severe insulin deficiency (Campbell-Thompson et al. 2016a), highlighting an important disconnect between measures of β-cell mass and function, especially during the peridiagnostic period (Oram et al. 2019).

The time point at which this reduction in β-cell mass begins during T1D evolution cannot be measured directly in living individuals; however, human pancreas studies may help to fill this gap. Diedisheim et al. (2016) reported that β-cell mass was not significantly different between AAb-positive donors at risk for T1D and AAb-negative controls. Surprisingly, no differences in β-cell mass were found between multiple and single AAb-positive donors. This observation differs from physiologic studies assessing β-cell function in living individuals (Felton et al. 2022), suggesting that very early changes in C-peptide secretion observed in clinical cohorts may emanate primarily from a change in β-cell function rather than alterations in mass. In contrast, studies in donors with long-standing T1D show that β-cell mass is markedly reduced by an estimated 88%–95% compared to controls, and β-cell area and mass declines with increasing disease duration (Campbell-Thompson et al. 2016a; Lam et al. 2017). Age has an important impact on the amount of residual β cells that remain in long-duration disease. Donors with an older age of T1D diagnosis have more remaining β cells and higher C-peptide levels compared to individuals with disease onset during childhood (Carr et al. 2022). The effects of age and disease duration observed in analysis of pancreata from organ donors are remarkably consistent with analysis of serum C-peptide in living T1D cohorts (Oram et al. 2014; Davis et al. 2015).

Analysis of nPOD tissues also has provided important insight into changes in proinsulin expression patterns and processing in both AAb-positive donors and donors with established T1D. In 2017, Wasserfall et al. (2017) reported the intriguing finding that proinsulin was present in pancreatic extract from donors with long-duration T1D even in the absence of mature insulin. These findings are remarkably consistent with analysis of serum proinsulin in individuals with long-standing T1D (Sims et al. 2019a; Leete et al. 2020). In addition, defects in prohormone processing appear to arise very early in the disease process. Analysis of nPOD tissues showed that islets from AAb-positive individuals have increases in absolute pancreatic proinsulin area and the proinsulin-to-insulin ratio, without significant reductions in the insulin-positive area or β-cell mass (Rodriguez-Calvo et al. 2017). Consistent with alterations in prohormone processing, reduced expression of *PCSK1* mRNA (Wasserfall et al. 2017) and decreased PC1/3 protein expression have been observed in nPOD tissues from donors with T1D (Sims et al. 2019b).

At present, it is unclear whether changes in prohormone processing are a cause or simply a consequence of autoimmunity. Altered proinsulin processing enzyme expression and impaired prohormone processing could be part of a larger phenotype of altered β-cell identity in T1D. Consistent with this idea, Wasserfall et al. (2017) identified reduced insulin mRNA expression and production in long-duration disease. Damond et al. (2019) analyzed nPOD tissues using imaging mass cytometry and found reduced expression of several key β-cell identity genes in the pancreas of T1D donors. Using pseudotime computational methods, they proposed a model of altered β-cell phenotype that precedes β-cell destruction. Others have described increased immune infiltration in islets that are β-cell-rich compared to islets lacking insulin (Campbell-Thompson et al. 2016a). Similarly, HLA class I overexpression appears to be limited to insulin-containing islets (Richardson et al. 2016).

In addition to alterations in the expression of genes associated with β-cell identity, interrogation of nPOD tissues has revealed modification of expression patterns of genes and proteins involved in several stress pathways including endoplasmic reticulum (ER) stress (Marhfour et al. 2012), autophagy (Muralidharan et al. 2021), alternative mRNA splicing (Wu et al. 2021), and senescence (Thompson et al. 2019). In aggregate, these data support a model whereby the β cell is complicit in diabetes development through activation of molecular pathways that increase β-cell immunogenicity and exacerbate autoimmunity. In the future, the use of viral lineage tracing methods in living pancreatic slices could facilitate studies aimed at addressing the timing and consequences of altered β-cell identity and the association of β-cell identity with immune activation (Qadir et al. 2020; Doke et al. 2023).

Functional Analysis of nPOD Tissues

nPOD's capacity to isolate islets and generate living pancreas slices from tissues of organ donors has enabled functional studies that have greatly enhanced our understanding of endocrine function during T1D. Panzer and colleagues generated live pancreas slices from four nPOD organ donors with T1D, with disease durations of 0, 1.5, 4, and 10 years, and compared insulin secretory characteristics to slices isolated from 19 organ donors without diabetes. They found that insulin secretion was significantly reduced in donors with T1D, and the extent of the reduction was correlated with disease duration (Panzer et al. 2020). Similar conclusions were reached in an analysis of tissues procured through the Human Pancreas Analysis Program (HPAP), where total amounts of insulin secretion were dramatically reduced in T1D donors. However, the authors concluded that the dynamics of responses to different stimuli were similar to nondiabetic controls, suggesting intact regulation of nutrient responses against a backdrop of reduced insulin content that may limit the magnitude of responses (Doliba et al. 2022). Additional findings from Brissova and colleagues (2022) described intact insulin secretory kinetics in islets isolated from a group of seven donors with T1D (disease duration spanning 2–31 years), including several nPOD donors.

A key takeaway from these studies is that results are likely influenced by the tissue type analyzed (i.e., islets vs. slices) and normalization techniques. Notably, there is no clear consensus in the field for how insulin secretion data should be analyzed and reported. For example, Panzer et al. (2020) normalized insulin secretion to β-cell mass, while Brissova and colleagues (2022) normalized secreted insulin to intracellular insulin content. Secondly, studies to date have described relatively small cohorts with heterogeneous donor characteristics, including disease duration. Thus, an integrated assessment comparing all available data using different normalization strategies from slices and islets could be extremely informative.

Notwithstanding this limitation, functional studies in both islets and pancreas slices have enabled analysis of other endocrine cell types outside of the β cell. Imaging studies have revealed important changes in the composition of islets within the T1D pancreas, where islets in individuals with T1D exhibit spatial disorganization that includes massive β-cell loss and a resulting predominance of α cells (Panzer et al. 2020). While these changes may or may not be associated with an overall change in α cell mass, they likely have important impacts on patterns of hormone secretion as well as changes in counterregulatory responses observed during disease evolution. Consistent with decades of studies in living individuals, glucagon secretory characteristics are altered in functional studies performed in tissues from donors with T1D (Carlsson et al. 2000, Arbelaez et al. 2014; Flatt et al. 2021). Brissova and colleagues (2022) described reduced glucagon secretion in isolated islets coupled with changes in α cell gene expression patterns in established diabetes. More recently, the HPAP consortium described alterations in glucagon secretory responses in a small cohort of nine GAD AAb (GADA)$^+$ donors, where insulin secretory responses were largely preserved, suggesting these changes arise early in the disease process (Doliba et al. 2022).

Glucagon release is regulated by hypoglycemia, amino acids, catecholamines, and neurotransmitters from both the parasympathetic and sympathetic branches of the autonomic nervous system. Thus, one potential etiology of impaired glucagon secretion in T1D could be altered pancreatic innervation. Consistent with this hypothesis, AAb-positive nPOD donors were found to have decreased islet sympathetic axon density and reduced tyrosine hydroxylase (TH)-positive axon numbers compared to donors with T1D. This same report found that α and δ cells were in close proximity to TH axons, indicating the possibility of direct sympathetic stimulation of these islet endocrine cell types, in addition to their known impact on β cells and nonendocrine islet cell types (Campbell-Thompson et al. 2021). It is worth noting that these changes were not confirmed in a separate analysis of T1D pancreata as part of the HPAP program (Richardson et al. 2023).

nPOD STUDIES HAVE REVEALED ABNORMALITIES OF ACCESSORY CELLS IN THE PANCREAS

Islet hormone secretion is also regulated by vascular tone, and not surprisingly, pancreata from donors with diabetes and AAb positivity exhibit alterations in islet vasculature. Donors with established T1D were found to have islet vessels with smaller diameter and higher density compared to control donors. Interestingly, these changes were not observed in islets with residual β cells, and exocrine vasculature was unaffected (Canzano et al. 2019). Importantly, Mateus Gonçalves et al. (2023) studied living pancreas slices to understand how changes in vascular phenotypes affect function. They found that islet pericyte and capillary responses to vasoactive stimuli were impaired in AAb-positive donors. Interestingly, microvascular dysfunction was associated with a switch in the phenotype of islet pericytes toward profibrotic myofibroblasts (Mateus Gonçalves et al. 2023). Along these lines, others have described significant alterations in the islet ECM in pancreata from donors with T1D, where hyaluronan (HA) was significantly increased both within and around the islet. Notably, this increased HA was in close proximity to islet microvessels, suggesting a potential influence on vascular responses (Bogdani et al. 2014; Nagy et al. 2015). More recently, increased HA deposition was observed in AAb-positive donors, the amount of HA staining in islets was associated with the number of AAb, and the most prominent HA deposits were colocalized with insulitis (Bogdani et al. 2020).

THE EXOCRINE PANCREAS IN T1D

Pancreas Size and Weight Are Abnormal in T1D

In normal human development, the pancreas increases in size with age, reaching a plateau by the mid- to late 20s with an eventual decrease in many individuals after 60 years of age (Saisho et al. 2007). Pancreas size is also influenced by body mass index (BMI) (Kou et al. 2014; Regnell et al. 2016). More than 100 years ago, autopsy studies noted that the pancreata of certain individuals with diabetes mellitus were reduced in size (Cecil 1909). With continued improvements in classifying the various forms of diabetes (i.e., insulin-dependent/T1D vs. non-insulin-dependent/T2D), it eventually became clear that these size modifications were largely restricted to those having T1D. The decrease in pancreas size was hypothesized to result from long-term insulinopenia, as the insulin produced by β-cells acts as a trophic factor to acini within the islet acinar portal system (Henderson et al. 1981). A lack of local elevations in insulin concentrations could, therefore, decrease acinar growth and enzyme production, while unopposed glucagon and somatostatin release would further contribute to an inhibition of exocrine pancreas function (Pandiri 2014; Foster et al. 2020). Thus, while the concept that exocrine abnormalities are associated with diabetes is not new, very few studies followed up on these initial observations.

Excitingly, studies emanating from the nPOD program have effectively rekindled research interest in older findings that the entire pancreas, rather than only the islets, may be of pathogenic significance in T1D. The long-held lack of research interest in the exocrine pancreas in T1D changed in 2012 with a publication using the transplant-quality tissues provided by nPOD (Campbell-Thompson et al. 2012d). This study validated the notion that pancreata from individuals with T1D were of reduced weight, thus adding to the previous efforts that assessed organs obtained at autopsy (Maclean and Ogilvie 1959; Löhr and Klöppel 1987). This effort also provided novel evidence that even subjects at increased risk for T1D (i.e., AAb-positive nondiabetic individuals) had reductions in pancreatic weight by ~25% (Campbell-Thompson et al. 2012d). Subsequent studies using nPOD tissues have confirmed and greatly expanded upon these initial efforts in terms of subject sample size and inclusion of additional anthropometric variables (Campbell-Thompson et al. 2016b).

These nPOD studies also provided support for in vivo pancreatic imaging in living subjects with or at varying levels of risk for T1D. More than a decade ago, imaging-based studies noted a reduced pancreas volume associated with T1D (Williams et al. 2012). Taken together with more recent investigations, findings now suggest reductions in pancreatic volume of ~20%–30% in recent-onset T1D cases and 30%–50% in long-standing disease in comparison to control subjects, usually matched for age and/or normalized for BMI (Williams et al. 2012; Gaglia et al. 2015; Campbell-Thompson et al. 2019; Virostko et al. 2019). Quite surprisingly, one magnetic resonance imaging (MRI)-based initiative demonstrated that AAb-negative first-degree relatives without diabetes, single AAb-positive individuals, and multiple AAb-positive individuals also had reduced pancreatic volume relative to general population controls (i.e., AAb-negative nonrelatives) (Campbell-Thompson et al. 2019), suggestive of potential genetic contributions to pancreatic size. Importantly, these efforts involving living subjects confirmed the nearly identical findings observed with nPOD tissues.

In T1D, the loss of β-cell mass is usually less severe in the pancreatic head and more dominant in the body and tail regions (Campbell-Thompson et al. 2016a). In concert with this observation, the aforementioned reduction in pancreas weight and volume is largely related to a reduction of the ventral portion of the organ, especially in the tail region (Campbell-Thompson et al. 2016b, 2019). Importantly, these and other reports (Fonseca et al. 1985; Lu et al. 2016; Augustine et al. 2020) show reduced pancreatic volume in T1D, irrespective of the imaging methodology used (e.g., computed tomography, MRI, ultrasound). These observations using assessments of pancreatic weight or pancreas volume in vivo are exceptionally important as they suggest that pancreatic size likely parallels the progressive loss-of-functional β-cell mass. This notion was recently confirmed through longitudinal MRI of subjects ranging from AAb-positive to stage 3 T1D and 12 months post-T1D onset (Virostko et al. 2019).

Insights into Changes in Pancreas Morphology and Function

Both the endocrine and exocrine compartments in the normal human pancreas are defined by notable morphological heterogeneity. This heterogeneity includes variations across pancreatic regions (i.e., head, body, tail) in terms of islet cell composition, size, and density (Hellman 1959). Similarly, acinar tissues typically display regionally distinct physiological and morphological variations (Kern and Ferner 1971). Such findings raise the question of whether either of these endocrine or exocrine variations occur in a unique form in settings of T1D. This notion is of particular importance because any relationship between the decline in pancreatic size and T1D cannot exclusively be attributed to β-cell loss, as islets comprise only 1%–2% of pancreas volume. Hence, a reduction in weight or volume of the pancreas must be ascribed to a loss in exocrine tissue (Gepts 1965).

To this end, studies comparing T1D pancreatic morphology in recent-onset cases, those with established disease, and persons with and without disease-associated AAb positivity have provided a series of intriguing findings. Specifically, nPOD studies have demonstrated that T1D donors lacking insulin-positive islet cells had reduced acinar tissue area compared to AAb-negative controls (Tang et al. 2021). Additional studies suggest that acinar cells are reduced in both size and number with loss of characteristic peri-islet amylase-negative cell clusters in T1D pancreata (Kusmartseva et al. 2020; Wright et al. 2020; Tang et al. 2021). Analysis of nPOD tissues identified that exocrine areas of the T1D pancreas are characterized by enhanced numbers of various immune cell types, supporting a model of generalized pancreatic inflammation. Specifically, elevations in the number of $CD4^+$ and $CD8^+$ T cells, macrophages, and dendritic cells have been observed (Rodriguez-Calvo et al. 2014). To date, preproinsulin-specific $CD8^+$ T cells have been identified in exocrine pancreas, but knowledge of additional antigenic specificities remains somewhat limited (Bender et al. 2020) relative to those identified from isolated islets (Babon et al. 2016). Moreover, it is not clear whether these immune cells have any functional ability to impart specific acinar cell destruction or dysfunction. Neutrophils and products of complement activation have also been observed throughout the tissues of some T1D pancreata, suggesting innate immune system involvement (Vecchio et al. 2018). The nonendocrine pancreas in T1D also displays increased fat infiltration, fibrosis (typically interacinar), and atherosclerosis (Atkinson et al. 2020). Multiple studies also report that atrophy in the acinar pancreas is often observed in those with long-standing durations of T1D. In one such report, the number of pancreatic acinar cells were decreased in T1D donors, regardless of the time of diabetes onset (Wright et al. 2020). A second study reported reduced size and increased density of acinar cells in T1D donor pancreas (Tang et al. 2021). Finally, pancreata from nPOD donors with T1D exhibit unique exocrine tissue transcriptomic and proteomic profiles (Woo et al. 2020; Välikangas et al. 2022), including elevation of antiviral immune response gene expression, altered exocrine function, activation of complement coagulation cascades, modification of ECM receptor interactions, and down-regulation of regenerating gene family genes. Despite these intriguing findings, it remains unclear how the cellular environment and morphology of the exocrine pancreas might contribute to T1D pathogenesis, thus stimulating a renewed interest in studies of exocrine function in T1D.

Volumetric and morphological findings on the human pancreas in T1D, including those emanating from nPOD, provided support to readdress long-standing observations involving exocrine function in this disease (Pollard et al. 1943; Frier et al. 1976, 1980; Lankisch et al. 1982; Landin-Olsson et al. 1990). These studies include initiatives to analyze serum or stool levels of pancreatic enzymes, a practice more routinely used for certain pediatric or adult disorders associated with pancreatic function (e.g., cystic fibrosis, meconium ileus, pancreatitis). It was noted that T1D is associated with reduced serum levels of trypsinogen and decreased fecal elastase-1 (Li et al. 2017; Campbell-Thompson et al. 2019; Augustine et al. 2020; Penno et al. 2020; Ross et al. 2021). Moreover, serological levels of lipase and trypsinogen are directly associated with pancreas size in subjects with T1D as well as in single and multiple AAb-positive relatives (Ross et al. 2021). Specifically, serum levels of enzymes reflective of exocrine function were low in T1D individuals, with multiple AAb-positive individuals also having reduced values compared to single AAb-positive subjects and AAb-negative controls. These data suggest that exocrine dysfunction may evolve as progression to T1D occurs, but these changes may not be clinically apparent until the late pre-T1D phase (Ross et al. 2021). Indeed, in the Australian Environmental Determinants of Islet Autoimmunity (ENDIA) study, fecal elastase-1 levels declined longitudinally in at-risk children during progression to islet autoimmunity and T1D diagnosis (Penno et al. 2020). Current studies within nPOD are using pancreatic slice cultures to determine the mechanisms underlying reduced exocrine function in T1D (Cohrs et al. 2024).

Key Questions to Be Addressed by nPOD Going Forward

After 17 years of program building and success, the next and most pressing goal for nPOD is to understand how the vast and diverse findings generated through research projects supported by nPOD can inform potential therapeutics. To this end, a number of future opportunities and key questions have been identified (Table 1). Moving forward, it is imperative that tissues and state-of-the art technologies be leveraged to address differences in diabetes between adults and children and to understand the role of prohormone processing defects, posttranslational antigenic processing defects, and changes in the exocrine pancreas during T1D development. To facilitate therapeutic discovery, a priority is to use live tissue platforms to advance immunotherapy and islet cell therapies. Two critical and guiding principles will be (1) to contextualize findings from these studies across diverse populations, and (2) to strengthen ties with key clinical trial networks to make nPOD discoveries and data available and accessible for clinical trial design. Analysis of heterogeneity will be an important undercurrent in these efforts, as there is increasing awareness of heterogeneity of clinical phenotypes, which may be driven by differences in genetic ancestry, geography (Kaddis et al. 2022), social determinants of health, as well as other etiologic factors (Battaglia et al. 2020). Similarly, nPOD studies have highlighted that heterogeneity exists at the macroscopic and microscopic level in the pancreas (Leete et al. 2016, 2020; Damond et al. 2019). What remains controversial and yet unexplained is whether observed heterogeneity represents random chance, is driven by simple baseline demographics, is the product of a limited sample size or biased donor pool, is reflective of distinct disease-associated phenotypes/endotypes (Battaglia et al. 2020), or can be explained by genetic differences. While large genome-wide association case-control studies have revealed the majority of heritable risk associated with T1D (Pociot and Lernmark 2016), the genetic contribution to heterogeneity within T1D is less well defined (McKeigue et al. 2019). Large sample sizes of T1D cases with detailed clinical phenotypes are needed for new genetic discovery, but progress in this area has been made by assessing variants already associated with diabetes (Redondo et al. 2023). The deposition of nPOD genetic data into the NIH database of Genotypes and Phenotypes (www.ncbi.nlm.nih.gov/projects/gap/cgi-bin/study.cgi?study_id=phs002861.v1.p1) (Perry et al. 2023) provides an opportunity for additional genotype–phenotype association studies to better understand heterogeneity and unique disease mechanisms (Perry et al. 2023). Furthermore, the data available in the nPOD repository will be an important resource to describe variation in T1D pathogenesis that may link clinical and pathological strands, and shed light on potential clusters or endotypes of T1D patients who may have distinct mechanisms amenable to specific treatments.

CONCLUSIONS

The evolution and progress of the nPOD program over the last 17 years has been remarkable. George Eisenbarth's dream of a comprehensive program to provide diabetes researchers with access to transplant-quality pancreata from organ donors with and at increased risk for T1D has transformed into an internationally recognized program that serves as a model system for other organ donor–based research programs. Moreover, the scientific findings and collaborations that have been made possible by nPOD have reshaped our understanding of human T1D pathophysiology. Our goal is that they can now be leveraged to pave the way for new disease-modifying and disease-preventative therapeutics. In closing, we want to acknowledge and thank the nPOD donors and their families for their incredible gifts. Without their selfless acts, nPOD would not exist.

ACKNOWLEDGMENTS

This research was performed with the support of the Network for Pancreatic Organ Donors with Diabetes (nPOD; RRID:SCR_014641), a collaborative T1D research project supported by the Juvenile Diabetes Research Foundation (JDRF) (nPOD: 5-SRA-2018-557-Q-R), and the Leona M. and Harry B. Helmsley Charitable Trust (Grant #2018PG-T1D053, G-2108-04793). Organ Procurement Organizations (OPOs) partnering with nPOD to provide research resources are listed at npod.org/for-partners/npod-partners. We also acknowledge the contributions of a large number of individuals whose collective efforts have helped build the nPOD program, including Clive Wasserfall, Desmond Schatz, Todd Brusko, Martha Campbell-Thompson, John Kaddis, and Maigan Brusko. We thank Emily Anderson-Baucum for her helpful comments and suggestions.

REFERENCES

Ahmed S, Cerosaletti K, James E, Long SA, Mannering S, Speake C, Nakayama M, Tree T, Roep BO, Herold KC, et al. 2019. Standardizing T-cell biomarkers in type 1 diabetes: challenges and recent advances. *Diabetes* **68:** 1366–1379. doi:10.2337/db19-0119

Anderson AM, Landry LG, Alkanani AA, Pyle L, Powers AC, Atkinson MA, Mathews CE, Roep BO, Michels AW, Nakayama M. 2021. Human islet T cells are highly reactive to preproinsulin in type 1 diabetes. *Proc Natl Acad Sci* **118:** e210720818. doi:10.1073/pnas.2107208118

Apaolaza PS, Balcacean D, Zapardiel-Gonzalo J, Rodriguez-Calvo T. 2023. The extent and magnitude of islet T cell infiltration as powerful tools to define the progression to type 1 diabetes. *Diabetologia* **66:** 1129–1141. doi:10.1007/s00125-023-05888-6

Arbelaez AM, Xing D, Cryer PE, Kollman C, Beck RW, Sherr J, Ruedy KJ, Tamborlane WV, Mauras N, Tsalikian E, et al. 2014. Blunted glucagon but not epinephrine responses to hypoglycemia occurs in youth with less than 1 yr duration of type 1 diabetes mellitus. *Pediatr Diabetes* **15:** 127–134. doi:10.1111/pedi.12070

Arif S, Leete P, Nguyen V, Marks K, Nor NM, Estorninho M, Kronenberg-Versteeg D, Bingley PJ, Todd JA, Guy C, et al. 2014. Blood and islet phenotypes indicate immunological heterogeneity in type 1 diabetes. *Diabetes* **63:** 3835–3845. doi:10.2337/db14-0365

Atkinson M, Mirmira R. 2023. The pathogenic "symphony" in type 1 diabetes: a disorder of the immune system, β cells, and exocrine pancreas. *Cell Metab* **35:** 1500–1518. doi:10.1016/j.cmet.2023.06.018

Atkinson MA, Campbell-Thompson M, Kusmartseva I, Kaestner KH. 2020. Organisation of the human pancreas in health and in diabetes. *Diabetologia* **63:** 1966–1973. doi:10.1007/s00125-020-05203-7

Augustine P, Gent R, Louise J, Taranto M, Penno M, Linke R, Couper JJ, ENDIA Study Group. 2020. Pancreas size and exocrine function is decreased in young children with recent-onset type 1 diabetes. *Diabet Med* **37:** 1340–1343. doi:10.1111/dme.13987

Babon JA, DeNicola ME, Blodgett DM, Crèvecoeur I, Buttrick TS, Maehr R, Bottino R, Naji A, Kaddis J, Elyaman W, et al. 2016. Analysis of self-antigen specificity of islet-infiltrating T cells from human donors with type 1 diabetes. *Nat Med* **22:** 1482–1487. doi:10.1038/nm.4203

Battaglia M, Ahmed S, Anderson MS, Atkinson MA, Becker D, Bingley PJ, Bosi E, Brusko TM, DiMeglio LA, Evans-Molina C, et al. 2020. Introducing the endotype concept to address the challenge of disease heterogeneity in type 1 diabetes. *Diabetes Care* **43:** 5–12. doi:10.2337/dc19-0880

Beam CA, Wasserfall C, Woodwyk A, Akers M, Rauch H, Blok T, Mason P, Vos D, Perry D, Brusko T, et al. 2020. Synchronization of the normal human peripheral immune system: a comprehensive circadian systems immunology analysis. *Sci Rep* **10:** 672. doi:10.1038/s41598-019-56951-5

Bender C, Rodriguez-Calvo T, Amirian N, Coppieters KT, von Herrath MG. 2020. The healthy exocrine pancreas contains preproinsulin-specific CD8 T cells that attack islets in type 1 diabetes. *Sci Adv* **6:** eabc5586. doi:10.1126/sciadv.abc5586

Bogdani M, Johnson PY, Potter-Perigo S, Nagy N, Day AJ, Bollyky PL, Wight TN. 2014. Hyaluronan and hyaluronan-binding proteins accumulate in both human type 1 diabetic islets and lymphoid tissues and associate with inflammatory cells in insulitis. *Diabetes* **63:** 2727–2743. doi:10.2337/db13-1658

Bogdani M, Speake C, Dufort MJ, Johnson PY, Larmore MJ, Day AJ, Wight TN, Lernmark Å, Greenbaum CJ. 2020. Hyaluronan deposition in islets may precede and direct the location of islet immune-cell infiltrates. *Diabetologia* **63:** 549–560. doi:10.1007/s00125-019-05066-7

Bogun MM, Bundy BN, Goland RS, Greenbaum CJ. 2020. C-peptide levels in subjects followed longitudinally before and after type 1 diabetes diagnosis in TrialNet. *Diabetes Care* **43:** 1836–1842. doi:10.2337/dc19-2288

Campbell-Thompson M, Wasserfall C, Kaddis J, Albanese-O'Neill A, Staeva T, Nierras C, Moraski J, Rowe P, Gianani R, Eisenbarth G, et al. 2012a. Network for pancreatic organ donors with diabetes (nPOD): developing a tissue biobank for type 1 diabetes. *Diabetes Metab Res Rev* **28:** 608–617. doi:10.1002/dmrr.2316

Campbell-Thompson ML, Heiple T, Montgomery E, Zhang L, Schneider L. 2012b. Staining protocols for human pancreatic islets. *J Vis Exp* **63:** e4068. doi:10.3791/4068

Campbell-Thompson ML, Montgomery EL, Foss RM, Kolheffer KM, Phipps G, Schneider L, Atkinson MA. 2012c. Collection protocol for human pancreas. *J Vis Exp* **63:** e4039. doi:10.3791/4039

Campbell-Thompson M, Wasserfall C, Montgomery EL, Atkinson MA, Kaddis JS. 2012d. Pancreas organ weight in individuals with disease-associated autoantibodies at risk for type 1 diabetes. *JAMA* **308:** 2337–2339. doi:10.1001/jama.2012.15008

Campbell-Thompson ML, Atkinson MA, Butler AE, Chapman NM, Frisk G, Gianani R, Giepmans BN, von Herrath MG, Hyöty H, Kay TW, et al. 2013. The diagnosis of insulitis in human type 1 diabetes. *Diabetologia* **56:** 2541–2543. doi:10.1007/s00125-013-3043-5

Campbell-Thompson M, Fu A, Kaddis JS, Wasserfall C, Schatz DA, Pugliese A, Atkinson MA. 2016a. Insulitis and β-cell mass in the natural history of type 1 diabetes. *Diabetes* **65:** 719–731. doi:10.2337/db15-0779

Campbell-Thompson ML, Kaddis JS, Wasserfall C, Haller MJ, Pugliese A, Schatz DA, Shuster JJ, Atkinson MA. 2016b. The influence of type 1 diabetes on pancreatic weight. *Diabetologia* **59:** 217–221. doi:10.1007/s00125-015-3752-z

Campbell-Thompson ML, Filipp SL, Grajo JR, Nambam B, Beegle R, Middlebrooks EH, Gurka MJ, Atkinson MA, Schatz DA, Haller MJ. 2019. Relative pancreas volume is reduced in first-degree relatives of patients with type 1 diabetes. *Diabetes Care* **42:** 281–287. doi:10.2337/dc18-1512

Campbell-Thompson M, Butterworth EA, Boatwright JL, Nair MA, Nasif LH, Nasif K, Revell AY, Riva A, Mathews CE, Gerling IC, et al. 2021. Islet sympathetic innervation and islet neuropathology in patients with type 1 diabetes. *Sci Rep* **11:** 6562. doi:10.1038/s41598-021-85659-8

Canzano JS, Nasif LH, Butterworth EA, Fu DA, Atkinson MA, Campbell-Thompson M. 2019. Islet microvasculature alterations with loss of β-cells in patients with type 1 diabetes. *J Histochem Cytochem* **67:** 41–52. doi:10.1369/0022155418778546

Carlsson A, Sundkvist G, Groop L, Tuomi T. 2000. Insulin and glucagon secretion in patients with slowly progressing autoimmune diabetes (LADA). *J Clin Endocrinol Metab* **85:** 76–80. doi:10.1210/jcem.85.1.6228

Carr ALJ, Inshaw JRJ, Flaxman CS, Leete P, Wyatt RC, Russell LA, Palmer M, Prasolov D, Worthington T, Hull B, et al. 2022. Circulating C-peptide levels in living children and young people and pancreatic β-cell loss in pancreas donors across type 1 diabetes disease duration. *Diabetes* **71:** 1591–1596. doi:10.2337/db22-0097

Cecil RL. 1909. A study of the pathological anatomy of the pancreas in ninety cases of diabetes mellitus. *J Exp Med* **11:** 266–290. doi:10.1084/jem.11.2.266

Chandra V, Ibrahim H, Halliez C, Prasad RB, Vecchio F, Dwivedi OP, Kvist J, Balboa D, Saarimäki-Vire J, Montaser H, et al. 2022. The type 1 diabetes gene TYK2 regulates β-cell development and its responses to interferon-α. *Nat Commun* **13:** 6363. doi:10.1038/s41467-022-34069-z

Chen J, Chernatynskaya AV, Li JW, Kimbrell MR, Cassidy RJ, Perry DJ, Muir AB, Atkinson MA, Brusko TM, Mathews CE. 2017. T cells display mitochondria hyperpolarization in human type 1 diabetes. *Sci Rep* **7:** 10835. doi:10.1038/s41598-017-11056-9

Cohrs CM, Chen C, Atkinson MA, Drotar DM, Speier S. 2024. Bridging the gap: pancreas tissue slices from organ and tissue donors for the study of diabetes pathogenesis. *Diabetes* **73:** 11–22. doi:10.2337/dbi20-0018

Coomans de Brachène A, Dos Santos RS, Marroqui L, Colli ML, Marselli L, Mirmira RG, Marchetti P, Eizirik DL. 2018. IFN-α induces a preferential long-lasting expression of MHC class I in human pancreatic β cells. *Diabetologia* **61:** 636–640. doi:10.1007/s00125-017-4536-4

Coomans de Brachène A, Castela A, Op de Beeck A, Mirmira RG, Marselli L, Marchetti P, Masse C, Miao W, Leit S, Evans-Molina C, et al. 2020. Preclinical evaluation of tyrosine kinase 2 inhibitors for human β-cell protection in type 1 diabetes. *Diabetes Obes Metab* **22:** 1827–1836. doi:10.1111/dom.14104

Coppieters KT, Dotta F, Amirian N, Campbell PD, Kay TW, Atkinson MA, Roep BO, von Herrath MG. 2012. Demonstration of islet-autoreactive CD8 T cells in insulitic lesions from recent onset and long-term type 1 diabetes patients. *J Exp Med* **209:** 51–60. doi:10.1084/jem.20111187

Damond N, Engler S, Zanotelli VRT, Schapiro D, Wasserfall CH, Kusmartseva I, Nick HS, Thorel F, Herrera PL, Atkinson MA, et al. 2019. A map of human type 1 diabetes progression by imaging mass cytometry. *Cell Metab* **29:** 755–768.e5. doi:10.1016/j.cmet.2018.11.014

Davis AK, DuBose SN, Haller MJ, Miller KM, DiMeglio LA, Bethin KE, Goland RS, Greenberg EM, Liljenquist DR, Ahmann AJ, et al. 2015. Prevalence of detectable C-peptide according to age at diagnosis and duration of type 1 diabetes. *Diabetes Care* **38:** 476–481. doi:10.2337/dc14-1952

Dean JW, Peters LD, Fuhrman CA, Seay HR, Posgai AL, Stimpson SE, Brusko MA, Perry DJ, Yeh WI, Newby BN, et al. 2020. Innate inflammation drives NK cell activation to impair Treg activity. *J Autoimmun* **108:** 102417. doi:10.1016/j.jaut.2020.102417

Delong T, Wiles TA, Baker RL, Bradley B, Barbour G, Reisdorph R, Armstrong M, Powell RL, Reisdorph N, Kumar N, et al. 2016. Pathogenic CD4 T cells in type 1 diabetes recognize epitopes formed by peptide fusion. *Science* **351:** 711–714. doi:10.1126/science.aad2791

Diedisheim M, Mallone R, Boitard C, Larger E. 2016. β-Cell mass in nondiabetic autoantibody-positive subjects: an analysis based on the network for pancreatic organ donors database. *J Clin Endocrinol Metab* **101:** 1390–1397. doi:10.1210/jc.2015-3756

Doke M, Álvarez-Cubela S, Klein D, Altilio I, Schulz J, Mateus Gonçalves L, Almaça J, Fraker CA, Pugliese A, Ricordi C, et al. 2023. Dynamic scRNA-seq of live human pancreatic slices reveals functional endocrine cell neogenesis through an intermediate ducto-acinar stage. *Cell Metab* **35:** 1944–1960.e7. doi:10.1016/j.cmet.2023.10.001

Doliba NM, Rozo AV, Roman J, Qin W, Traum D, Gao L, Liu J, Manduchi E, Liu C, Golson ML, et al. 2022. α Cell dysfunction in islets from nondiabetic, glutamic acid decarboxylase autoantibody-positive individuals. *J Clin Invest* **132:** e156243. doi:10.1172/JCI156243

Driver JP, Racine JJ, Ye C, Lamont DJ, Newby BN, Leeth CM, Chapman HD, Brusko TM, Chen YG, Mathews CE, et al. 2017. Interferon-γ limits diabetogenic CD8$^+$ T-cell effector responses in type-1 diabetes. *Diabetes* **66:** 710–721. doi:10.2337/db16-0846

Felton JL, Cuthbertson D, Warnock M, Lohano K, Meah F, Wentworth JM, Sosenko J, Evans-Molina C; Type 1 Diabetes TrialNet Study Group. 2022. HOMA2-B enhances assessment of type 1 diabetes risk among TrialNet Pathway to Prevention participants. *Diabetologia* **65:** 88–100. doi:10.1007/s00125-021-05573-6

Flatt AJS, Greenbaum CJ, Shaw JAM, Rickels MR. 2021. Pancreatic islet reserve in type 1 diabetes. *Ann NY Acad Sci* **1495:** 40–54. doi:10.1111/nyas.14572

Fonseca V, Berger LA, Beckett AG, Dandona P. 1985. Size of pancreas in diabetes mellitus: a study based on ultrasound. *Br Med J (Clin Res Ed)* **291:** 1240–1241. doi:10.1136/bmj.291.6504.1240

Foster TP, Bruggeman B, Campbell-Thompson M, Atkinson MA, Haller MJ, Schatz DA. 2020. Exocrine pancreas dysfunction in type 1 diabetes. *Endocr Pract* **26:** 1505–1513. doi:10.4158/EP-2020-0295

Foulis AK, Liddle CN, Farquharson MA, Richmond JA, Weir RS. 1986. The histopathology of the pancreas in type 1 (insulin-dependent) diabetes mellitus: a 25-year review of deaths in patients under 20 years of age in the United Kingdom. *Diabetologia* **29:** 267–274. doi:10.1007/BF00452061

Frier BM, Saunders JH, Wormsley KG, Bouchier IA. 1976. Exocrine pancreatic function in juvenile-onset diabetes mellitus. *Gut* **17:** 685–691. doi:10.1136/gut.17.9.685

Frier BM, Adrian TE, Saunders JH, Bloom SR. 1980. Serum trypsin concentration and pancreatic trypsin secretion in insulin-dependent diabetes mellitus. *Clin Chim Acta* **105:** 297–300. doi:10.1016/0009-8981(80)90472-6

Fuhrman CA, Yeh WI, Seay HR, Saikumar Lakshmi P, Chopra G, Zhang L, Perry DJ, McClymont SA, Yadav M, Lopez MC, et al. 2015. Divergent phenotypes of human regulatory T cells expressing the receptors TIGIT and CD226. *J Immunol* **195:** 145–155. doi:10.4049/jimmunol.1402381

Gaglia JL, Harisinghani M, Aganj I, Wojtkiewicz GR, Hedgire S, Benoist C, Mathis D, Weissleder R. 2015. Noninvasive mapping of pancreatic inflammation in recent-onset type-1 diabetes patients. *Proc Natl Acad Sci* **112:** 2139–2144. doi:10.1073/pnas.1424993112

Gepts W. 1965. Pathologic anatomy of the pancreas in juvenile diabetes mellitus. *Diabetes* **14:** 619–633. doi:10.2337/diab.14.10.619

Guyer P, Arribas-Layton D, Manganaro A, Speake C, Lord S, Eizirik DL, Kent SC, Mallone R, James EA. 2023. Recognition of mRNA splice variant and secretory granule epitopes by CD4$^+$ T cells in type 1 diabetes. *Diabetes* **72:** 85–96. doi:10.2337/db22-0191

Haller MJ, Gitelman SE, Gottlieb PA, Michels AW, Perry DJ, Schultz AR, Hulme MA, Shuster JJ, Zou B, Wasserfall CH, et al. 2016. Antithymocyte globulin plus G-CSF combination therapy leads to sustained immunomodulatory and metabolic effects in a subset of responders with established type 1 diabetes. *Diabetes* **65:** 3765–3775. doi:10.2337/db16-0823

Hellman B. 1959. Actual distribution of the number and volume of the islets of Langerhans in different size classes in non-diabetic humans of varying ages. *Nature* **184:** 1498–1499. doi:10.1038/1841498a0

Henderson JR, Daniel PM, Fraser PA. 1981. The pancreas as a single organ: the influence of the endocrine upon the exocrine part of the gland. *Gut* **22:** 158–167. doi:10.1136/gut.22.2.158

Huber MK, Drotar DM, Hiller H, Beery ML, Joseph P, Kusmartseva I, Speier S, Atkinson MA, Mathews CE, Phelps EA. 2021. Observing islet function and islet-immune cell interactions in live pancreatic tissue slices. *J Vis Exp* **170:** 10.3791/62207. doi:10.3791/62207

HuBMAP Consortium. 2019. The human body at cellular resolution: the NIH Human Biomolecular Atlas Program. *Nature* **574:** 187–192. doi:10.1038/s41586-019-1629-x

Hunt MS, Yang SJ, Mortensen E, Boukhris A, Buckner J, Cook PJ, Rawlings DJ. 2023. Dual-locus, dual-HDR editing permits efficient generation of antigen-specific regulatory T cells with robust suppressive activity. *Mol Ther* **31:** 2872–2886. doi:10.1016/j.ymthe.2023.07.016

Insel RA, Dunne JL, Atkinson MA, Chiang JL, Dabelea D, Gottlieb PA, Greenbaum CJ, Herold KC, Krischer JP, Lernmark Å, et al. 2015. Staging presymptomatic type 1 diabetes: a scientific statement of JDRF, the Endocrine Society, and the American Diabetes Association. *Diabetes Care* **38:** 1964–1974. doi:10.2337/dc15-1419

Kaddis JS, Pugliese A, Atkinson MA. 2015. A run on the biobank: what have we learned about type 1 diabetes from the nPOD tissue repository? *Curr Opin Endocrinol Diabetes Obes* **22:** 290–295. doi:10.1097/MED.0000000000000171

Kaddis JS, Perry DJ, Vu AN, Rich SS, Atkinson MA, Schatz DA, Roep BO, Brusko TM. 2022. Improving the prediction of type 1 diabetes across ancestries. *Diabetes Care* **45:** e48–e50. doi:10.2337/dc21-1254

Kaestner KH, Powers AC, Naji A; HPAP Consortium; Atkinson MA. 2019. NIH initiative to improve understanding of the pancreas, islet, and autoimmunity in type 1 diabetes: the Human Pancreas Analysis Program (HPAP). *Diabetes* **68:** 1394–1402. doi:10.2337/db19-0058

Kern H, Ferner H. 1971. Fine structure of the exocrine pancreas tissue of man. *Z Zellforsch Mikrosk Anat* **113:** 322–343. doi:10.1007/BF00968543

Khosravi-Maharlooei M, Obradovic A, Misra A, Motwani K, Holzl M, Seay HR, DeWolf S, Nauman G, Danzl N, Li H, et al. 2019. Crossreactive public TCR sequences undergo positive selection in the human thymic repertoire. *J Clin Invest* **129:** 2446–2462. doi:10.1172/JCI124358

Korpos É, Kadri N, Loismann S, Findeisen CR, Arfuso F, Burke GW, Richardson SJ, Morgan NG, Bogdani M, Pugliese A, et al. 2021. Identification and characterisation of tertiary lymphoid organs in human type 1 diabetes. *Diabetologia* **64:** 1626–1641. doi:10.1007/s00125-021-05453-z

Kou K, Saisho Y, Jinzaki M, Itoh H. 2014. Relationship between body mass index and pancreas volume in Japanese people. *JOP* **15:** 626–627. doi:10.6092/1590-8577/2858

Kusmartseva I, Beery M, Hiller H, Padilla M, Selman S, Posgai A, Nick HS, Campbell-Thompson M, Schatz DA, Haller MJ, et al. 2020. Temporal analysis of amylase expression in control, autoantibody-positive, and type 1 diabetes pancreatic tissues. *Diabetes* **69:** 60–66. doi:10.2337/db19-0554

Lam CJ, Jacobson DR, Rankin MM, Cox AR, Kushner JA. 2017. β Cells persist in T1D pancreata without evidence of ongoing β-cell turnover or neogenesis. *J Clin Endocrinol Metab* **102:** 2647–2659. doi:10.1210/jc.2016-3806

Landin-Olsson M, Borgström A, Blom L, Sundkvist G, Lernmark A. 1990. Immunoreactive trypsin(ogen) in the sera of children with recent-onset insulin-dependent diabetes and matched controls. The Swedish Childhood Diabetes Group. *Pancreas* **5:** 241–247. doi:10.1097/00006676-199005000-00001

Lankisch PG, Manthey G, Otto J, Koop H, Talaulicar M, Willms B, Creutzfeldt W. 1982. Exocrine pancreatic function in insulin-dependent diabetes mellitus. *Digestion* **25:** 211–216. doi:10.1159/000198833

Leete P, Willcox A, Krogvold L, Dahl-Jørgensen K, Foulis AK, Richardson SJ, Morgan NG. 2016. Differential insulitic profiles determine the extent of β-cell destruction and the age at onset of type 1 diabetes. *Diabetes* **65:** 1362–1369. doi:10.2337/db15-1615

Leete P, Oram RA, McDonald TJ, Shields BM, Ziller C; TIGI Study Team; Hattersley AT, Richardson SJ, Morgan NG. 2020. Studies of insulin and proinsulin in pancreas and serum support the existence of aetiopathological endotypes of type 1 diabetes associated with age at diagnosis. *Diabetologia* **63:** 1258–1267. doi:10.1007/s00125-020-05115-6

Li X, Campbell-Thompson M, Wasserfall CH, McGrail K, Posgai A, Schultz AR, Brusko TM, Shuster J, Liang F, Muir A, et al. 2017. Serum trypsinogen levels in type 1 diabetes. *Diabetes Care* **40:** 577–582. doi:10.2337/dc16-1774

Linsley P, Nakayama M, Balmas E, Chen J, Pour F, Bansal S, Serti E, Speake C, Pugliese A, Cerosaletti K. 2023. Self-reactive germline-like TCR α chains shared between blood and pancreas. *Res Sq* doi:10.21203/rs.3.rs-3446917/v1

Löhr M, Klöppel G. 1987. Residual insulin positivity and pancreatic atrophy in relation to duration of chronic type 1 (insulin-dependent) diabetes mellitus and microangiopathy. *Diabetologia* **30:** 757–762. doi:10.1007/BF00275740

Lu J, Hou X, Pang C, Zhang L, Hu C, Zhao J, Bao Y, Jia W. 2016. Pancreatic volume is reduced in patients with latent autoimmune diabetes in adults. *Diabetes Metab Res Rev* **32:** 858–866. doi:10.1002/dmrr.2806

Maclean N, Ogilvie R. 1959. Observations on the pancreatic islet tissue of young diabetic subjects. *Diabetes* **8:** 83–91. doi:10.2337/diab.8.2.83

Marhfour I, Lopez XM, Lefkaditis D, Salmon I, Allagnat F, Richardson SJ, Morgan NG, Eizirik DL. 2012. Expression of endoplasmic reticulum stress markers in the islets of patients with type 1 diabetes. *Diabetologia* **55:** 2417–2420. doi:10.1007/s00125-012-2604-3

Mateus Gonçalves L, Fahd Qadir MM, Boulina M, Makhmutova M, Pereira E, Almaça J. 2023. Pericyte dysfunction and impaired vasomotion are hallmarks of islets during the pathogenesis of type 1 diabetes. *Cell Rep* **42:** 112913. doi:10.1016/j.celrep.2023.112913

McGinty JW, Marré ML, Bajzik V, Piganelli JD, James EA. 2015. T cell epitopes and post-translationally modified epitopes in type 1 diabetes. *Curr Diab Rep* **15:** 90. doi:10.1007/s11892-015-0657-7

McKeigue PM, Spiliopoulou A, McGurnaghan S, Colombo M, Blackbourn L, McDonald TJ, Onengut-Gomuscu S, Rich SS, Palmer CNA, McKnight JA, et al. 2019. Persistent C-peptide secretion in type 1 diabetes and its relationship to the genetic architecture of diabetes. *BMC Med* **17:** 165. doi:10.1186/s12916-019-1392-8

Michels AW, Landry LG, McDaniel KA, Yu L, Campbell-Thompson M, Kwok WW, Jones KL, Gottlieb PA, Kappler JW, Tang Q, et al. 2017. Islet-derived CD4 T cells targeting proinsulin in human autoimmune diabetes. *Diabetes* **66:** 722–734. doi:10.2337/db16-1025

Motwani K, Peters LD, Vliegen WH, El-Sayed AG, Seay HR, Lopez MC, Baker HV, Posgai AL, Brusko MA, Perry DJ, et al. 2020. Human regulatory T cells from umbilical cord blood display increased repertoire diversity and lineage stability relative to adult peripheral blood. *Front Immunol* **11:** 611. doi:10.3389/fimmu.2020.00611

Muralidharan C, Conteh AM, Marasco MR, Crowder JJ, Kuipers J, de Boer P, Linnemann AK. 2021. Pancreatic β cell autophagy is impaired in type 1 diabetes. *Diabetologia* **64:** 865–877. doi:10.1007/s00125-021-05387-6

Nagy N, Kaber G, Johnson PY, Gebe JA, Preisinger A, Falk BA, Sunkari VG, Gooden MD, Vernon RB, Bogdani M, et al. 2015. Inhibition of hyaluronan synthesis restores immune tolerance during autoimmune insulitis. *J Clin Invest* **125:** 3928–3940. doi:10.1172/JCI79271

Newby BN, Brusko TM, Zou B, Atkinson MA, Clare-Salzler M, Mathews CE. 2017. Type 1 interferons potentiate human $CD8^+$ T cell cytotoxicity through a STAT4- and granzyme B-dependent pathway. *Diabetes* **66:** 3061–3071. doi:10.2337/db17-0106

Obarorakpor N, Patel D, Boyarov R, Amarsaikhan N, Cepeda JR, Eastes D, Robertson S, Johnson T, Yang K, Tang Q, et al. 2023. Regulatory T cells targeting a pathogenic MHC class II: insulin peptide epitope postpone spontaneous autoimmune diabetes. *Front Immunol* **14:** 1207108. doi:10.3389/fimmu.2023.1207108

Olehnik SK, Fowler JL, Avramovich G, Hara M. 2017. Quantitative analysis of intra- and inter-individual variability of human β-cell mass. *Sci Rep* **7:** 16398. doi:10.1038/s41598-017-16300-w

Oram RA, Jones AG, Besser RE, Knight BA, Shields BM, Brown RJ, Hattersley AT, McDonald TJ. 2014. The majority of patients with long-duration type 1 diabetes are insulin microsecretors and have functioning β cells. *Diabetologia* **57:** 187–191. doi:10.1007/s00125-013-3067-x

Oram RA, Sims EK, Evans-Molina C. 2019. β Cells in type 1 diabetes: mass and function; sleeping or dead? *Diabetologia* **62:** 567–577. doi:10.1007/s00125-019-4822-4

Pandiri A. 2014. Overview of exocrine pancreatic pathobiology. *Toxicol Pathol* **42:** 207–216. doi:10.1177/0192623313509907

Panzer JK, Hiller H, Cohrs CM, Almaça J, Enos SJ, Beery M, Cechin S, Drotar DM, Weitz JR, Santini J, et al. 2020. Pancreas tissue slices from organ donors enable in situ analysis of type 1 diabetes pathogenesis. *JCI Insight* **5:** e13452. doi:10.1172/jci.insight.134525

Penno MAS, Oakey H, Augustine P, Taranto M, Barry SC, Colman PG, Craig ME, Davis EA, Giles LC, Harris M, et al. 2020. Changes in pancreatic exocrine function in young at-risk children followed to islet autoimmunity and type 1 diabetes in the ENDIA study. *Pediatr Diabetes* **21:** 945–949. doi:10.1111/pedi.13056

Perry DJ, Shapiro MR, Chamberlain SW, Kusmartseva I, Chamala S, Balzano-Nogueira L, Yang M, Brant JO, Brusko M, Williams MD, et al. 2023. A genomic data archive from the Network for Pancreatic Organ donors with Diabetes. *Sci Data* **10:** 323. doi:10.1038/s41597-023-02244-6

Peters L, Posgai A, Brusko T. 2019. Islet–immune interactions in type 1 diabetes: the nexus of β cell destruction. *Clin Exp Immunol* **198:** 326–340. doi:10.1111/cei.13349

Pociot F, Lernmark A. 2016. Genetic risk factors for type 1 diabetes. *Lancet* **387:** 2331–2339. doi:10.1016/S0140-6736(16)30582-7

Pollard HM, Miller L, Brewer WA. 1943. The external secretion of the pancreas and diabetes mellitus. *AJDD* **10:** 20–23. doi:10.1007/BF02997405

Pugliese A, Yang M, Kusmarteva I, Heiple T, Vendrame F, Wasserfall C, Rowe P, Moraski JM, Ball S, Jebson L, et al. 2014. The Juvenile Diabetes Research Foundation Network for Pancreatic Organ Donors with Diabetes (nPOD) Program: goals, operational model and emerging findings. *Pediatr Diabetes* **15:** 1–9. doi:10.1111/pedi.12097

Qadir MMF, Álvarez-Cubela S, Weitz J, Panzer JK, Klein D, Moreno-Hernández Y, Cechin S, Tamayo A, Almaça J, Hiller H, et al. 2020. Long-term culture of human pancreatic slices as a model to study real-time islet regeneration. *Nat Commun* **11:** 3265. doi:10.1038/s41467-020-17040-8

Quesada-Masachs E, Zilberman S, Rajendran S, Chu T, McArdle S, Kiosses WB, Lee JM, Yesildag B, Benkahla MA, Pawlowska A, et al. 2022. Upregulation of HLA class II in pancreatic β cells from organ donors with type 1 diabetes. *Diabetologia* **65:** 387–401. doi:10.1007/s00125-021-05619-9

Redondo MJ, Richardson SJ, Perry D, Minard CG, Carr ALJ, Brusko T, Kusmartseva I, Pugliese A, Atkinson MA. 2023. Milder loss of insulin-containing islets in individuals with type 1 diabetes and type 2 diabetes-associated TCF7L2 genetic variants. *Diabetologia* **66:** 127–131. doi:10.1007/s00125-022-05818-y

Regnell SE, Peterson P, Trinh L, Broberg P, Leander P, Lernmark Å, Månsson S, Elding Larsson H. 2016. Pancreas volume and fat fraction in children with type 1 diabetes. *Diabet Med* **33:** 1374–1379. doi:10.1111/dme.13115

Richardson SJ, Rodriguez-Calvo T, Gerling IC, Mathews CE, Kaddis JS, Russell MA, Zeissler M, Leete P, Krogvold L, Dahl-Jørgensen K, et al. 2016. Islet cell hyperexpression of HLA class I antigens: a defining feature in type 1 diabetes. *Diabetologia* **59:** 2448–2458. doi:10.1007/s00125-016-4067-4

Richardson TM, Saunders DC, Haliyur R, Shrestha S, Cartailler JP, Reinert RB, Petronglo J, Bottino R, Aramandla R, Bradley AM, et al. 2023. Human pancreatic capillaries and nerve fibers persist in type 1 diabetes despite β cell loss. *Am J Physiol Endocrinol Metab* **324:** E251–E267. doi:10.1152/ajpendo.00246.2022

Rodriguez-Calvo T, Ekwall O, Amirian N, Zapardiel-Gonzalo J, von Herrath MG. 2014. Increased immune cell infiltration of the exocrine pancreas: a possible contribution to the pathogenesis of type 1 diabetes. *Diabetes* **63:** 3880–3890. doi:10.2337/db14-0549

Rodriguez-Calvo T, Zapardiel-Gonzalo J, Amirian N, Castillo E, Lajevardi Y, Krogvold L, Dahl-Jørgensen K, von Herrath MG. 2017. Increase in pancreatic proinsulin and preservation of β-cell mass in autoantibody-positive donors prior to type 1 diabetes onset. *Diabetes* **66:** 1334–1345. doi:10.2337/db16-1343

Ross JJ, Wasserfall CH, Bacher R, Perry DJ, McGrail K, Posgai AL, Dong X, Muir A, Li X, Campbell-Thompson M, et al. 2021. Exocrine pancreatic enzymes are a serological biomarker for type 1 diabetes staging and pancreas size. *Diabetes* **70:** 944–954. doi:10.2337/db20-0995

Russell MA, Redick SD, Blodgett DM, Richardson SJ, Leete P, Krogvold L, Dahl-Jørgensen K, Bottino R, Brissova M, Spaeth JM, et al. 2019. HLA class II antigen processing and presentation pathway components demonstrated by transcriptome and protein analyses of islet β-cells from donors with type 1 diabetes. *Diabetes* **68:** 988–1001. doi:10.2337/db18-0686

Saisho Y, Butler AE, Meier JJ, Monchamp T, Allen-Auerbach M, Rizza RA, Butler PC. 2007. Pancreas volumes in humans from birth to age one hundred taking into account sex, obesity, and presence of type-2 diabetes. *Clin Anat* **20:** 933–942. doi:10.1002/ca.20543

Seay HR, Yusko E, Rothweiler SJ, Zhang L, Posgai AL, Campbell-Thompson M, Vignali M, Emerson RO, Kaddis JS, Ko D, et al. 2016. Tissue distribution and clonal diversity of the T and B cell repertoire in type 1 diabetes. *JCI Insight* **1:** e88242. doi:10.1172/jci.insight.88242

Seay HR, Putnam AL, Cserny J, Posgai AL, Rosenau EH, Wingard JR, Girard KF, Kraus M, Lares AP, Brown HL, et al. 2017. Expansion of human tregs from cryopreserved umbilical cord blood for GMP-compliant autologous adoptive cell transfer therapy. *Mol Ther Methods Clin Dev* **4:** 178–191. doi:10.1016/j.omtm.2016.12.003

Sebastiani G, Ventriglia G, Stabilini A, Socci C, Morsiani C, Laurenzi A, Nigi L, Formichi C, Mfarrej B, Petrelli A, et al. 2017. Regulatory T-cells from pancreatic lymphnodes of patients with type-1 diabetes express increased levels of microRNA miR-125a-5p that limits CCR2 expression. *Sci Rep* **7:** 6897. doi:10.1038/s41598-017-07172-1

Shapira SN, Naji A, Atkinson MA, Powers AC, Kaestner KH. 2022. Understanding islet dysfunction in type 2 diabetes through multidimensional pancreatic phenotyping: the Human Pancreas Analysis Program. *Cell Metab* **34:** 1906–1913. doi:10.1016/j.cmet.2022.09.013

Shapiro M, Atkinson M, Brusko T. 2019. Pleiotropic roles of the insulin-like growth factor axis in type 1 diabetes. *Curr Opin Endocrinol Diabetes Obes* **26:** 188–194. doi:10.1097/MED.0000000000000484

Shapiro MR, Wasserfall CH, McGrail SM, Posgai AL, Bacher R, Muir A, Haller MJ, Schatz DA, Wesley JD, von Herrath M, et al. 2020a. Insulin-like growth factor dysregulation both preceding and following type 1 diabetes diagnosis. *Diabetes* **69:** 413–423. doi:10.2337/db19-0942

Shapiro MR, Yeh WI, Longfield JR, Gallagher J, Infante CM, Wellford S, Posgai AL, Atkinson MA, Campbell-Thompson M, Lieberman SM, et al. 2020b. CD226 deletion reduces type 1 diabetes in the NOD mouse by impairing thymocyte development and peripheral T cell activation. *Front Immunol* **11:** 2180. doi:10.2337/db19-0942

Shapiro MR, Peters LD, Brown ME, Cabello-Kindelan C, Posgai AL, Bayer AL, Brusko TM. 2023. Insulin-like growth factor-1 synergizes with IL-2 to induce homeostatic proliferation of regulatory T cells. *J Immunol* **211:** 1108–1122. doi:10.4049/jimmunol.2200651

Sims EK, Bahnson HT, Nyalwidhe J, Haataja L, Davis AK, Speake C, DiMeglio LA, Blum J, Morris MA, Mirmira RG, et al. 2019a. Proinsulin secretion is a persistent feature of type 1 diabetes. *Diabetes Care* **42:** 258–264. doi:10.2337/dc17-2625

Sims EK, Syed F, Nyalwidhe J, Bahnson HT, Haataja L, Speake C, Morris MA, Balamurugan AN, Mirmira RG, Nadler J, et al. 2019b. Abnormalities in proinsulin processing in islets from individuals with longstanding T1D. *Transl Res* **213:** 90–99. doi:10.1016/j.trsl.2019.08.001

Smith MJ, Packard TA, O'Neill SK, Henry Dunand CJ, Huang M, Fitzgerald-Miller L, Stowell D, Hinman RM, Wilson PC, Gottlieb PA, et al. 2015. Loss of anergic B cells in prediabetic and new-onset type 1 diabetic patients. *Diabetes* **64:** 1703–1712. doi:10.2337/db13-1798

Spanier JA, Fung V, Wardell CM, Alkhatib MH, Chen Y, Swanson LA, Dwyer AJ, Weno ME, Silva N, Mitchell JS, et al. 2023. Tregs with an MHC class II peptide-specific chimeric antigen receptor prevent autoimmune diabetes in mice. *J Clin Invest* **133:** e168601. doi:10.1172/JCI168601

Stensland ZC, Magera CA, Broncucia H, Gomez BD, Rios-Guzman NM, Wells KL, Nicholas CA, Rihanek M, Hunter MJ, Toole KP, et al. 2023. Identification of an anergic BND cell-derived activated B cell population (BND2) in young-onset type 1 diabetes patients. *J Exp Med* **220:** e20221604. doi:10.1084/jem.20221604

Tang X, Kusmartseva I, Kulkarni S, Posgai A, Speier S, Schatz DA, Haller MJ, Campbell-Thompson M, Wasserfall CH, Roep BO, et al. 2021. Image-based machine learning algorithms for disease characterization in the human type 1 diabetes pancreas. *Am J Pathol* **191:** 454–462. doi:10.1016/j.ajpath.2020.11.010

Thompson PJ, Shah A, Ntranos V, Van Gool F, Atkinson M, Bhushan A. 2019. Targeted elimination of senescent β cells prevents type 1 diabetes. *Cell Metab* **29:** 1045–1060.e10. doi:10.1016/j.cmet.2019.01.021

Välikangas T, Lietzén N, Jaakkola MK, Krogvold L, Eike MC, Kallionpää H, Tuomela S, Mathews C, Gerling IC, Oikarinen S, et al. 2022. Pancreas whole tissue transcriptomics highlights the role of the exocrine pancreas in patients with recently diagnosed type 1 diabetes. *Front Endocrinol* **13:** 861985. doi:10.3389/fendo.2022.861985

Vecchio F, Lo Buono N, Stabilini A, Nigi L, Dufort MJ, Geyer S, Rancoita PM, Cugnata F, Mandelli A, Valle A, et al. 2018. Abnormal neutrophil signature in the blood and pancreas of presymptomatic and symptomatic type 1 diabetes. *JCI Insight* **3:** e122146. doi:10.1172/jci.insight.122146

Vendrame F, Pileggi A, Laughlin E, Allende G, Martin-Pagola A, Molano RD, Diamantopoulos S, Standifer N, Geubtner K, Falk BA, et al. 2010. Recurrence of type 1 diabetes after simultaneous pancreas-kidney transplantation, despite immunosuppression, is associated with autoantibodies and pathogenic autoreactive CD4T-cells. *Diabetes* **59:** 947–957. doi:10.2337/db09-0498

Virostko J, Williams J, Hilmes M, Bowman C, Wright JJ, Du L, Kang H, Russell WE, Powers AC, Moore DJ. 2019. Pancreas volume declines during the first year after diagnosis of type 1 diabetes and exhibits altered diffusion at disease onset. *Diabetes Care* **42:** 248–257. doi:10.2337/dc18-1507

Waibel M, Wentworth JM, So M, Couper JJ, Cameron FJ, MacIsaac RJ, Atlas G, Gorelik A, Litwak S, Sanz-Villanueva L, et al. 2023. Baricitinib and β-cell function in patients with new-onset type 1 diabetes. *N Engl J Med* **389:** 2140–2150. doi:10.1056/NEJMoa2306691

Wang YJ, Traum D, Schug J, Gao L, Liu C; HPAP Consortium; Atkinson MA, Powers AC, Feldman MD, Naji A, et al. 2019. Multiplexed in situ imaging mass cytometry analysis of the human endocrine pancreas and immune system in type 1 diabetes. *Cell Metab* **29:** 769–783.e4. doi:10.1016/j.cmet.2019.01.003

Wasserfall C, Nick HS, Campbell-Thompson M, Beachy D, Haataja L, Kusmartseva I, Posgai A, Beery M, Rhodes C, Bonifacio E, et al. 2017. Persistence of pancreatic insulin mRNA expression and proinsulin protein in type 1 diabetes pancreata. *Cell Metab* **26:** 568–575.e3. doi:10.1016/j.cmet.2017.08.013

Williams AJ, Thrower SL, Sequeiros IM, Ward A, Bickerton AS, Triay JM, Callaway MP, Dayan CM. 2012. Pancreatic volume is reduced in adult patients with recently diagnosed type 1 diabetes. *J Clin Endocrinol Metab* **97:** E2109–E2113. doi:10.1210/jc.2012-1815

Woo J, Sudhir P, Zhang Q. 2020. Pancreatic tissue proteomics unveils key proteins, pathways, and networks associated with type 1 diabetes. *Proteomics Clin Appl* **14:** e2000053. doi:10.1002/prca.202000053

Wright JJ, Saunders DC, Dai C, Poffenberger G, Cairns B, Serreze DV, Harlan DM, Bottino R, Brissova M, Powers AC. 2020. Decreased pancreatic acinar cell number in type 1 diabetes. *Diabetologia* **63:** 1418–1423. doi:10.1007/s00125-020-05155-y

Wu W, Syed F, Simpson E, Lee CC, Liu J, Chang G, Dong C, Seitz C, Eizirik DL, Mirmira RG, et al. 2021. The impact of pro-inflammatory cytokines on alternative splicing patterns in human islets. *Diabetes* **71:** 116–127. doi:10.2337/db20-0847

Yang SJ, Singh AK, Drow T, Tappen T, Honaker Y, Barahmand-Pour-Whitman F, Linsley PS, Cerosaletti K, Mauk K, Xiang Y, et al. 2022. Pancreatic islet-specific engineered T_{regs} exhibit robust antigen-specific and bystander immune suppression in type 1 diabetes models. *Sci Transl Med* **14:** eabn1716. doi:10.1126/scitranslmed.abn1716

Yeh WI, Seay HR, Newby B, Posgai AL, Moniz FB, Michels A, Mathews CE, Bluestone JA, Brusko TM. 2017. Avidity and bystander suppressive capacity of human regulatory T cells expressing de novo autoreactive T-cell receptors in type 1 diabetes. *Front Immunol* **8:** 1313. doi:10.3389/fimmu.2017.01313

The Role of B Lymphocytes in Type 1 Diabetes

Mia J. Smith,[1] Joanne Boldison,[2] and F. Susan Wong[3]

[1]Department of Pediatrics, Barbara Davis Center for Diabetes, The University of Colorado Anschutz Medical Campus, Aurora, Colorado 80045, USA

[2]Institute of Biomedical and Clinical Science, College of Medicine and Health, University of Exeter, Exeter EX2 5DW, United Kingdom

[3]Division of Infection and Immunity and Systems Immunity University Research Institute, School of Medicine, Cardiff University, Cardiff CF14 4XN, United Kingdom

Correspondence: mia.smith@cuanschutz.edu; j.boldison@exeter.ac.uk

While autoreactive T cells are known to induce β-cell death in type 1 diabetes (T1D), self-reactive B cells also play an important role in the pathogenesis of T1D. Studies have shown that individuals living with T1D have an increased frequency of self-reactive B cells that escape from the bone marrow and populate peripheral organs, become activated, and participate in disease. These failed tolerance mechanisms may be attributed to genetic risk alleles that are associated with the development of T1D. Once in the periphery, these self-reactive B cells act as important antigen-presenting cells to autoreactive T cells and produce autoantibodies that are used to predict individuals at risk for or diagnosed with T1D. Here, we discuss the evidence that B cells are important in the pathogenesis of T1D, how these cells escape normal tolerance mechanisms, their role in disease progression, and how targeting these cells and/or monitoring them as biomarkers for response to therapy will be of clinical benefit.

Autoimmunity generally ensues in the setting of genetic susceptibility, occurring in response to an environmental trigger, leading to a loss of central and peripheral immune tolerance. Type 1 diabetes (T1D) has been predominantly considered an autoimmune condition in which T cells play a prominent pathogenic role in the destruction of the insulin-producing β cells of the pancreas, but B cells and other antigen-presenting cells are also required in a complex network for autoimmunity to occur. The pathogenic process occurs over many years, with autoantibodies being one of the earliest markers of this disease. It is relatively difficult to study aspects of the pathogenesis of T1D, as the target organ—the β cells of the pancreatic islets of Langerhans, are inaccessible, lying deep within the human body abdominal cavity. Our insights into many aspects of the pathogenesis have been signposted by the nonobese diabetic (NOD) mouse model, which has remarkably similar features to some of the human clinical aspects of the disease, including both high genetic susceptibility with the major histocompatibility complex contributing a large proportion of risk, as well as the influence of the environment in the development of diabetes, although the actual factors are different.

Cite this article as *Cold Spring Harb Perspect Med* doi: 10.1101/cshperspect.a041593

In this article, the focus on the role of B cells in diabetes development will be discussed, with insights gained from the NOD mouse model highlighted alongside the observations that these have led to in humans. The many B-cell functions will be explored, with consideration of the various ways in which B cells may contribute to the autoimmunity in T1D, including antigen presentation and diversification of the immune response, cytokine production, autoantibody production, development of follicular dendritic cells, and alteration in immune regulation.

What is the evidence that B cells are involved in the pathogenic processes leading to T1D? NOD mice that have a targeted IgM gene deletion ($\mu MT^{-/-}$), resulting in B-cell developmental arrest (Serreze et al. 1996; Akashi et al. 1997; Wong et al. 1998), or B cells depleted by the administration of antibodies at a very early age (Noorchashm et al. 1997) have a very low incidence of autoimmune diabetes. This has been even more strongly emphasized by the depletion of B cells in NOD mice with agents that have included anti-CD20 (Hu et al. 2007; Xiu et al. 2008), toxin Calicheamicin conjugated to anti-CD22 (Fiorina et al. 2008), neutralization of the B-cell growth factor BAFF (Zekavat et al. 2008), and BCMA–huFc fusion protein (Mariño et al. 2009) to more specifically deplete follicular and marginal zone B cells, which have all resulted in protection against the development of autoimmune diabetes. Importantly, studies in recently diagnosed individuals with T1D demonstrated that depletion of B cells using anti-CD20 (Rituximab) preserved β-cell function (i.e., decreased rate of C-peptide loss) and reduced exogenous insulin needs up to 1 year following treatment (Pescovitz et al. 2009). However, these benefits were no longer seen by the end of the second year once B-cell numbers had been restored to normal levels following the initial course of treatment (Pescovitz et al. 2014). Thus, these lines of evidence provide strong support for the proposition that autoreactive B cells play an important role in the etiology and/or progression of T1D and that targeting B cells may have therapeutic potential. However, there are practical considerations in the choice of the therapy that could be used (see below).

BREAKDOWN OF B-CELL TOLERANCE IN T1D

Previous studies have shown that as many as 70% of B cells generated in the bone marrow are autoreactive (Wardemann et al. 2003). In healthy individuals, these self-reactive B cells are normally tolerized (silenced) by one of three mechanisms: (1) receptor editing, (2) clonal deletion, or (3) anergy (Fig. 1A). Central tolerance in the bone marrow encompasses both receptor editing and clonal deletion, whereas peripheral tolerance includes anergy. B cells that bind self-antigen with high avidity in the bone marrow undergo receptor editing, in which strong B-cell receptor (BCR) signals induce rearrangement of the antigen receptor light chain genes, silencing one allele and expressing a second. If the new antigen receptor lacks self-reactivity, the B cell can continue development and populate the periphery as a naive B cell capable of responding to pathogenic insults (Halverson et al. 2004; Meffre and Wardemann 2008). For many B cells, this process is successful, but when it is not, death by clonal deletion/apoptosis occurs. If the BCR has a moderate avidity for self-antigen, the B cell can exit the bone marrow and enter the periphery but is suppressed via anergy (Bluestone et al. 2010; Jeker et al. 2012). Anergic B cells are characterized by an inability to become activated, proliferate, and differentiate into antibody-secreting cells (Gauld et al. 2005, 2006; Merrell et al. 2006; Cambier et al. 2007; Duty et al. 2009). Chronic stimulation by self-antigen (signal 1) in the absence of T-cell help (signal 2) is critical for the induction and maintenance of B-cell anergy. Anergic B cells down-regulate their BCR, particularly surface IgM, and increase activation of negative regulatory signaling molecules, such as PTEN and SHIP-1 (O'Neill et al. 2011; Getahun et al. 2016, 2017). Importantly, anergy is reversible if the autoantigen dissociates from the BCR or the autoreactive B cell receives help from a cognate T cell.

A breakdown in the tolerance mechanisms discussed above likely contributes to the development of T1D. Menard et al. (2011) found that self-reactive B cells, as defined by the binding of

 Cite this article as *Cold Spring Harb Perspect Med* doi: 10.1101/cshperspect.a041593

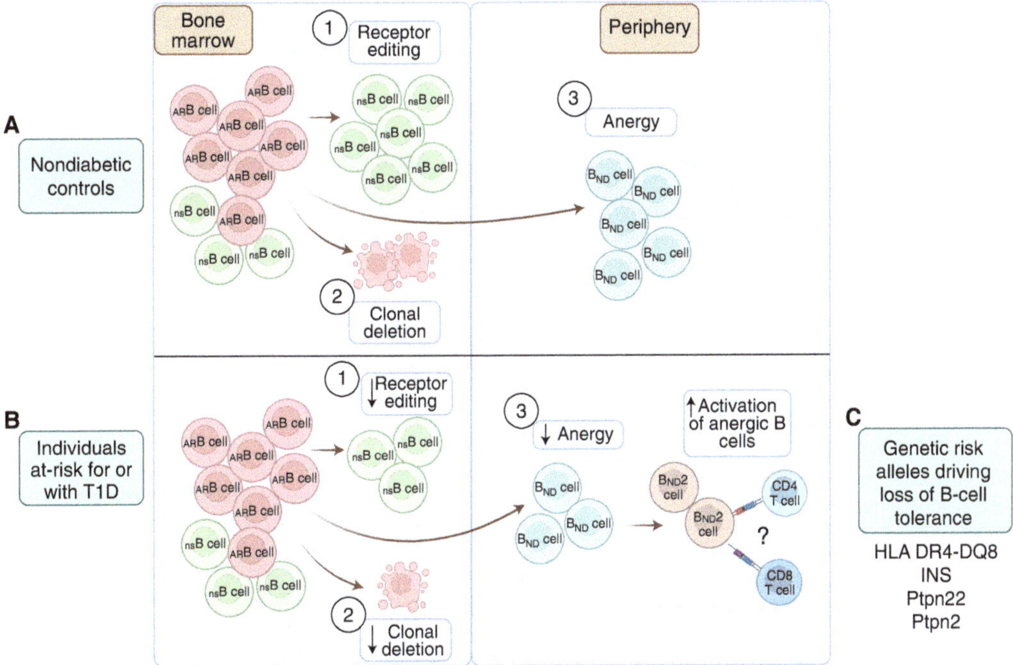

Figure 1. Failed B lymphocyte tolerance mechanisms in type 1 diabetes (T1D). (*A*) Central tolerance occurs in the bone marrow and includes receptor editing and clonal deletion, while peripheral tolerance occurs in the periphery and includes anergy. It has been shown that ~70% of B cells made in the bone marrow are autoreactive ($_{AR}$B cell). In nondiabetic individuals, $_{AR}$B cells with high affinity for self-antigen will undergo (1) receptor editing. If these cells fail to edit their B-cell receptor (BCR) to a nonautoreactive BCR, they will then undergo (2) clonal deletion/apoptosis. $_{AR}$B cells with low-to-moderate affinity can escape into the periphery, where they will undergo B-cell anergy, becoming a B_{ND} cell. Together, these B-cell tolerance mechanisms help prevent the development of autoimmunity. (*B*) In individuals at risk for or with T1D, it has been shown that $_{AR}$B cells fail to undergo proper silencing by receptor editing, clonal deletion, and anergy. Autoreactive B cells that escape into the periphery become activated, becoming $B_{ND}2$ cells, and likely interact with cognate $CD4^+$ and $CD8^+$ T cells to help drive the development of T1D. (*C*) Loss of these B-cell tolerance mechanisms in T1D is associated with high-risk genetic risk alleles, including expression of the human leukocyte antigen (HLA) DR4–DQ8 haplotype and polymorphisms in INS, Ptpn22, and Ptpn2.

their antibody to permeabilized Hep-2 cells, are increased among the new emigrant/transitional and mature naive B cells in individuals with T1D (Table 1), suggesting impairment of both central (receptor editing or clonal deletion) and peripheral (anergy) B-cell tolerance. Importantly, these autoreactive B cells were found to be polyreactive, binding also to lipopolysaccharide (LPS) and insulin. Furthermore, the frequency of recombining sequence (RS) rearrangements in lambda-positive B cells, which is a surrogate measure of receptor editing, is decreased in T1D subjects compared to healthy control individuals (Panigrahi et al. 2008). Taken together, these results demonstrate T1D subjects exhibit a breakdown in central tolerance mechanisms, which likely allows escape of autoreactive B cells into the periphery.

If central tolerance mechanisms fail, B cells that enter the periphery should undergo a state of anergy or unresponsiveness. However, studies indicate that individuals with T1D have an impaired ability to maintain self-reactive B cells via anergy. Analyzing the frequency of total anergic B cells (termed B_{ND}) versus insulin-binding anergic B cells along a continuum of diabetes development, it was found that autoantibody-positive first-degree relatives and recently

Table 1. B-cell subsets that have been shown to be altered in human type 1 diabetes (T1D) and nonobese diabetic (NOD) mouse

B-cell subset	Phenotype	Mechanism(s) of action	Change in tissue	References
Human T1D				
New emigrant/ transitional	Poly/autoreactive $CD19^+$ $CD27^-$ IgM^{hi} $CD24^{hi}$	Unknown	↑ in blood	Menard et al. 2011
Mature naive	Poly/autoreactive $CD19^+$ $CD27^-$ IgM^+ IgD^+	Unknown	↑ in blood	Menard et al. 2011
Anergic (B_{ND})	$CD19^+$ $CD27^-$ $IgM^{-/lo}$ IgD^+ +/− Insulin-binding	Tolerized/ unresponsive self-reactive	↓ in blood	Smith et al. 2015; Habib et al. 2019
Activated previously anergic ($B_{ND}2$)	Insulin-binding $CD19^+$ $CD27^-$ IgM^- IgD^+ $CD21^-$ $CXCR5^-$	Unknown	↑ in blood in young-onset (≤10 yr old)	Stensland et al. 2023
Breg	$CD25^{hi}$ Breg	Inhibit T cell and APC responses	↓ in blood	Zhang et al. 2022
	Memory Breg ($CD24^{hi}$ $CD27^+$)	Inhibit T cell and APC responses	↓ in blood	Tompa and Faresjo 2024
	$CD5^+$ Breg	Inhibit T cell and APC responses	↑ in blood	Tompa and Faresjo 2024
NOD mouse				
B1a	$CD5^+$	Innate-like; can activate pDCs	↑ in pancreas (at 2 wk of age)	Diana et al. 2013
Plasmablasts	$CD138^+$ $CD44^{hi}$	Antibody-secreting cells	↑ in pancreas when diabetic	Boldison et al. 2021; Ling et al. 2022
Follicular B cell	IgD^+ $CD138^+$	Unknown	↑ in pancreas when diabetic	Ryan et al. 2010; Serreze et al. 2011; Boldison et al. 2019
Inflammatory B cells (via gene expression)	↑ Expression of IFN-α-related and proinflammatory genes	Unknown	↑ in the pancreatic lymph node	Boldison et al. 2023
$TLR7^+$ B cells	$TLR7^+$ B cells	Unknown	↑ in the pancreas	Boldison et al. 2023

(<1 yr) diagnosed individuals with T1D have a significant decrease in total and insulin-reactive anergic B cells in their peripheral blood compared to healthy controls and individuals living with long-standing diabetes (Table 1; Smith et al. 2015; Habib et al. 2019). Interestingly, some autoantibody-negative first-degree relatives display a similar loss of insulin-reactive anergic B cells in their peripheral blood, suggesting that loss of anergy may precede activation and differentiation of these cells into autoantibody-secreting cells. Recent studies have identified a subset of B_{ND} cells, termed $B_{ND}2$, which expresses increased markers of activation, including the T-cell costimulatory molecules CD80 and CD86, and are functionally no longer anergic in T1D donors (Table 1). Importantly, insulin-binding $B_{ND}2$ cells were increased in the peripheral blood and pancreatic lymph nodes (PLNs) of young-onset T1D donors, suggesting activation of previously anergic autoreactive B cells occurs at an increased frequency in individuals with T1D (Fig. 1B). Given that insulin-binding $B_{ND}2$ cells have increased surface expression of CD80 and CD86, it is tempting to speculate that previously islet-specific anergic B cells may participate in pathogenic responses (Stensland et al. 2023).

Cite this article as *Cold Spring Harb Perspect Med* doi: 10.1101/cshperspect.a041593

ASSOCIATION OF GENETIC RISK ALLELES WITH B CELLS IN T1D

It has long been known that human leukocyte antigen (HLA) alleles play a major role in susceptibility to T1D, but there are many other contributory genetic loci, with currently more than 90 gene regions identified by genome-wide association studies (GWASs) (Redondo et al. 2023). Fine mapping to genetic loci that are associated with the development of T1D indicates that these susceptibility loci are shared with other autoimmune conditions and involve genes associated with immune cell function. These include loci that influence B- and T-cell responses, immunoregulatory cell activity, as well as some that play a role in innate immunity.

Given that the development of T1D is driven in part by genetic risk alleles, it seems likely that these factors could mediate their effects by promoting loss of central and peripheral B-cell tolerance. The T1D risk allele most affecting the odds ratio for disease development is HLA class II. DR4–DQ8 followed by DR3–DQ2 confer the greatest risk (Erlich et al. 2008; Concannon et al. 2009). CD4 T cells recognizing self-peptides in the context of DR4–DQ8 could evoke loss of B-cell tolerance. In line with this, the loss of anergic insulin-binding B cells and acquisition of $B_{ND}2$ cells is associated with carriers of the DR4–DQ8 haplotype (Smith et al. 2015; Stensland et al. 2023). The genetic polymorphism conferring the second highest risk is in the VNTR region of the insulin (*INS*) gene (Concannon et al. 2009). This polymorphism is thought to increase the number of insulin-specific T cells in the periphery due to impaired T-cell tolerance induction in the thymus (Pugliese et al. 1997). Hence, an increase in insulin-specific T cells would promote the activation of insulin-reactive B cells, driving them to participate in the disease. Indeed, studies have found that loss of anergic insulin-binding B cells is associated with insulin allotypes, suggesting T cells are likely driving the loss of B-cell anergy (Smith et al. 2018b).

In addition, impaired B-cell tolerance is associated with polymorphisms in the genes encoding the phosphatases, *PTPN22* and *PTPN2*, both of which are expressed in B and T cells and involved in the regulation of B- and T-cell receptor signaling (Cerosaletti and Buckner 2012). Mutations in *PTPN22*, which encodes the lymphoid tyrosine phosphatase, Lyp, confer the third highest contributor to T1D risk, after HLA and the *INS* genes (Concannon et al. 2009). Individuals who express the R620W variant of *PTPN22* have reduced signaling through the BCR, and this is suggested to increase the release of autoreactive B cells into the periphery (Rieck et al. 2007). The R620W variant also predicts that, in those individuals who become positive for insulin autoantibodies, these insulin autoantibodies will appear first (Steck et al. 2014). This variant, which is also found in other autoimmune conditions, increases the frequency of autoreactive and polyreactive B cells in the peripheral blood that have recently emigrated from the bone marrow (Menard et al. 2011). Targeted ectopic expression of the risk allele in B cells in vivo leads to autoimmunity (Dai et al. 2013).

The *PTPN2* gene encodes another protein tyrosine phosphatase that has been shown to have a range of functions, including negative regulation of JAK/STAT signaling (Simoncic et al. 2002) and T-cell receptor signaling (Wiede et al. 2011). A study in which *Ptpn2* was deleted in the hematopoietic compartment of adult mice demonstrated that these mice developed autoimmunity characterized by an increase in the number of B cells, including germinal center (GC) B cells, as well as antinuclear autoantibody production (Wiede et al. 2017). Studies in the Smith laboratory have shown that B-cell-specific deletion of *Ptpn2* in C57BL/6 mice leads to activation of B cells, a hyperresponsive phenotype, and autoantibody production (B Alexander and M Smith, unpubl.). Thus, polymorphisms in genes whose products function as negative regulators of BCR signaling may confer T1D risk by impairing central and peripheral B-cell tolerance. Other T1D-associated allelic variants of genes expressed in B cells, such as *BACH2* and *SH2B3*, may also in time be proven to impair B-cell tolerance.

While no genetic risk alleles are known to exist for PTEN, a negative regulator of the PI3-kinase pathway, it has been shown that total B cells from individuals with new-onset T1D exhibit decreased expression of PTEN compared to control subjects (Smith et al. 2019). Defects in the regulation of the PI3-kinase pathway (i.e., gain-of-function [GOF] mutations) can lead to increased infections, cancer, and autoimmunity (Fruman et al. 2017; Michalovich and Nejentsev 2018). Hence one might speculate that decreased expression of a negative regulator, such as PTEN, in all B cells would alter signaling thresholds, allowing rogue activation of autoreactive B cells. Further studies are needed to support this idea.

B CELLS AND AUTOANTIBODIES

Autoantibodies recognizing antigens expressed in the islets were one of the earliest indications of T1D having an autoimmune basis—with antibodies to insulin (Palmer et al. 1983), glutamic acid decarboxylase (GAD) (Baekkeskov et al. 1990), tyrosine phosphatase like protein I-A2 (Payton et al. 1995), Zinc transporter 8 (ZnT8) (Wenzlau et al. 2007), and most recently tetrapanin-7 (McLaughlin et al. 2016).

In humans, the presence of autoantibodies to GAD, IA-2, and insulin has been used to predict the future development of T1D (Ziegler et al. 2013). Indeed, T1D is now staged; prediabetes, or stage 1 and stage 2, is recognized as the presence of 2 or more diabetes autoantibodies without dysglycemia (stage 1) or with dysglycemia (stage 2), as proposed by Insel et al. (2015) and adopted for screening programs. Although these autoantibodies are now recognized as very important biomarkers for the future development of T1D and for diagnosing an individual with T1D, current dogma suggests they are not pathogenic.

There are multiple lines of evidence from the NOD mouse that suggest that autoantibodies are not necessary for the development of autoimmune diabetes, although some studies have suggested a modulating role. The direct transfer of human serum antibodies into SCID mice (Petersen et al. 1993) or NOD mouse serum into NOD mice (Serreze et al. 1998) does not induce diabetes, nor is the transfer of antibodies through milk important (Washburn et al. 2007). However, when B-cell-sufficient offspring are born to B-cell-deficient mice, the incidence of diabetes is reduced, implying that maternally transmitted antibodies may be important in mice (Greeley et al. 2002). Furthermore, through embryo transfer experiments, NOD offspring born to nondiabetes susceptible mothers developed insulitis but had reduced diabetes (Kagohashi et al. 2005). Additionally, mice that have B cells that express surface antibody but are lacking in soluble antibody production are able to develop diabetes, albeit at a much lower rate (Wong et al. 2004). In humans, it is interesting that offspring of mothers who have diabetes autoantibodies are not at increased risk of future development of T1D (Koczwara et al. 2004), and there is a greater risk of development of diabetes in offspring where fathers have diabetes compared with mothers (Warram et al. 1984). Indeed, in a subset of individuals (HLA DR3^{+} but DR4/DQ8^{-}), the presence of autoantibodies appeared to be protective (Koczwara et al. 2004). These studies indicate that soluble antibodies likely do not play a major role in causing diabetes, but is this lack of pathogenic effect absolute?

There are a number of observations that suggest that autoantibodies may impact disease pathogenesis. Autoantibodies can play a pathogenic role through FcR-mediated antigen–antibody uptake and activation by dendritic cells and macrophages that then present antigen to self-reactive T cells. It has been demonstrated that FcR-deficient NOD mice are protected from diabetes and insulitis is alleviated (Inoue et al. 2007). Moreover, the secretion of anti-islet autoantibodies acts in an FcR-mediated fashion to enhance the expansion of islet-reactive CD4 T cells in mice (Silva et al. 2011). Studies in humans indicate a tight correlation with the number of autoantibody specificities present and the progression to diabetes. Importantly, of all the possible autoantibodies that an individual can develop, it has only been shown for anti-insulin antibodies that higher titer levels correlate with disease progression (Steck et al. 2011, 2016), suggesting a pathogenic role for anti-insulin antibodies in T1D. Hence, the current dogma that autoantibodies are likely not pathogenic remains uncertain. Nevertheless, other aspects of

B-cell function, such as antigen presentation to T cells, may be more important.

B CELLS AS ANTIGEN-PRESENTING CELLS

Much evidence suggests that of the many functions of B cells, their ability to present antigens to T cells, is of considerable importance (see Fig. 2; Serreze et al. 1998; Silveira et al. 2002; Mariño et al. 2012). B cells are the only antigen-specific APCs that recognize antigen via the more than 10^5 BCRs on their cell surface, making them very potent and efficient at processing and presenting self-antigen to cognate autoreactive $CD4^+$ (Kendall et al. 2013; Pearson et al. 2020) and $CD8^+$ T cells (Mariño et al. 2012; Boldison et al. 2020). In the NOD mouse model, if B cells are prevented from presenting antigen via either class I or class II, diabetes development is reduced, demonstrating the importance of B cells to present antigen to both $CD4^+$ and $CD8^+$ T cells (Noorchashm et al. 1999; Mariño et al. 2012). In addition, BCR specificity is particularly important as NOD mice that have a reduced antigen-specific BCR repertoire also develop a reduced incidence of diabetes (Silveira et al. 2002; Wong et al. 2004). Conversely, accelerated autoimmune diabetes occurs in NOD mice that express an anti-insulin heavy chain gene (VH125Tg.NOD), rendering ~1%–2% of peripheral B cells insulin binding (Hulbert et al. 2001; Kendall et al. 2013). The same increased rate and penetrance of diabetes development is seen in the V_H125^{SD}.NOD mouse, in which the VH125 gene is directly targeted into the IgH locus, enabling class-switch recombination to occur (Felton et al. 2018). In both models, the heavy chain is fixed but can pair with a variety of endogenous light chains. Thus, most peripheral B cells are non-insulin-reactive, but the 1%–2% of B cells that are insulin-reactive are sufficient to drive accelerated diabetes development. These anti-insulin B cells are from the VH125.NOD mouse models can act as antigen-presenting cells to insulin-reactive T cells (Kendall et al. 2013; Fel-

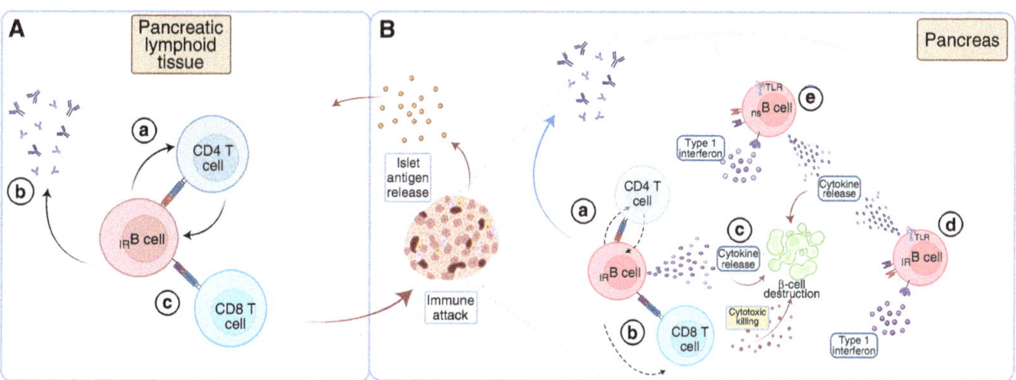

Figure 2. B lymphocyte involvement in type 1 diabetes (T1D). (*A*) In the peripheral lymphoid tissue islet-reactive B cells ($_{IR}$B cells) process and present islet antigens to CD4 T cells (*a*) and receive CD4 T cell help to produce islet autoantibodies (*b*), which are used as a biomarker in T1D. $_{IR}$B cells will also cross present antigen to CD8 T cells leading to activation and islet immune attack. (*B*) In the pancreatic tissue it is still unknown which B cells are present during β-cell destruction, and how they perpetuate β-cell demise. We have suggested several roles that may occur in the tissue during T1D: (*a*) $_{IR}$B cells present islet antigens to CD4 T cells. (*b*) $_{IR}$B cells cross present islet antigens to CD8 T cells, which may lead to further cytotoxic CD8 T-cell activation and B cells to (*c*) release pro-inflammatory cytokines due to the altered environment and received signals. (*d*) $_{IR}$B cells may undergo activation without T cell help, activated by cytokines such as IFN-α or an innate signal through the Toll-like receptor (TLR) pathways leading to cytokine release and possible antibody production. (*e*) Nonspecific B cells ($_{ns}$B cells) could be part of the pancreatic immune repertoire and undergo similar activation discussed in (*d*). As B cells are more prominent in the islet tissue in individuals with young-onset diabetes, this scheme of events would be more likely to be operative in those individuals.

ton et al. 2018; Boldison et al. 2019). Reciprocal effects of insulin-specific $CD4^+$ T cells on insulin-reactive B cells have been studied in transgenic mice in which increased levels of both T and B insulin-reactive cells are expressed. The pathogenic $CD4^+$ T cells, 8F10, recognizing insulin amino acids B12–20, when expressed as a transgene in the NOD mouse do not cause disease, but accelerate diabetes when the T-cell transgene is on the NOD $RAG1^{-/-}$ genetic background (Mohan et al. 2013). When the 8F10 transgenic NOD mouse was crossed with the V_H125^{SD}.NOD mouse, which develops accelerated disease, diabetes incidence was considerably reduced. Interestingly, however, when naive 8F10 $CD4^+$ T cells were cotransferred with V_H125^{SD}.NOD B cells into $RAG^{-/-}$ mice, diabetes was accelerated compared to naive 8F10 $CD4^+$ T cells alone or with nontransgenic B cells (Wan et al. 2016). In the presence of the 8F10 T cells, the frequency of GCs in PLNs was considerably increased, and these GC were also increased in the mesenteric, inguinal, and axillary lymph nodes, with concomitant high production of insulin autoantibodies, which were class-switched. These GC responses were also found when 8F10 and V_H125^{SD} were cotransferred into the $RAG^{-/-}$ mice (Wan et al. 2016). Thus, the insulin-specific $CD4^+$ T cells increased the autoantibody production from the insulin-reactive B cells, which in turn were also able to activate the antigen-specific $CD4^+$ T cells. In a different model, the regulatory insulin-specific $CD4^+$ T cells 2H6 (Du et al. 2006), which play a suppressive/regulatory role on recognition of insulin B9–23, when crossed with VH125 BCR transgenic mice to generate 2H6VH125 double transgenic mice, also develop reduced spontaneous diabetes (Pearson et al. 2020). The regulation promoted by the 2H6 cells, which produce TGF-β, reduced the expression of MHC class II and costimulatory molecules on the VH125 B cells, and reduced antigen presentation. Reciprocally, the 2H6 cells also demonstrated weaker proliferation when activated by the VH125 B cells but the presence of the B cells from the VH125 BCR did not affect the regulatory phenotype of the 2H6 $CD4^+$ T cells (Pearson et al. 2020). Furthermore, the expression of these 2H6 regulatory T cells reduced the GCs seen in the PLNs of the VH125 BCR transgenic mice. Thus, the antigen-specific $CD4^+$ T cells will modulate the pathogenic antigen-specific B cells, by altering GC responses and concomitant autoantibody responses, dependent on their phenotype. Reciprocally, the antigen-specific B cells also reinforce the phenotypes of the $CD4^+$ T cells.

Due to the inherent difficulties of demonstrating directly that islet-reactive B cells are presenting antigen to cognate islet-reactive T cells in stage 1, 2, or 3 T1D individuals, most evidence that B cells act as important antigen-presenting cells to T cells has come from studies in mice. Nevertheless, studies of the pancreas from donors with T1D (discussed in more detail below) have demonstrated a strong correlation with the number and proximity of B cells found in inflamed islets with $CD8^+$ T cells, suggesting B cells may be acting as antigen-presenting cells to $CD8^+$ T cells in the pancreas (Willcox et al. 2009). Future studies are needed to expand upon these findings to determine the role of B cells more conclusively in the pancreatic islets.

REGULATORY B CELLS IN T1D

As we have discussed above, it is well established that B cells are associated with a pathogenic role in disease; however, it is important to note that under specific circumstances and environments, B cells can exert regulatory effects. Regulatory B cells (Bregs) in T1D have recently been extensively reviewed (Ben Nasr et al. 2021; Boldison and Wong 2021) and so in this paper we will only provide a brief overview, highlighting some recent observations. Many Breg subsets suppress inflammation via the production of IL-10. However, unlike regulatory T cells, there are no definitive markers of Bregs, and therefore, without assessing IL-10 (or other anti-inflammatory cytokines such as TGF-β and IL-35), it is difficult to define a Breg. However, with increased multiparameter flow cytometric capabilities, many distinct subsets of Bregs, distinguished by the expression of a selection of immune markers, have been identified. These Breg populations suppress inflammatory responses from T cells, DCs, and monocytes in both mice and humans, although it should be noted that in permissive environments, most B cells can differentiate into Bregs (Rosser and Mauri 2015). In T1D, there is evidence for both numerical and functional defects in specific Breg populations; however, some disparity exists between studies (which is extensively discussed in Boldison and Wong [2021]), likely due to the use of different markers, lack of IL-10 assessment or different donor cohorts. More recent studies have reported a decrease in $CD25^{hi}$ Bregs, a population high in IL-10 and TGF-β production (Kessel et al. 2012), in T1D donors compared to healthy controls (Zhang et al. 2022). Tompa and Faresjo characterized Bregs in children with T1D (and/or celiac disease) and demonstrated a decrease in memory Bregs ($CD24^{hi}$ $CD27^{+}$) but an increase in $CD5^{+}$ Bregs (Table 1; Tompa and Faresjo 2024). Additional studies will be required to fully elucidate the complex network of Breg subsets and allow an understanding of the relationship between the changes we observe and different donor demographics.

Recent experiments in NOD mice have shown that a unique $CD103^{+}$ B-cell population with immunosuppressive properties are expanded in the NLRP6-deficient mouse and can protect from diabetes development (Pearson et al. 2023). $CD103^{+}$ Bregs produced IL-10 and TGF-β, reduced antigen-specific CD4 T-cell responses, and were controlled by the presence of NLRP6. This work supports the notion that in some environments B cells can play a vital role in maintaining immunity. Furthermore, antigen-specific engineered B cells have the capacity to protect from autoimmune diabetes induced by both insulin-reactive $CD8^{+}$ T cells and antigen-specific $CD4^{+}$ T cells (Chen et al. 2023). These studies suggest that B cells could be manipulated to enhance their regulatory capacity to suppress autoimmunity. Additional research is required to fully elucidate the importance of Bregs in the development of diabetes and whether we can harness their regulatory capacity.

B CELLS IN THE PANCREATIC TISSUE

So far, many of the studies evaluating B lymphocytes in the pancreas have used immunohistochemical techniques on fixed tissue collected postmortem from individuals diagnosed with T1D. However, early studies on pancreatic biopsy specimens from donors with newly diagnosed T1D observed the presence of B cells in inflamed pancreatic islets (Itoh et al. 1993). Pancreatic samples from individuals with a T1D diagnosis are still relatively rare, and samples from donors who have had a recent diagnosis or are at risk of developing diabetes are rarer still (Leete 2023). Therefore, much of the research on B-cell phenotype and function within the pancreatic tissue has relied on T1D mouse models. In the NOD mouse, B-1a cells, which are innate-like B cells that mainly reside in the peritoneal cavity, can be detected as early as 2 weeks of age in the pancreas, and these cells can activate plasmacytoid DCs via dsDNA-specific IgG immune complexes resulting in IFN-α production and the initiation of diabetes (Table 1; Diana et al. 2013). Depletion of B-1a cells in the NOD model can inhibit the diabetogenic T-cell response and protects the mice from the development of disease (Kendall et al. 2004; Ryan et al. 2010; Diana et al. 2013). During the development of diabetes in the NOD model, B-1a cells are replaced with a more follicular B-cell phenotype in the pancreas, which is characterized by the expression of IgD, the up-regulation of CD138 (Ryan et al. 2010; Serreze et al. 2011; Boldison et al. 2019) and an increase in $CD138^{+}$ $CD44^{hi}$ plasmablasts (Table 1; Boldison et al. 2021; Ling et al. 2022). However, in human T1D pancreatic tissue, very few $CD138^{+}$ or $Ki67^{+}$ B cells are observed (Arif et al. 2014), indicating that, so far, in the donors assessed, the presence of blasting or plasmablast-like B cells is rare.

Studies from the VH125 BCR transgenic mouse demonstrate specific recruitment of insulin-reactive B cells to both the PLN and pancreas (Smith et al. 2018a; Boldison et al. 2019). Importantly, these insulin-reactive B cells in the target tissue and draining lymph nodes have increased expression of CD86, a marker of B-cell activation and an important costimulatory molecule necessary for T-cell activation (Henry et al. 2012; Smith et al. 2018a). Studies from mice have now been translated to humans. Recently, it was shown that insulin-reactive B cells are also found in increased frequencies in the PLN of donors with T1D compared to nondiabetic controls (Stensland et al. 2023).

Gene studies in NOD mice, comparing $CD19^+$ B-cell populations in the pancreas and the PLNs, when the pancreas has extensive insulitis, have demonstrated that B cells are transcriptionally different to the PLN, with induction of an innate immune signature characterized by IFN-α-related genes (i.e., *Irf7* and *Tlr7*) alongside proinflammatory cytokine-related genes such as *Il6* and *Il1b* (Table 1; Boldison et al. 2023). In this same study, TLR7 protein expression in $CD20^+$ B cells in the NOD mouse pancreas, was possibly induced by the presence of IFN-α and could play a role in promoting damage through cytokine production (Boldison et al. 2023). Moreover, the deletion of TLR7 in the NOD mouse model suppresses diabetes development (Debreceni et al. 2020; Huang et al. 2021), specifically by altering the functional responses of B cells and inhibiting cytotoxic $CD8^+$ T-cell activation (Huang et al. 2021). It is not yet known if $CD20^+$ B cells in human T1D pancreatic tissue adopt an IFN signature, but it is well-established that IFN-α is expressed by the β cells of individuals with T1D (Foulis et al. 1987) and IFN-associated genes are overexpressed in the islets of new-onset T1D donors (Lundberg et al. 2016). Currently, little phenotyping has been performed on $CD20^+$ B cells found in human T1D pancreatic tissue, and, therefore, it is still unknown whether specific subsets of B cells are recruited to the tissue, how early they are found in the pancreas during the development of T1D or whether they are altered within the inflamed pancreatic environment. However, a new body of evidence is now accumulating indicating that B cells may play a crucial role in approaches to new therapeutic strategies, which will be discussed below.

EVIDENCE FOR B-CELL-TARGETED TREATMENT STRATIFICATION

Several ground-breaking studies have recently proposed that there are distinct immune phenotypes or endotypes in T1D, with age of diagnosis being the major factor. Seminal work by Willcox et al. (2009) identified $CD20^+$ B cells in the pancreas of recent-onset donors, with the most abundant frequencies observed at the later stages of β-cell destruction. These B cells were strongly associated with the presence of $CD8^+$ T cells (Willcox et al. 2009), suggesting B-cell presentation of antigen and B cell–CD8 T-cell cross talk (see Fig. 2). Further immunohistological analysis in this T1D donor cohort (Exeter Archival Diabetes Biobank [EADB]) noted that recent-onset donors, diagnosed at a young age, had significantly larger numbers of $CD20^+$ B cells as part of their insulitic pancreas profile. Donors who were diagnosed at older ages had fewer immune cells, and very few $CD20^+$ B cells were present in the pancreas (Arif et al. 2014). The follow-up in-depth study by Leete et al. (2016) on a larger number of donors from the EADB, DiViD (Diabetes Virus Detection study), and nPOD (Network for Pancreatic Organ Donors with Diabetes) confirmed the earlier observations. In this follow-up study, using the age of diagnosis and the ratio of $CD20^+$ B cells to $CD4^+$ T cells present in inflamed pancreatic islets, it was evident that donors diagnosed with T1D when <7 yr of age had a high $CD20^+$ B cell: $CD4^+$ T-cell ratio, compared to donors diagnosed >13 years of age and above, and this was correlated with fewer insulin-containing islets. Furthermore, a detailed study using imaging mass cytometry reported that one of four recent-onset T1D donors who were diagnosed at a young age displayed a prominent $CD20^+$ B-cell profile in the pancreas (Damond et al. 2019). Recent gene expression studies were performed in a select number of donors from the EADB cohort (diagnosed young with an increased frequency of $CD20^+$ B cells [T1DE1] and diagnosed >7 yr of age and with fewer $CD20^+$ B cells [T1DE2]). These studies demonstrated a number of genes overexpressed in T1DE1 donors associated with lymphocyte regulation, including *IKZF3* (Torabi et al. 2023), which is involved in B-cell differentiation and activation (Schmitt et al. 2002). Other gene expression studies using whole blood RNA sequencing from new-onset T1D donors revealed fast progressors, characterized by a rapid loss of C-peptide, is predicted by the age of diagnosis and associated with a B-cell gene signature (Linsley et al. 2019b).

 Cite this article as *Cold Spring Harb Perspect Med* doi: 10.1101/cshperspect.a041593

B-CELL-TARGETED THERAPEUTIC STRATEGIES

In NOD mice, a number of therapies targeting B cells were shown to protect the mice from developing autoimmune diabetes, both when given before overt disease, or even after diabetes had developed as discussed earlier (Hu et al. 2007; Xiu et al. 2008). In humans, the early studies using a single course of Rituximab (anti-CD20) (Fig. 3A) showed that the treatment clearly depleted B cells for the first 6 months following treatment, but B-cell numbers returned to normal levels by 12–18 months post-therapy. As mentioned above, individuals with T1D who were treated with Rituximab showed reduced requirement for insulin and preserved C-peptide 1 year following treatment, which was not sustained at the 2-year follow-up visit. Hence, like many other therapies given at the time of overt stage 3 T1D, the Rituximab trial showed B-cell depletion after sufficient β-cell mass has been destroyed to require exogenous insulin administration does not have a lasting effect, and therefore, may have been too little, too late (Pescovitz et al. 2009, 2014). One year following treatment, the study showed a reduction of IgM antibodies, which may take longer than 1 year to return to pretreatment levels, with a corresponding reduction in the B-cell response to new antigens during this time. However, IgG responses were maintained. In addition, the ability of B cells to respond to a previously encountered antigen (recall response), as well as new antigens, was restored once the B cells recovered, with naive B cells recovering more rapidly than memory B cells (Pescovitz et al. 2011). Following treatment with Rituximab, the newly generated B cells included just as many autoreactive cells as at the baseline visit (Chamberlain et al. 2016; Linsley

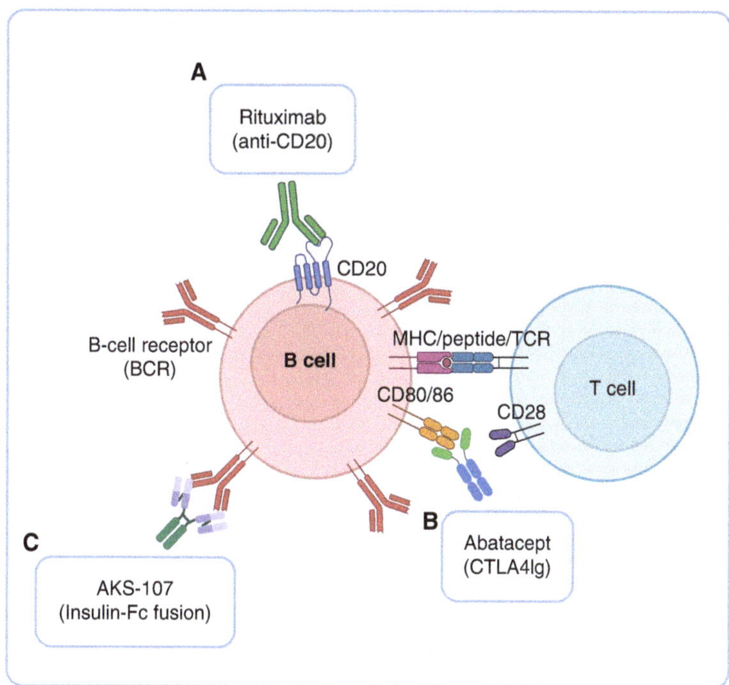

Figure 3. Examples of B-cell-targeted therapies. A variety of B-cell-targeted therapies have been used to delay or treat human type 1 diabetes (T1D) and autoimmune diabetes in the nonobese diabetic (NOD) mouse. These include (*A*) Rituximab, which targets CD20 expressed on B lymphocytes, (*B*) Abatacept, which blocks the interaction of CD80/86 and CD28, preventing stimulation of T cells, and (*C*) antigen-specific therapies, such as AKS-107, which is a fusion protein comprising insulin, and the human IgG1 Fc region, which selectively binds to and depletes insulin-reactive B cells.

et al. 2019a), which implies that there was not a fundamental change in the mechanisms that prevent the generation and/or release of autoreactive B cells from the bone marrow. Therefore, to be effective in the long term, further treatment would be required.

However, as a pan-B-cell depletion therapy, there are elements of immunosuppression that may limit the use of Rituximab, especially if it requires further courses of administration. Since Rituximab is an early generation chimeric anti-B-cell antibody, the likelihood of antichimeric antibodies developing is increased. The possibility of using second-generation humanized anti-B-cell antibodies may, therefore, be a useful strategy. Thus, while targeting B cells using Rituximab had obvious C-peptide preserving effects, there is clearly scope for improving on the current outcomes. For example, initiating treatment early in the course of the disease, such as in stage 1 when autoantibodies are first detected, may be superior. In addition, future studies are needed to help identify which individuals are likely to be a responder versus a nonresponder. For example, it was found that a subgroup of individuals treated with Rituximab had an increase in T-cell proliferative response to antigens, including islet autoantigens, earlier after treatment, suggesting that these individuals may have more potential for further islet β-cell damage, and are less likely to respond favorably to Rituximab treatment (Linsley et al. 2019a). It may also be important to identify and target other cell types that treatment with Rituximab has uncovered. These include T follicular helper cells ($CD4^+CXCR5^+ICOS^+$ T cells) that are increased in individuals with T1D and that were shown to decrease with Rituximab treatment (Xu et al. 2013). It is also worth noting other B-cell-targeted therapies, such as a BAFF blockade, which may be more effective at mediating T1D protection (Wang et al. 2017) and circumvents the possibility that the CD20 molecule is down-regulated on B cells upon entry into the pancreas (Serreze et al. 2011). Similarly, recent studies using CD19-targeting chimeric antigen receptor (CAR) T cells to deplete B cells in various autoimmune conditions, such as SLE, idiopathic inflammatory myositis, and systemic sclerosis, have demonstrated they are safe and effective, and therefore may warrant testing in the treatment or prevention of T1D (Mackensen et al. 2022; Müller et al. 2024).

CTLA4Ig (Abatacept), which blocks costimulatory molecules CD80 and CD86 that are expressed on antigen-presenting cells such as B cells, has been transiently effective when given to individuals at the time of overt clinical presentation (Orban et al. 2011), although not when administered earlier in stage 1 (Fig. 3B; Russell et al. 2023). Further analysis of the effects of Abatacept suggests that individuals who respond less well to treatment had an increase in the number of B cells at baseline, and an increase in gene expression of alternative costimulatory ligands *ICOSLG* (interacting with ICOS) and *CD40* (interacting with CD154), which are both strongly expressed on B cells. These findings suggest that these B cells may preferentially use other ligands when CD80 and CD86 are blocked (Linsley et al. 2019b), making this treatment less effective.

Given the potential for immunosuppression that general depletion of B cells may cause, a recent study in NOD mice showed that targeting insulin-specific B cells may be effective in reducing autoimmune diabetes. Alleva and colleagues used a metabolically inactive recombinant Fc fusion protein, AKS-107, comprising the human insulin A and B chains linked to human IgG1 Fc fragment, which binds to and depletes insulin-specific B cells (Fig. 3C). They demonstrated that treatment in prediabetic VH125Tg.NOD mice, as well as wild-type (WT) NOD mice, reduced the development of diabetes (Alleva et al. 2024). Recent work has further indicated the importance of insulin-specific B cells in human T1D, particularly in young-onset T1D (Stensland et al. 2023). Other antigen-specific B-cell-targeted therapies have been tested in the NOD mouse and have shown promising results (Henry et al. 2012; Leon et al. 2019; Zhang et al. 2019). It would potentially be an interesting type of reagent to trial in humans at risk of T1D, perhaps together with another agent.

Collectively, there is now increasing evidence that B-cell-targeted therapy will be most effective in patients that develop T1D at a young age. Indeed, in pediatric T1D patients, combined therapy of Rituximab and autologous Tregs was superior to Treg monotherapy alone (Zieliński et al. 2022). In addition, in the early Rituximab trial, the participants who were youngest in age tended to respond better than those who were older at onset (Pescovitz et al. 2009). Furthermore, it may also be true of other demographics, aside from age, which are associated with a B-cell-immune phenotype that we have not yet explored. For more effective B-cell-targeted therapies, it will be necessary to understand who would benefit most from a B-cell intervention, and which B-cell intervention strategy is likely to be the most successful. Lastly, combination therapies will likely be needed to provide the most robust targeting of the immune system to prevent ultimate progression to T1D.

REFERENCES

Akashi T, Nagafuchi S, Anzai K, Kondo S, Kitamura D, Wakana S, Ono J, Kikuchi M, Niho Y, Watanabe T. 1997. Direct evidence for the contribution of B cells to the progression of insulitis and the development of diabetes in non-obese diabetic mice. *Int Immunol* **9:** 1159–1164. doi:10.1093/intimm/9.8.1159

Alleva DG, Delpero AR, Sathiyaseelan T, Murikipudi S, Lancaster TM, Atkinson MA, Wasserfall CH, Yu L, Ragupathy R, Bonami RH, et al. 2024. An antigen-specific immunotherapeutic, AKS-107, deletes insulin-specific B cells and prevents murine autoimmune diabetes. *Front Immunol* **15:** 1367514. doi:10.3389/fimmu.2024.1367514

Arif S, Leete P, Nguyen V, Marks K, Nor NM, Estorninho M, Kronenberg-Versteeg D, Bingley PJ, Todd JA, Guy C, et al. 2014. Blood and islet phenotypes indicate immunological heterogeneity in type 1 diabetes. *Diabetes* **63:** 3835–3845. doi:10.2337/db14-0365

Baekkeskov S, Aanstoot HJ, Christgau S, Reetz A, Solimena M, Cascalho M, Folli F, Richter-Olesen H, Camilli PD. 1990. Identification of the 64 K autoantigen in insulin-dependent diabetes as the GABA-synthesizing enzyme glutamic acid decarboxylase. *Nature* **347:** 151–156. doi:10.1038/347151a0

Ben Nasr M, Usuelli V, Seelam AJ, D'Addio F, Abdi R, Markmann JF, Fiorina P. 2021. Regulatory B cells in autoimmune diabetes. *J Immunol* **206:** 1117–1125. doi:10.4049/jimmunol.2001127

Bluestone JA, Herold K, Eisenbarth G. 2010. Genetics, pathogenesis and clinical interventions in type 1 diabetes. *Nature* **464:** 1293–1300. doi:10.1038/nature08933

Boldison J, Wong FS. 2021. Regulatory B cells: role in type 1 diabetes. *Front Immunol* **12:** 746187. doi:10.3389/fimmu.2021.746187

Boldison J, Da Rosa LC, Buckingham L, Davies J, Wen L, Wong FS. 2019. Phenotypically distinct anti-insulin B cells repopulate pancreatic islets after anti-CD20 treatment in NOD mice. *Diabetologia* **62:** 2052–2065. doi:10.1007/s00125-019-04974-y

Boldison J, Da Rosa LC, Davies J, Wen L, Wong FS. 2020. Dendritic cells license regulatory B cells to produce IL-10 and mediate suppression of antigen-specific CD8 T cells. *Cell Mol Immunol* **17:** 843–855. doi:10.1038/s41423-019-0324-z

Boldison J, Thayer TC, Davies J, Wong FS. 2021. Natural protection from type 1 diabetes in NOD mice is characterized by a unique pancreatic islet phenotype. *Diabetes* **70:** 955–965. doi:10.2337/db20-0945

Boldison J, Hopkinson JR, Davies J, Pearson JA, Leete P, Richardson S, Morgan NG, Wong FS. 2023. Gene expression profiling in NOD mice reveals that B cells are highly educated by the pancreatic environment during autoimmune diabetes. *Diabetologia* **66:** 551–566. doi:10.1007/s00125-022-05839-7

Cambier JC, Gauld SB, Merrell KT, Vilen BJ. 2007. B-cell anergy: from transgenic models to naturally occurring anergic B cells? *Nat Rev Immunol* **7:** 633–643. doi:10.1038/nri2133

Cerosaletti K, Buckner JH. 2012. Protein tyrosine phosphatases and type 1 diabetes: genetic and functional implications of PTPN2 and PTPN22. *Rev Diabet Stud* **9:** 188–200. doi:10.1900/RDS.2012.9.188

Chamberlain N, Massad C, Oe T, Cantaert T, Herold KC, Meffre E. 2016. Rituximab does not reset defective early B cell tolerance checkpoints. *J Clin Invest* **126:** 282–287. doi:10.1172/JCI83840

Chen D, Kakabadse D, Fishman S, Weinstein-Marom H, Davies J, Boldison J, Thayer TC, Wen L, Gross G, Wong FS. 2023. Novel engineered B lymphocytes targeting islet-specific T cells inhibit the development of type 1 diabetes in non-obese diabetic Scid mice. *Front Immunol* **14:** 1227133. doi:10.3389/fimmu.2023.1227133

Concannon P, Rich SS, Nepom GT. 2009. Genetics of type 1A diabetes. *N Engl J Med* **360:** 1646–1654. doi:10.1056/NEJMra0808284

Dai X, James RG, Habib T, Singh S, Jackson S, Khim S, Moon RT, Liggitt D, Wolf-Yadlin A, Buckner JH, et al. 2013. A disease-associated PTPN22 variant promotes systemic autoimmunity in murine models. *J Clin Invest* **123:** 2024–2036. doi:10.1172/JCI66963

Damond N, Engler S, Zanotelli VRT, Schapiro D, Wasserfall CH, Kusmartseva I, Nick HS, Thorel F, Herrera PL, Atkinson MA, et al. 2019. A map of human type 1 diabetes progression by imaging mass cytometry. *Cell Metab* **29:** 755–768.e5. doi:10.1016/j.cmet.2018.11.014

Debreceni IL, Chimenti MS, Serreze DV, Geurts AM, Chen YG, Lieberman SM. 2020. Toll-like receptor 7 is required for lacrimal gland autoimmunity and type 1 diabetes development in male nonobese diabetic mice. *Int J Mol Sci* **21:** 9478. doi:10.3390/ijms21249478

Diana J, Simoni Y, Furio L, Beaudoin L, Agerberth B, Barrat F, Lehuen A. 2013. Crosstalk between neutrophils, B-1a cells and plasmacytoid dendritic cells initiates autoimmune diabetes. *Nat Med* **19:** 65–73. doi:10.1038/nm.3042

Du W, Wong FS, Li MO, Peng J, Qi H, Flavell RA, Sherwin R, Wen L. 2006. TGF-β signaling is required for the function of insulin-reactive T regulatory cells. *J Clin Invest* **116:** 1360–1370. doi:10.1172/JCI27030

Duty JA, Szodoray P, Zheng NY, Koelsch KA, Zhang Q, Swiatkowski M, Mathias M, Garman L, Helms C, Nakken B, et al. 2009. Functional anergy in a subpopulation of naive B cells from healthy humans that express autoreactive immunoglobulin receptors. *J Exp Med* **206:** 139–151. doi:10.1084/jem.20080611

Erlich H, Valdes AM, Noble J, Carlson JA, Varney M, Concannon P, Mychaleckyj JC, Todd JA, Bonella P, Fear AL, et al. 2008. HLA DR-DQ haplotypes and genotypes and type 1 diabetes risk: analysis of the type 1 diabetes genetics consortium families. *Diabetes* **57:** 1084–1092. doi:10.2337/db07-1331

Felton JL, Maseda D, Bonami RH, Hulbert C, Thomas JW. 2018. Anti-insulin B cells are poised for antigen presentation in type 1 diabetes. *J Immunol* **201:** 861–873. doi:10.4049/jimmunol.1701717

Fiorina P, Vergani A, Dada S, Jurewicz M, Wong M, Law K, Wu E, Tian Z, Abdi R, Guleria I, et al. 2008. Targeting CD22 reprograms B-cells and reverses autoimmune diabetes. *Diabetes* **57:** 3013–3024. doi:10.2337/db08-0420

Foulis AK, Farquharson MA, Meager A. 1987. Immunoreactive α-interferon in insulin-secreting β cells in type 1 diabetes mellitus. *Lancet* **2:** 1423–1427. doi:10.1016/S0140-6736(87)91128-7

Fruman DA, Chiu H, Hopkins BD, Bagrodia S, Cantley LC, Abraham RT. 2017. The PI3K pathway in human disease. *Cell* **170:** 605–635. doi:10.1016/j.cell.2017.07.029

Gauld SB, Benschop RJ, Merrell KT, Cambier JC. 2005. Maintenance of B cell anergy requires constant antigen receptor occupancy and signaling. *Nat Immunol* **6:** 1160–1167. doi:10.1038/ni1256

Gauld SB, Merrell KT, Cambier JC. 2006. Silencing of autoreactive B cells by anergy: a fresh perspective. *Curr Opin Immunol* **18:** 292–297. doi:10.1016/j.coi.2006.03.015

Getahun A, Beavers NA, Larson SR, Shlomchik MJ, Cambier JC. 2016. Continuous inhibitory signaling by both SHP-1 and SHIP-1 pathways is required to maintain unresponsiveness of anergic B cells. *J Exp Med* **213:** 751–769. doi:10.1084/jem.20150537

Getahun A, Wemlinger SM, Rudra P, Santiago ML, van Dyk LF, Cambier JC. 2017. Impaired B cell function during viral infections due to PTEN-mediated inhibition of the PI3K pathway. *J Exp Med* **214:** 931–941. doi:10.1084/jem.20160972

Greeley SA, Katsumata M, Yu L, Eisenbarth GS, Moore DJ, Goodarzi H, Barker CF, Naji A, Noorchashm H. 2002. Elimination of maternally transmitted autoantibodies prevents diabetes in nonobese diabetic mice. *Nat Med* **8:** 399–402. doi:10.1038/nm0402-399

Habib T, Long SA, Samuels PL, Brahmandam A, Tatum M, Funk A, Hocking AM, Cerosaletti K, Mason MT, Whalen E, et al. 2019. Dynamic immune phenotypes of B and T helper cells mark distinct stages of T1D progression. *Diabetes* **68:** 1240–1250. doi:10.2337/db18-1081

Halverson R, Torres RM, Pelanda R. 2004. Receptor editing is the main mechanism of B cell tolerance toward membrane antigens. *Nat Immunol* **5:** 645–650. doi:10.1038/ni1076

Henry RA, Kendall PL, Thomas JW. 2012. Autoantigen-specific B-cell depletion overcomes failed immune tolerance in type 1 diabetes. *Diabetes* **61:** 2037–2044. doi:10.2337/db11-1746

Hu CY, Rodriguez-Pinto D, Du W, Ahuja A, Henegariu O, Wong FS, Shlomchik MJ, Wen L. 2007. Treatment with CD20-specific antibody prevents and reverses autoimmune diabetes in mice. *J Clin Invest* **117:** 3857–3867. doi:10.1172/JCI32405

Huang J, Peng J, Pearson JA, Efthimiou G, Hu Y, Tai N, Xing Y, Zhang L, Gu J, Jiang J, et al. 2021. Toll-like receptor 7 deficiency suppresses type 1 diabetes development by modulating B-cell differentiation and function. *Cell Mol Immunol* **18:** 328–338. doi:10.1038/s41423-020-00590-8

Hulbert C, Riseili B, Rojas M, Thomas JW. 2001. B cell specificity contributes to the outcome of diabetes in nonobese diabetic mice. *J Immunol* **167:** 5535–5538. doi:10.4049/jimmunol.167.10.5535

Inoue Y, Kaifu T, Sugahara-Tobinai A, Nakamura A, Miyazaki J, Takai T. 2007. Activating Fcγ receptors participate in the development of autoimmune diabetes in NOD mice. *J Immunol* **179:** 764–774. doi:10.4049/jimmunol.179.2.764

Insel RA, Dunne JL, Atkinson MA, Chiang JL, Dabelea D, Gottlieb PA, Greenbaum CJ, Herold KC, Krischer JP, Lernmark Å, et al. 2015. Staging presymptomatic type 1 diabetes: a scientific statement of JDRF, the Endocrine Society, and the American Diabetes Association. *Diabetes Care* **38:** 1964–1974. doi:10.2337/dc15-1419

Itoh N, Hanafusa T, Miyazaki A, Miyagawa J, Yamagata K, Yamamoto K, Waguri M, Imagawa A, Tamura S, Inada M, et al. 1993. Mononuclear cell infiltration and its relation to the expression of major histocompatibility complex antigens and adhesion molecules in pancreas biopsy specimens from newly diagnosed insulin-dependent diabetes mellitus patients. *J Clin Invest* **92:** 2313–2322. doi:10.1172/JCI116835

Jeker LT, Bour-Jordan H, Bluestone JA. 2012. Breakdown in peripheral tolerance in type 1 diabetes in mice and humans. *Cold Spring Harb Perspect Med* **2:** a007807. doi:10.1101/cshperspect.a007807

Kagohashi Y, Udagawa J, Abiru N, Kobayashi M, Moriyama K, Otani H. 2005. Maternal factors in a model of type 1 diabetes differentially affect the development of insulitis and overt diabetes in offspring. *Diabetes* **54:** 2026–2031. doi:10.2337/diabetes.54.7.2026

Kendall PL, Woodward EJ, Hulbert C, Thomas JW. 2004. Peritoneal B cells govern the outcome of diabetes in nonobese diabetic mice. *Eur J Immunol* **34:** 2387–2395. doi:10.1002/eji.200324744

Kendall PL, Case JB, Sullivan AM, Holderness JS, Wells KS, Liu E, Thomas JW. 2013. Tolerant anti-insulin B cells are effective APCs. *J Immunol* **190:** 2519–2526. doi:10.4049/jimmunol.1202104

Kessel A, Haj T, Peri R, Snir A, Melamed D, Sabo E, Toubi E. 2012. Human $CD19^+CD25^{high}$ B regulatory cells suppress proliferation of $CD4^+$ T cells and enhance Foxp3 and CTLA-4 expression in T-regulatory cells. *Autoimmun Rev* **11:** 670–677. doi:10.1016/j.autrev.2011.11.018

Koczwara K, Bonifacio E, Ziegler AG. 2004. Transmission of maternal islet antibodies and risk of autoimmune diabetes in offspring of mothers with type 1 diabetes. *Diabetes* **53:** 1–4. doi:10.2337/diabetes.53.1.1

Leete P. 2023. Type 1 diabetes in the pancreas: a histological perspective. *Diabet Med* **40:** e15228. doi:10.1111/dme.15228

Leete P, Willcox A, Krogvold L, Dahl-Jørgensen K, Foulis AK, Richardson SJ, Morgan NG. 2016. Differential insulitic profiles determine the extent of β-cell destruction and the age at onset of type 1 diabetes. *Diabetes* **65:** 1362–1369. doi:10.2337/db15-1615

Leon MA, Wemlinger SM, Larson NR, Ruffalo JK, Sestak JO, Middaugh CR, Cambier JC, Berkland C. 2019. Soluble antigen arrays for selective desensitization of insulin-reactive B cells. *Mol Pharm* **16:** 1563–1572. doi:10.1021/acs.molpharmaceut.8b01250

Ling Q, Shen L, Zhang W, Qu D, Wang H, Wang B, Liu Y, Lu J, Zhu D, Bi Y. 2022. Increased plasmablasts enhance T cell-mediated beta cell destruction and promote the development of type 1 diabetes. *Mol Med* **28:** 18. doi:10.1186/s10020-022-00447-y

Linsley PS, Greenbaum CJ, Rosasco M, Presnell S, Herold KC, Dufort MJ. 2019a. Elevated T cell levels in peripheral blood predict poor clinical response following rituximab treatment in new-onset type 1 diabetes. *Genes Immun* **20:** 293–307. doi:10.1038/s41435-018-0032-1

Linsley PS, Greenbaum CJ, Speake C, Long SA, Dufort MJ. 2019b. B lymphocyte alterations accompany abatacept resistance in new-onset type 1 diabetes. *JCI Insight* **4:** e126136. doi:10.1172/jci.insight.126136

Lundberg M, Krogvold L, Kuric E, Dahl-Jørgensen K, Skog O. 2016. Expression of interferon-stimulated genes in insulitic pancreatic islets of patients recently diagnosed with type 1 diabetes. *Diabetes* **65:** 3104–3110. doi:10.2337/db16-0616

Mackensen A, Müller F, Mougiakakos D, Böltz S, Wilhelm A, Aigner M, Völkl S, Simon D, Kleyer A, Munoz L, et al. 2022. Anti-CD19 CAR T cell therapy for refractory systemic lupus erythematosus. *Nat Med* **28:** 2124–2132. doi:10.1038/s41591-022-02017-5

Mariño E, Villanueva J, Walters S, Liuwantara D, Mackay F, Grey ST. 2009. $CD4^+CD25^+$ T-cells control autoimmunity in the absence of B-cells. *Diabetes* **58:** 1568–1577. doi:10.2337/db08-1504

Mariño E, Tan B, Binge L, Mackay CR, Grey ST. 2012. B-cell cross-presentation of autologous antigen precipitates diabetes. *Diabetes* **61:** 2893–2905. doi:10.2337/db12-0006

McLaughlin KA, Richardson CC, Ravishankar A, Brigatti C, Liberati D, Lampasona V, Piemonti L, Morgan D, Feltbower RG, Christie MR. 2016. Identification of tetraspanin-7 as a target of autoantibodies in type 1 diabetes. *Diabetes* **65:** 1690–1698. doi:10.2337/db15-1058

Meffre E, Wardemann H. 2008. B-cell tolerance checkpoints in health and autoimmunity. *Curr Opin Immunol* **20:** 632–638. doi:10.1016/j.coi.2008.09.001

Menard L, Saadoun D, Isnardi I, Ng YS, Meyers G, Massad C, Price C, Abraham C, Motaghedi R, Buckner JH, et al. 2011. The PTPN22 allele encoding an R620W variant interferes with the removal of developing autoreactive B cells in humans. *J Clin Invest* **121:** 3635–3644. doi:10.1172/JCI45790

Merrell KT, Benschop RJ, Gauld SB, Aviszus K, Decote-Ricardo D, Wysocki LJ, Cambier JC. 2006. Identification of anergic B cells within a wild-type repertoire. *Immunity* **25:** 953–962. doi:10.1016/j.immuni.2006.10.017

Michalovich D, Nejentsev S. 2018. Activated PI3 kinase δ syndrome: from genetics to therapy. *Front Immunol* **9:** 369. doi:10.3389/fimmu.2018.00369

Mohan JF, Calderon B, Anderson MS, Unanue ER. 2013. Pathogenic $CD4^+$ T cells recognizing an unstable peptide of insulin are directly recruited into islets bypassing local lymph nodes. *J Exp Med* **210:** 2403–2414. doi:10.1084/jem.20130582

Müller F, Taubmann J, Bucci L, Wilhelm A, Bergmann C, Volkl S, Aigner M, Rothe T, Minopoulou I, Tur C, et al. 2024. CD19 CAR T-cell therapy in autoimmune disease—a case series with follow-up. *N Engl J Med* **390:** 687–700. doi:10.1056/NEJMoa2308917

Noorchashm H, Noorchashm N, Kern J, Rostami SY, Barker CF, Naji A. 1997. B-cells are required for the initiation of insulitis and sialitis in nonobese diabetic mice. *Diabetes* **46:** 941–946. doi:10.2337/diab.46.6.941

Noorchashm H, Lieu YK, Noorchashm N, Rostami SY, Greeley SA, Schlachterman A, Song HK, Noto LE, Jevnikar AM, Barker CF, et al. 1999. I-Ag7-mediated antigen presentation by B lymphocytes is critical in overcoming a checkpoint in T cell tolerance to islet β cells of nonobese diabetic mice. *J Immunol* **163:** 743–750. doi:10.4049/jimmunol.163.2.743

O'Neill SK, Getahun A, Gauld SB, Merrell KT, Tamir I, Smith MJ, Dal Porto JM, Li QZ, Cambier JC. 2011. Monophosphorylation of CD79a and CD79b ITAM motifs initiates a SHIP-1 phosphatase-mediated inhibitory signaling cascade required for B cell anergy. *Immunity* **35:** 746–756. doi:10.1016/j.immuni.2011.10.011

Orban T, Bundy B, Becker DJ, DiMeglio LA, Gitelman SE, Goland R, Gottlieb PA, Greenbaum CJ, Marks JB, Monzavi R, et al. 2011. Co-stimulation modulation with abatacept in patients with recent-onset type 1 diabetes: a randomised, double-blind, placebo-controlled trial. *Lancet* **378:** 412–419. doi:10.1016/S0140-6736(11)60886-6

Palmer JP, Asplin CM, Clemons P, Lyen K, Tatpati O, Raghu PK, Paquette TL. 1983. Insulin antibodies in insulin-dependent diabetics before insulin treatment. *Science* **222:** 1337–1339. doi:10.1126/science.6362005

Panigrahi AK, Goodman NG, Eisenberg RA, Rickels MR, Naji A, Luning Prak ET. 2008. RS rearrangement frequency as a marker of receptor editing in lupus and type 1 diabetes. *J Exp Med* **205:** 2985–2994. doi:10.1084/jem.20082053

Payton MA, Hawkes CJ, Christie MR. 1995. Relationship of the 37,000- and 40,000-M(r) tryptic fragments of islet antigens in insulin-dependent diabetes to the protein tyrosine phosphatase-like molecule IA-2 (ICA512). *J Clin Invest* **96:** 1506–1511. doi:10.1172/JCI118188

Pearson JA, Li Y, Majewska-Szczepanik M, Guo J, Zhang L, Liu Y, Wong FS, Wen L. 2020. Insulin-reactive T cells convert diabetogenic insulin-reactive VH125 B cells into tolerogenic cells by reducing germinal center T:B cell interactions in NOD mice. *Front Immunol* **11:** 585886. doi:10.3389/fimmu.2020.585886

Pearson JA, Peng J, Huang J, Yu X, Tai N, Hu Y, Sha S, Flavell RA, Zhao H, Wong FS, et al. 2023. NLRP6 deficiency expands a novel $CD103^+$ B cell population that confers immune tolerance in NOD mice. *Front Immunol* **14:** 1147925. doi:10.3389/fimmu.2023.1147925

Pescovitz MD, Greenbaum CJ, Krause-Steinrauf H, Becker DJ, Gitelman SE, Goland R, Gottlieb PA, Marks JB, McGee PF, Moran AM, et al. 2009. Rituximab, B-lymphocyte depletion, and preservation of β-cell function. *N Engl J Med* **361:** 2143–2152. doi:10.1056/NEJMoa 0904452

Pescovitz MD, Torgerson TR, Ochs HD, Ocheltree E, McGee P, Krause-Steinrauf H, Lachin JM, Canniff J, Greenbaum C, Herold KC, et al. 2011. Effect of rituximab on human in vivo antibody immune responses. *J Allergy Clin Immunol* **128:** 1295–1302.e5. doi:10.1016/j.jaci.2011.08.008

Pescovitz MD, Greenbaum CJ, Bundy B, Becker DJ, Gitelman SE, Goland R, Gottlieb PA, Marks JB, Moran A, Raskin P, et al. 2014. B-lymphocyte depletion with rituximab and β-cell function: two-year results. *Diabetes Care* **37:** 453–459. doi:10.2337/dc13-0626

Petersen JS, Marshall MO, Baekkeskov S, Hejnæs KR, Høier-Madsen M, Dyrberg T. 1993. Transfer of type 1 (insulin-dependent) diabetes mellitus associated autoimmunity to mice with severe combined immunodeficiency (SCID). *Diabetologia* **36:** 510–515. doi:10.1007/BF02743266

Pugliese A, Zeller M, Fernandez A Jr, Zalcberg LJ, Bartlett RJ, Ricordi C, Pietropaolo M, Eisenbarth GS, Bennett ST, Patel DD. 1997. The insulin gene is transcribed in the human thymus and transcription levels correlated with allelic variation at the INS VNTR-IDDM2 susceptibility locus for type 1 diabetes. *Nat Genet* **15:** 293–297. doi:10 .1038/ng0397-293

Redondo MJ, Onengut-Gumuscu S, Gaulton KJ. 2023. Genetics of type 1 diabetes. In *Diabetes in America* (ed. Lawrence JM, Casagrande SS, Herman WH, Wexler DJ, Cefalu WT). National Institute of Diabetes and Digestive and Kidney Diseases, Bethesda, Maryland.

Rieck M, Arechiga A, Onengut-Gumuscu S, Greenbaum C, Concannon P, Buckner JH. 2007. Genetic variation in PTPN22 corresponds to altered function of T and B lymphocytes. *J Immunol* **179:** 4704–4710. doi:10.4049/jimmu nol.179.7.4704

Rosser EC, Mauri C. 2015. Regulatory B cells: origin, phenotype, and function. *Immunity* **42:** 607–612. doi:10 .1016/j.immuni.2015.04.005

Russell WE, Bundy BN, Anderson MS, Cooney LA, Gitelman SE, Goland RS, Gottlieb PA, Greenbaum CJ, Haller MJ, Krischer JP, et al. 2023. Abatacept for delay of type 1 diabetes progression in stage 1 relatives at risk: a randomized, double-masked, controlled trial. *Diabetes Care* **46:** 1005–1013. doi:10.2337/dc22-2200

Ryan GA, Wang CJ, Chamberlain JL, Attridge K, Schmidt EM, Kenefeck R, Clough LE, Dunussi-Joannopoulos K, Toellner KM, Walker LS. 2010. B1 cells promote pancreas infiltration by autoreactive T cells. *J Immunol* **185:** 2800–2807. doi:10.4049/jimmunol.1000856

Schmitt C, Tonnelle C, Dalloul A, Chabannon C, Debré P, Rebollo A. 2002. Aiolos and Ikaros: regulators of lymphocyte development, homeostasis and lymphoproliferation. *Apoptosis* **7:** 277–284. doi:10.1023/A:1015372322419

Serreze DV, Chapman HD, Varnum DS, Hanson MS, Reifsnyder PC, Richard SD, Fleming SA, Leiter EH, Shultz LD. 1996. B lymphocytes are essential for the initiation of T cell-mediated autoimmune diabetes: analysis of a new "speed congenic" stock of NOD.Ig mu null mice. *J Exp Med* **184:** 2049–2053. doi:10.1084/jem.184.5.2049

Serreze DV, Fleming SA, Chapman HD, Richard SD, Leiter EH, Tisch RM. 1998. B lymphocytes are critical antigen-presenting cells for the initiation of T cell-mediated autoimmune diabetes in nonobese diabetic mice. *J Immunol* **161:** 3912–3918. doi:10.4049/jimmunol.161.8.3912

Serreze DV, Chapman HD, Niens M, Dunn R, Kehry MR, Driver JP, Haller M, Wasserfall C, Atkinson MA. 2011. Loss of intra-islet CD20 expression may complicate efficacy of B-cell-directed type 1 diabetes therapies. *Diabetes* **60:** 2914–2921. doi:10.2337/db11-0705

Silva DG, Daley SR, Hogan J, Lee SK, Teh CE, Hu DY, Lam KP, Goodnow CC, Vinuesa CG. 2011. Anti-islet autoantibodies trigger autoimmune diabetes in the presence of an increased frequency of islet-reactive CD4 T cells. *Diabetes* **60:** 2102–2111. doi:10.2337/db10-1344

Silveira PA, Johnson E, Chapman HD, Bui T, Tisch RM, Serreze DV. 2002. The preferential ability of B lymphocytes to act as diabetogenic APC in NOD mice depends on expression of self-antigen-specific immunoglobulin receptors. *Eur J Immunol* **32:** 3657–3666. doi:10 .1002/1521-4141(200212)32:12<3657::AID-IMMU3657> 3.0.CO;2-E

Simoncic PD, Lee-Loy A, Barber DL, Tremblay ML, McGlade CJ. 2002. The T cell protein tyrosine phosphatase is a negative regulator of Janus family kinases 1 and 3. *Curr Biol* **12:** 446–453. doi:10.1016/S0960-9822(02)00 697-8

Smith MJ, Packard TA, O'Neill SK, Henry Dunand CJ, Huang M, Fitzgerald-Miller L, Stowell D, Hinman RM, Wilson PC, Gottlieb PA, et al. 2015. Loss of anergic B cells in prediabetic and new-onset type 1 diabetic patients. *Diabetes* **64:** 1703–1712. doi:10.2337/db13-1798

Smith MJ, Hinman RM, Getahun A, Kim S, Packard TA, Cambier JC. 2018a. Silencing of high-affinity insulin-reactive B lymphocytes by anergy and impact of the NOD genetic background in mice. *Diabetologia* **61:** 2621–2632. doi:10.1007/s00125-018-4730-z

Smith MJ, Rihanek M, Wasserfall C, Mathews CE, Atkinson MA, Gottlieb PA, Cambier JC. 2018b. Loss of B-cell anergy in type 1 diabetes is associated with high-risk HLA and non-HLA disease susceptibility alleles. *Diabetes* **67:** 697–703. doi:10.2337/db17-0937

Smith MJ, Ford BR, Rihanek M, Coleman BM, Getahun A, Sarapura VD, Gottlieb PA, Cambier JC. 2019. Elevated PTEN expression maintains anergy in human B cells and reveals unexpectedly high repertoire autoreactivity. *JCI Insight* **4:** e123384. doi:10.1172/jci.insight.123384

Steck AK, Johnson K, Barriga KJ, Miao D, Yu L, Hutton JC, Eisenbarth GS, Rewers MJ. 2011. Age of islet autoantibody appearance and mean levels of insulin, but not GAD or IA-2 autoantibodies, predict age of diagnosis of type 1 diabetes: diabetes autoimmunity study in the young. *Diabetes Care* **34:** 1397–1399. doi:10.2337/dc10-2088

Steck AK, Dong F, Wong R, Fouts A, Liu E, Romanos J, Wijmenga C, Norris JM, Rewers MJ. 2014. Improving prediction of type 1 diabetes by testing non-HLA genetic variants in addition to HLA markers. *Pediatr Diabetes* **15:** 355–362. doi:10.1111/pedi.12092

Steck AK, Fouts A, Miao D, Zhao Z, Dong F, Sosenko J, Gottlieb P, Rewers MJ, Yu L. 2016. ECL-IAA and ECL-GADA can identify high-risk single autoantibody-positive relatives in the TrialNet Pathway to Prevention Study.

Diabetes Technol Ther **18:** 410–414. doi:10.1089/dia.2015.0316

Stensland ZC, Magera CA, Broncucia H, Gomez BD, Rios-Guzman NM, Wells KL, Nicholas CA, Rihanek M, Hunter MJ, Toole KP, et al. 2023. Identification of an anergic BND cell-derived activated B cell population (BND2) in young-onset type 1 diabetes patients. *J Exp Med* **220:** e20221604. doi:10.1084/jem.20221604

Tompa A, Faresjö M. 2024. Shift in the B cell subsets between children with type 1 diabetes and/or celiac disease. *Clin Exp Immunol* **216:** 36–44. doi:10.1093/cei/uxad136

Torabi F, Vadakekolathu J, Wyatt R, Leete P, Tombs MA, Richardson CC, Boocock DJ, Turner MD, Morgan NG, Richardson SJ, et al. 2023. Differential expression of genes controlling lymphocyte differentiation and migration in two distinct endotypes of type 1 diabetes. *Diabet Med* **40:** e15155. doi:10.1111/dme.15155

Wan X, Thomas JW, Unanue ER. 2016. Class-switched anti-insulin antibodies originate from unconventional antigen presentation in multiple lymphoid sites. *J Exp Med* **213:** 967–978. doi:10.1084/jem.20151869

Wang Q, Racine JJ, Ratiu JJ, Wang S, Ettinger R, Wasserfall C, Atkinson MA, Serreze DV. 2017. Transient BAFF blockade inhibits type 1 diabetes development in nonobese diabetic mice by enriching immunoregulatory B lymphocytes sensitive to deletion by anti-CD20 cotherapy. *J Immunol* **199:** 3757–3770. doi:10.4049/jimmunol.1700822

Wardemann H, Yurasov S, Schaefer A, Young JW, Meffre E, Nussenzweig MC. 2003. Predominant autoantibody production by early human B cell precursors. *Science* **301:** 1374–1377. doi:10.1126/science.1086907

Warram JH, Krolewski AS, Gottlieb MS, Kahn CR. 1984. Differences in risk of insulin-dependent diabetes in offspring of diabetic mothers and diabetic fathers. *N Engl J Med* **311:** 149–152. doi:10.1056/NEJM198407193110304

Washburn LR, Dang H, Tian J, Kaufman DL. 2007. The postnatal maternal environment influences diabetes development in nonobese diabetic mice. *J Autoimmun* **28:** 19–23. doi:10.1016/j.jaut.2006.11.006

Wenzlau JM, Juhl K, Yu L, Moua O, Sarkar SA, Gottlieb P, Rewers M, Eisenbarth GS, Jensen J, Davidson HW, et al. 2007. The cation efflux transporter ZnT8 (Slc30A8) is a major autoantigen in human type 1 diabetes. *Proc Natl Acad Sci* **104:** 17040–17045. doi:10.1073/pnas.0705894104

Wiede F, Shields BJ, Chew SH, Kyparissoudis K, van Vliet C, Galic S, Tremblay ML, Russell SM, Godfrey DI, Tiganis T. 2011. T cell protein tyrosine phosphatase attenuates T cell signaling to maintain tolerance in mice. *J Clin Invest* **121:** 4758–4774. doi:10.1172/JCI59492

Wiede F, Sacirbegovic F, Leong YA, Yu D, Tiganis T. 2017. PTPN2-deficiency exacerbates T follicular helper cell and B cell responses and promotes the development of autoimmunity. *J Autoimmun* **76:** 85–100. doi:10.1016/j.jaut.2016.09.004

Willcox A, Richardson SJ, Bone AJ, Foulis AK, Morgan NG. 2009. Analysis of islet inflammation in human type 1 diabetes. *Clin Exp Immunol* **155:** 173–181. doi:10.1111/j.1365-2249.2008.03860.x

Wong FS, Visintin I, Wen L, Granata J, Flavell R, Janeway CA. 1998. The role of lymphocyte subsets in accelerated diabetes in nonobese diabetic-rat insulin promoter-B7-1 (NOD-RIP-B7-1) mice. *J Exp Med* **187:** 1985–1993. doi:10.1084/jem.187.12.1985

Wong FS, Wen L, Tang M, Ramanathan M, Visintin I, Daugherty J, Hannum LG, Janeway CA, Shlomchik MJ. 2004. Investigation of the role of B-cells in type 1 diabetes in the NOD mouse. *Diabetes* **53:** 2581–2587. doi:10.2337/diabetes.53.10.2581

Xiu Y, Wong CP, Bouaziz JD, Hamaguchi Y, Wang Y, Pop SM, Tisch RM, Tedder TF. 2008. B lymphocyte depletion by CD20 monoclonal antibody prevents diabetes in nonobese diabetic mice despite isotype-specific differences in FcγR effector functions. *J Immunol* **180:** 2863–2875. doi:10.4049/jimmunol.180.5.2863

Xu X, Shi Y, Cai Y, Zhang Q, Yang F, Chen H, Gu Y, Zhang M, Yu L, Yang T. 2013. Inhibition of increased circulating Tfh cell by anti-CD20 monoclonal antibody in patients with type 1 diabetes. *PLoS ONE* **8:** e79858. doi:10.1371/journal.pone.0079858

Zekavat G, Rostami SY, Badkerhanian A, Parsons RF, Koeberlein B, Yu M, Ward CD, Migone TS, Yu L, Eisenbarth GS, et al. 2008. In vivo BLyS/BAFF neutralization ameliorates islet-directed autoimmunity in nonobese diabetic mice. *J Immunol* **181:** 8133–8144. doi:10.4049/jimmunol.181.11.8133

Zhang L, Sosinowski T, Cox AR, Cepeda JR, Sekhar NS, Hartig SM, Miao D, Yu L, Pietropaolo M, Davidson HW. 2019. Chimeric antigen receptor (CAR) T cells targeting a pathogenic MHC class II:peptide complex modulate the progression of autoimmune diabetes. *J Autoimmun* **96:** 50–58. doi:10.1016/j.jaut.2018.08.004

Zhang J, Fu Q, He Y, Lv H, Qian Y, Zhang Y, Chen H, Xu X, Yang T, Xu K. 2022. Differences of circulating $CD25^{hi}$ Bregs and their correlations with CD4 effector and regulatory T cells in autoantibody-positive T1D compared with age-matched healthy individuals. *J Immunol Res* **2022:** 2269237. doi:10.1155/2022/2269237

Ziegler AG, Rewers M, Simell O, Simell T, Lempainen J, Steck A, Winkler C, Ilonen J, Veijola R, Knip M, et al. 2013. Seroconversion to multiple islet autoantibodies and risk of progression to diabetes in children. *J Am Med Assoc* **309:** 2473–2479. doi:10.1001/jama.2013.6285

Zieliński M, Żalińska M, Iwaszkiewicz-Grześ D, Gliwiński M, Hennig M, Jaźwińska-Curyłło A, Kamińska H, Sakowska J, Wołoszyn-Durkiewicz A, Owczuk R, et al. 2022. Combined therapy with $CD4^+$ $CD25highCD127^-$ T regulatory cells and anti-CD20 antibody in recent-onset type 1 diabetes is superior to monotherapy: randomized phase I/II trial. *Diabetes Obes Metab* **24:** 1534–1543. doi:10.1111/dom.14723

Innate Immunity in Type 1 Diabetes

Léo Bertrand,[1,2] Alexander V. Chervonsky,[3] and Agnès Lehuen[1,2]

[1]Université Paris Cité, Institut Cochin, INSERM, CNRS, 75014 Paris, France

[2]Laboratoire d'Excellence Inflamex, Université Paris Cité, 75014 Paris, France

[3]Department of Pathology, Committee on Immunology, Committee on Microbiology, The University of Chicago, Chicago, Illinois 60637, USA

Correspondence: agnes.lehuen@inserm.fr

Type 1 diabetes (T1D) results from the destruction of pancreatic β cells by the immune system, to which both pancreatic β-cell dysfunction and pathological activation of the immune system contribute. This paper is focused on understanding the modalities of this activation, and the genetic and environmental factors increasing its risk. Innate immunity has a critical role in the loss of self-tolerance and promotion of inflammation either directly using innate effector mechanisms or by providing activation signals to anti-islet adaptive autoimmunity. We provide an overview of various deleterious and protective roles of innate immunity in T1D inside pancreatic islets, regional lymph nodes, and distant locations such as the gut.

Type 1 diabetes (T1D) is an autoimmune disease characterized by the selective destruction of pancreatic β cells by the immune system. The resulting hyperglycemia requires patients to follow a lifelong insulin replacement therapy, and despite treatment patients remain vulnerable to multiple disease complications. Studies in human patients and animal models of the disease have demonstrated that, while β-cell destruction requires the cytotoxic activity of adaptive T cells, innate immune cells are involved during all stages of pathogenesis. Whereas these cells are very diverse in shape and functions, they all share common properties, including a spontaneous reactivity to signals of microbial invasion and tissue damage, a rapid response to such stimuli, and the ability to support adaptive immune responses by priming and release of appropriate cytokines. Therefore, understanding why and how innate immunity is involved in T1D pathogenesis is essential to comprehend its onset, particularly with regard to known genetic and environmental risk factors of T1D. In this article, we describe the direct immune effector functions of innate immunity in the pancreatic islets during T1D, before describing how innate cells are critical in modulating the autoimmune and tolerogenic adaptive immune responses against β cells. Finally, we discuss how innate immune reactions at locations distant from the pancreas, such as the gut, may contribute to disease progression.

INNATE CELLS AS DIRECT IMMUNE EFFECTORS IN PANCREAS

Early Recruitment of Innate Effectors to Islets

Most knowledge on pancreatic islet infiltration by innate immune cells comes from studies in

Cite this article as *Cold Spring Harb Perspect Med* doi: 10.1101/cshperspect.a041595

the Bio-Breeding (BB) rat and nonobese diabetic (NOD) mouse T1D models. Macrophages and conventional dendritic cells (cDCs) are the first innate cells to infiltrate pancreatic islets early during the prediabetic stages (Lee et al. 1988; Walker et al. 1988; Voorbij et al. 1989; Reddy et al. 1993; Jansen et al. 1994). Plasmacytoid DCs (pDCs) and neutrophils are also present in NOD mice islets (Diana et al. 2013; Diana and Lehuen 2014). Regarding innate lymphoid cells (ILCs), natural killer (NK) cells infiltrate the islets of NOD mice (Flodström et al. 2002; Poirot et al. 2004; Alba et al. 2008; Brauner et al. 2010); but infiltration by non-NK ILC1s, ILC2s, or ILC3s has not yet been reported. Infiltration of innate cells starts early during the weaning period and can occur in NOD.SCID mice lacking B and T cells (Dahlén et al. 1998). Moreover, such early infiltration initiates further pancreatic inflammation by adaptive immune cells with rearranged antigen receptors. Among those, there are some with limited antigen receptor diversity, innate-like cells such as invariant natural killer T (iNKT), γδT, mucosal-associated invariant T (MAIT), and B-1a cells (Simoni et al. 2011; Diana et al. 2013; Markle et al. 2013b; Rouxel et al. 2017).

Comparatively, reported human islet infiltration by innate immune cells seems to be moderate (Willcox et al. 2009). Analyses on pancreatic tissues confirmed the sparse presence of $CD68^+$ macrophages and DCs at various stages of insulitis (Uno et al. 2007; Willcox et al. 2009). Interestingly, macrophages were the most frequent immune cell type in insulin-deficient islets (Willcox et al. 2009). NK cells were also significantly detected in human islets of recent-onset T1D patients, although that was found alongside Coxsackievirus infection (Dotta et al. 2007). Neutrophils were also detected in pancreatic islets in both at-risk and recent-onset T1D patients (Vecchio et al. 2018). Concerning innate-like T cells, the presence of $CD4^-$ $CD8^-$ γδT cells has been reported in human islets (Santamaria et al. 1994). While one study reported an absence of MAIT cells in human pancreatic islets, they were detected in exocrine tissue (Kuric et al. 2018). Of note, this analysis was performed in adult patients where the reduced blood frequency and increased activation and cytotoxicity of MAIT cells are much more moderate compared to children (Rouxel et al. 2017; Nel et al. 2021). The determination of precise infiltration kinetics in humans remains a challenge, as most human pancreatic samples were collected several years after T1D onset, therefore, long after the first innate immune infiltration (Willcox et al. 2009; Campbell-Thompson et al. 2012). Thus, it is possible that transient and rare infiltrating innate immune cell subsets are long gone from human islets at these later stages, which overall feature a lesser degree of immune infiltration.

Infiltrating innate immune cells in the pancreas are recruited from the blood, and β cells can themselves promote the first waves of recruitment through the secretion of chemokines (Fig. 1). Most islet-infiltrating macrophages are former migrating blood monocytes, recruited notably by early β-cell-produced CCL2 and CXCL10 (Chen et al. 2001; Cardozo et al. 2003; Martin et al. 2008). This migration is critical in T1D pathogenesis as blocking it with an anti-CD11b/CD18 antibody is sufficient to protect NOD mice against disease onset (Hutchings et al. 1990). Interestingly, some inflammatory macrophages are likely originated from resident macrophages that underwent a proinflammatory polarization due to the islet micro-environment during disease progression (Arnush et al. 1998; Zakharov et al. 2020). These macrophages are likely to have a critical negative role, as their depletion significantly impairs disease progression (Carrero et al. 2017). Infiltrating blood monocytes form the bulk of most infiltrating cDCs/monocyte-derived (mo)-DCs, recruited through increased CCL5/CCL8 and CCL19/21 expression in pancreatic islets (Bouma et al. 2005; Klementowicz et al. 2017).

Initiation and Amplification of Pancreatic Inflammation

How exactly innate immune cells are activated in T1D remains incompletely understood. Due to the polygenic nature of the disease, one cannot exclude a contribution from the patient's genetics that manifests in the absence of exogenous stimuli. At the same time, both human and mouse β cells express pattern-recognition receptors (PRRs), including Toll-like receptor (TLR)2, TLR3, TLR4, and TLR9 (Wen et al. 2004). These receptors can recognize exogenous pathogen-associated molecular patterns (PAMPs), as well as damage-associated molecular patterns (DAMPs).

The importance of exogenous PAMPs has been demonstrated when NOD mice lacking the shared TLR adaptor MyD88 and housed under specific-pathogen-free (SPF) conditions were found to be protected against diabetes development (Wen et al. 2008). Similarly, deletions of individual PRRs led to clear effects in SPF conditions: *Tlr2*$^{-/-}$ NOD mice were partially protected against T1D (Kim et al. 2007, 2011; Burrows et al. 2015), whereas *Tlr4*$^{-/-}$ mice had accelerated T1D under the same housing conditions (Burrows et al. 2015). These effects of MyD88, TLR2, and TLR4 deficiency were lost under germ-free (GF) conditions, supporting the role of microbiota and TLR interactions (Wen et al. 2008; Chervonsky 2013; Burrows et al. 2015).

Innate response triggers are not necessarily of bacterial origin. The presence of viruses capable of infecting β cells, particularly enteroviruses, has been linked to T1D (Yoon et al. 1979; Dotta et al. 2007). Viral dsRNA detection through TLR and RIG-I-like (RLR) pathways can induce apoptosis and strong production of chemokines, IL-15, and type I interferons (IFNs) in β cells (Fig. 1; Liu et al. 2002; Dogusan et al. 2008; Colli et al. 2010). The studies on pancreatic samples reported between half and all human T1D pancreatic samples had evidence of Coxsackievirus B infection, compared to <20% for controls (Dotta et al. 2007; Krogvold et al. 2015). An even greater amplification of innate responses by viral presence in the pancreas might be the mechanism behind the fulminant T1D onset. Indeed, pancreata of such patients are characterized by massive macrophage infiltration, high TLR and RLR expression, and the presence of enterovirus RNA (Shibasaki et al. 2010; Aida et al. 2011).

Successful development of T1D in GF NOD mice and BB rats (Patrick et al. 2013; Burrows et al. 2015), suggested that innate immunity could be triggered by endogenous signals. It was hypothesized that an early wave of β-cell physiological apoptosis can precipitate an uncontrolled release of DAMPs in the islet environment (Turley et al. 2003; Diana et al. 2013). This early wave is present in humans (Kassem et al. 2000), and might contribute to late-onset T1D in adults, since blocking caspase activity in NOD mice at 1 week of age led to a long-term prevention of T1D onset in adult animals (Diana et al. 2013). Apoptosis of β cells might also be initiated due to endogenous dysfunction of β cells, which are very sensitive to endoplasmic reticulum (ER) stress (Meyerovich et al. 2016). Cytokines increase ER stress (Cardozo et al. 2005). Mechanisms of compensation of such stress, namely, the unfolded protein response, might be as detrimental for T1D onset as the ER stress itself (Lee et al. 2023). DAMPs can be carriers of endogenous DNA and can be recognized by pDCs through TLR9, triggering their activation (Diana et al. 2013). In fact, *Tlr9*$^{-/-}$ NOD mice have delayed diabetes onset, lower pDC frequency, and IFN-α levels in pancreatic lymph nodes (pLNs) (Wong et al. 2008; Zhang et al. 2010). Other PRR pathways sensing nucleic acids, such as TLR7, might be involved as well (Lee et al. 2011).

Conjunction of both β-cell endogenous damage signals and direct foreign material detection by innate immune cells may trigger their strong activation. Increased presence of bacterial DNA in pLNs in diabetic NOD mice suggested a potential similar bacterial trigger of β cells and innate immune cells in islets (Rouxel et al. 2017). Therefore, whereas β cells are likely to be the main driver of early innate immune cell recruitment and activation in pancreatic islets (Roep et al. 2021), this process may be further amplified by microbial signals in case of infection.

There are also several considerations that need to be recognized when interpreting the results of genetic manipulations. Most of the studies trying to identify individual PRRs associated with T1D were performed in complete gene knocked-out mice, which does not allow to single out the gene's role specifically in innate cells or β cells in the islets. Moreover, most of such knockouts were done in a pre-CRISPR-Cas9 era leaving a possibility that the carryover genes

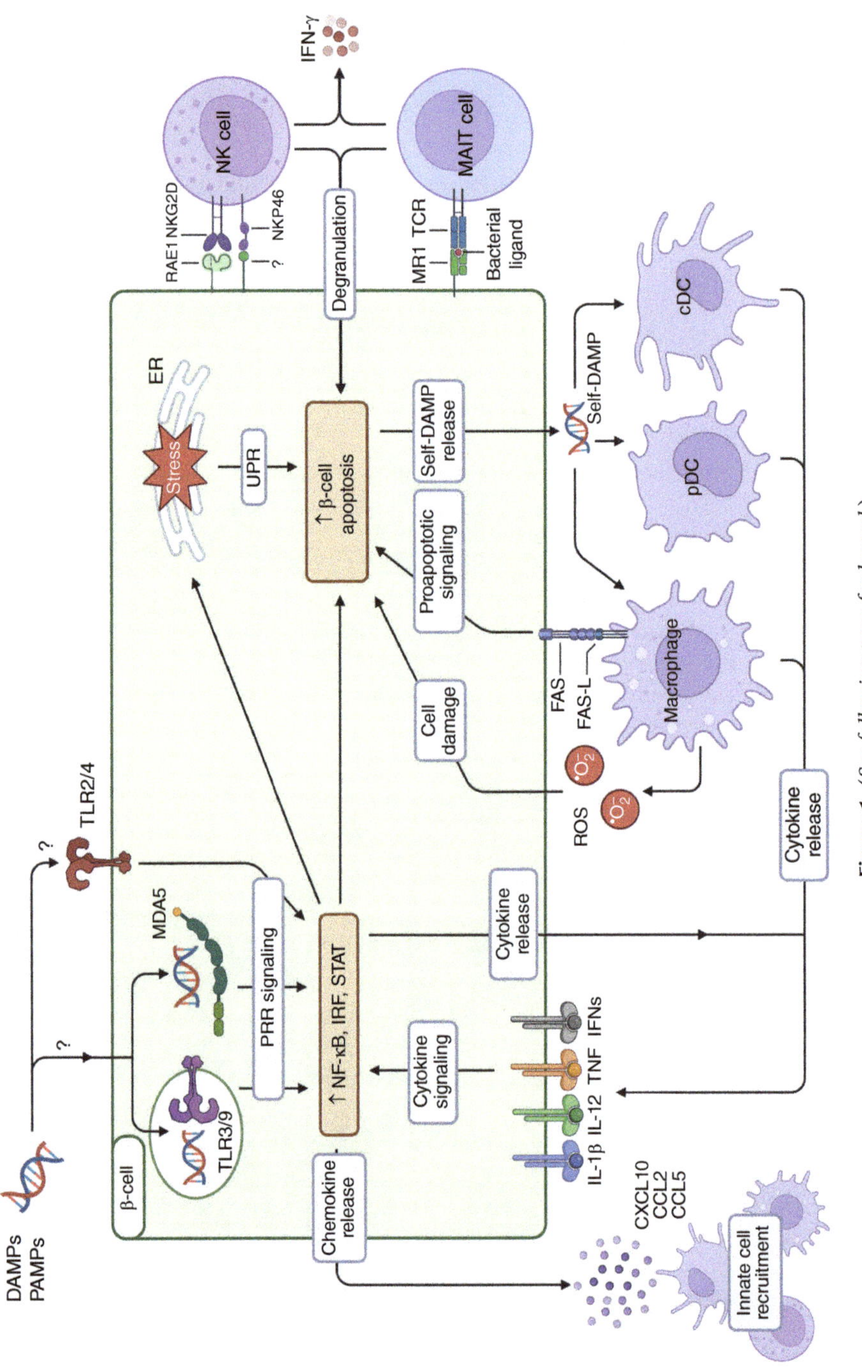

Figure 1. *(See following page for legend.)*

from other backgrounds contributed to the phenotype. Additionally, extrapolation of the rodent findings to humans should be done at the pathway level and not only on orthologous genes.

Innate Effector Mechanisms Contributing to the Inflammatory Response in the Islets

Once activated, innate immune cells locally proliferate and produce large amounts of proinflammatory cytokines, dramatically amplifying insulitis (Figs. 1 and 2). Macrophages and cDCs produce proinflammatory cytokines including TNF, IL-1β, and IL-6 (Arnush et al. 1998; Dahlén et al. 1998; Wachlin et al. 2003; Uno et al. 2007). An increase of macrophage-associated cytokine levels can even be detected in peripheral blood before disease onset (Hussain et al. 1996). Infiltrating pDCs produce large amounts of IFN-α that increase β-cell stress and support cDC maturation, a key step in initiating disease (Li et al. 2008; Li and McDevitt 2011; Diana et al. 2013). Macrophages, as well as DCs themselves also support their own maturation through IL-12 production. Moreover, even before any T-cell insulitis, Th1/17 cytokines traditionally associated with adaptive lymphocytes are already produced by innate-like cells. Secretion of IFN-γ by NK and MAIT cells was directly observed in islets of NOD mice (Feuerer et al. 2009; Brauner et al. 2010; Rouxel et al. 2017), and might also be performed by intraislets $CD27^+$ $CD44^{lo}$ γδT cells as those cells infiltrate islets and are skewed toward IFN-γ production (Markle et al. 2013b). Intraislet $CD4^-$ $CD8^-$ iNKT17 cells spontaneously produce IL-17 that can promote T1D (Simoni et al. 2011). A similar secretion of IL-17 by $CD27^-$ $CD44^{hi}$ γδT cells has been suggested based on their ability to produce IL-17 and their preferential accumulation but was not observed directly (Markle et al. 2013b). Early production of Th1 and Th17 cytokines by these cells, although limited compared to later adaptive lymphocyte production, is nonetheless likely critical in amplifying and sustaining local innate autoimmunity.

While most chemokines are produced by β cells themselves, inflammatory macrophages directly secrete CXCL1/CXCL2 that attract neutrophils (Diana and Lehuen 2014). Infiltrated neutrophils in both NOD mice and humans secrete components of neutrophil extracellular traps, particularly neutrophil elastase that further increases macrophage recruitment into islets (Diana et al. 2013; Shu et al. 2020). Murine neutrophils also release cathelicidin-related antimicrobial peptide (CRAMP) able to bind self-DNA released by dying β cells (Diana et al. 2013). Same self-DNA is also targeted by IgGs secreted by B-1a cells infiltrating the pancreas of NOD mice, and in conjunction with CRAMP is critical in initiating disease progression, as these IgGs

Figure 1. Onset of pancreatic inflammation is mediated by both pancreatic β cells and innate immune cells. Pancreatic β cells express several pattern recognition receptors (PRRs), including Toll-like receptors (TLRs) and RIG-I-like receptors (RLRs). A recognition by these PRRs (TLR2, 3, 4, 9, MDA5) of endogenous and exogenous pathogen-associated and damage-associated molecular patterns (PAMPs and DAMPs) can trigger activation of key transcriptional factors (NF-κB, IRF, STAT). Expression of these transcription factors increases ER stress and proapoptotic signaling. Most importantly, it promotes the release of multiple cytokines and chemokines by β cells, which recruit and activate innate immune cells into the islets. Infiltrating immune cells produce additional cytokines including type I interferons (IFNs), interleukin (IL)-1β, IL-12, tumor necrosis factor (TNF), and IFN-γ that increase local inflammation and β-cell stress. Ultimately, macrophages, natural killer (NK) and mucosal-associated invariant T (MAIT) cells can directly destroy pancreatic β cells, either through reactive oxygen species (ROS) production, FAS (CD95) signaling, or granzyme–perforin degranulation. Death of β cells in such an inflammatory environment leads to further release of immune-stimulating self-DAMPs, that maintain and amplify the cascade described, in both neighboring β cells and innate immune cells. (cDC) Conventional dendritic cell, (ER) endoplasmic reticulum, (CCL) CC-chemokine ligand, (CXCL) CXC-chemokine ligand, (IRF) interferon response factor, (MR1) major histocompatibility complex, class I-related protein, (NKG2D) natural killer group 2, member D, (NKp46) natural killer p46, (pDC) plasmacytoid dendritic cell, (RAE1) retinoic acid early transcript 1, (TCR) T-cell receptor, (UPR) unfolded protein response.

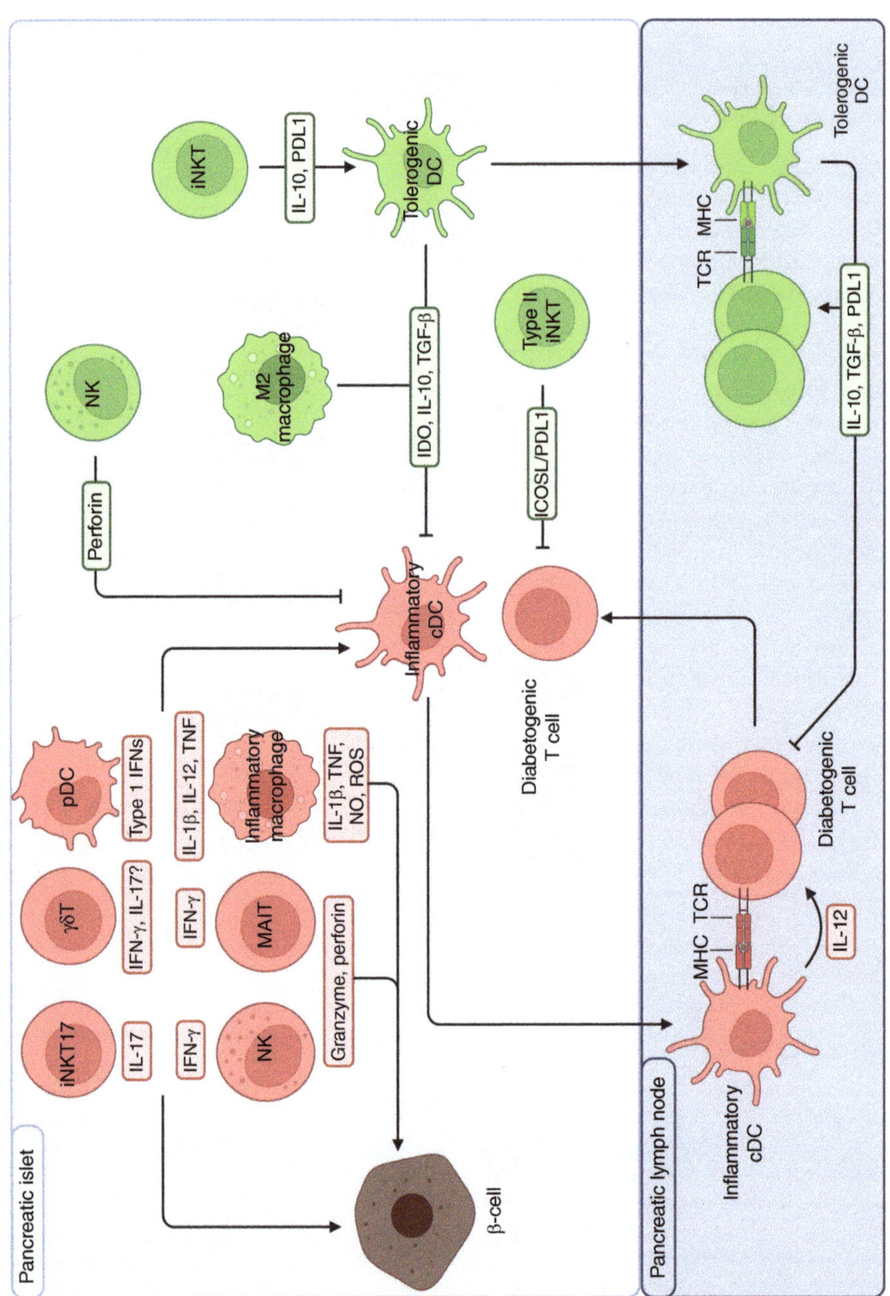

Figure 2. *(See following page for legend.)*

Cite this article as *Cold Spring Harb Perspect Med* doi: 10.1101/cshperspect.a041595

can be bound by Fc receptors on neutrophils, triggering their activation (Diana et al. 2013). It is currently not known whether the human equivalent of CRAMP, LL-37, plays a similar role. Of note, cDC and NK cell activation might be also initiated through Fc recognition (Inoue et al. 2007).

Innate immune cells can also directly induce β-cell death, first by indirect damage through cellular stress (Fig. 1). TNF, IL-1β, IL-6, and IFN-γ significantly decrease β-cell function and insulin release, increase intracellular DNA damage and surface expression of the death receptor FAS (Chervonsky et al. 1997; Stassi et al. 1997; Savinov et al. 2003a; Wachlin et al. 2003). TNF can induce cell death through the TNFR1 pathway (Kägi et al. 1999), most likely through arming resident macrophages (Varanasi et al. 2012). Infiltrated macrophages also synthesize radical oxygen species and stimulate nitric oxide production that further damage β cells (Kaneto et al. 1995; Suarez-Pinzon et al. 1997). Innate immune cells can also directly exercise cytotoxicity. Macrophages reportedly express FAS-L molecules in pancreatic islets (Moriwaki et al. 1999). In NOD mice, islet destruction increased with the presence of infiltrating granzyme B-positive MAIT cells. Additionally, they are able to kill human β cells in vitro (Rouxel et al. 2017). Similarly, the presence of infiltrating NK cells, which are known for their cytotoxic activity, correlates with islet lesion severity (Poirot et al. 2004). They express high levels of CD107a, indicating degranulation, and can kill after NKP46 engagement (Brauner et al. 2010; Gur et al. 2010, 2011). NKP46 blockade reduced NK cell cytotoxicity and successfully delayed T1D onset in NOD mice (Gur et al. 2010). However, several reports have also highlighted defects in cytotoxic capacity and general hyporesponsiveness of NK cells in NOD mice (Brauner et al. 2010). Increased PD1 expression suggests NK cells might display functional exhaustion, in line with extensive activation and cytotoxicity in islets. While direct innate immune cell cytotoxicity is minor in total β-cell destruction, this early killing by innate cells may significantly increase self-antigen release and the likelihood to transition to a deleterious autoreactive adaptive immune response.

Genetic Dysfunctions of Innate Immune Cells in T1D

Some features of innate immunity in organisms susceptible to T1D could be attributed to genetic variations, whereas the others suggest a genetic component. The first group is identified by large-scale genetic studies. Several polymorphisms were found in innate immune genes potentially associated with T1D. Susceptible and protective variants were found for the RLR receptor *MDA5* (Smyth et al. 2006; Nejentsev et al. 2009), whereas activating *KIR* receptor polymorphisms were positively associated with T1D cases (Soltani et al. 2020). *TLR2* and *TLR3* alleles were also associated with T1D (Bjørnvold et al. 2009; Assmann et al. 2014).

Figure 2. Deleterious and protective innate immune cell cross talk in the pancreas in type 1 diabetes. Multiple innate immune cells, including invariant natural killer T 17 (iNKT17) cells, γδT, natural killer (NK), mucosal-associated invariant T (MAIT) cells, plasmacytoid DCs (pDCs), and macrophages exert direct pathological functions on β cells through the establishment of a proinflammatory environment in the islets and direct β-cell killing. Importantly, it promotes the uptake of pancreatic self-antigens by conventional DCs (cDCs), their activation, and their migration into the pancreatic lymph nodes (pLNs) where they subsequently initiate the adaptive immune response against β cells. However, innate immune cells, such as iNKT, NK, and regulatory macrophages can also limit autoimmunity, by suppressing or killing diabetogenic cDCs, by inducing the recruitment of tolerogenic DCs and regulatory T cells (Tregs), or by inactivating autoimmune T cells through programmed death ligand 1 (PDL1) or inducible T-cell costimulator ligand (ICOSL) presentation. Balance between these deleterious and protective features of innate cells is critical in β-cell survival or destruction. (IFN) Interferon, (IL) interleukin, (MHC) major histocompatibility complex, (NO) nitric oxide, (ROS) reactive oxygen species, (TCR) T-cell receptor, (TGF) transforming growth factor, (TNF) tumor necrosis factor, (Treg) regulatory T cell.

The second group (suggested genetic component) is larger, but not yet linked to particular genes. Strong and various anomalies of frequency and phenotype of blood innate immune cells are observed in relatives and autoantibody-positive patients (Hussain et al. 1987; Lang et al. 1991; Takahashi et al. 1998; Krętowski et al. 1999; Peng et al. 2003; Valle et al. 2013; Kayserova et al. 2014; Xia et al. 2014; Beristain-Covarrubias et al. 2015; Rouxel et al. 2017; Vecchio et al. 2018). Such dysfunctions may be not only linked to disease progression but might precede it and contribute to the disease through various mechanisms. First is a potential deficiency in the clearing functions of innate immunity. Proper disposal of apoptotic immune cells is mainly mediated by macrophages, without initiating inflammation. However, NOD mouse macrophages display a deficiency in capability and consequently fail to properly dispose of apoptotic β-cell remains (O'Brien et al. 2002, 2006). On the contrary, they react very aggressively with high secretion of proinflammatory cytokines, which likely favors autoimmune reactivity (Stoffels et al. 2004). Notably, IL-12 secretion by macrophages in response to lipopolysaccharide (LPS) or CD40 ligand is higher in NOD mice compared to other strains (Alleva et al. 2000; Stoffels et al. 2004). In NOD mice, cDCs are generated from myeloid progenitors at a higher rate (Steptoe et al. 2002), and display higher activation of the NF-κB pathway (Poligone et al. 2002; Mollah et al. 2008). In cases where infection may serve as trigger for T1D initiation or progression, innate immunity deficiencies, such as defects in the IFN-α pathway, may also contribute. Cross talk between iNKT and pDCs through OX40 participates in the clearing of pancreatic infection, while preventing diabetogenic cytotoxic responses (Diana et al. 2009). A failure of infection control by innate immunity may lead to increased adaptive responses, stimulating autoimmunity, and bystander damage of β cells. The relative contribution of these or other potential mechanisms to the pathogenic roles of innate immunity in T1D and the demonstration of their genetic basis remains a critical avenue for future explorations.

INNATE CELLS AS MODULATORS OF ADAPTIVE IMMUNITY IN THE PANCREAS

Antigen Presentation Function

A significant cross talk between innate and adaptive immune responses is involved in the pathogenesis of T1D (Fig. 2). Indeed, cDCs are essential in the induction of adaptive autoimmune responses against β-cell antigens. This was first shown in RIP-LCMV mice, in which β cells express a lymphocytic choriomeningitis virus (LCMV) antigen (Ohashi et al. 1991; Oldstone et al. 1991). Repeated injections of cDCs constitutively expressing this LCMV antigen in these mice were sufficient to trigger destructive insulitis and diabetes onset (Ludewig et al. 1998). It is now established that upon physiological, stress/inflammation-mediated or infection-mediated death of β cells, cDCs uptake pancreatic self-antigens (Turley et al. 2003; Horwitz et al. 2004). They can process those into highly immunogenic-modified autoantigens (McLaughlin et al. 2016). Activated cDCs express CCR7, a step requiring IL-21, and then migrate into pLNs (Turley et al. 2003; Van Belle et al. 2012). In the pLNs, especially former islet-resident CD103$^+$ DCs, they present antigens to CD4$^+$ and CD8$^+$ T cells (Höglund et al. 1999; Ferris et al. 2014). Activation of diabetogenic T cells in at-risk subjects may be favored by the presentation of an altered immune repertoire by cDCs. The highest-risk MHC alleles associated with T1D were found to share a common nonaspartic acid residue at position 57 in the class II β-chain, modifying their ability to bind peptides (Todd et al. 1987). These high-risk MHC alleles thus may favor binding of islet self-antigens, increasing the likelihood of cDC-mediated diabetogenic T-cell activation (van Lummel et al. 2016). Other intermediaries of the MHC-II presentation pathway are also dysregulated in cDCs, with increased proteic expression of HLA-CLIP, HLA-DM, and HLA-DO (Gilles et al. 2023). However, diabetes development was not affected by the loss of H2-O in NOD mice (Lee et al. 2021). Various other innate cells can present self-antigens and activate naive T cells. Marginal zone B cells invade pLNs in NOD mice during disease progression and can present insulin to diabetogenic T cells (Mariño et al. 2008). pDCs may also participate, as they were shown to better present immune complexes to autoreactive T cells compared to cDCs (Allen et al. 2009).

Secondary Activation Signals

Activation can also be increased through secondary signals from cDCs. Interestingly, multiple studies reported conflicting results on costimulatory molecule expression, such as CD86, by cDCs in patients and animal models compared to controls (Jansen et al. 1995; Dahlén et al. 2000; Marleau and Singh 2002; Poligone et al. 2002; Steptoe et al. 2002). These discrepancies may be due to strain diversity, tissue origin, and activation status of cDCs analyzed in these studies. Taken together, it is likely that while naive DCs display a maturation deficiency, activated cDCs carrying pancreatic self-antigens have an increased capacity to provide costimulation signals to diabetogenic T cells (Marleau and Singh 2002; Poligone et al. 2002; Steptoe et al. 2002). Marginal zone B cells present in pLNs of NOD mice have a high expression of CD80/86 as well (Mariño et al. 2008). T-cell differentiation also requires cytokines. cDCs produce higher levels of IL-12 compared to controls, increasing their ability to activate T cells and promoting differentiation toward a Th1 phenotype (Marleau and Singh 2002; Poligone et al. 2002). Of note, IL-12 production by macrophages participates also in Th1 differentiation and promotion of anti-islet cytotoxicity (Jun et al. 1999). An increased frequency of Th17 cells was observed in pLNs from patients with T1D (Ferraro et al. 2011), although their role in T1D pathogenesis is uncertain. Nevertheless, this suggests the existence of pro-Th17 cDCs in the pLNs, able to produce pro-Th17 cytokines such as IL-1β and IL-6, which have other proinflammatory properties as well. Although not directly observed, these cDCs might preferentially be mo-DCs, as blood monocytes display spontaneous increased secretion of both IL-1β and IL-6 in patients with T1D (Bradshaw et al. 2009; Devaraj et al. 2009). Roughly 10% of observed cDCs in the pancreas from human patients reportedly expressed IL-1β (Uno et al. 2007).

Intraislet Adaptive Immunity Support by Innate Cells

Innate immune cells also directly support effector adaptive T cells after their differentiation. They promote their migration and recruitment into pancreatic islets. Exposed to IL-1β, TNF, and IFN-γ, β cells express CCL2, CCL5, as well as CXCL9 and CXCL10 that promote the recruitment of adaptive T cells into islets. High CXCL10 expression has been reported in insulitic lesions in human islets (Roep et al. 2010). In mice, deletion of CXCR3 (CXCL9/10 receptor) significantly delays islet infiltration and destruction by T cells (Frigerio et al. 2002). Therefore, the early production of IFN-γ by NK and innate-like T cells is likely critical for CXCL9/10 production and recruitment of the first adaptive autoreactive lymphocytes into islets (Savinov et al. 2001). CCL21 is also required for T-cell migration into the islets, but whether innate immune cells stimulate its production is not precisely known (Savinov et al. 2003b; Bouma et al. 2005). DCs interacting with the endothelium of the postcapillary venules were shown to promote the transmigration of $CD4^+$ T cells into the islets (Calderon et al. 2011). In the islet microenvironment, cDCs and macrophages are able to present captured self-antigens to both $CD4^+$ and $CD8^+$ T cells and restimulate these cells, enhancing their cytokine production and cytotoxicity against β cells. Taken together, innate immune cells are essential in promoting adaptive diabetogenic responses, from early activation in the pLNs to supporting effector functions in the islets.

Promotion of Adaptive Immune Tolerance against β Cells by Innate Cells in the pLNs

Despite their role in promoting inflammatory adaptive immune responses, innate immune cells are also involved in generating tolerogenic adaptive immune responses (Fig. 2). Early experiments showed that transfer of DCs in NOD mice could prevent disease onset (Clare-Salzler et al. 1992), suggesting that tolerance could be enforced by innate immune cells during activation of autoreactive T cells in the pLNs. Protective effects from DCs were first associated with their ability to stimulate the generation of $CD4^+$ Th2 lymphocytes able to prevent disease (Feili-Hariri et al. 2003). In NOD mice, this protective effect was further suggested with models of parasitic infections that both increased Th2 responses and protection against T1D (Zaccone et al. 2003). Production of the Th2 cytokine IL-4 or IL-13 by iNKT cells in pLNs was also first believed to directly mediate the protective effects of this cell population (Hong et al. 2001; Laloux et al. 2001; Sharif et al. 2001; Forestier et al. 2007; Usero et al. 2016). However, studies showed that the protective pLN tolerance was directly enforced by tolerogenic cDCs and pDCs, whose generation was promoted notably by iNKT cells, explaining their protective role (Chen et al. 2005; Wang et al. 2008; Diana et al. 2011; Beaudoin et al. 2014). iNKT cells can directly induce TGF-β-producing tolerogenic pDCs in the pLNs, through the production of IL-10 by iNKT cells and a PD-1/PD-L1 interaction between iNKT cells and pDCs, respectively (Chen et al. 2005; Diana et al. 2011; Beaudoin et al. 2014). Tolerogenic cDCs and pDCs are characterized by lower levels of MHC class II, costimulatory CD80/CD86, IL-12, and IFN-α expression (Kared et al. 2005; Gaudreau et al. 2007; Beaudoin et al. 2014). Therefore, these DCs are less effective in stimulating diabetogenic T cells, and promote functional anergy of those cells (Gaudreau et al. 2007), a process that can be also mediated by iNKT cells (Beaudoin et al. 2002). The effect of tolerogenic cDCs and pDCs is likely indirect, coming from the induction of $CD4^+$ $CD25^+$ $FOXP3^+$ regulatory T cells (Tregs), up-regulating their conversion and proliferation in pLNs (Chilton et al. 2004; Diana et al. 2011; Beaudoin et al. 2014; Ferreira et al. 2014). At the later stages, tolerogenic cDCs promote Treg survival through IL-7 production (Harnaha et al. 2006), and upscale the future production of IL-10 by mature Tregs (Ferreira et al. 2014). In cooperation with iNKT cells, tolerogenic pDCs also increase CXCR3 expression on Tregs, allowing their subsequent migration into the inflamed pancreatic islets (Beaudoin et al. 2014).

These protective effects of tolerogenic DCs and iNKT cells against disease through Treg generation suggest natural defects of those cells in animal models and patients with T1D. In NOD mice, iNKT cells display several anomalies of both frequency and function (Gombert et al. 1996; Lehuen et al. 1998). Moreover, all the protective effects previously described required a treatment with the most potent iNKT cell ligand, α-galactosylceramide, suggesting a deficient or dysfunctional activation of those cells in T1D. Compared to mice, evidence of iNKT cell frequency anomalies in humans remains unclear (Oikawa et al. 2002; Kis et al. 2007). However, blood iNKT cells tend to display an increased Th1 bias that might reduce their Th2 or tolerogenic properties (Wilson et al. 1998; Kis et al. 2007; Usero et al. 2016). Regarding DCs, several studies highlighted a failure of these cells to trigger induction of tolerance or activation-induced cell death in autoreactive T cells due to incorrect costimulation and resistance from diabetogenic T cells (Jansen et al. 1995; Dahlén et al. 2000). Deficiencies in tolerogenic DC generation and maturation were reported as well. In the pancreas, the generation of tolerogenic DCs, as well as anti-inflammatory macrophages, is decreased due to reduced CRAMP secretion by β cells (Sun et al. 2015). Treatments with cytokines involved in DC maturation, including FLT3-L, G-CSF, or GM-CSF rescued expansion of functional tolerogenic cDCs and protected NOD mice against disease (Chilton et al. 2004; Kared et al. 2005; Gaudreau et al. 2007). Supplementation of NOD mice with metabolites known to increase tolerogenic cDC expansion and maturation, such as vitamin D (1,25-Dihydroxyvitamin D3) and microbiota-derived short-chain fatty acids (SCFAs), also provided protection against disease onset (Ferreira et al. 2014; Mariño et al. 2017). Treatment with FLT3-L was protective only at the early stages of the disease before detecting anti-islet T cells in peripheral blood (Van Belle et al. 2010). At later stages, this treatment accelerated T1D onset. This suggests the existence of an early limited time window during which the migratory DC phenotype is decided

 Cite this article as *Cold Spring Harb Perspect Med* doi: 10.1101/cshperspect.a041595

between tolerance or inflammatory in at-risk subjects, with long-lasting consequences.

Enforcement of Immune Tolerance by Innate Cells in Pancreatic Islets

Innate cells can also directly enforce tolerance in the pancreatic islets, through various mechanisms (Fig. 2). DCs from NOD mice previously infected by *Salmonella typhimurium* block anti-islet T-cell homing into the pancreatic islets, by altering chemokine expression patterns of CXCL10 and CCL21a (Raine et al. 2006). In pancreatic islets, $CD4^+$ type II iNKT cells suppress the effector function of autoreactive T cells through ICOS and PD1 immune checkpoints (Kadri et al. 2012). Additionally, innate immune cells can release immunomodulating factors. Tolerogenic cDCs directly produce immunosuppressive IL-10 (Gaudreau et al. 2007; Kriegel et al. 2012), as do transferred myeloid-derived suppressor cells (MDSCs) or M2 macrophages (Yin et al. 2010; Parsa et al. 2012). These cells were also able to inhibit autoimmune responses in the pancreatic islets by secreting indoleamine 2,3-dioxygenase (IDO) (Yin et al. 2010; Parsa et al. 2012; Ghazarian et al. 2013). This enzyme dampens immune responses by catabolizing tryptophan, a key amino acid for effector T cells (Alexander et al. 2002). Secretion of IDO by pDCs was also sufficient to inhibit insulitis in the pancreatic islets (Saxena et al. 2007). Finally, NK cells are able to delay autoimmunity against islet grafts by killing diabetogenic cDCs (Beilke et al. 2005). It is important to stress that all these intraislet tolerance-inducing pathways participate in the homeostatic tolerance in islets, preventing disease. However, their effect is likely far from sufficient to compete against high pancreatic inflammation in patients and animal models developing the disease, even more so that strong inflammation directly inhibits these tolerance mechanisms.

The balance between tolerance and inflammation by pancreatic innate immunity is, therefore, key in whether β cells will be targeted or protected against destructive autoimmunity. It is now, however, clearly evident that the involvement of innate immunity in T1D does not limit itself to the pancreas and pLNs and extends to other digestive organs, especially the gut.

DISTANT INNATE IMMUNITY CAN AFFECT ISLET AUTOIMMUNITY

Innate Immune Dysfunction in the Gut

Observations of innate immunity dysfunction in the gut of diabetes-prone or diabetic animals and humans are plentiful. For example, an estimated 4%–9% of T1D patients suffer from celiac disease compared to 1% of the general population, which suggests an increased risk of those patients to develop gut inflammation (Kahaly and Hansen 2016). Early reports on human biopsies highlighted increased HLA-DR and HLA-DQ expression patterns in the villi, as well as increased frequency of IL-$1\alpha^+$ and IL-4^+ jejunal cells (Savilahti et al. 1999; Westerholm-Ormio et al. 2003). Further studies highlighted an up-regulation of inflammatory gene expression in duodenal mucosa biopsies of T1D patients (Pellegrini et al. 2017), including cytokines (*TNF, IL1β*), chemokines (*CCL13, CCL19, CCL20, CCL22*), and their receptors (*IL4R, CCR2, CCR7, CCR8*). In NOD mice, before disease development, gene expression of *Il6, Il12, Tnf*, and *Il1β* is increased in the gut; compared to BALB/c and nonobese resistant (NOR) mice that do not develop the disease (Miranda et al. 2019; Sorini et al. 2019). Moreover, histological analysis in T1D patients showed dense areas of inflammatory infiltrate that were notably populated by an increased $CD68^+$ monocyte/macrophage cell lineage (Pellegrini et al. 2017). Interestingly, this infiltrate was not observed in biopsies from patients suffering from celiac disease, suggesting a unique intestinal innate proinflammatory signature in T1D patients (Westerholm-Ormio et al. 2003; Pellegrini et al. 2017).

Protective gut immunity is affected as well. Th17 immunity is critical for the maintenance of gut integrity as IL-17 and IL-22 promote the secretion of antimicrobial peptides and enterocyte fucosylation and defense (Liang et al. 2006; Pickard et al. 2014). In NOD mice, intestinal ILCs, iNKT and γδT cells, display a general loss

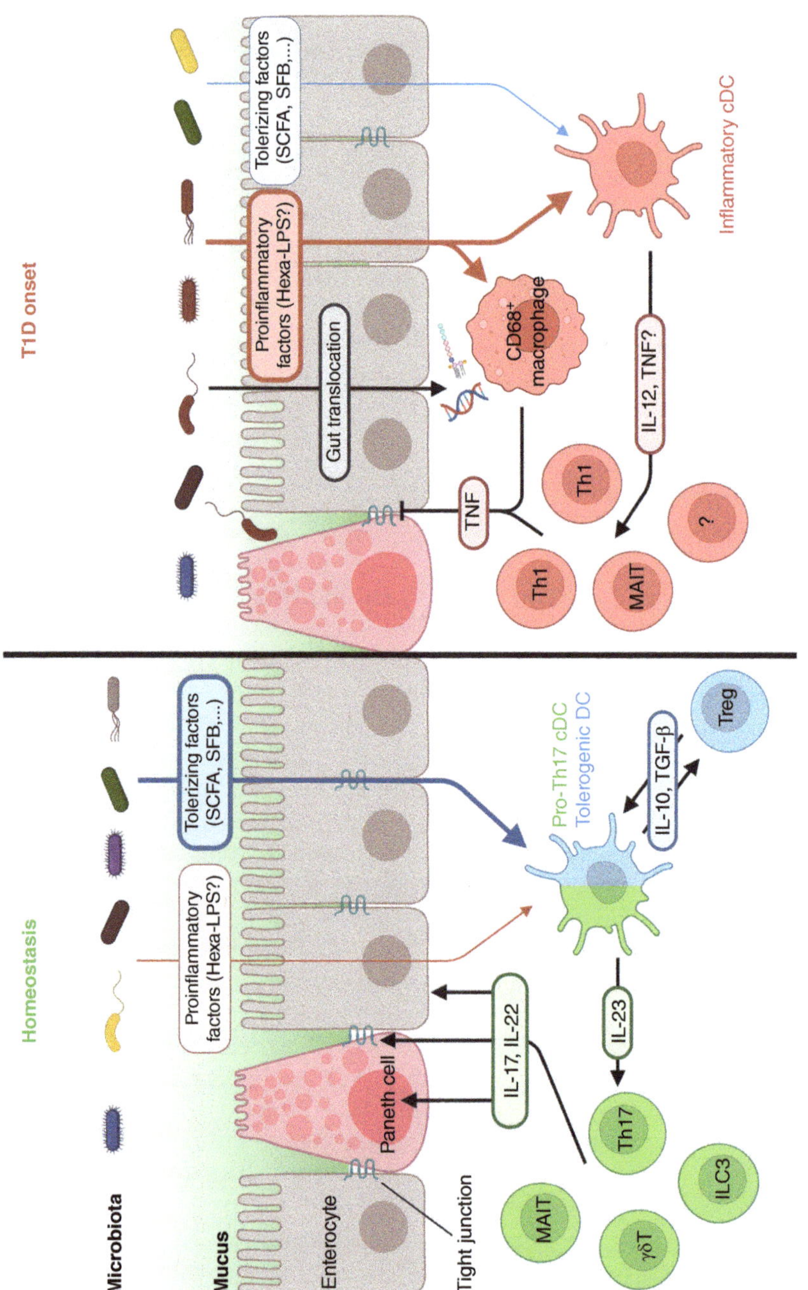

Figure 3. (*See following page for legend.*)

of both IL-17 production and ROR-γT expression at diabetes onset compared to younger prediabetic NOD mice (Rouland et al. 2022; Saksida et al. 2023). Defects in IL-17$^+$ γδT cells in the lamina propria of the ileum and colon have also been associated with accelerated disease onset (Candon et al. 2015). MAIT cell frequency is significantly reduced at disease onset along with expression of ROR-γT, IL-17, and IL-22 (Rouxel et al. 2017; Rouland et al. 2022). Levels of *Il17* and *Il23* mRNA levels are increased in young NOD mice compared to BALB/c (Sorini et al. 2019), but are strongly diminished in older, diabetic mice, as well as in B6 mice that received low-dose streptozotocin (Rouland et al. 2022). Therefore, despite a strain-specific increased Th17 immunity in young NOD mice, disease progression likely leads to loss of Th17 immunity capacity in innate and innate-like cells. Regarding intestinal cDCs, their pro-Th17 capabilities during T1D progression remain unexplored. Loss of *Il17* and *Il23* gene expression, as well as IL-17 production from T cells as disease progresses indirectly suggests a loss of pro-Th17 cDCs in NOD mice. These observations may point at increased antimicrobial responses early in life that may promote the development of autoimmunity to the point where such responses are no longer important for the disease progression. However, one study reported that the frequency of Th17 cells is increased in human biopsies, although several months had passed since onset for most of the studied patients (Lo Conte et al. 2023). To understand the importance of such observations and their connection to diabetogenesis, further analyses, particularly of human gut biopsies from recent-onset and at-risk subjects would be required. Finally, immune tolerance is affected as well, as the frequency of CD103$^+$ tolerogenic DCs in diabetic and prediabetic NOD mice in the mesenteric lymph nodes is reduced compared to NOR mice (Coombes et al. 2007; Miranda et al. 2019). In patients with T1D, tolerogenic DCs in the lamina propria of the small intestine are defective as they fail to induce Tregs (Badami et al. 2011). The origin and course of these alterations may be linked to pancreatic autoimmunity. Massive production of TNF by diabetogenic T cells that infiltrate the intestines was sufficient to initiate loss of intestinal Th17 immunity in NOD mice (Rouland et al. 2022). Increasing evidence, however, suggests that these intestinal innate immune alterations are intimately associated with alterations of the intestinal microbiota (Fig. 3).

A Link with the Gut Microbiota

The existence of such a link with intestinal innate immunity was first established by showing that MyD88$^{-/-}$ SPF NOD mice were protected against T1D, but not MyD88$^{-/-}$ GF NOD mice (Wen et al. 2008). This study, along with similar findings in GF BB rats made an important point, that organ-specific autoimmunity did not require microbes for its progression (Wen et al. 2008; Patrick et al. 2013). Treatments with large-spectrum antibiotics also accelerated and increased disease onset in NOD mice (Candon et al. 2015; Livanos et al. 2016). This led to the hypothesis that specific protective bacterial species (specific lineage hypothesis) could prevent

Figure 3. Alterations of intestinal innate immunity in type 1 diabetes (T1D). At homeostasis, a diverse and healthy gut microbiota results in a balance shifted toward a greater production of tolerizing factors compared to pro-diabetes proinflammatory factors. Conventional dendritic cell (cDC) phenotype is likely to be mostly either tolerogenic or pro-Th17 through interleukin (IL)-23 production. Innate immune cells, including mucosal-associated invariant T (MAIT) cells, γδT, and innate lymphoid cells (ILCs) participate in the maintenance of the gut barrier by secreting IL-17 and IL-22 that stimulate Paneth and epithelial cell functions. Tolerance is also maintained through the generation of regulatory T cells (Tregs). However, in patients and animal models of T1D, at onset, dysbiosis in the microbiota and leaky gut favor the exposure of immune cells, particularly dendritic cells (DCs), to greater amounts of microbiota-derived proinflammatory factors. Infiltration of diabetogenic Th1 cells and CD68$^+$ macrophages results in sustained intestinal inflammation through tumor necrosis factor (TNF) release that further weakens epithelial integrity. (LPS) Lipopolysaccharide, (TGF) transforming growth factor, (SCFAs) short-chain fatty acids, (SFB) segmented filamentous bacteria.

disease onset through TLR and innate immunity stimulation (Wen et al. 2008; Chervonsky 2013). However, it is more likely that microbiota, as a consortium, provides both protective and deleterious signaling through innate immunity (balanced signal hypothesis), with a disbalance toward proinflammatory signals during progression toward T1D, potentially through various TLRs (Fig. 3; Burrows et al. 2015). TIR-domain-containing adaptor-inducing IFN-β (TRIF) and TLR4 can mediate microbiota tolerance against T1D, whereas prodiabetogenic signals can be sent from the microbiota through TLR2 signaling (Burrows et al. 2015). However, the microbial ligands involved remain to be identified. Recent studies have started to unveil microbiota signals involved in this balance. Reduction of protolerogenic SCFA levels has been reported in both patients and animal models of T1D (Sun et al. 2015; Mariño et al. 2017; Vatanen et al. 2018; Huang et al. 2020). Supplementation with SCFA rescues intestinal tolerance and protects NOD mice against T1D (Mariño et al. 2017; Huang et al. 2020).

Effects of microbiota on T1D also depend on sex hormones. The long-known sexual dimorphism of T1D in NOD mice (females have higher incidence) is lifted in GF conditions (Wen et al. 2008; Markle et al. 2013a; Yurkovetskiy et al. 2013). Since several unrelated bacterial lineages were capable to protect males without affecting female disease (Yurkovetskiy et al. 2013), it is likely that they provide a general innate immunity-activating signal that complements signaling from the sex hormones. The details of these interactions remain unknown, and it is not clear how it translates to human T1D where sexual dimorphism is lacking unless it is associated with polyglandular autoimmunity (Hansen et al. 2015).

Thus, the question of the contribution of commensal and pathogenic microbiota to T1D pathogenesis, versus the mostly protective role of those became the central point of the studies in the field. One direction of the studies of the microbiota-T1D connection is the search for microbial "perpetrators." Although human studies are rather correlative in nature, they became a major undertaking in the recent years. Several large-scale studies have demonstrated that patients progressing toward or with T1D display a significant loss of microbiota diversity but did not uncover such microbial "perpetrators" (de Goffau et al. 2013, 2014; Dunne et al. 2014; Alkanani et al. 2015; Kostic et al. 2015; Pellegrini et al. 2017; Stewart et al. 2018; Vatanen et al. 2018). However, studies in NOD mice have highlighted the segmented filamentous bacteria (SFB) as a protective species, as SFB colonization was associated with protection against T1D through likely its ability to stimulate protective intestinal Th17 immunity (Gaboriau-Routhiau et al. 2009; Ivanov et al. 2009; Kriegel et al. 2011; Rouland et al. 2022).

It is important to appreciate that microbial products can elicit different effects on disease development depending on (1) their physical and chemical properties (such as acylation and aggregation of LPS), (2) location within the gut, and (3) gut's permeability. For example, levels of intestinal bacteria producing LPS with higher innate immune activation capabilities (hexa-acylated LPS) are decreased in children belonging to populations with high T1D incidence (Vatanen et al. 2016) suggesting that it may be protective in children with higher abundance of *Enterobacteriae*. However, hexa-acylated LPS, different from the prevalent penta-acylated LPS in mammals and released from dietary gluten digestion by *Enterococcus faecalis*, increased diabetes onset in NOD mice in a TLR4-dependent manner (Funsten et al. 2023).

A Distant Effect on Pancreatic Autoimmunity?

Intestinal innate immunity, through its dysfunction, may indirectly modulate pancreatic autoimmune responses (Vaarala et al. 2008). Loss of gut immune barrier strength results in a loss of gut integrity (Fig. 3). Thickness of intestinal tight junctions, as well as expression of their constitutive proteins, is decreased at disease onset (Secondulfo et al. 2004; Neu et al. 2005; Rouland et al. 2022). Loss of fucosylation also decreases epithelial cell protection (Pickard et al. 2014; Rouland et al. 2022). Functional tests using mannitol or fluorescein isothiocyanate–dextran showed an increased transepithelial passage of these compounds from the gut to blood and urine, even before disease onset (Neu et al. 2005; Bosi et al. 2006; Rouland et al. 2022). Bacterial translocation across the intestinal barrier is increased into the portal vein and the liver (Rouland et al. 2022). $Mr1^{-/-}$ NOD mice that do not possess intestinal MAIT cells display a further increase of gut permeability, with greater levels of bacterial 16S DNA in pLNs and increased T1D frequency (Rouxel et al. 2017). Such a result is unexpected, as more bacteria are likely to be more protective, but may lead to the identification of specific microbial lineage(s) characteristic of a given colony that may serve as T1D promoters. On the other hand, passive transportation by the lymph of bacterial or viral antigens from the gut to pLNs has long been suspected to potentially stimulate disease through bystander activation (Turley et al. 2005; Rouxel et al. 2017). At the same time, protective factors such as SCFA can also be transported to islets (Sun et al. 2015). Both the increased translocation due to gut leakiness, and a disbalance in the compounds transported, reflecting the one in the gut microbiota, are likely at play in this increased bystander effect in the islets (Fig. 4).

Recent studies have strengthened the early notion that this transportation could be active and mediated by intestinal cDCs (Turley et al. 2005), directly promoting pancreatic autoimmunity. The pLNs not only drain lymph from the pancreas but also from the liver, duodenum (Brown et al. 2023), and potentially from the colon where drainage to pLNs was noted during

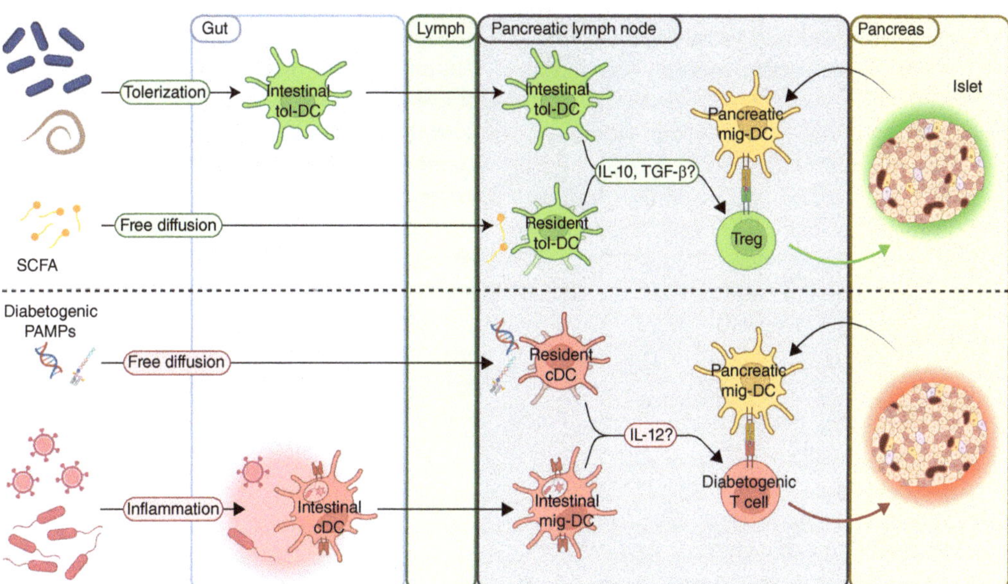

Figure 4. Mediation of pancreatic autoimmunity by intestinal and pancreatic innate immune cells. Pancreatic lymph nodes (pLNs) drain lymph from the pancreas and the gut, allowing microbiota and infectious mediators to modulate local immune responses against β cells. Gut tolerizing factors, such as short-chain fatty acids (SCFAs), can induce intestinal tolerogenic dendritic cells (tol-DCs) that can be drained toward the pLNs, where they promote the induction of regulatory T (Treg) cells. These factors can also freely reach the pLN through the lymph drainage, directly promoting tolerance in DCs present in the pLNs. This cross talk between gut and pLNs can turn detrimental in type 1 diabetes (T1D). Intestinal inflammation and infection can lead to the migration of inflammatory conventional dendritic cells (cDCs) in the pLNs, where they likely stimulate the activation of diabetogenic T cells through bystander effects. The free diffusion of diabetogenic pathogen-associated molecular patterns (PAMPs), such as microbial DNA, is increased due to gut leakiness, while the drainage of tolerizing factors is likely diminished. This increased drainage of proinflammatory factors from the gut to the pancreas might also stimulate bystander activation by resident DCs in the pLNs. (IL) Interleukin, (TGF) transforming growth factor, (SCFAs) short-chain fatty acids.

infection with *Citrobacter rodentium* (Pöysti et al. 2022). Adaptive T cells entering pLNs can encounter cDCs that migrated from the pancreas, but also from the liver and intestines (Turley et al. 2005; Pöysti et al. 2022; Brown et al. 2023). According to their tissue of origin, these cDCs display a variable proinflammatory capacity, with cDCs from the liver or pancreas promoting conventional Th1 responses, while cDCs from duodenal origin promote more Th2, Th17, and tolerogenic adaptive responses (Brown et al. 2023). However, viral intestinal infection temporarily switches intestinal cDCs toward a proinflammatory phenotype, which tips the scales toward the pro-Th1 environment in the pLNs. A similar mechanism is observed during *C. rodentium* infection, where colonic cDCs uptake bacterial antigens, activate, and migrate into the pLNs (Lee et al. 2010; Pöysti et al. 2022). Reversal of this homeostatic tolerogenicity of cDCs drained from the infected gut also promotes autoimmunity and activation of diabetogenic T cells in the pLNs (Pöysti et al. 2022; Brown et al. 2023). Therefore, intestinal innate inflammation can propagate through migratory cDCs to pLNs (Fig. 4). Bystander IL-12 secretion may support the activation of diabetogenic T cells by incoming proinflammatory pancreatic cDCs loaded with self-antigens. This also provides an interesting explanation to why enteroviral infections have long been associated with T1D development (Wang et al. 2021). Mechanistical explanations of this link involved both a direct pancreatic infection by the pathogen and the requirement of an already existing immune response (Serreze et al. 2000; Ghazarian et al. 2013). However, a restricted infection in the gut only, in at-risk patients already progressing toward disease, could dramatically accelerate and promote the onset of T1D, as intestinal DCs propagate inflammation from the gut to pLNs (Pöysti et al. 2022; Brown et al. 2023). Of note, this propagation mechanism has been highlighted during an acute intestinal inflammation in response to pathogen infection, which is different from the low-grade, chronic intestinal inflammation described in patients and animal models of T1D. The same mechanism might also promote protection against T1D after intestinal parasite infection that enforces local intestinal tolerance (Saunders et al. 2007). Taken together, it is likely that innate immunity in the gut influences pancreatic autoimmunity through their shared lymphatic network. In T1D, the conjunction of a nascent autoimmune reaction in the pancreas with intestinal inflammation can trigger a deleterious circle, where each reinforce alterations of the other, and where gut exposure to environmental factors such as infections becomes a vulnerability for the pancreas.

CONCLUDING REMARKS

Innate immunity in T1D has a complex role, with the potential to promote and maintain tolerance that is deficient or lost during progression toward disease and replaced with a strong capacity to support the destruction of β cells. Still, there is also evidence that these protective functions can be rescued with exogenous immune stimulation that could re-envigorate these cells or favor tolerance if given during a precise window during which the immune response remains malleable. Further studies on innate immune mechanisms and their sequence are warranted and may provide new targets for the prevention of T1D, while the majority of clinical trials have focused on adaptive immunity. Most importantly, evidence from the global roles of innate immunity in T1D supports its characterization as a multiorgan pathology in which the pancreas, the gut, and perhaps the liver are involved, as all share the same lymphatic networks and close exposure to the gut microbiota.

ACKNOWLEDGMENTS

L.B., A.V.C., and A.L. designed figures and wrote the present review. L.B. is supported by grants from the Fondation pour la Recherche Médicale (FRM) (FDT202204015005) and Aide aux Jeunes Diabétiques. A.V.C. is supported by National Institutes of Health (NIH) grants R01AI158744, R01AI127411, and P30DK042086. A.L. is supported by grants from ANR-18-IDEX-0001, ANR-19-CE14-0041-01, ANR-20-CE14-0044, and FRM EQU20190300 7779.

REFERENCES

Aida K, Nishida Y, Tanaka S, Maruyama T, Shimada A, Awata T, Suzuki M, Shimura H, Takizawa S, Ichijo M, et al. 2011. RIG-I- and MDA5-initiated innate immunity linked with adaptive immunity accelerates β-cell death in fulminant type 1 diabetes. *Diabetes* **60:** 884–889. doi:10.2337/db10-0795

Alba A, Planas R, Clemente X, Carrillo J, Ampudia R, Puertas MC, Pastor X, Tolosa E, Pujol-Borrell R, Verdaguer J, et al. 2008. Natural killer cells are required for accelerated type 1 diabetes driven by interferon-β. *Clin Exp Immunol* **151:** 467–475. doi:10.1111/j.1365-2249.2007.03580.x

Alexander AM, Crawford M, Bertera S, Rudert WA, Takikawa O, Robbins PD, Trucco M. 2002. Indoleamine 2,3-dioxygenase expression in transplanted NOD islets prolongs graft survival after adoptive transfer of diabetogenic splenocytes. *Diabetes* **51:** 356–365. doi:10.2337/diabetes.51.2.356

Alkanani AK, Hara N, Gottlieb PA, Ir D, Robertson CE, Wagner BD, Frank DN, Zipris D. 2015. Alterations in intestinal microbiota correlate with susceptibility to type 1 diabetes. *Diabetes* **64:** 3510–3520. doi:10.2337/db14-1847

Allen JS, Pang K, Skowera A, Ellis R, Rackham C, Lozanoska-Ochser B, Tree T, Leslie RDG, Tremble JM, Dayan CM, et al. 2009. Plasmacytoid dendritic cells are proportionally expanded at diagnosis of type 1 diabetes and enhance islet autoantigen presentation to T-cells through immune complex capture. *Diabetes* **58:** 138–145. doi:10.2337/db08-0964

Alleva DG, Pavlovich RP, Grant C, Kaser SB, Beller DI. 2000. Aberrant macrophage cytokine production is a conserved feature among autoimmune-prone mouse strains: elevated interleukin (IL)-12 and an imbalance in tumor necrosis factor-α and IL-10 define a unique cytokine profile in macrophages from young nonobese diabetic mice. *Diabetes* **49:** 1106–1115. doi:10.2337/diabetes.49.7.1106

Arnush M, Scarim AL, Heitmeier MR, Kelly CB, Corbett JA. 1998. Potential role of resident islet macrophage activation in the initiation of autoimmune diabetes. *J Immunol* **160:** 2684–2691. doi:10.4049/jimmunol.160.6.2684

Assmann TS, de Almeida Brondani L, Bauer AC, Canani LH, Crispim D. 2014. Polymorphisms in the TLR3 gene are associated with risk for type 1 diabetes mellitus. *Eur J Endocrinol* **170:** 519–527. doi:10.1530/EJE-13-0963

Badami E, Sorini C, Coccia M, Usuelli V, Molteni L, Bolla AM, Scavini M, Mariani A, King C, Bosi E, et al. 2011. Defective differentiation of regulatory FoxP3$^+$ T cells by small-intestinal dendritic cells in patients with type 1 diabetes. *Diabetes* **60:** 2120–2124. doi:10.2337/db10-1201

Beaudoin L, Laloux V, Novak J, Lucas B, Lehuen A. 2002. NKT cells inhibit the onset of diabetes by impairing the development of pathogenic T cells specific for pancreatic β cells. *Immunity* **17:** 725–736. doi:10.1016/s1074-7613(02)00473-9

Beaudoin L, Diana J, Ghazarian L, Simoni Y, Boitard C, Lehuen A. 2014. Plasmacytoid dendritic cells license regulatory T cells, upon iNKT-cell stimulation, to prevent autoimmune diabetes. *Eur J Immunol* **44:** 1454–1466. doi:10.1002/eji.201343910

Beilke JN, Kuhl NR, Van Kaer L, Gill RG. 2005. NK cells promote islet allograft tolerance via a perforin-dependent mechanism. *Nat Med* **11:** 1059–1065. doi:10.1038/nm1296

Beristain-Covarrubias N, Canche-Pool E, Gomez-Diaz R, Sanchez-Torres LE, Ortiz-Navarrete V. 2015. Reduced iNKT cells numbers in type 1 diabetes patients and their first-degree relatives. *Immun Inflamm Dis* **3:** 411–419. doi:10.1002/iid3.79

Bjørnvold M, Munthe-Kaas MC, Egeland T, Joner G, Dahl-Jørgensen K, Njølstad PR, Akselsen HE, Gervin K, Carlsen KCL, Carlsen KH, et al. 2009. A TLR2 polymorphism is associated with type 1 diabetes and allergic asthma. *Genes Immun* **10:** 181–187. doi:10.1038/gene.2008.100

Bosi E, Molteni L, Radaelli MG, Folini L, Fermo I, Bazzigaluppi E, Piemonti L, Pastore MR, Paroni R. 2006. Increased intestinal permeability precedes clinical onset of type 1 diabetes. *Diabetologia* **49:** 2824–2827. doi:10.1007/s00125-006-0465-3

Bouma G, Coppens JMC, Mourits S, Nikolic T, Sozzani S, Drexhage HA, Versnel MA. 2005. Evidence for an enhanced adhesion of DC to fibronectin and a role of CCL19 and CCL21 in the accumulation of DC around the pre-diabetic islets in NOD mice. *Eur J Immunol* **35:** 2386–2396. doi:10.1002/eji.200526251

Bradshaw EM, Raddassi K, Elyaman W, Orban T, Gottlieb PA, Kent SC, Hafler DA. 2009. Monocytes from patients with type 1 diabetes spontaneously secrete proinflammatory cytokines inducing Th17 cells. *J Immunol* **183:** 4432–4439. doi:10.4049/jimmunol.0900576

Brauner H, Elemans M, Lemos S, Broberger C, Holmberg D, Flodström-Tullberg M, Kärre K, Höglund P. 2010. Distinct phenotype and function of NK cells in the pancreas of nonobese diabetic mice. *J Immunol* **184:** 2272–2280. doi:10.4049/jimmunol.0804358

Brown H, Komnick MR, Brigleb PH, Dermody TS, Esterházy D. 2023. Lymph node sharing between pancreas, gut, and liver leads to immune crosstalk and regulation of pancreatic autoimmunity. *Immunity* **56:** 2070–2085.e11. doi:10.1016/j.immuni.2023.07.008

Burrows MP, Volchkov P, Kobayashi KS, Chervonsky AV. 2015. Microbiota regulates type 1 diabetes through Toll-like receptors. *Proc Natl Acad Sci* **112:** 9973–9977. doi:10.1073/pnas.1508740112

Calderon B, Carrero JA, Miller MJ, Unanue ER. 2011. Entry of diabetogenic T cells into islets induces changes that lead to amplification of the cellular response. *Proc Natl Acad Sci* **108:** 1567–1572. doi:10.1073/pnas.1018975108

Campbell-Thompson M, Wasserfall C, Kaddis J, Albanese-O'Neill A, Staeva T, Nierras C, Moraski J, Rowe P, Gianani R, Eisenbarth G, et al. 2012. Network for Pancreatic Organ Donors with Diabetes (nPOD): developing a tissue biobank for type 1 diabetes. *Diabetes Metab Res Rev* **28:** 608–617. doi:10.1002/dmrr.2316

Candon S, Perez-Arroyo A, Marquet C, Valette F, Foray AP, Pelletier B, Milani C, Ventura M, Bach JF, Chatenoud L. 2015. Antibiotics in early life alter the gut microbiome and increase disease incidence in a spontaneous mouse model of autoimmune insulin-dependent diabetes. *PLoS ONE* **10:** e0125448. doi:10.1371/journal.pone.0125448

Cardozo AK, Proost P, Gysemans C, Chen MC, Mathieu C, Eizirik DL. 2003. IL-1β and IFN-γ induce the expression of diverse chemokines and IL-15 in human and rat pancreatic islet cells, and in islets from pre-diabetic NOD mice. *Diabetologia* **46:** 255–266. doi:10.1007/s00125-002-1017-0

Cardozo AK, Ortis F, Storling J, Feng YM, Rasschaert J, Tonnesen M, Van Eylen F, Mandrup-Poulsen T, Herchuelz A, Eizirik DL. 2005. Cytokines downregulate the sarcoendoplasmic reticulum pump Ca^{2+} ATPase 2b and deplete endoplasmic reticulum Ca^{2+}, leading to induction of endoplasmic reticulum stress in pancreatic β-cells. *Diabetes* **54:** 452–461. doi:10.2337/diabetes.54.2.452

Carrero JA, McCarthy DP, Ferris ST, Wan X, Hu H, Zinselmeyer BH, Vomund AN, Unanue ER. 2017. Resident macrophages of pancreatic islets have a seminal role in the initiation of autoimmune diabetes of NOD mice. *Proc Natl Acad Sci* **114:** E10418–E10427. doi:10.1073/pnas.1713543114

Chen MC, Proost P, Gysemans C, Mathieu C, Eizirik DL. 2001. Monocyte chemoattractant protein-1 is expressed in pancreatic islets from prediabetic NOD mice and in interleukin-1β-exposed human and rat islet cells. *Diabetologia* **44:** 325–332. doi:10.1007/s001250051622

Chen YG, Choisy-Rossi CM, Holl TM, Chapman HD, Besra GS, Porcelli SA, Shaffer DJ, Roopenian D, Wilson SB, Serreze DV. 2005. Activated NKT cells inhibit autoimmune diabetes through tolerogenic recruitment of dendritic cells to pancreatic lymph nodes. *J Immunol* **174:** 1196–1204. doi:10.4049/jimmunol.174.3.1196

Chervonsky AV. 2013. Microbiota and autoimmunity. *Cold Spring Harb Perspect Biol* **5:** a007294. doi:10.1101/cshperspect.a007294

Chervonsky AV, Wang Y, Wong FS, Visintin I, Flavell RA, Janeway CA, Matis LA. 1997. The role of Fas in autoimmune diabetes. *Cell* **89:** 17–24. doi:10.1016/s0092-8674(00)80178-6

Chilton PM, Rezzoug F, Fugier-Vivier I, Weeter LA, Xu H, Huang Y, Ray MB, Ildstad ST. 2004. Flt3-ligand treatment prevents diabetes in NOD mice. *Diabetes* **53:** 1995–2002. doi:10.2337/diabetes.53.8.1995

Clare-Salzler MJ, Brooks J, Chai A, Van Herle K, Anderson C. 1992. Prevention of diabetes in nonobese diabetic mice by dendritic cell transfer. *J Clin Invest* **90:** 741–748. doi:10.1172/JCI115946

Colli ML, Moore F, Gurzov EN, Ortis F, Eizirik DL. 2010. MDA5 and PTPN2, two candidate genes for type 1 diabetes, modify pancreatic β-cell responses to the viral by-product double-stranded RNA. *Hum Mol Genet* **19:** 135–146. doi:10.1093/hmg/ddp474

Coombes JL, Siddiqui KRR, Arancibia-Cárcamo CV, Hall J, Sun CM, Belkaid Y, Powrie F. 2007. A functionally specialized population of mucosal $CD103^+$ DCs induces $Foxp3^+$ regulatory T cells via a TGF-β and retinoic acid-dependent mechanism. *J Exp Med* **204:** 1757–1764. doi:10.1084/jem.20070590

Dahlén E, Dawe K, Ohlsson L, Hedlund G. 1998. Dendritic cells and macrophages are the first and major producers of TNF-α in pancreatic islets in the nonobese diabetic mouse. *J Immunol* **160:** 3585–3593. doi:10.4049/jimmunol.160.7.3585

Dahlén E, Hedlund G, Dawe K. 2000. Low CD86 expression in the nonobese diabetic mouse results in the impairment of both T cell activation and CTLA-4 up-regulation. *J Immunol* **164:** 2444–2456. doi:10.4049/jimmunol.164.5.2444

de Goffau MC, Luopajärvi K, Knip M, Ilonen J, Ruohtula T, Härkönen T, Orivuori L, Hakala S, Welling GW, Harmsen HJ, et al. 2013. Fecal microbiota composition differs between children with β-cell autoimmunity and those without. *Diabetes* **62:** 1238–1244. doi:10.2337/db12-0526

de Goffau MC, Fuentes S, van den Bogert B, Honkanen H, de Vos WM, Welling GW, Hyöty H, Harmsen HJM. 2014. Aberrant gut microbiota composition at the onset of type 1 diabetes in young children. *Diabetologia* **57:** 1569–1577. doi:10.1007/s00125-014-3274-0

Devaraj S, Dasu MR, Park SH, Jialal I. 2009. Increased levels of ligands of Toll-like receptors 2 and 4 in type 1 diabetes. *Diabetologia* **52:** 1665–1668. doi:10.1007/s00125-009-1394-8

Diana J, Lehuen A. 2014. Macrophages and β-cells are responsible for CXCR2-mediated neutrophil infiltration of the pancreas during autoimmune diabetes. *EMBO Mol Med* **6:** 1090–1104. doi:10.15252/emmm.201404144

Diana J, Griseri T, Lagaye S, Beaudoin L, Autrusseau E, Gautron AS, Tomkiewicz C, Herbelin A, Barouki R, von Herrath M, et al. 2009. NKT cell-plasmacytoid dendritic cell cooperation via OX40 controls viral infection in a tissue-specific manner. *Immunity* **30:** 289–299. doi:10.1016/j.immuni.2008.12.017

Diana J, Brezar V, Beaudoin L, Dalod M, Mellor A, Tafuri A, von Herrath M, Boitard C, Mallone R, Lehuen A. 2011. Viral infection prevents diabetes by inducing regulatory T cells through NKT cell-plasmacytoid dendritic cell interplay. *J Exp Med* **208:** 729–745. doi:10.1084/jem.20101692

Diana J, Simoni Y, Furio L, Beaudoin L, Agerberth B, Barrat F, Lehuen A. 2013. Crosstalk between neutrophils, B-1a cells and plasmacytoid dendritic cells initiates autoimmune diabetes. *Nat Med* **19:** 65–73. doi:10.1038/nm.3042

Dogusan Z, García M, Flamez D, Alexopoulou L, Goldman M, Gysemans C, Mathieu C, Libert C, Eizirik DL, Rasschaert J. 2008. Double-stranded RNA induces pancreatic β-cell apoptosis by activation of the Toll-like receptor 3 and interferon regulatory factor 3 pathways. *Diabetes* **57:** 1236–1245. doi:10.2337/db07-0844

Dotta F, Censini S, van Halteren AGS, Marselli L, Masini M, Dionisi S, Mosca F, Boggi U, Muda AO, Del Prato S, et al. 2007. Coxsackie B4 virus infection of β cells and natural killer cell insulitis in recent-onset type 1 diabetic patients. *Proc Natl Acad Sci* **104:** 5115–5120. doi:10.1073/pnas.0700442104

Dunne JL, Triplett EW, Gevers D, Xavier R, Insel R, Danska J, Atkinson MA. 2014. The intestinal microbiome in type 1 diabetes. *Clin Exp Immunol* **177:** 30–37. doi:10.1111/cei.12321

Feili-Hariri M, Falkner DH, Gambotto A, Papworth GD, Watkins SC, Robbins PD, Morel PA. 2003. Dendritic cells transduced to express interleukin-4 prevent diabetes in nonobese diabetic mice with advanced insulitis. *Hum Gene Ther* **14:** 13–23. doi:10.1089/10430340360464679

Ferraro A, Socci C, Stabilini A, Valle A, Monti P, Piemonti L, Nano R, Olek S, Maffi P, Scavini M, et al. 2011. Expansion of Th17 cells and functional defects in T regulatory cells are key features of the pancreatic lymph nodes in patients with type 1 diabetes. *Diabetes* **60:** 2903–2913. doi:10.2337/db11-0090

Ferreira GB, Gysemans CA, Demengeot J, da Cunha JPMCM, Vanherwegen AS, Overbergh L, Van Belle TL, Pauwels F, Verstuyf A, Korf H, et al. 2014. 1,25-Dihydroxyvitamin d3 promotes tolerogenic dendritic cells with functional migratory properties in NOD mice. *J Immunol* **192:** 4210–4220. doi:10.4049/jimmunol.1302350

Ferris ST, Carrero JA, Mohan JF, Calderon B, Murphy KM, Unanue ER. 2014. A minor subset of Batf3-dependent antigen-presenting cells in islets of Langerhans is essential for the development of autoimmune diabetes. *Immunity* **41:** 657–669. doi:10.1016/j.immuni.2014.09.012

Feuerer M, Shen Y, Littman DR, Benoist C, Mathis D. 2009. How punctual ablation of regulatory T cells unleashes an autoimmune lesion within the pancreatic islets. *Immunity* **31:** 654–664. doi:10.1016/j.immuni.2009.08.023

Flodström M, Maday A, Balakrishna D, Cleary MM, Yoshimura A, Sarvetnick N. 2002. Target cell defense prevents the development of diabetes after viral infection. *Nat Immunol* **3:** 373–382. doi:10.1038/ni771

Forestier C, Takaki T, Molano A, Im JS, Baine I, Jerud ES, Illarionov P, Ndonye R, Howell AR, Santamaria P, et al. 2007. Improved outcomes in NOD mice treated with a novel Th2 cytokine-biasing NKT cell activator. *J Immunol* **178:** 1415–1425. doi:10.4049/jimmunol.178.3.1415

Frigerio S, Junt T, Lu B, Gerard C, Zumsteg U, Holländer GA, Piali L. 2002. β Cells are responsible for CXCR3-mediated T-cell infiltration in insulitis. *Nat Med* **8:** 1414–1420. doi:10.1038/nm1202-792

Funsten MC, Yurkovetskiy LA, Kuznetsov A, Reiman D, Hansen CHF, Senter KI, Lee J, Ratiu J, Dahal-Koirala S, Antonopoulos DA, et al. 2023. Microbiota-dependent proteolysis of gluten subverts diet-mediated protection against type 1 diabetes. *Cell Host Microbe* **31:** 213–227.e9. doi:10.1016/j.chom.2022.12.009

Gaboriau-Routhiau V, Rakotobe S, Lécuyer E, Mulder I, Lan A, Bridonneau C, Rochet V, Pisi A, De Paepe M, Brandi G, et al. 2009. The key role of segmented filamentous bacteria in the coordinated maturation of gut helper T cell responses. *Immunity* **31:** 677–689. doi:10.1016/j.immuni.2009.08.020

Gaudreau S, Guindi C, Ménard M, Besin G, Dupuis G, Amrani A. 2007. Granulocyte-macrophage colony-stimulating factor prevents diabetes development in NOD mice by inducing tolerogenic dendritic cells that sustain the suppressive function of $CD4^+CD25^+$ regulatory T cells. *J Immunol* **179:** 3638–3647. doi:10.4049/jimmunol.179.6.3638

Ghazarian L, Diana J, Beaudoin L, Larsson PG, Puri RK, van Rooijen N, Flodström-Tullberg M, Lehuen A. 2013. Protection against type 1 diabetes upon coxsackievirus B4 infection and iNKT-cell stimulation: role of suppressive macrophages. *Diabetes* **62:** 3785–3796. doi:10.2337/db12-0958

Gilles A, Hu L, Virdis F, Sant'Angelo DB, Dimitrova N, Hedrick JA, Denzin LK. 2023. The MHC class II antigen-processing and presentation pathway is dysregulated in type 1 diabetes. *J Immunol* **211:** 1630–1642. doi:10.4049/jimmunol.2300213

Gombert JM, Herbelin A, Tancrède-Bohin E, Dy M, Carnaud C, Bach JF. 1996. Early quantitative and functional deficiency of $NK1^+$-like thymocytes in the NOD mouse. *Eur J Immunol* **26:** 2989–2998. doi:10.1002/eji.1830261226

Gur C, Porgador A, Elboim M, Gazit R, Mizrahi S, Stern-Ginossar N, Achdout H, Ghadially H, Dor Y, Nir T, et al. 2010. The activating receptor NKp46 is essential for the development of type 1 diabetes. *Nat Immunol* **11:** 121–128. doi:10.1038/ni.1834

Gur C, Enk J, Kassem SA, Suissa Y, Magenheim J, Stolovich-Rain M, Nir T, Achdout H, Glaser B, Shapiro J, et al. 2011. Recognition and killing of human and murine pancreatic β cells by the NK receptor NKp46. *J Immunol* **187:** 3096–3103. doi:10.4049/jimmunol.1101269

Hansen MP, Matheis N, Kahaly GJ. 2015. Type 1 diabetes and polyglandular autoimmune syndrome: a review. *World J Diabetes* **6:** 67–79. doi:10.4239/wjd.v6.i1.67

Harnaha J, Machen J, Wright M, Lakomy R, Styche A, Trucco M, Makaroun S, Giannoukakis N. 2006. Interleukin-7 is a survival factor for $CD4^+$ $CD25^+$ T-cells and is expressed by diabetes-suppressive dendritic cells. *Diabetes* **55:** 158–170. doi:10.2337/diabetes.55.01.06.db05-0340

Höglund P, Mintern J, Waltzinger C, Heath W, Benoist C, Mathis D. 1999. Initiation of autoimmune diabetes by developmentally regulated presentation of islet cell antigens in the pancreatic lymph nodes. *J Exp Med* **189:** 331–339. doi:10.1084/jem.189.2.331

Hong S, Wilson MT, Serizawa I, Wu L, Singh N, Naidenko OV, Miura T, Haba T, Scherer DC, Wei J, et al. 2001. The natural killer T-cell ligand α-galactosylceramide prevents autoimmune diabetes in non-obese diabetic mice. *Nat Med* **7:** 1052–1056. doi:10.1038/nm0901-1052

Horwitz MS, Ilic A, Fine C, Balasa B, Sarvetnick N. 2004. Coxsackieviral-mediated diabetes: induction requires antigen-presenting cells and is accompanied by phagocytosis of β cells. *Clin Immunol* **110:** 134–144. doi:10.1016/j.clim.2003.09.014

Huang J, Pearson JA, Peng J, Hu Y, Sha S, Xing Y, Huang G, Li X, Hu F, Xie Z, et al. 2020. Gut microbial metabolites alter IgA immunity in type 1 diabetes. *JCI Insight* **5:** 135718. doi:10.1172/jci.insight.135718

Hussain MJ, Alviggi L, Millward BA, Leslie RD, Pyke DA, Vergani D. 1987. Evidence that the reduced number of natural killer cells in type 1 (insulin-dependent) diabetes may be genetically determined. *Diabetologia* **30:** 907–911. doi:10.1007/BF00295872

Hussain MJ, Peakman M, Gallati H, Lo SS, Hawa M, Viberti GC, Watkins PJ, Leslie RD, Vergani D. 1996. Elevated serum levels of macrophage-derived cytokines precede and accompany the onset of IDDM. *Diabetologia* **39:** 60–69. doi:10.1007/BF00400414

Hutchings P, Rosen H, O'Reilly L, Simpson E, Gordon S, Cooke A. 1990. Transfer of diabetes in mice prevented by blockade of adhesion-promoting receptor on macrophages. *Nature* **348:** 639–642. doi:10.1038/348639a0

Inoue Y, Kaifu T, Sugahara-Tobinai A, Nakamura A, Miyazaki JI, Takai T. 2007. Activating Fcγ receptors participate in the development of autoimmune diabetes in NOD mice. *J Immunol* **179:** 764–774. doi:10.4049/jimmunol.179.2.764

Ivanov II, Atarashi K, Manel N, Brodie EL, Shima T, Karaoz U, Wei D, Goldfarb KC, Santee CA, Lynch SV, et al. 2009. Induction of intestinal Th17 cells by segmented filamentous bacteria. *Cell* **139:** 485–498. doi:10.1016/j.cell.2009.09.033

Jansen A, Homo-Delarche F, Hooijkaas H, Leenen PJ, Dardenne M, Drexhage HA. 1994. Immunohistochemical characterization of monocytes-macrophages and dendritic cells involved in the initiation of the insulitis and β-cell destruction in NOD mice. *Diabetes* **43:** 667–675. doi:10.2337/diab.43.5.667

Jansen A, van Hagen M, Drexhage HA. 1995. Defective maturation and function of antigen-presenting cells in type 1 diabetes. *Lancet* **345:** 491–492. doi:10.1016/s0140-6736(95)90586-3

Jun HS, Yoon CS, Zbytnuik L, van Rooijen N, Yoon JW. 1999. The role of macrophages in T cell-mediated autoimmune diabetes in nonobese diabetic mice. *J Exp Med* **189:** 347–358. doi:10.1084/jem.189.2.347

Kadri N, Korpos E, Gupta S, Briet C, Löfbom L, Yagita H, Lehuen A, Boitard C, Holmberg D, Sorokin L, et al. 2012. $CD4^+$ type II NKT cells mediate ICOS and programmed death-1-dependent regulation of type 1 diabetes. *J Immunol* **188:** 3138–3149. doi:10.4049/jimmunol.1101390

Kägi D, Ho A, Odermatt B, Zakarian A, Ohashi PS, Mak TW. 1999. TNF receptor 1-dependent β cell toxicity as an effector pathway in autoimmune diabetes. *J Immunol* **162:** 4598–4605. doi:10.4049/jimmunol.162.8.4598

Kahaly GJ, Hansen MP. 2016. Type 1 diabetes associated autoimmunity. *Autoimmun Rev* **15:** 644–648. doi:10.1016/j.autrev.2016.02.017

Kaneto H, Fujii J, Seo HG, Suzuki K, Matsuoka T, Nakamura M, Tatsumi H, Yamasaki Y, Kamada T, Taniguchi N. 1995. Apoptotic cell death triggered by nitric oxide in pancreatic β-cells. *Diabetes* **44:** 733–738. doi:10.2337/diab.44.7.733

Kared H, Masson A, Adle-Biassette H, Bach JF, Chatenoud L, Zavala F. 2005. Treatment with granulocyte colony-stimulating factor prevents diabetes in NOD mice by recruiting plasmacytoid dendritic cells and functional $CD4^+CD25^+$ regulatory T-cells. *Diabetes* **54:** 78–84. doi:10.2337/diabetes.54.1.78

Kassem SA, Ariel I, Thornton PS, Scheimberg I, Glaser B. 2000. β-Cell proliferation and apoptosis in the developing normal human pancreas and in hyperinsulinism of infancy. *Diabetes* **49:** 1325–1333. doi:10.2337/diabetes.49.8.1325

Kayserova J, Vcelakova J, Stechova K, Dudkova E, Hromadkova H, Sumnik Z, Kolouskova S, Spisek R, Sediva A. 2014. Decreased dendritic cell numbers but increased TLR9-mediated interferon-α production in first degree relatives of type 1 diabetes patients. *Clin Immunol* **153:** 49–55. doi:10.1016/j.clim.2014.03.018

Kim HS, Han MS, Chung KW, Kim S, Kim E, Kim MJ, Jang E, Lee HA, Youn J, Akira S, et al. 2007. Toll-like receptor 2 senses β-cell death and contributes to the initiation of autoimmune diabetes. *Immunity* **27:** 321–333. doi:10.1016/j.immuni.2007.06.010

Kim DH, Lee JC, Kim S, Oh SH, Lee MK, Kim KW, Lee MS. 2011. Inhibition of autoimmune diabetes by TLR2 tolerance. *J Immunol* **187:** 5211–5220. doi:10.4049/jimmunol.1001388

Kis J, Engelmann P, Farkas K, Richman G, Eck S, Lolley J, Jalahej H, Borowiec M, Kent SC, Treszl A, et al. 2007. Reduced $CD4^+$ subset and Th1 bias of the human iNKT cells in type 1 diabetes mellitus. *J Leukoc Biol* **81:** 654–662. doi:10.1189/jlb.1106654

Klementowicz JE, Mahne AE, Spence A, Nguyen V, Satpathy AT, Murphy KM, Tang Q. 2017. Cutting edge: origins, recruitment, and regulation of $CD11c^+$ cells in inflamed islets of autoimmune diabetes mice. *J Immunol* **199:** 27–32. doi:10.4049/jimmunol.1601062

Kostic AD, Gevers D, Siljander H, Vatanen T, Hyötyläinen T, Hämäläinen AM, Peet A, Tillmann V, Pöhö P, Mattila I, et al. 2015. The dynamics of the human infant gut microbiome in development and in progression toward type 1 diabetes. *Cell Host Microbe* **17:** 260–273. doi:10.1016/j.chom.2015.01.001

Krętowski A, Mysliwiec J, Szelachowska M, Turowski D, Wysocka J, Kowalska I, Kinalska I. 1999. γδ T-cells alterations in the peripheral blood of high risk diabetes type 1 subjects with subclinical pancreatic B-cells impairment. *Immunol Lett* **68:** 289–293. doi:10.1016/s0165-2478(99)00066-8

Kriegel MA, Sefik E, Hill JA, Wu HJ, Benoist C, Mathis D. 2011. Naturally transmitted segmented filamentous bacteria segregate with diabetes protection in nonobese diabetic mice. *Proc Natl Acad Sci* **108:** 11548–11553. doi:10.1073/pnas.1108924108

Kriegel MA, Rathinam C, Flavell RA. 2012. Pancreatic islet expression of chemokine CCL2 suppresses autoimmune diabetes via tolerogenic $CD11c^+$ $CD11b^+$ dendritic cells. *Proc Natl Acad Sci* **109:** 3457–3462. doi:10.1073/pnas.1115308109

Krogvold L, Edwin B, Buanes T, Frisk G, Skog O, Anagandula M, Korsgren O, Undlien D, Eike MC, Richardson SJ, et al. 2015. Detection of a low-grade enteroviral infection in the islets of Langerhans of living patients newly diagnosed with type 1 diabetes. *Diabetes* **64:** 1682–1687. doi:10.2337/db14-1370

Kuric E, Krogvold L, Hanssen KF, Dahl-Jørgensen K, Skog O, Korsgren O. 2018. No evidence for presence of mucosal-associated invariant T cells in the insulitic lesions in patients recently diagnosed with type 1 diabetes. *Am J Pathol* **188:** 1744–1748. doi:10.1016/j.ajpath.2018.04.009

Laloux V, Beaudoin L, Jeske D, Carnaud C, Lehuen A. 2001. NK T cell-induced protection against diabetes in vα14-jα281 transgenic nonobese diabetic mice is associated with a Th2 shift circumscribed regionally to the islets and functionally to islet autoantigen. *J Immunol* **166:** 3749–3756. doi:10.4049/jimmunol.166.6.3749

Lang FP, Schatz DA, Pollock BH, Riley WJ, Maclaren NK, Dumont-Driscoll M, Barrett DJ. 1991. Increased T lymphocytes bearing the γδ T cell receptor in subjects at high risk for insulin dependent diabetes. *J Autoimmun* **4:** 925–933. doi:10.1016/0896-8411(91)90055-h

Lee KU, Kim MK, Amano K, Pak CY, Jaworski MA, Mehta JG, Yoon JW. 1988. Preferential infiltration of macrophages during early stages of insulitis in diabetes-prone BB rats. *Diabetes* **37:** 1053–1058. doi:10.2337/diab.37.8.1053

Lee AS, Gibson DL, Zhang Y, Sham HP, Vallance BA, Dutz JP. 2010. Gut barrier disruption by an enteric bacterial pathogen accelerates insulitis in NOD mice. *Diabetologia* **53:** 741–748. doi:10.1007/s00125-009-1626-y

Lee AS, Ghoreishi M, Cheng WK, Chang TYE, Zhang YQ, Dutz JP. 2011. Toll-like receptor 7 stimulation promotes autoimmune diabetes in the NOD mouse. *Diabetologia* **54:** 1407–1416. doi:10.1007/s00125-011-2083-y

Lee J, Cullum E, Stoltz K, Bachmann N, Strong Z, Millick DD, Denzin LK, Chang A, Tarakanova V, Chervonsky AV, et al. 2021. Mouse homologue of human HLA-DO does not preempt autoimmunity but controls murine γ-herpesvirus MHV68. *J Immunol* **207:** 2944–2951. doi:10.4049/jimmunol.2100650

Lee H, Sahin GS, Chen CW, Sonthalia S, Cañas SM, Oktay HZ, Duckworth AT, Brawerman G, Thompson PJ, Hatzoglou M, et al. 2023. Stress-induced β cell early senescence confers protection against type 1 diabetes. *Cell Metab* **35:** 2200–2215.e9. doi:10.1016/j.cmet.2023.10.014

Lehuen A, Lantz O, Beaudoin L, Laloux V, Carnaud C, Bendelac A, Bach JF, Monteiro RC. 1998. Overexpression of natural killer T cells protects Vα14-Jα281 transgenic non-obese diabetic mice against diabetes. *J Exp Med* **188:** 1831–1839. doi:10.1084/jem.188.10.1831

Li Q, McDevitt HO. 2011. The role of interferon α in initiation of type I diabetes in the NOD mouse. *Clin Immunol* **140:** 3–7. doi:10.1016/j.clim.2011.04.010

Li Q, Xu B, Michie SA, Rubins KH, Schreriber RD, McDevitt HO. 2008. Interferon-α initiates type 1 diabetes in non-obese diabetic mice. *Proc Natl Acad Sci* **105:** 12439–12444. doi:10.1073/pnas.0806439105

Liang SC, Tan XY, Luxenberg DP, Karim R, Dunussi-Joannopoulos K, Collins M, Fouser LA. 2006. Interleukin (IL)-22 and IL-17 are coexpressed by Th17 cells and cooperatively enhance expression of antimicrobial peptides. *J Exp Med* **203:** 2271–2279. doi:10.1084/jem.20061308

Liu D, Cardozo AK, Darville MI, Eizirik DL. 2002. Double-stranded RNA cooperates with interferon-γ and IL-1β to induce both chemokine expression and nuclear factor-κβ-dependent apoptosis in pancreatic β-cells: potential mechanisms for viral-induced insulitis and β-cell death in type 1 diabetes mellitus. *Endocrinology* **143:** 1225–1234. doi:10.1210/endo.143.4.8737

Livanos AE, Greiner TU, Vangay P, Pathmasiri W, Stewart D, McRitchie S, Li H, Chung J, Sohn J, Kim S, et al. 2016. Antibiotic-mediated gut microbiome perturbation accelerates development of type 1 diabetes in mice. *Nat Microbiol* **1:** 16140. doi:10.1038/nmicrobiol.2016.140

Lo Conte M, Cosorich I, Ferrarese R, Antonini Cencicchio M, Nobili A, Palmieri V, Massimino L, Lamparelli LA, Liang W, Riba M, et al. 2023. Alterations of the intestinal mucus layer correlate with dysbiosis and immune dysregulation in human type 1 diabetes. *EBioMedicine* **91:** 104567. doi:10.1016/j.ebiom.2023.104567

Ludewig B, Odermatt B, Landmann S, Hengartner H, Zinkernagel RM. 1998. Dendritic cells induce autoimmune diabetes and maintain disease via de novo formation of local lymphoid tissue. *J Exp Med* **188:** 1493–1501. doi:10.1084/jem.188.8.1493

Mariño E, Batten M, Groom J, Walters S, Liuwantara D, Mackay F, Grey ST. 2008. Marginal-zone B-cells of non-obese diabetic mice expand with diabetes onset, invade the pancreatic lymph nodes, and present autoantigen to diabetogenic T-cells. *Diabetes* **57:** 395–404. doi:10.2337/db07-0589

Mariño E, Richards JL, McLeod KH, Stanley D, Yap YA, Knight J, McKenzie C, Kranich J, Oliveira AC, Rossello FJ, et al. 2017. Gut microbial metabolites limit the frequency of autoimmune T cells and protect against type 1 diabetes. *Nat Immunol* **18:** 552–562. doi:10.1038/ni.3713

Markle JGM, Frank DN, Mortin-Toth S, Robertson CE, Feazel LM, Rolle-Kampczyk U, von Bergen M, McCoy KD, Macpherson AJ, Danska JS. 2013a. Sex differences in the gut microbiome drive hormone-dependent regulation of autoimmunity. *Science* **339:** 1084–1088. doi:10.1126/science.1233521

Markle JGM, Mortin-Toth S, Wong ASL, Geng L, Hayday A, Danska JS. 2013b. Γδ T cells are essential effectors of type 1 diabetes in the nonobese diabetic mouse model. *J Immunol* **190:** 5392–5401. doi:10.4049/jimmunol.1203502

Marleau AM, Singh B. 2002. Myeloid dendritic cells in non-obese diabetic mice have elevated costimulatory and T helper-1-inducing abilities. *J Autoimmun* **19:** 23–35. doi:10.1006/jaut.2002.0597

Martin AP, Rankin S, Pitchford S, Charo IF, Furtado GC, Lira SA. 2008. Increased expression of CCL2 in insulin-producing cells of transgenic mice promotes mobilization of myeloid cells from the bone marrow, marked insulitis, and diabetes. *Diabetes* **57:** 3025–3033. doi:10.2337/db08-0625

McLaughlin RJ, de Haan A, Zaldumbide A, de Koning EJ, de Ru AH, van Veelen PA, van Lummel M, Roep BO. 2016. Human islets and dendritic cells generate post-translationally modified islet autoantigens. *Clin Exp Immunol* **185:** 133–140. doi:10.1111/cei.12775

Meyerovich K, Ortis F, Allagnat F, Cardozo AK. 2016. Endoplasmic reticulum stress and the unfolded protein response in pancreatic islet inflammation. *J Mol Endocrinol* **57:** R1–R17. doi:10.1530/JME-15-0306

Miranda MCG, Oliveira RP, Torres L, Aguiar SLF, Pinheiro-Rosa N, Lemos L, Guimarães MA, Reis D, Silveira T, Ferreira Ê, et al. 2019. Frontline science: abnormalities in the gut mucosa of non-obese diabetic mice precede the onset of type 1 diabetes. *J Leukoc Biol* **106:** 513–529. doi:10.1002/JLB.3HI0119-024RR

Mollah ZUA, Pai S, Moore C, O'Sullivan BJ, Harrison MJ, Peng J, Phillips K, Prins JB, Cardinal J, Thomas R. 2008. Abnormal NF-κB function characterizes human type 1 diabetes dendritic cells and monocytes. *J Immunol* **180:** 3166–3175. doi:10.4049/jimmunol.180.5.3166

Moriwaki M, Itoh N, Miyagawa J, Yamamoto K, Imagawa A, Yamagata K, Iwahashi H, Nakajima H, Namba M, Nagata S, et al. 1999. Fas and Fas ligand expression in inflamed islets in pancreas sections of patients with recent-onset type I diabetes mellitus. *Diabetologia* **42:** 1332–1340. doi:10.1007/s001250051446

Nejentsev S, Walker N, Riches D, Egholm M, Todd JA. 2009. Rare variants of *IFIH1*, a gene implicated in antiviral responses, protect against type 1 diabetes. *Science* **324:** 387–389. doi:10.1126/science.1167728

Nel I, Beaudoin L, Gouda Z, Rousseau C, Soulard P, Rouland M, Bertrand L, Boitard C, Larger E, Lehuen A. 2021. MAIT cell alterations in adults with recent-onset and long-term type 1 diabetes. *Diabetologia* **64:** 2306–2321. doi:10.1007/s00125-021-05527-y

Neu J, Reverte CM, Mackey AD, Liboni K, Tuhacek-Tenace LM, Hatch M, Li N, Caicedo RA, Schatz DA, Atkinson M. 2005. Changes in intestinal morphology and permeability in the biobreeding rat before the onset of type 1 diabetes. *J*

Pediatr Gastroenterol Nutr **40:** 589–595. doi:10.1097/01.mpg.0000159636.19346.c1

O'Brien BA, Huang Y, Geng X, Dutz JP, Finegood DT. 2002. Phagocytosis of apoptotic cells by macrophages from NOD mice is reduced. *Diabetes* **51:** 2481–2488. doi:10.2337/diabetes.51.8.2481

O'Brien BA, Geng X, Orteu CH, Huang Y, Ghoreishi M, Zhang Y, Bush JA, Li G, Finegood DT, Dutz JP. 2006. A deficiency in the in vivo clearance of apoptotic cells is a feature of the NOD mouse. *J Autoimmun* **26:** 104–115. doi:10.1016/j.jaut.2005.11.006

Ohashi PS, Oehen S, Buerki K, Pircher H, Ohashi CT, Odermatt B, Malissen B, Zinkernagel RM, Hengartner H. 1991. Ablation of "tolerance" and induction of diabetes by virus infection in viral antigen transgenic mice. *Cell* **65:** 305–317. doi:10.1016/0092-8674(91)90164-t

Oikawa Y, Shimada A, Yamada S, Motohashi Y, Nakagawa Y, Irie JI, Maruyama T, Saruta T. 2002. High frequency of $v\alpha24^+$ $v\beta11^+$ T-cells observed in type 1 diabetes. *Diabetes Care* **25:** 1818–1823. doi:10.2337/diacare.25.10.1818

Oldstone MB, Nerenberg M, Southern P, Price J, Lewicki H. 1991. Virus infection triggers insulin-dependent diabetes mellitus in a transgenic model: role of anti-self (virus) immune response. *Cell* **65:** 319–331. doi:10.1016/0092-8674(91)90165-u

Parsa R, Andresen P, Gillett A, Mia S, Zhang XM, Mayans S, Holmberg D, Harris RA. 2012. Adoptive transfer of immunomodulatory M2 macrophages prevents type 1 diabetes in NOD mice. *Diabetes* **61:** 2881–2892. doi:10.2337/db11-1635

Patrick C, Wang GS, Lefebvre DE, Crookshank JA, Sonier B, Eberhard C, Mojibian M, Kennedy CR, Brooks SPJ, Kalmokoff ML, et al. 2013. Promotion of autoimmune diabetes by cereal diet in the presence or absence of microbes associated with gut immune activation, regulatory imbalance, and altered cathelicidin antimicrobial peptide. *Diabetes* **62:** 2036–2047. doi:10.2337/db12-1243

Pellegrini S, Sordi V, Bolla AM, Saita D, Ferrarese R, Canducci F, Clementi M, Invernizzi F, Mariani A, Bonfanti R, et al. 2017. Duodenal mucosa of patients with type 1 diabetes shows distinctive inflammatory profile and microbiota. *J Clin Endocrinol Metab* **102:** 1468–1477. doi:10.1210/jc.2016-3222

Peng R, Li Y, Brezner K, Litherland S, Clare-Salzler MJ. 2003. Abnormal peripheral blood dendritic cell populations in type 1 diabetes. *Ann NY Acad Sci* **1005:** 222–225. doi:10.1196/annals.1288.031

Pickard JM, Maurice CF, Kinnebrew MA, Abt MC, Schenten D, Golovkina TV, Bogatyrev SR, Ismagilov RF, Pamer EG, Turnbaugh PJ, et al. 2014. Rapid fucosylation of intestinal epithelium sustains host-commensal symbiosis in sickness. *Nature* **514:** 638–641. doi:10.1038/nature13823

Poirot L, Benoist C, Mathis D. 2004. Natural killer cells distinguish innocuous and destructive forms of pancreatic islet autoimmunity. *Proc Natl Acad Sci* **101:** 8102–8107. doi:10.1073/pnas.0402065101

Poligone B, Weaver DJ, Sen P, Baldwin AS, Tisch R. 2002. Elevated NF-κB activation in nonobese diabetic mouse dendritic cells results in enhanced APC function. *J Immunol* **168:** 188–196. doi:10.4049/jimmunol.168.1.188

Pöysti S, Toivonen R, Takeda A, Silojärvi S, Yatkin E, Miyasaka M, Hänninen A. 2022. Infection with the enteric pathogen *C. rodentium* promotes islet-specific autoimmunity by activating a lymphatic route from the gut to pancreatic lymph node. *Mucosal Immunol* **15:** 471–479. doi:10.1038/s41385-022-00490-2

Raine T, Zaccone P, Mastroeni P, Cooke A. 2006. *Salmonella typhimurium* infection in nonobese diabetic mice generates immunomodulatory dendritic cells able to prevent type 1 diabetes. *J Immunol* **177:** 2224–2233. doi:10.4049/jimmunol.177.4.2224

Reddy S, Liu W, Elliott RB. 1993. Distribution of pancreatic macrophages preceding and during early insulitis in young NOD mice. *Pancreas* **8:** 602–608. doi:10.1097/00006676-199309000-00012

Roep BO, Kleijwegt FS, van Halteren AGS, Bonato V, Boggi U, Vendrame F, Marchetti P, Dotta F. 2010. Islet inflammation and CXCL10 in recent-onset type 1 diabetes. *Clin Exp Immunol* **159:** 338–343. doi:10.1111/j.1365-2249.2009.04087.x

Roep BO, Thomaidou S, van Tienhoven R, Zaldumbide A. 2021. Type 1 diabetes mellitus as a disease of the β-cell (do not blame the immune system?) *Nat Rev Endocrinol* **17:** 150–161. doi:10.1038/s41574-020-00443-4

Rouland M, Beaudoin L, Rouxel O, Bertrand L, Cagninacci L, Saffarian A, Pedron T, Gueddouri D, Guilmeau S, Burnol AF, et al. 2022. Gut mucosa alterations and loss of segmented filamentous bacteria in type 1 diabetes are associated with inflammation rather than hyperglycaemia. *Gut* **71:** 296–308. doi:10.1136/gutjnl-2020-323664

Rouxel O, Da Silva J, Beaudoin L, Nel I, Tard C, Cagninacci L, Kiaf B, Oshima M, Diedisheim M, Salou M, et al. 2017. Cytotoxic and regulatory roles of mucosal-associated invariant T cells in type 1 diabetes. *Nat Immunol* **18:** 1321–1331. doi:10.1038/ni.3854

Saksida T, Paunović V, Koprivica I, Mićanović D, Jevtić B, Jonić N, Stojanović I, Pejnović N. 2023. Development of type 1 diabetes in mice is associated with a decrease in IL-2-producing ILC3 and $FoxP3^+$ Treg in the small intestine. *Molecules* **28:** 3366. doi:10.3390/molecules28083366

Santamaria P, Lewis C, Jessurun J, Sutherland DE, Barbosa JJ. 1994. Skewed T-cell receptor usage and junctional heterogeneity among isletitis αβ and γδ T-cells in human IDDM [corrected]. *Diabetes* **43:** 599–606. doi:10.2337/diab.43.4.599

Saunders KA, Raine T, Cooke A, Lawrence CE. 2007. Inhibition of autoimmune type 1 diabetes by gastrointestinal helminth infection. *Infect Immun* **75:** 397–407. doi:10.1128/IAI.00664-06

Savilahti E, Örmälä T, Saukkonen T, Sandini-Pohjavuori U, Kantele JM, Arato A, Ilonen J, Akerblom HK. 1999. Jejuna of patients with insulin-dependent diabetes mellitus (IDDM) show signs of immune activation. *Clin Exp Immunol* **116:** 70–77. doi:10.1046/j.1365-2249.1999.00860.x

Savinov AY, Wong FS, Chervonsky AV. 2001. IFN-γ affects homing of diabetogenic T cells. *J Immunol* **167:** 6637–6643. doi:10.4049/jimmunol.167.11.6637

Savinov AY, Tcherepanov A, Green EA, Flavell RA, Chervonsky AV. 2003a. Contribution of Fas to diabetes development. *Proc Natl Acad Sci* **100:** 628–632. doi:10.1073/pnas.0237359100

Savinov AY, Wong FS, Stonebraker AC, Chervonsky AV. 2003b. Presentation of antigen by endothelial cells and chemoattraction are required for homing of insulin-specific CD8+ T cells. *J Exp Med* **197:** 643–656. doi:10.1084/jem.20021378

Saxena V, Ondr JK, Magnusen AF, Munn DH, Katz JD. 2007. The countervailing actions of myeloid and plasmacytoid dendritic cells control autoimmune diabetes in the nonobese diabetic mouse. *J Immunol* **179:** 5041–5053. doi:10.4049/jimmunol.179.8.5041

Secondulfo M, Iafusco D, Carratù R, deMagistris L, Sapone A, Generoso M, Mezzogiomo A, Sasso FC, Cartenì M, De Rosa R, et al. 2004. Ultrastructural mucosal alterations and increased intestinal permeability in non-celiac, type I diabetic patients. *Dig Liver Dis* **36:** 35–45. doi:10.1016/j.dld.2003.09.016

Serreze DV, Ottendorfer EW, Ellis TM, Gauntt CJ, Atkinson MA. 2000. Acceleration of type 1 diabetes by a coxsackievirus infection requires a preexisting critical mass of autoreactive T-cells in pancreatic islets. *Diabetes* **49:** 708–711. doi:10.2337/diabetes.49.5.708

Sharif S, Arreaza GA, Zucker P, Mi QS, Sondhi J, Naidenko OV, Kronenberg M, Koezuka Y, Delovitch TL, Gombert JM, et al. 2001. Activation of natural killer T cells by α-galactosylceramide treatment prevents the onset and recurrence of autoimmune type 1 diabetes. *Nat Med* **7:** 1057–1062. doi:10.1038/nm0901-1057

Shibasaki S, Imagawa A, Tauriainen S, Iino M, Oikarinen M, Abiru H, Tamaki K, Seino H, Nishi K, Takase I, et al. 2010. Expression of toll-like receptors in the pancreas of recent-onset fulminant type 1 diabetes. *Endocr J* **57:** 211–219. doi:10.1507/endocrj.k09e-291

Shu L, Zhong L, Xiao Y, Wu X, Liu Y, Jiang X, Tang T, Hoo R, Zhou Z, Xu A. 2020. Neutrophil elastase triggers the development of autoimmune diabetes by exacerbating innate immune responses in pancreatic islets of non-obese diabetic mice. *Clin Sci (Lond)* **134:** 1679–1696. doi:10.1042/CS20200021

Simoni Y, Gautron AS, Beaudoin L, Bui LC, Michel ML, Coumoul X, Eberl G, Leite-de-Moraes M, Lehuen A. 2011. NOD mice contain an elevated frequency of iNKT17 cells that exacerbate diabetes. *Eur J Immunol* **41:** 3574–3585. doi:10.1002/eji.201141751

Smyth DJ, Cooper JD, Bailey R, Field S, Burren O, Smink LJ, Guja C, Ionescu-Tirgoviste C, Widmer B, Dunger DB, et al. 2006. A genome-wide association study of nonsynonymous SNPs identifies a type 1 diabetes locus in the interferon-induced helicase (IFIH1) region. *Nat Genet* **38:** 617–619. doi:10.1038/ng1800

Soltani S, Mostafaei S, Aslani S, Farhadi E, Mahmoudi M. 2020. Association of KIR gene polymorphisms with type 1 diabetes: a meta-analysis. *J Diabetes Metab Disord* **19:** 1777–1786. doi:10.1007/s40200-020-00569-2

Sorini C, Cosorich I, Lo Conte M, De Giorgi L, Facciotti F, Lucianò R, Rocchi M, Ferrarese R, Sanvito F, Canducci F, et al. 2019. Loss of gut barrier integrity triggers activation of islet-reactive T cells and autoimmune diabetes. *Proc Natl Acad Sci* **116:** 15140–15149. doi:10.1073/pnas.1814558116

Stassi G, De Maria R, Trucco G, Rudert W, Testi R, Galluzzo A, Giordano C, Trucco M. 1997. Nitric oxide primes pancreatic β cells for Fas-mediated destruction in insulin-dependent diabetes mellitus. *J Exp Med* **186:** 1193–1200. doi:10.1084/jem.186.8.1193

Steptoe RJ, Ritchie JM, Harrison LC. 2002. Increased generation of dendritic cells from myeloid progenitors in autoimmune-prone nonobese diabetic mice. *J Immunol* **168:** 5032–5041. doi:10.4049/jimmunol.168.10.5032

Stewart CJ, Ajami NJ, O'Brien JL, Hutchinson DS, Smith DP, Wong MC, Ross MC, Lloyd RE, Doddapaneni H, Metcalf GA, et al. 2018. Temporal development of the gut microbiome in early childhood from the TEDDY study. *Nature* **562:** 583–588. doi:10.1038/s41586-018-0617-x

Stoffels K, Overbergh L, Giulietti A, Kasran A, Bouillon R, Gysemans C, Mathieu C. 2004. NOD macrophages produce high levels of inflammatory cytokines upon encounter of apoptotic or necrotic cells. *J Autoimmun* **23:** 9–15. doi:10.1016/j.jaut.2004.03.012

Suarez-Pinzon WL, Szabó C, Rabinovitch A. 1997. Development of autoimmune diabetes in NOD mice is associated with the formation of peroxynitrite in pancreatic islet β-cells. *Diabetes* **46:** 907–911. doi:10.2337/diab.46.5.907

Sun J, Furio L, Mecheri R, van der Does AM, Lundeberg E, Saveanu L, Chen Y, van Endert P, Agerberth B, Diana J. 2015. Pancreatic β-cells limit autoimmune diabetes via an immunoregulatory antimicrobial peptide expressed under the influence of the gut microbiota. *Immunity* **43:** 304–317. doi:10.1016/j.immuni.2015.07.013

Takahashi K, Honeyman MC, Harrison LC. 1998. Impaired yield, phenotype, and function of monocyte-derived dendritic cells in humans at risk for insulin-dependent diabetes. *J Immunol* **161:** 2629–2635. doi:10.4049/jimmunol.161.5.2629

Todd JA, Bell JI, McDevitt HO. 1987. HLA-DQβ gene contributes to susceptibility and resistance to insulin-dependent diabetes mellitus. *Nature* **329:** 599–604. doi:10.1038/329599a0

Turley S, Poirot L, Hattori M, Benoist C, Mathis D. 2003. Physiological β cell death triggers priming of self-reactive T cells by dendritic cells in a type-1 diabetes model. *J Exp Med* **198:** 1527–1537. doi:10.1084/jem.20030966

Turley SJ, Lee JW, Dutton-Swain N, Mathis D, Benoist C. 2005. Endocrine self and gut non-self intersect in the pancreatic lymph nodes. *Proc Natl Acad Sci* **102:** 17729–17733. doi:10.1073/pnas.0509006102

Uno S, Imagawa A, Okita K, Sayama K, Moriwaki M, Iwahashi H, Yamagata K, Tamura S, Matsuzawa Y, Hanafusa T, et al. 2007. Macrophages and dendritic cells infiltrating islets with or without β cells produce tumour necrosis factor-α in patients with recent-onset type 1 diabetes. *Diabetologia* **50:** 596–601. doi:10.1007/s00125-006-0569-9

Usero L, Sánchez A, Pizarro E, Xufré C, Martí M, Jaraquemada D, Roura-Mir C. 2016. Interleukin-13 pathway alterations impair invariant natural killer T-cell-mediated regulation of effector T cells in type 1 diabetes. *Diabetes* **65:** 2356–2366. doi:10.2337/db15-1350

Vaarala O, Atkinson MA, Neu J. 2008. The "perfect storm" for type 1 diabetes: the complex interplay between intestinal microbiota, gut permeability, and mucosal immunity. *Diabetes* **57:** 2555–2562. doi:10.2337/db08-0331

Valle A, Giamporcaro GM, Scavini M, Stabilini A, Grogan P, Bianconi E, Sebastiani G, Masini M, Maugeri N, Porretti L, et al. 2013. Reduction of circulating neutrophils precedes and accompanies type 1 diabetes. *Diabetes* **62:** 2072–2077. doi:10.2337/db12-1345

Van Belle TL, Juntti T, Liao J, von Herrath MG. 2010. Preexisting autoimmunity determines type 1 diabetes outcome after Flt3-ligand treatment. *J Autoimmun* **34:** 445–452. doi:10.1016/j.jaut.2009.11.010

Van Belle TL, Nierkens S, Arens R, von Herrath MG. 2012. Interleukin-21 receptor-mediated signals control autoreactive T cell infiltration in pancreatic islets. *Immunity* **36:** 1060–1072. doi:10.1016/j.immuni.2012.04.005

van Lummel M, van Veelen PA, de Ru AH, Janssen GMC, Pool J, Laban S, Joosten AM, Nikolic T, Drijfhout JW, Mearin ML, et al. 2016. Dendritic cells guide islet autoimmunity through a restricted and uniquely processed peptidome presented by high-risk HLA-DR. *J Immunol* **196:** 3253–3263. doi:10.4049/jimmunol.1501282

Varanasi V, Avanesyan L, Schumann DM, Chervonsky AV. 2012. Cytotoxic mechanisms employed by mouse T cells to destroy pancreatic β-cells. *Diabetes* **61:** 2862–2870. doi:10.2337/db11-1784

Vatanen T, Kostic AD, d'Hennezel E, Siljander H, Franzosa EA, Yassour M, Kolde R, Vlamakis H, Arthur TD, Hämäläinen AM, et al. 2016. Variation in microbiome LPS immunogenicity contributes to autoimmunity in humans. *Cell* **165:** 842–853. doi:10.1016/j.cell.2016.04.007

Vatanen T, Franzosa EA, Schwager R, Tripathi S, Arthur TD, Vehik K, Lernmark Å, Hagopian WA, Rewers MJ, She JX, et al. 2018. The human gut microbiome in early-onset type 1 diabetes from the TEDDY study. *Nature* **562:** 589–594. doi:10.1038/s41586-018-0620-2

Vecchio F, Lo Buono N, Stabilini A, Nigi L, Dufort MJ, Geyer S, Rancoita PM, Cugnata F, Mandelli A, Valle A, et al. 2018. Abnormal neutrophil signature in the blood and pancreas of presymptomatic and symptomatic type 1 diabetes. *JCI Insight* **3:** e122146. doi:10.1172/jci.insight.122146

Voorbij HA, Jeucken PH, Kabel PJ, De Haan M, Drexhage HA. 1989. Dendritic cells and scavenger macrophages in pancreatic islets of prediabetic BB rats. *Diabetes* **38:** 1623–1629. doi:10.2337/diab.38.12.1623

Wachlin G, Augstein P, Schröder D, Kuttler B, Klöting I, Heinke P, Schmidt S. 2003. IL-1β, IFN-γ and TNF-α increase vulnerability of pancreatic β cells to autoimmune destruction. *J Autoimmun* **20:** 303–312. doi:10.1016/s0896-8411(03)00039-8

Walker R, Bone AJ, Cooke A, Baird JD. 1988. Distinct macrophage subpopulations in pancreas of prediabetic BB/E rats: possible role for macrophages in pathogenesis of IDDM. *Diabetes* **37:** 1301–1304. doi:10.2337/diab.37.9.1301

Wang J, Cho S, Ueno A, Cheng L, Xu BY, Desrosiers MD, Shi Y, Yang Y. 2008. Ligand-dependent induction of noninflammatory dendritic cells by anergic invariant NKT cells minimizes autoimmune inflammation. *J Immunol* **181:** 2438–2445. doi:10.4049/jimmunol.181.4.2438

Wang K, Ye F, Chen Y, Xu J, Zhao Y, Wang Y, Lan T. 2021. Association between enterovirus infection and type 1 diabetes risk: a meta-analysis of 38 case-control studies. *Front Endocrinol (Lausanne)* **12:** 706964. doi:10.3389/fendo.2021.706964

Wen L, Peng J, Li Z, Wong FS. 2004. The effect of innate immunity on autoimmune diabetes and the expression of Toll-like receptors on pancreatic islets. *J Immunol* **172:** 3173–3180. doi:10.4049/jimmunol.172.5.3173

Wen L, Ley RE, Volchkov PY, Stranges PB, Avanesyan L, Stonebraker AC, Hu C, Wong FS, Szot GL, Bluestone JA, et al. 2008. Innate immunity and intestinal microbiota in the development of type 1 diabetes. *Nature* **455:** 1109–1113. doi:10.1038/nature07336

Westerholm-Ormio M, Vaarala O, Pihkala P, Ilonen J, Savilahti E. 2003. Immunologic activity in the small intestinal mucosa of pediatric patients with type 1 diabetes. *Diabetes* **52:** 2287–2295. doi:10.2337/diabetes.52.9.2287

Willcox A, Richardson SJ, Bone AJ, Foulis AK, Morgan NG. 2009. Analysis of islet inflammation in human type 1 diabetes. *Clin Exp Immunol* **155:** 173–181. doi:10.1111/j.1365-2249.2008.03860.x

Wilson SB, Kent SC, Patton KT, Orban T, Jackson RA, Exley M, Porcelli S, Schatz DA, Atkinson MA, Balk SP, et al. 1998. Extreme Th1 bias of invariant Vα24JαQ T cells in type 1 diabetes. *Nature* **391:** 177–181. doi:10.1038/34419

Wong FS, Hu C, Zhang L, Du W, Alexopoulou L, Flavell RA, Wen L. 2008. The role of Toll-like receptors 3 and 9 in the development of autoimmune diabetes in NOD mice. *Ann NY Acad Sci* **1150:** 146–148. doi:10.1196/annals.1447.039

Xia CQ, Peng R, Chernatynskaya AV, Yuan L, Carter C, Valentine J, Sobel E, Atkinson MA, Clare-Salzler MJ. 2014. Increased IFN-α-producing plasmacytoid dendritic cells (pDCs) in human Th1-mediated type 1 diabetes: pDCs augment Th1 responses through IFN-α production. *J Immunol* **193:** 1024–1034. doi:10.4049/jimmunol.1303230

Yin B, Ma G, Yen CY, Zhou Z, Wang GX, Divino CM, Casares S, Chen SH, Yang WC, Pan PY. 2010. Myeloid-derived suppressor cells prevent type 1 diabetes in murine models. *J Immunol* **185:** 5828–5834. doi:10.4049/jimmunol.0903636

Yoon JW, Austin M, Onodera T, Notkins AL. 1979. Virus-induced diabetes mellitus—isolation of a virus from the pancreas of a child with diabetic ketoacidosis. *N Engl J Med* **300:** 1173–1179. doi:10.1056/NEJM197905243002102

Yurkovetskiy L, Burrows M, Khan AA, Graham L, Volchkov P, Becker L, Antonopoulos D, Umesaki Y, Chervonsky AV. 2013. Gender bias in autoimmunity is influenced by microbiota. *Immunity* **39:** 400–412. doi:10.1016/j.immuni.2013.08.013

Zaccone P, Fehérvári Z, Jones FM, Sidobre S, Kronenberg M, Dunne DW, Cooke A. 2003. *Schistosoma mansoni* antigens modulate the activity of the innate immune response and prevent onset of type 1 diabetes. *Eur J Immunol* **33:** 1439–1449. doi:10.1002/eji.200323910

Zakharov PN, Hu H, Wan X, Unanue ER. 2020. Single-cell RNA sequencing of murine islets shows high cellular complexity at all stages of autoimmune diabetes. *J Exp Med* **217:** e20192362. doi:10.1084/jem.20192362

Zhang Y, Lee AS, Shameli A, Geng X, Finegood D, Santamaria P, Dutz JP. 2010. TLR9 blockade inhibits activation of diabetogenic CD8^{+} T cells and delays autoimmune diabetes. *J Immunol* **184:** 5645–5653. doi:10.4049/jimmunol.0901814

T Cell Differentiation in Autoimmune Type 1 Diabetes

Andrea Schietinger,[1,2] Ian T. McBain,[2] Katrina M. Hawley,[1] and Svetlana Miakicheva[2]

[1]Immunology Program, Memorial Sloan Kettering Cancer Center, New York, New York 10065, USA

[2]Immunology and Microbial Pathogenesis Program, Weill Cornell Graduate School of Medical Sciences, New York, New York 10065, USA

Correspondence: schietia@mskcc.org

Type 1 diabetes (T1D) is a progressive T cell–mediated autoimmune disease that results from the breakdown of tolerance mechanisms in β-cell-specific T cells. Although CD8 T cells are primarily responsible for the destruction of insulin-producing β cells, intriguingly, HLA class II allelic polymorphisms confer the greatest genetic risk for the development of T1D, suggesting a critical role of CD4 T cells in disease initiation and progression. Many aspects of autoimmune T cell differentiation remain enigmatic, including where and how autoimmune CD8 and CD4 T cells arise, which molecular programs control autoimmune T cell differentiation, and how CD8 T cells sustain β-cell destruction in the face of persistent self-antigen encounter. In this work, we summarize our current understanding of β-cell-specific CD8 and CD4 T cell differentiation and function, the role of autoimmune stem-like progenitor CD8 T cells in initiating and sustaining disease, and molecular programs and key transcription factors associated with the diabetogenic T cell response.

The pathogenesis of autoimmune T1D is complex and involves immune cell infiltration of the pancreas: self-reactive β-cell-specific CD8 T cells destroy insulin-producing β cells in the pancreatic islets of Langerhans, leading to insulin deficiency and loss of glucose homeostasis (Bluestone et al. 2010; Herold et al. 2024). Although β-cell-specific CD8 T cells are thought to be the primary pathogenic population that eliminates β cells, MHC class II allelic polymorphisms (including HLA-DR3/4 and HLA-DQ2/8) confer the greatest genetic risk for the development of T1D, suggesting a critical role of CD4 T cells in T1D pathogenesis (Rich et al. 1984; Redondo et al. 2018). Despite notable advances in antigen discovery (Delong et al. 2016; Pugliese 2017; Purcell et al. 2019; James et al. 2020; Mannering et al. 2021), many aspects of autoimmune β-cell-specific T cell differentiation and programming remain elusive, including (1) where and how autoimmune T cells arise, (2) how β-cell-specific CD8 T cells avoid functional "exhaustion" and sustain β-cell destruction in the face of persistent self-antigen, and (3) how CD4 T cells facilitate the pathogenic CD8 T cell response.

Many T cell–mediated autoimmune diseases, including T1D, are caused by the break-

Cite this article as *Cold Spring Harb Perspect Med* doi: 10.1101/cshperspect.a041592

down of peripheral tolerance mechanisms, allowing self-reactive T cells to acquire cytotoxic effector function and destroy self-tissues. Genetic predisposition combined with environmental factors (e.g., viral infections) has been implicated in triggering the breakdown of T cell tolerance to β-cell antigens (Gamble et al. 1969; Yeung et al. 2011; Coppieters et al. 2012; Knip and Simell 2012). More than 100 genome-wide regions (encompassing ~50 genes) have been linked to T1D-risk (Robertson et al. 2021), many of which are defined by single-nucleotide polymorphisms (SNPs) predominantly found within genes involved in immune regulation such as T cell activation, function, and differentiation (e.g., kinases/phosphatases [*PTPN22*], transcription factors [*BACH2*], cytokines and cytokine receptors [*IL-2RA*, *IL-2*, *IL-10*, *PRF1*], and costimulatory/inhibitory molecules [*CTLA4*]). Given the significant genetic risk conferred by variations in HLA loci and immune-related genes, T cell–self-antigen interactions are considered the main drivers of T1D pathogenesis.

CD8 T cells specific for numerous β-cell antigens have been identified in the pancreas, pancreatic lymph node (pLN), and peripheral blood of patients with T1D, and include specificities against insulin (INS) and islet-associated glucose-6-phosphatase catalytic subunit-related protein (IGRP) (James et al. 2020). Interestingly, β-cell-specific CD8 T cells are also found in the peripheral blood of healthy individuals, with similar frequencies to those found in patients with T1D (Mallone et al. 2007; Culina et al. 2018). Due to the inaccessibility of the pancreas, most studies have been limited to sampling T cells in circulation; T cells in the blood, however, do not accurately reflect the phenotypes of T cells in the pancreas (Culina et al. 2018). Thus, mechanistic insights into human autoimmune β-cell-specific T cell differentiation and functional states remain limited.

Most of our knowledge on the mechanistic underpinnings of T1D pathogenesis has come from studies in the nonobese diabetic (NOD) mouse, a spontaneous clinically relevant mouse model of T1D. The NOD mouse recapitulates many aspects of the human disease, including CD4 and CD8 T cell responses to many of the same β-cell antigens and similar T1D risk-associated genes (Anderson and Bluestone 2005; Unanue 2014). Technological advances, such as single-cell transcriptional and epigenetic analyses, spatial transcriptomics, and analyses of T cell receptor (TCR) repertoires of T cells from pLN and pancreas of NOD mice as well as human tissues have allowed us to begin to dissect differentiation state dynamics, phenotypes, and molecular programs of β-cell-specific CD8 and CD4 T cells involved in T1D pathogenesis (Ito et al. 2018; Gioia et al. 2019; Abdelsamed et al. 2020; Zakharov et al. 2020; Fasolino et al. 2022; Gearty et al. 2022; Grebinoski et al. 2022; Kasmani et al. 2022; Collier et al. 2023; Patil et al. 2023, 2024; Mitchell et al. 2024).

In this work, we summarize our current understanding of T cell differentiation, function, and population heterogeneity of β-cell-specific CD8 and CD4 T cells in T1D. We discuss the molecular programs and key transcription factors (TFs) associated with the diabetogenic T cell response, the role of stem-like progenitor CD8 T cells in initiating and sustaining disease, and the role of CD4 T cells in β-cell-specific CD8 T cell differentiation and function.

β-CELL-SPECIFIC CD8 AND CD4 T CELLS: CELLULAR PLAYERS IN T1D PATHOGENESIS

β-Cell destruction in NOD mice begins at an early age, with infiltration of innate immune cells (e.g., macrophages) into the pancreatic islets (Lee et al. 1988), causing sufficient β-cell damage leading to antigen presentation in the pLN. Disease initiation in NOD mice requires CD8 T cell priming in the pLN and reactivity to insulin by CD4 T cells (Höglund et al. 1999; Ferris et al. 2016; Gagnerault et al. 2022): (1) removal of the pLN in young NOD mice protects against insulitis and T1D (Levisetti et al. 2004; Gagnerault et al. 2022), and (2) a single-point mutation in the CD4 T cell epitope InsB9:23 (insulin B chain) completely prevents T1D of NOD mice (Nakayama et al. 2005). *Batf3*-dependent $CD103^+$ dendritic cells (DCs), a DC subset that accumulates in NOD islets and migrates to the pLN, are essential for β-cell-specific CD8 and CD4 T cell priming and migration to the pancreas; *Batf3*-deficient NOD mice (which lack CD103$^+$ DC) are completely protected from T1D (Ferris et al. 2014). Thus, an interdependent relationship between DC, CD4 T cells, and CD8 T cells in pLN initiates autoimmune T1D. How precisely CD4 T cells and DC prime β-cell-specific CD8 T cells and initiate autoimmune CD8 T cell differentiation in pLN remains unclear.

While innate immune cells and CD4 T cells are required to prime and initiate pancreatic infiltration of CD8 T cells, CD8 T cells act as the major T cell population driving pancreatic islet destruction. The appearance of certain CD8 T cell specificities in pancreatic islets is not random; antigens from insulin are generally considered to be the earliest antigens targeted by CD8 T cells in NOD mice and T1D patients, with epitope spreading to other antigens occurring over time (Dubois-LaForgue et al. 1999; Wong et al. 1999). CD8 T cells recognizing the β-cell antigen IGRP represent a major pathogenic population in later disease stages in mice and humans (DiLorenzo et al. 2002; Lieberman et al. 2003). CD8 T cells are able to directly kill β cells in an antigen-dependent manner, primarily via the release of cytolytic granules containing granzymes and perforin, cytokine IFN-γ, and to a lesser extent FasL/Fas (Thomas et al. 2010; Mollah et al. 2012; Trivedi et al. 2016; De George et al. 2023). NOD mice lacking MHC class I on β cells fail to develop diabetes, and mice depleted of CD8 T cells during insulitis are protected (Wang et al. 1996; Hamilton-Williams et al. 2003).

Although adoptive transfer studies utilizing monoclonal TCR transgenic β-cell-specific CD4 T cells showed that CD4 T cells can transfer disease independently of CD8 T cells (Haskins and McDuffie 1990; Katz et al. 1993; Mitchell et al. 2024), numerous studies have demonstrated a codependence of CD4 and CD8 T cells for disease, but underlying mechanisms remain incompletely understood (Christianson et al. 1993; Burton et al. 2008; Phillips et al. 2009). CD4 T cell and CD8 T cell codependency has been shown in two ways: (1) antibody-mediated depletion of CD4 or CD8 T cells in NOD wild-type (WT) mice prevents T1D (Miller et al. 1988; Shizuru et al. 1988), and (2) adoptive transfer of β-cell-specific CD8 T cells into NOD SCID mice (which lack endogenous T and B cells) requires cotransfer of CD4 T cells for pancreatic infiltration and disease onset (e.g., polyclonal CD4 T cells from spleens of prediabetic NOD WT mice) (Christianson et al. 1993). T1D involves two sequential steps at two anatomically distinct sites: the pLN, where CD4 T cells initiate autoimmune CD8 T cell priming and programming, and the pancreas/islets, where CD4 T cells may be required for maintaining diabetogenic CD8 T cell function and cytotoxicity. For each step, we will discuss possible mechanisms as to how CD8 and CD4 T cells exert their function(s).

β-CELL-SPECIFIC CD8 T CELLS: PHENOTYPES AND FUNCTIONAL STATES

CD8 T cell differentiation and functional states are determined by the nature, context, and duration of antigen encounter (Fig. 1; Phillip and Schietinger 2022). In acute, inflammatory settings (e.g., acute infection), naive antigen-specific CD8 T cells differentiate into highly functional cytotoxic effector T cells and ultimately form memory T cells. In settings where CD8 T cells are exposed to persistent antigen and receive chronic TCR stimulation, such as in the context of tumors or chronic infections, CD8 T cells generally enter a hyporesponsive state referred to as T cell exhaustion or dysfunction (Philip and Schietinger 2022); exhausted/dysfunctional T cells express numerous inhibitory molecules, such as PD1, CTLA4, LAG3, CD39, 2B4, TIM3, TIGIT, and are unable to produce effector cytokines (IFN-γ, TNF-α) and/or cytotoxic molecules (perforin, granzyme). In autoimmune T1D, β-cell-specific CD8 T cells express inhibitory receptors, the same as those expressed by antigen-specific exhausted/dysfunctional CD8 T cells in tumors and chronic infections (Fig. 1; McKinney et al. 2015; Abdelsamed et al. 2020; Ciecko et al. 2021; Gearty et al. 2022; Grebinoski et al. 2022; Kasmani et al. 2022; Collier et al. 2023; Selck et al. 2024). Paradoxically, despite presumed "chronic" β-cell-/self-antigen exposure and acquisition of an "exhausted" phenotype, β-cell-specific T cells do not become dysfunctional and instead retain

Settings of persistent antigen encounter

Context	Antigen load	Specificity	Affinity (TCR/pMHC)	Functional state	Inhibitory receptors	Transcription factors	
Autoimmune type 1 diabetes		Self	Low	Functional	Yes	TCF1^hi (Stem-like) TCF1^lo (Diff)	TOX+
Tumor		Self or neo/ foreign	Low and high (depending on antigen specificity)	Dysfunctional (also referred to as anergic, exhausted)	Yes	TCF1^hi (Stem-like) TCF1^lo (Diff)	TOX+
Chronic infection		Foreign	High	Exhausted	Yes	TCF1^hi (Stem-like) TCF1^lo (Diff)	TOX+
Acute infection		Foreign	High	Functional	Low/no and transient	TCF1^lo (Effector) TCF1^hi (Memory)	Transiently TOX^lo/+

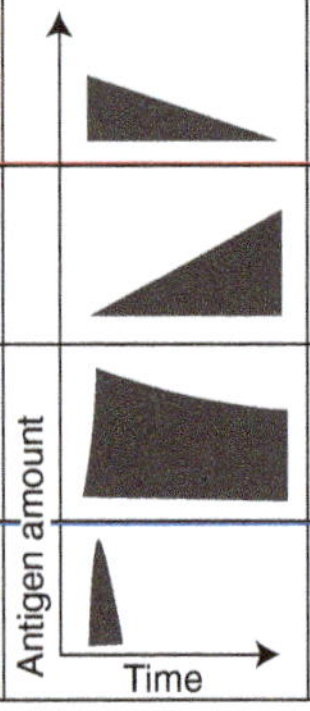

Antigen amount
Time

Figure 1. Autoimmune CD8 T cells in type 1 diabetes represent a unique differentiation state with features distinct from and shared with T cell states in other contexts and diseases. Antigen specificities, CD8 T cell receptor (TCR) affinities, functional states, phenotypes (inhibitory receptor expression), and transcription factor profiles (expression of TCF1 and TOX) across contexts of persistent antigen encounter and acute/inflammatory antigen encounter: autoimmune T1D (red; *top*), tumor (blue), chronic infection (purple), acute infection (green). In contexts and diseases of persistent antigen encounter, antigen-specific CD8 T cell responses are sustained by stem-like $TCF1^{hi}$ T cells, which self-renew and give rise to differentiated $TCF1^{lo}$ progeny (Diff). In settings of acute antigen encounters, CD8 T cells differentiate into effector and memory T cell populations.

effector functions capable of progressively destroying β cells. Why autoimmune β-cell-specific CD8 T cells in T1D resist dysfunction in the face of persistent self-antigen remains enigmatic. Comparisons of transcriptional and epigenetic programs of autoimmune β-cell-specific CD8 T cells with effector CD8 T cells in acute infections or exhausted CD8 T cells in chronic infections show that autoimmune T cells represent a unique T cell differentiation state (Fig. 1; Abdelsamed et al. 2020; Gearty et al. 2022).

Studies in humans demonstrated a link between the exhaustion phenotype, function, and disease progression. For example, a study by the Long group showed that islet-specific CD8 T cell phenotypes in T1D subjects predicted the rate of disease progression (Wiedeman et al. 2020): in patients with slow disease progression, islet-specific CD8 T cells displayed an increased exhaustion phenotype with the expression of multiple inhibitory receptors (PD1, 2B4, TIGIT), limited cytokine production, and reduced proliferative capacity, in contrast to patients who progressed rapidly. An increased exhaustion phenotype (EOMES, KLRG1, TIGIT) of peripheral blood CD8 T cells similarly correlated with slow rates of disease in at-risk individuals treated with anti-CD3 monoclonal antibody (teplizumab) (Long et al. 2016; Herold et al. 2019). Congruent with these findings, transcriptional signatures associated with CD8 T cell exhaustion have been shown to predict better prognosis in multiple autoimmune and inflammatory diseases, including T1D (McKinney et al. 2015). Autoreactive CD8 T cells harboring an exhaustion-like program and expressing inhibitory receptors have been considered "restrained," as deficiency in distinct inhibitory receptor genes (e.g., *Lag3* [encoding LAG3]), results in the accelerated onset of T1D in NOD mice (Grebinoski et al. 2022). Moreover, deficiency or blockade of PD1 signaling (through genetic ablation of PD1 or PDL1, or treatment with anti-PD1 and/or PDL1 mAb) dramatically accelerates T1D onset in mice (Ansari et al. 2003; Wang et al. 2005; Guleria et al. 2007; Collier et al. 2023). Importantly, cancer patients treated with immune checkpoint blockade antibodies (ICB; PD1/PDL1/CTLA4) have been shown to develop immune-related adverse events (IRAEs), and the development of T1D has been observed in a subset of ICB-treated cancer patients (Akturk et al. 2019; Singh et al. 2023). Thus, inhibitory receptor signaling appears to be required to maintain peripheral self-tolerance to β-cell antigens as well as to dampen effector function and cytotoxicity of autoimmune β-cell-specific T cells.

MOLECULAR PROGRAMS AND FACTORS ASSOCIATED WITH THE AUTOIMMUNE CD8 T CELL STATE

One TF critical for peripheral CD8 T cell differentiation and associated with T cell exhaustion is TOX, a high mobility group (HMG) box protein thought to bind DNA in a sequence-independent yet structure-dependent manner (O'Flaherty and Kaye 2003; Aliahmad et al. 2012). TOX is induced in CD8 T cells following antigen encounter/TCR stimulation: during acute stimulation/activation (e.g., acute infection), TOX expression is low and transient, disappearing when antigen is cleared (Alfei et al. 2019; Khan et al. 2019; Scott et al. 2019). However, when antigen persists, as in tumors or chronic infections, TOX expression progressively increases with time, driven by chronic antigen encounter and TCR stimulation (Alfei et al. 2019; Khan et al. 2019; Scott et al. 2019; Seo et al. 2019; Yao et al. 2019). TOX induces a transcriptional and epigenetic program associated with exhaustion and regulates the expression of numerous inhibitory receptors (Alfei et al. 2019; Khan et al. 2019; Scott et al. 2019; Seo et al. 2019; Yao et al. 2019).

Inhibitory receptors act as a physiological negative feedback mechanism to prevent overstimulation of activated CD8 T cells; consequently, *Tox*-deficiency in CD8 T cells results in the loss of inhibitory receptor expression, and subsequently activation-induced cell death (Fig. 1; Alfei et al. 2019; Khan et al. 2019; Scott et al. 2019; Yao et al. 2019). Thus, TOX is absolutely required for T cell survival and persistence in settings of chronic antigen/TCR stimulation. Autoimmune β-cell-specific T cells also express TOX (Abdelsamed et al. 2020; Ciecko et al. 2021; Gearty et al. 2022; Grebinoski et al. 2022; Kasmani et al. 2022; Selck et al. 2024). Unlike in tumors and chronic infections where TOX and inhibitory receptor expression are associated with functional hyporesponsiveness, in autoimmune β-cell-specific T cells TOX and inhibitory receptor expression are not linked to dysfunction. Whether TOX is required for the persistence and survival of autoimmune β-cell-specific T cells remains to be seen.

An important and unresolved question is which factors define the pathogenic autoimmune T cell state. One T cell–intrinsic factor that determines T cell differentiation and functional states is TCR affinity, the signal strength of the interaction between TCR and peptide-bound MHC (pMHC), as has been extensively demonstrated in vitro and in vivo in acute infection models (Altan-Bonnet and Germain 2005; Skokos et al. 2007; Zehn et al. 2009; Denton et al. 2011; King et al. 2012; Conley et al. 2016; Ozga et al. 2016; Balyan et al. 2017; Richard et al. 2018). The TCR affinity of peripheral T cells specific to foreign (neo-) antigens is generally high, while the TCR affinity to self-antigens is low (Stone et al. 2009). Studies assessing the impact of TCR affinity on T cell phenotype and function in settings of persistent antigen (e.g., tumor and chronic infection) demonstrated that high TCR signal strength results in T cell exhaustion and dysfunction, while low(er) signal strength retains T cell effector function (Lin and Welsh 1998; Probst et al. 2003; Ueno et al. 2004; Schober et al. 2020; Sim et al. 2020); this was associated with low(er) expression of TOX, low(er) expression of inhibitory receptors and distinct transcriptional and epigenetic programs (Shakiba et al. 2022). Thus, varying TCR signal strengths drive distinct TOX and inhibitory receptor expression levels and are associated with distinct functional states. Interestingly, autoimmune β-cell-specific CD8 T cells express lower levels of TOX and inhibitory receptors, compared to exhausted/dysfunctional CD8 T cells in tumors or chronic infection. Thus, β-cell-specific CD8 T cells may harbor a "Goldilocks" level of TCR affinity to self-antigens that allows autoimmune β-cell-specific T cells to persist as well as maintain effector function in the face of persistent self-antigen to progressively destroy β cells (Samassa and Mallone 2022).

POPULATION HETEROGENEITY, STEMNESS, AND DIFFERENTIATION OF β-CELL-SPECIFIC CD8 T CELLS

In settings of persistent (self or foreign) antigen encounter, the current paradigm is that antigen-specific CD8 T cell responses are sustained by a stem-like, progenitor T cell pool that self-renews and gives rise to differentiated progeny. Since the initial reports describing progenitor "stem-like" CD8 T cells in chronic infection (Paley et al. 2012; He et al. 2016; Im et al. 2016; Leong et al. 2016; Utzschneider et al. 2016; Wu et al. 2016), a plethora of studies followed, describing similar progenitor T cells in other contexts of persistent antigen encounter, such as cancer (Wu et al. 2016; Brummelman et al. 2018; Sade-Feldman et al. 2018; Jansen et al. 2019; Siddiqui et al. 2019; Connolly et al. 2021; Philip and Schietinger 2022) and inflammatory and autoimmune diseases, including T1D (Abdelsamed et al. 2020; Ciecko et al. 2021; Gearty et al. 2022; Grebinoski et al. 2022). T cell factor 1 (TCF1, encoded by *Tcf7*), an HMG box TF and member of the T cell factor/lymphoid enhancer factor (Tcf/Lef) family, has emerged as a key regulatory TF in stem-like T cells. In peripheral T cells, TCF1 promotes T cell stemness, self-renewal, and memory formation, largely through the suppression of *Prdm1* (BLIMP1), a TF that drives differentiation (Escobar et al. 2020; Gounari and Khazaie 2022; Zhao et al. 2022). Several recent studies have investigated T cell heterogeneity, stemness, and differentiation in T1D in mouse and human (Abdelsamed et al. 2020; Ciecko et al. 2021; Gearty et al. 2022; Grebinoski et al. 2022). A study by the Youngblood group demonstrated that islet-reactive peripheral blood CD8 T cells in patients with T1D harbor transcriptional and epigenetic programs associated with stem-like features and are epigenetically distinct from memory T cells and exhausted CD8 T cells in chronic infection, for example, HIV (Abdelsamed et al. 2020). In NOD mice, stem-like, self-renewing β-cell-specific TCF1^{hi} CD8 T cells have been identified in pLN (Gearty et al. 2022); pLN TCF1^{hi} stem-like T cells give rise to TCF1^{lo} differentiated progeny that migrate to the pancreas and destroy β cells (Fig. 2). Importantly, stem-like TCF1^{hi} T cells in the pLN must continuously seed the pancreas with differentiated TCF1^{lo} T cells to sustain β-cell destruction. NOD mice treated with FTY720, an S1P receptor agonist that blocks LN egress, were protected from disease (Morris et al. 2011; Gearty et al. 2022). These findings suggest that pLN provides a reservoir of stem-like T cells, which initiate and sustain tissue destruction through the continuous generation of pathogenic TCF1^{lo} T cells. Thus, the β-cell-specific autoimmune T cell pool comprises three distinct T cell subsets: pLN TCF1^{hi}, pLN TCF1^{lo}, and pancreatic TCF1^{lo} cells (Fig. 2). The three populations harbor distinct transcriptional programs, with pLN TCF1^{hi} expressing genes associated with T cell survival, proliferation and self-renewal, and TCF1^{lo} from pLN and pancreas expressing genes associated with effector function, terminal differentiation, and apoptosis (Gearty et al. 2022). The phenotypic bifurcation into TCF1^{hi} and TCF1^{lo} populations is unique to β-cell-specific CD8 T cells in the pLN, as those

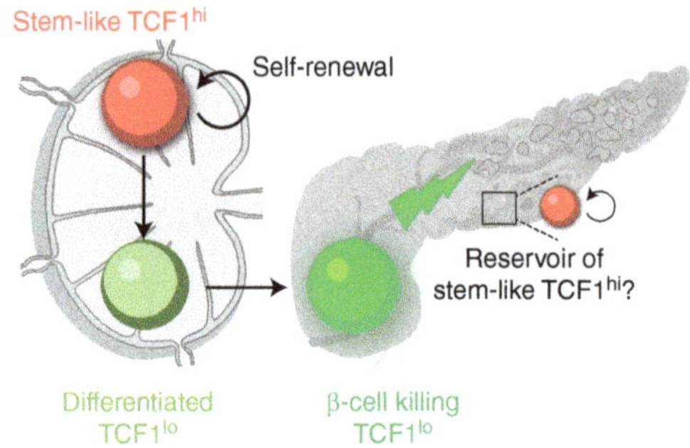

Figure 2. Proposed model of autoimmune β-cell-specific CD8 T cell differentiation in type 1 diabetes. TCF1^{hi} β-cell-specific CD8 T cells in the pancreatic lymph node represent a stem-like T cell pool that self-renews and gives rise to differentiated TCF1^{lo} T cells, which migrate to the pancreas and kill β cells in islets; stem-like T cells in pancreatic lymph nodes must continuously seed the pancreas with new differentiated T cells to sustain β-cell destruction and induce T1D in the clinically relevant nonobese diabetic mouse model. A reservoir of self-renewing stem-like T cells may exist in the pancreas (e.g., in specialized niches). Whether self-renewing stem-like CD8 T cells exist in lymph nodes and/or pancreas of patients with T1D remains to be seen.

in other LN or spleen express high levels of TCF1 but lack a distinct TCF1^{lo} population, suggesting that β-cell antigens that drain from the pancreas and are presented in pLN drive β-cell-specific CD8 T cell differentiation.

T cell differentiation and function in lymph nodes is generally spatially restricted and established through distinct intranodal positioning of CD45^{-} stromal (e.g., lymphatic endothelial cells, fibroblast reticular cells [FRCs]) and CD45^{+} myeloid cells (e.g., DCs), which establish specialized microenvironments with qualitatively and quantitatively distinct cytokines/chemokines, costimulatory/-inhibitory signals, and antigenic contents (Eisenbarth 2019). For example, during acute infections, effector and memory CD8 T cell fates are determined in distinct LN regions: CXCR3-expressing effector CD8 T cells localize at the LN periphery through DC-derived CXCL9/CXCL10 binding, while CCR7-expressing memory precursors are confined to the T cell zone through binding to FRC-derived CCL19/CCL21 (Duckworth et al. 2021). Interestingly, organ donors with T1D exhibit cellular and phenotypic differences in their lymph node stromal cell compartment compared to healthy individuals (Postigo-Fernandez et al. 2019). For topics on myeloid and stromal cell populations in pLN and their functional roles in T1D, we refer readers to excellent reviews (Creusot et al. 2018; Postigo-Fernandez et al. 2019).

β-Cell-specific stem-like TCF1^{hi} and differentiated TCF1^{lo} CD8 T cells in pLN of NOD mice harbor distinct expression patterns of integrins and chemokine receptors (e.g., CCR7, CXCR3, CXCR6, very late antigen-4 [VLA4]), suggesting that autoimmune β-cell-specific CD8 T cell differentiation is associated with distinct intranodal positioning mediated through distinct chemokine/chemokine receptor axes (Gearty et al. 2022). Notably, antibody blockades targeting the CXCL10/CXCR3 axis (Lasch et al. 2015) or VLA4 (Baron et al. 1994) reduces T1D progression in mice, and NOD mice deficient of CCR7 are protected from disease (Martin et al. 2009). While blockade of these and other integrins and chemokine receptor-ligand pathways have been thought to mitigate disease by blocking T cell trafficking and recruitment to the pancreatic islets (Sandor et al. 2019), they might also function in pLN by disrupting T cell differentiation and preventing the generation of differentiated, diabetogenic T cells.

Studies in other disease contexts demonstrated that TCF1^{hi} stem-like and TCF1^{lo} terminally differentiated populations are similarly spatially segregated, with TCF1^{hi} progenitor T cells generally found in secondary lymphoid tissues, while differentiated TCF1^{lo} T cells are predominantly found in peripheral tissues (He et al. 2016; Im et al. 2016; Connolly et al. 2021; Schnell et al. 2021). Intriguingly, self-renewing TCF1^{hi} CD8 T cells have been found in the pancreas in NOD mice, undergoing IL-27-dependent differentiation to become TCF1^{lo} terminal effectors during the progression of T1D (Fig. 2; Ciecko et al. 2021). Specialized microenvironments or niches (e.g., ectopic lymphoid-like or tertiary lymphoid structures) within the pancreas may facilitate the maintenance of TCF1^{hi} β-cell-specific progenitor-like CD8 T cells. Tertiary lymphoid structures are clusters of CD4 T cells, B cells, and DCs, which develop in nonlymphoid tissues at sites of chronic inflammation and resemble follicles found in secondary lymphoid organs (Dong et al. 2024). In tumors, tertiary lymphoid structures and specialized niches have been shown to represent a reservoir of stem-like TCF1^{hi} CD8 T cells that generate effector-like, differentiated TCF1^{lo} T cells following ICB treatment (Jansen et al. 2019; Peng et al. 2021; Chen et al. 2024). While lymphoid-like structures have been described in the pancreas of NOD mice (Kendall et al. 2007), their presence and functional role in individuals with T1D remain unclear (Korpos et al. 2021).

Taken together, β-cell-specific stem-like, progenitor CD8 T cells appear to represent a critical T cell population and differentiation state that initiates and sustains β-cell destruction. Critical questions remain: (1) how do stem-like TCF1^{hi} T cells form, (2) what are the factors and signals that determine the maintenance of TCF1^{hi} progenitor T cells and promote their differentiation, and (3) do β-cell-specific stem-like CD8 T cells exist in patients with T1D?

The existence of a disease-driving stem-like T cell population in T1D makes it an attractive target for therapeutic intervention. A recent clinical study demonstrated that a single course of anti-CD3 mAb, teplizumab, conferred long-term protection from T1D in at-risk individuals, but the specific mechanisms responsible remain incompletely explained (Herold et al. 2019; Sims et al. 2021). Similarly, in NOD mice, anti-CD3 mAb treatment has been shown to result in long-term protection from T1D, but the mechanisms at play are also unclear (Chatenoud et al. 1992a; Chatenoud and Bluestone 2007); studies have suggested that anti-CD3 mAb treatment induces short- and long-term effects persisting for months after treatment (Chatenoud et al. 1992b, 1997). Both cell-extrinsic and cell-intrinsic changes have been implicated in the long-term response to anti-CD3 mAb therapy, including the induction of regulatory T cells and CD8 and CD4 T cell tolerance (Chatenoud et al. 1997; Belghith et al. 2003). Thus, anti-CD3 treatment likely targets multiple T cell populations to induce long-term T1D remission. An accumulation of polyclonal CD8 T cells with an exhaustion-like phenotype was observed in the blood of responders a few months after treatment, suggesting that anti-CD3 mAb treatment-induced tolerance might be mediated through a β-cell-intrinsic reprogramming and the induction of an enhanced exhaustion phenotype that correlates with, or results in, diminished T cell function and cytotoxicity (Long et al. 2016; Herold et al. 2019; Sims et al. 2021). Additionally, given the necessity of stem-like T cells for disease initiation and progression in NOD mice, it is tempting to speculate whether one of the underlying mechanisms of anti-CD3-mediated long-term tolerance includes the targeting and tolerization of the autoimmune stem-like T cell pool.

CD4 T CELLS IN T1D

The strong genetic HLA II association with T1D risk, together with the results of targeted genetic and antibody-mediated CD4 T cell depletion studies in mice, support a critical role for CD4 T cells in disease initiation and progression (Miller et al. 1988; Shizuru et al. 1988). The NOD MHC class II molecule I-Ag^7 contains a polymorphism in position 57 of the MHC class II β-chain (similar to the β-chain of human HLA II), which profoundly affects the MHC class II peptidome and CD4 T cell repertoire, and a mutation at position 57 prevents T1D in NOD mice (Suri et al. 2005; Stadinski et al. 2023). Studies in infection, transplantation, and cancer have demonstrated that CD4 T cells are required during all phases of CD8 T cell differentiation for proper CD8 T cell effector function, including (1) priming, (2) recruitment into peripheral tissues, and (3) licensing CD8 T cell cytotoxicity during the effector phase. However, less is known about the functional roles of CD4 T cells in T1D, and at which stages CD4 T cells promote β-cell-specific CD8 T cell differentiation, or how CD4 T cells exert direct pathogenic functions.

ANTIGEN SPECIFICITIES AND CD4 T CELL POLARIZATION STATES

Numerous islet-specific CD4 T cell epitopes have been identified, encompassing both genetically and nongenetically encoded epitopes (Amdare et al. 2021). While genetically encoded epitopes are derived from self-proteins (e.g., [pro]insulin, chromogranin A), nongenetically encoded (neo)epitopes are classified as hybrid insulin peptides (HIPs) that were first identified by the Haskins group and found in both mice and humans during homeostasis and disease (Jung et al. 2015; Delong et al. 2016; Wiles et al. 2017, 2019; Parras et al. 2021; Crawford et al. 2022; Wenzlau et al. 2022; Callebaut et al. 2024). HIPs are created through peptide bond formation between the carboxylic acid group of C-peptide fragments of proinsulin and the amino terminus of peptide fragments from β-cell secretory granule proteins such as chromogranin A (Ins:ChgA; murine 2.5 HIP, also found in humans) or islet amyloid polypeptide (Ins:IAPP; 6.9 HIP) (Delong et al. 2016; Wan et al. 2018; Wiles et al. 2019, 2021a,b; Callebaut et al. 2024). HIP-specific CD4 T cells have been found in the pancreas of organ donors with T1D as well as in the peripheral blood of recently diagnosed patients with T1D (Babon et al. 2016; Baker et al. 2019; Mitchell et al. 2021). In NOD mice, HIP-specific CD4 T cells are pathogenic and mediate disease in adoptive transfer studies utilizing TCR transgenic HIP-specific CD4 T cells, including 2.5 and 6.9 HIP TCR CD4 T cells (Haskins and McDuffie 1990; Katz et al. 1993; Burton et al. 2008; Mitchell et al. 2024).

In NOD mice, insulin-specific CD4 T cells are the first T cells to infiltrate into the pancreas, and a single amino acid substitution at position 16 in the insulin B chain completely prevents T1D induction, highlighting a key role of insulin-specific CD4 T cells in disease initiation (Nakayama et al. 2005; Gioia et al. 2019; Costanzo et al. 2024). CD4 T cells reactive to 2.5 or 6.9 HIP appear in later disease stages in mice and humans, with numbers of insulin-reactive CD4 T cells declining (Baker et al. 2018; Gioia et al. 2019).

TCR signal strength and cytokine milieu determine CD4 T cell differentiation and polarization to distinct T helper (T_H) lineages, including T_H1, T_H2, T_H17, T follicular helper (T_{FH}), or T regulatory (T_{REG}) (Zhu 2018). Each CD4 T_H lineage is determined by its lineage-specific master TF and associated with a unique lineage-defining effector cytokine (e.g., for T_H1, TBET and IFN-γ; T_H2, GATA3 and IL-4/IL-5/IL-13; T_H17, RORγt and IL-17/IL-22T_{FH}, BCL6, and IL-21; T_{REG}, FOXP3 and TGFβ, IL-10, and IL-35) (Zhou et al. 2009a; Zhu 2018). In T1D, proinflammatory T_H1 as well as T_{FH} are important for pathogenesis, while T_H2 CD4 T cells as well as T_{REG} have been shown to exert protective or suppressive roles, respectively (Walker and von Herrath 2016). Although there is some evidence for a pathogenic role of T_H17 CD4 T cells in T1D (Arif et al. 2011; Ferraro et al. 2011; Li et al. 2015), in this section, we focus on T_H1, T_{FH}, and T_{REG} CD4 T cells, and describe their potential roles in T1D pathogenesis (Fig. 3).

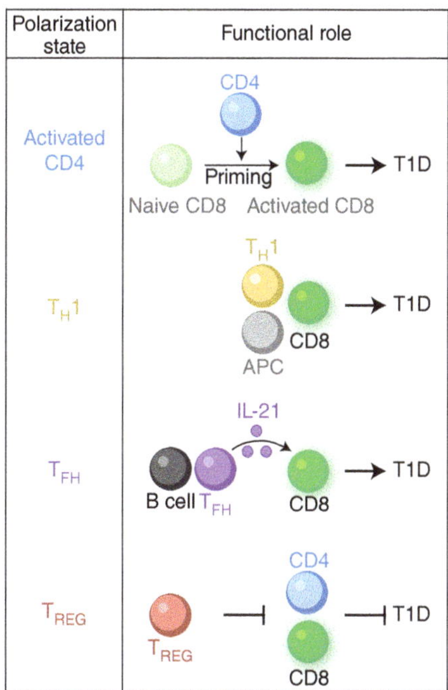

Figure 3. Polarization states and functional roles of CD4 T cells during autoimmune β-cell-specific CD8 T cell differentiation in type 1 diabetes (T1D). Activated CD4 T cells facilitate the priming of autoreactive naive β-cell-specific CD8 T cells in pancreatic lymph nodes (*top*). T helper 1 (T_H1) promotes effector function and cytotoxicity of β-cell-specific CD8 T cells in the pancreas (*top middle*). T follicular helper (T_{FH}) and their interaction with B cells drive IL-21 production, a critical cytokine that promotes the differentiation and cytotoxic function of IL-21R-expressing β-cell-specific CD8 T cells (*bottom middle*). Regulatory CD4 T cells (T_{REG}) restrain autoreactive CD8 and CD4 T cells and mitigate T1D (*bottom*).

THE ROLE OF CD4 T CELLS DURING THE PRIMING AND EFFECTOR PHASE OF CD8 T CELLS

In antigen-draining lymph nodes, CD4 T cells "license" DC through CD40-CD40L (Bennett et al. 1998; Ridge et al. 1998; Schoenberger et al. 1998) resulting in increased antigen-presentation (MHC I and II), production of inflammatory cytokines IL-12/IL-15, and induction of costimulatory molecules (CD80/86, CD70, 41BBL). In T1D, several loci associated with antigen processing and presentation, costimulation, and APC maturation are genetically linked with risk for T1D in mice and humans and are implicated in defective induction and/or maintenance of immune tolerance (Creusot et al. 2018). A critical role of CD4 T cells in DC maturation and β-cell-specific CD8 T cell priming has been demonstrated in various studies: *CD40Lg*$^{-/-}$ NOD mice are protected from

T1D, and CD4 T cells from *CD40Lg*$^{-/-}$ NOD mice fail to induce T1D in CD8 T cell cotransfer studies (Eshima et al. 2003). Furthermore, antibody-mediated blockade of CD40L of young (3- to 4-wk old) NOD mice prevents insulitis and subsequent onset of T1D, but not of older (9-wk-old) mice (Balasa et al. 1997). Congruent with these findings, adoptive transfer of previously primed autoreactive T cells into secondary hosts led to rapid induction of T1D even in the absence of CD40/CD40L signaling (Balasa et al. 1997). Together, these studies highlight the importance of CD4 T cells and CD40/CD40L signaling for DC licensing, CD8 T cell activation, and disease initiation (Fig. 3).

T_H1 CD4 T cells have been suggested to be required within pancreatic islets for licensing and sustaining cytotoxicity of diabetogenic CD8 T cells and β-cell killing (Espinosa-Carrasco et al. 2018). In a genetic mouse model of T1D, in which β cells express a model antigen, it was shown that T_H1 antigen-specific CD4 T cells empowered antigen-specific CD8 T cells to maintain effector function and eliminate β cells. CD8 T cells deprived of continuous CD4 T cell help at the target site failed to maintain optimal effector functions, resulting in a significant delay of disease onset. Within islets, CD4 T cells and CD8 T cells were shown to co-engage with APC (macrophages, DCs), forming a three-cell-type cluster. Interestingly, CD4 T cell::CD8 T cell::APC three-cell-type clusters were also shown to be required for the cytolytic response of CD8 T cells in allogeneic transplant settings, and more recently in the context of tumors for cancer cell elimination (Mitchison and O'Malley 1987; Espinosa-Carrasco et al. 2024). Thus, T_H1-like CD4 T cells appear to be required together with APC within islets to promote CD8 T cell cytolytic effector function and β-cell elimination (Fig. 3).

Other mechanisms of how T_H1 CD4 T cells may contribute to T1D pathogenesis include (1) recruitment and activation of macrophages for β-cell elimination, (2) increasing MHC class I expression on β cells to promote CD8 T cell recognition and elimination of β cells, and (3) direct interaction with MHC class II on β cells (shown to be up-regulated by proinflammatory cytokines) (Thomas et al. 1998; Cantor and Haskins 2007; Calderon et al. 2011; Zhao et al. 2015; Russell et al. 2019; Hu et al. 2020; Quesada-Masachs et al. 2022).

THE ROLE OF T_{FH} CD4 T CELLS AND IL-21 SIGNALING IN T1D PATHOGENESIS

T_{FH} enables B cells to form germinal centers in secondary lymphoid organs to generate high-affinity and class-switched antibodies. In patients with T1D, the frequencies of circulating insulin-specific and polyclonal CD4 T cells with a T_{FH} phenotype are elevated along with increased IL-21 levels (Ferreira et al. 2015; Kenefeck et al. 2015; Viisanen et al. 2017; Vecchione et al. 2021; Sharma et al. 2023). It is well established that T_{FH} development requires B cells, and B cells are required for T1D initiation. One of the first diagnostic markers to determine at-risk T1D patients is islet-specific autoantibodies, including both IgM and class-switched IgG subtypes (Millward et al. 1988; Dozio et al. 1994; Couper et al. 1998; Hawa et al. 2000; Lohmann et al. 2000; Hoppu et al. 2004). Intriguingly, numbers of insulin-specific CD4 T cells and polyclonal T_{FH} directly correlate with insulin-reactive antibody titers, suggesting insulin-specific T (T_{FH}) and B-cell interactions may be the first step in driving the disease (Ferreira et al. 2015; Kenefeck et al. 2015; Spanier et al. 2017; Viisanen et al. 2017).

In NOD mice, T_{FH} and/or IL-21-producing islet-specific CD4 T cells have been found in the pLN and islets (Wan et al. 2016; Ito et al. 2018). The importance of IL-21 in driving T1D is highlighted by several observations: (1) in vivo neutralization of IL-21 in NOD mice, (2) *IL-21*-deficient NOD mice, and (3) *IL-21r*-deficient NOD mice are all protected from T1D (Spolski et al. 2008; McGuire et al. 2011a; Allred et al. 2021). At a cellular level, deficiency of IL-21 in CD4 T cells completely abrogates T1D onset and, interestingly, lack of the IL-21R on β-cell-specific CD8 T cells prevents disease, suggesting CD4 T cell–derived IL-21 is required the pathogenic CD8 T cell responses (McGuire et al. 2011b).

Interestingly, T_{FH} and cognate germinal center B-cell interactions have recently been shown to be critical for CD8 T cell cytotoxicity and target elimination in the contexts of tumors and chronic infections: cognate B-cell–T_{FH} interactions promote T_{FH}-IL-21 production, which then binds to IL-21R-expressing antigen-specific CD8 T cells, sustaining their cytolytic programs and effector functions (Yi et al. 2009; Cui et al. 2021; Zander et al. 2022). In T1D, similar cell–cell interactions and mechanisms could be driving β-cell destruction: islet-specific T_{FH} and B cell interactions lead to IL-21 secretion, which acts on β-cell-specific CD8 T cells to sustain cytotoxicity and the pathogenic response (Fig. 3). While T_{FH} are likely the primary source of IL-21, T_H1 CD4 T cells in murine islets have also been shown to produce IL-21 (Ciecko et al. 2023). Blockade of the IL-21-signaling axis has emerged as an attractive therapeutic intervention for the treatment of T1D (von Herrath et al. 2021).

DEVELOPMENT AND DIFFERENTIATION OF T_{REG} CD4 T CELLS IN T1D

Although the frequency of polyclonal FOXP3$^+$ T_{REG} in the blood of patients with T1D is comparable to healthy individuals, there is a substantial decrease in the frequency of insulin-specific FOXP3$^+$ T_{REG} (McClymont et al. 2011; Sharma et al. 2023). Defective IL-2R signaling has been proposed as the underlying mechanism for reduced FOXP3 expression, T_{REG} instability, and dysfunction in T1D (Long et al. 2010; McClymont et al. 2011; Garg et al. 2012). T_{REG} has been shown to delay T1D in NOD mice. For instance, NOD mice depleted of FOXP3$^+$ T_{REG}, or *Cd28*-deficient NOD mice (which largely lack a FOXP3-compartment) present with accelerated induction of T1D (Salomon et al. 2000; Feuerer et al. 2009; Watts et al. 2021).

Two types of T_{REG} exist, thymically derived (tT_{REG}) and peripheral T_{REG} (pT_{REG}) (Shevach and Thornton 2014; Li and Rudensky 2016). tT_{REG} are thought to represent the major suppressive T_{REG} population in T1D. TCR-based lineage tracing and FOXP3$^+$ fate-mapping studies in NOD mice report limited pT_{REG} conversion (Wong et al. 2007; Zhou et al. 2009b). In addition, genetic mouse models preventing pT_{REG} induction reveal no significant impact on the overall numbers of FOXP3$^+$ CD4 T cells and minimal or no acceleration of T1D incidence (Wong et al. 2007; Schuster et al. 2018). An intriguing observation supporting the lack of pT_{REG} induction in T1D is that HIP-specific CD4 T cells, whose antigens are thought to be exclusively generated in the islets and are not presented in the thymus, largely lack a FOXP3$^+$ T_{REG} compartment (Baker et al. 2018; Ito et al. 2018).

Several lines of evidence suggest an active differentiation process of FOXP3$^+$ T_{REG} cells within islets: FOXP3$^+$ CD4 T cells can either differentiate into pathogenic ex-FOXP3 CD4 T cells, or into a TBET-expressing FOXP3$^+$ T_{REG} with increased suppressor function. Genetic fate mapping studies showed ex-FOXP3-expressing CD4 T cells were enriched in islets in NOD mice (Zhou et al. 2009b). Moreover, TCR sequencing identified that a significant population of ex-FOXP3 "conventional" CD4 T cells shared TCR clonality with FOXP3$^+$ T_{REG} cells (Zhou et al. 2009b). Interestingly, in adoptive transfer studies, ex-FOXP3 CD4 T cells were found to be pathogenic and induced T1D. Conversely, FOXP3$^+$ Treg cells can also up-regulate TBET, differentiating into TBET$^+$ FOXP3$^+$ T cells in islets, mitigating proliferation and IFN-γ production of CD4 and CD8 T cells, as well as APC activation (Tan et al. 2016). Consequently, genetic deletion of *Tbet* in FOXP3$^+$ T_{REG} results in accelerated onset of T1D despite maintaining overall numbers of FOXP3$^+$ T_{REG}. High TCR signal strength and/or exposure to IFN-γ have been proposed to drive differentiation into TBET$^+$ T_{REG} (Kornete et al. 2015; Sprouse et al. 2018). This differentiation process is not exclusive to islets and has been reported in pLN as well (Tan et al. 2016).

Multiple therapeutic interventions are being pursued to enhance suppressor function and/or frequencies of FOXP3$^+$ T_{REG} cells for the prevention and/or treatment of T1D (Bluestone et al. 2023): (1) low-dose IL-2 therapy, which was shown to result in increased FOXP3$^+$ tT_{REG} numbers and reduced IL-21$^+$ T_{FH} (with no impact on expansion and activation of conventional effector CD4 or CD8 T cells) (Dwyer et al.

2016; Rosenzwajg et al. 2020; Zhang et al. 2022), (2) tolerance induction of islet-specific CD4 T cells via delivery of islet-antigen loaded nanoparticles or other approaches (Writing Committee for the Type 1 Diabetes TrialNet Oral Insulin Study Group et al. 2017; Prasad et al. 2018; Jamison et al. 2019; Hannelius et al. 2020; DiLisio and Haskins 2021; Wesley et al. 2022; Firdessa Fite et al. 2023), (3) islet-specific CAR T_{REG} engineering (Spanier et al. 2023), and (4) adoptive transfer of engineered T_{REG} (Yang et al. 2022; Uenishi et al. 2024) or in vitro expanded T_{REG} (although a recent phase II clinical trial demonstrated limited efficacy) (Bender et al. 2024).

CONCLUDING REMARKS AND OUTSTANDING QUESTIONS

Despite the considerable advances in our understanding of the underlying mechanisms defining the autoimmune β-cell-specific T cell state in mouse and human, several important questions remain. An unresolved question is why autoimmune β-cell-specific CD8 T cells resist functional exhaustion. The prevailing paradigm is that persistent antigen/TCR stimulation leads to hyporesponsiveness and functional exhaustion, which strikingly contrasts observations in T1D; autoimmune β-cell-specific CD8 T cells express TOX, PD1, and other inhibitory receptors, yet retain effector function and cytotoxic capabilities. Recent studies now demonstrate despite the association between TOX and inhibitory receptor expression (exhaustion phenotype) and functional hyporesponsiveness, T cell phenotypes, and functional states of CD8 T cells are not coregulated. More work is required to understand the mechanisms that drive the expression of TOX and inhibitory receptors and determine their functional consequences, as well as identify which signals and mechanisms control effector function and cytotoxicity of CD8 T cells.

The recent identification of autoimmune stem-like CD8 T cells in mice and humans could explain this paradox (Abdelsamed et al. 2020; Ciecko et al. 2021; Gearty et al. 2022; Grebinoski et al. 2022). Pathogenic, differentiated CD8 T cells do not persist long enough in the pancreas to undergo chronic antigen stimulation and are constantly replenished by the autoimmune stem-like T cell pool, leading to sustained β-cell destruction and induction of T1D. In addition, TOX and inhibitory receptors, which are induced by antigen encounter, are expressed at lower levels by autoimmune β-cell-specific T cells, reflecting a key distinction between autoimmune and exhausted/dysfunctional CD8 T cells in chronic infections and tumors. Moreover, as discussed above, TCR signal strength determines TOX-mediated differentiation and functional states. Thus, it will be important to elucidate whether the lower TCR affinity to (self-) β-cell antigens allow autoimmune T cells to maintain effector function. Understanding the relationships between antigen chronicity, TCR signal strength, functional states, and the role of TOX, will inform the design of new therapeutic interventions.

Other outstanding questions include the following. Where and how are autoimmune stem-like CD8 T cells generated and sustained? What factors and signals drive their differentiation into pathogenic autoimmune CD8 T cells? Do specialized microanatomical sites or "niches" in secondary lymphoid tissues or within the pancreas preserve autoimmune T cell stemness and self-renewal capacity while blocking terminal differentiation? Moreover, given the critical role of CD4 T cells in the initiation and progression of T1D, it would be interesting to explore whether CD4 T cells are required for the generation and/or maintenance of autoimmune stem-like CD8 T cells or their differentiation. Numerous mechanisms have been proposed to explain how CD4 T cells may modulate autoimmune CD8 T cell differentiation, including T_H1 and T_{FH} during the effector phase. Additionally, the fact that T_{REG} are able to further differentiate into either pathogenic or more suppressive phenotypes, leads back to the broader, less explored question of how naive CD4 T cells choose their identity and polarization states in T1D. Interestingly, stem-like CD4 T cells have recently been identified in numerous inflammatory and autoimmune diseases in mice and humans, including multiple sclerosis (Schnell et al. 2021), autoimmune vasculitis (Sato et al. 2023), ulcerative colitis (Li et al. 2024), allergic diseases

(Kratchmarov et al. 2024), as well as in chronic infection (Xia et al. 2022) and allograft rejection (Zou et al. 2024). Thus, an intriguing question is whether stem-like CD4 T cells exist in T1D.

Continued advances in single-cell technologies, including multiplexed protein imaging, spatially mapped chromatin accessibility, transcriptomics as well as metabolomics and single-cell TCR sequencing (Cao et al. 2018; Thornton et al. 2021; Wu et al. 2024), combined with the integration of basic immunology insights and clinical observations and data, will allow us to continue to gain mechanistic insights into the spatiotemporal factors determining autoimmune β-cell-specific T cell differentiation, imperative for the design of effective strategies for the prevention and treatment of T1D and other T cell–mediated autoimmune diseases.

ACKNOWLEDGMENTS

This work was supported by NIH R01AI173249 (A.S.), Juvenile Diabetes Research Foundation JDRF SRA-2023-1410-S-B (A.S.), Lloyd Old STAR Award of the Cancer Research Institute (A.S.), MSKCC Basic Research Innovation Award (BRIA) (A.S.), the Hearst Foundation (K.M.H.), and NIH F31DK141119 (S.M.).

REFERENCES

Abdelsamed HA, Zebley CC, Nguyen H, Rutishauser RL, Fan Y, Ghoneim HE, Crawford JC, Alfei F, Alli S, Ribeiro SP, et al. 2020. β-Cell-specific CD8$^+$ T cells maintain stem cell memory-associated epigenetic programs during type 1 diabetes. *Nat Immunol* **21:** 578–587. doi:10.1038/s41590-020-0633-5

Akturk HK, Kahramangil D, Sarwal A, Hoffecker L, Murad MH, Michels AW. 2019. Immune checkpoint inhibitor-induced type 1 diabetes: a systematic review and meta-analysis. *Diabet Med* **36:** 1075–1081. doi:10.1111/dme.14050

Alfei F, Kanev K, Hofmann M, Wu M, Ghoneim HE, Roelli P, Utzschneider DT, von Hoesslin M, Cullen JG, Fan Y, et al. 2019. TOX reinforces the phenotype and longevity of exhausted T cells in chronic viral infection. *Nature* **571:** 265–269. doi:10.1038/s41586-019-1326-9

Aliahmad P, Seksenyan A, Kaye J. 2012. The many roles of TOX in the immune system. *Curr Opin Immunol* **24:** 173–177. doi:10.1016/j.coi.2011.12.001

Allred MG, Chimenti MS, Ciecko AE, Chen YG, Lieberman SM. 2021. Characterization of type I interferon-associated chemokines and cytokines in lacrimal glands of nonobese diabetic mice. *Int J Mol Sci* **22:** 3767. doi:10.3390/ijms22073767

Altan-Bonnet G, Germain RN. 2005. Modeling T cell antigen discrimination based on feedback control of digital ERK responses. *PLoS Biol* **3:** e356. doi:10.1371/journal.pbio.0030356

Amdare N, Purcell AW, DiLorenzo TP. 2021. Noncontiguous T cell epitopes in autoimmune diabetes: from mice to men and back again. *J Biol Chem* **297:** 100827. doi:10.1016/j.jbc.2021.100827

Anderson MS, Bluestone JA. 2005. The NOD mouse: a model of immune dysregulation. *Annu Rev Immunol* **23:** 447–485. doi:10.1146/annurev.immunol.23.021704.115643

Ansari MJ, Salama AD, Chitnis T, Smith RN, Yagita H, Akiba H, Yamazaki T, Azuma M, Iwai H, Khoury SJ, et al. 2003. The programmed death-1 (PD-1) pathway regulates autoimmune diabetes in nonobese diabetic (NOD) mice. *J Exp Med* **198:** 63–69. doi:10.1084/jem.20022125

Arif S, Moore F, Marks K, Bouckenooghe T, Dayan CM, Planas R, Vives-Pi M, Powrie J, Tree T, Marchetti P, et al. 2011. Peripheral and islet interleukin-17 pathway activation characterizes human autoimmune diabetes and promotes cytokine-mediated β-cell death. *Diabetes* **60:** 2112–2119. doi:10.2337/db10-1643

Babon JA, DeNicola ME, Blodgett DM, Crèvecoeur I, Buttrick TS, Maehr R, Bottino R, Naji A, Kaddis J, Elyaman W, et al. 2016. Analysis of self-antigen specificity of islet-infiltrating T cells from human donors with type 1 diabetes. *Nat Med* **22:** 1482–1487. doi:10.1038/nm.4203

Baker RL, Jamison BL, Wiles TA, Lindsay RS, Barbour G, Bradley B, Delong T, Friedman RS, Nakayama M, Haskins K. 2018. CD4 T cells reactive to hybrid insulin peptides are indicators of disease activity in the NOD mouse. *Diabetes* **67:** 1836–1846. doi:10.2337/db18-0200

Baker RL, Rihanek M, Hohenstein AC, Nakayama M, Michels A, Gottlieb PA, Haskins K, Delong T. 2019. Hybrid insulin peptides are autoantigens in type 1 diabetes. *Diabetes* **68:** 1830–1840. doi:10.2337/db19-0128

Balasa B, Krahl T, Patstone G, Lee J, Tisch R, McDevitt HO, Sarvetnick N. 1997. CD40 ligand–CD40 interactions are necessary for the initiation of insulitis and diabetes in nonobese diabetic mice. *J Immunol* **159:** 4620–4627. doi:10.4049/jimmunol.159.9.4620

Balyan R, Gund R, Ebenezer C, Khalsa JK, Verghese DA, Krishnamurthy T, George A, Bal V, Rath S, Chaudhry A. 2017. Modulation of naive CD8 T cell response features by ligand density, affinity, and continued signaling via internalized TCRs. *J Immunol* **198:** 1823–1837. doi:10.4049/jimmunol.1600083

Baron JL, Reich EP, Visintin I, Janeway CA Jr. 1994. The pathogenesis of adoptive murine autoimmune diabetes requires an interaction between α 4-integrins and vascular cell adhesion molecule-1. *J Clin Invest* **93:** 1700–1708. doi:10.1172/JCI117153

Belghith M, Bluestone JA, Barriot S, Mégret J, Bach JF, Chatenoud L. 2003. TGF-β-dependent mechanisms mediate restoration of self-tolerance induced by antibodies to CD3 in overt autoimmune diabetes. *Nat Med* **9:** 1202–1208. doi:10.1038/nm924

Bender C, Wiedeman AE, Hu A, Ylescupidez A, Sietsema WK, Herold KC, Griffin KJ, Gitelman SE, Long SA; T-Rex Study Group, et al. 2024. A phase 2 randomized trial with autologous polyclonal expanded regulatory T cells in children with new-onset type 1 diabetes. *Sci Transl Med* **16:** eadn2404. doi:10.1126/scitranslmed.adn2404

Bennett SR, Carbone FR, Karamalis F, Flavell RA, Miller JF, Heath WR. 1998. Help for cytotoxic-T-cell responses is mediated by CD40 signalling. *Nature* **393:** 478–480. doi:10.1038/30996

Bluestone JA, Herold K, Eisenbarth G. 2010. Genetics, pathogenesis and clinical interventions in type 1 diabetes. *Nature* **464:** 1293–1300. doi:10.1038/nature08933

Bluestone JA, McKenzie BS, Beilke J, Ramsdell F. 2023. Opportunities for Treg cell therapy for the treatment of human disease. *Front Immunol* **14:** 1166135. doi:10.3389/fimmu.2023.1166135

Brummelman J, Mazza EMC, Alvisi G, Colombo FS, Grilli A, Mikulak J, Mavilio D, Alloisio M, Ferrari F, Lopci E, et al. 2018. High-dimensional single cell analysis identifies stem-like cytotoxic $CD8^+$ T cells infiltrating human tumors. *J Exp Med* **215:** 2520–2535. doi:10.1084/jem.20180684

Burton AR, Vincent E, Arnold PY, Lennon GP, Smeltzer M, Li CS, Haskins K, Hutton J, Tisch RM, Sercarz EE, et al. 2008. On the pathogenicity of autoantigen-specific T-cell receptors. *Diabetes* **57:** 1321–1330. doi:10.2337/db07-1129

Calderon B, Carrero JA, Miller MJ, Unanue ER. 2011. Entry of diabetogenic T cells into islets induces changes that lead to amplification of the cellular response. *Proc Natl Acad Sci* **108:** 1567–1572. doi:10.1073/pnas.1018975108

Callebaut A, Guyer P, Baker RL, Gallegos JB, Hohenstein AC, Gottlieb PA, Mathieu C, Overbergh L, Haskins K, James EA. 2024. An insulin-chromogranin a hybrid peptide activates DR11-restricted T cells in human type 1 diabetes. *Diabetes* **73:** 743–750. doi:10.2337/db23-0622

Cantor J, Haskins K. 2007. Recruitment and activation of macrophages by pathogenic CD4 T cells in type 1 diabetes: evidence for involvement of CCR8 and CCL1. *J Immunol* **179:** 5760–5767. doi:10.4049/jimmunol.179.9.5760

Cao J, Cusanovich DA, Ramani V, Aghamirzaie D, Pliner HA, Hill AJ, Daza RM, McFaline-Figueroa JL, Packer JS, Christiansen L, et al. 2018. Joint profiling of chromatin accessibility and gene expression in thousands of single cells. *Science* **361:** 1380–1385. doi:10.1126/science.aau0730

Chatenoud L, Bluestone JA. 2007. CD3-specific antibodies: a portal to the treatment of autoimmunity. *Nat Rev Immunol* **7:** 622–632. doi:10.1038/nri2134

Chatenoud L, Thervet E, Primo J, Bach JF. 1992a. Rémission de la maladie établie chez la souris NOD diabétique par l'anticorps monoclonal anti-CD3 [Remission of established disease in diabetic NOD mice induced by anti-CD3 monoclonal antibody]. *C R Acad Sci III* **315:** 225–228.

Chatenoud L, Thervet E, Primo J, Bach JF. 1992b. Anti-CD3 antibody induces long-term remission of overt autoimmunity in nonobese diabetic mice. *Proc Natl Acad Sci* **91:** 123–127. doi:10.1073/pnas.91.1.123

Chatenoud L, Primo J, Bach JF. 1997. CD3 antibody-induced dominant self tolerance in overtly diabetic NOD mice. *J Immunol* **158:** 2947–2954. doi:10.4049/jimmunol.158.6.2947

Chen JH, Nieman LT, Spurrell M, Jorgji V, Elmelech L, Richieri P, Xu KH, Madhu R, Parikh M, Zamora I, et al. 2024. Human lung cancer harbors spatially organized stem-immunity hubs associated with response to immunotherapy. *Nat Immunol* **25:** 644–658. doi:10.1038/s41590-024-01792-2

Christianson SW, Shultz LD, Leiter EH. 1993. Adoptive transfer of diabetes into immunodeficient NOD-*scid/scid* mice. Relative contributions of $CD4^+$ and $CD8^+$ T-cells from diabetic versus prediabetic NOD.NON-*Thy*-1a donors. *Diabetes* **42:** 44–55. doi:10.2337/diab.42.1.44

Ciecko AE, Schauder DM, Foda B, Petrova G, Kasmani MY, Burns R, Lin CW, Drobyski WR, Cui W, Chen YG. 2021. Self-renewing islet $TCF1^+$ CD8 T cells undergo IL-27-controlled differentiation to become $TCF1^-$ terminal effectors during the progression of type 1 diabetes. *J Immunol* **207:** 1990–2004. doi:10.4049/jimmunol.2100362

Collier JL, Pauken KE, Lee CAA, Patterson DG, Markson SC, Conway TS, Fung ME, France JA, Mucciarone KN, Lian CG, et al. 2023. Single-cell profiling reveals unique features of diabetogenic T cells in anti-PD-1-induced type 1 diabetes mice. *J Exp Med* **220:** e20221920. doi:10.1084/jem.20221920

Conley JM, Gallagher MP, Berg LJ. 2016. T cells and gene regulation: the switching on and turning up of genes after T cell receptor stimulation in CD8 T cells. *Front Immunol* **7:** 76. doi:10.3389/fimmu.2016.00076

Connolly KA, Kuchroo M, Venkat A, Khatun A, Wang J, William I, Hornick NI, Fitzgerald BL, Damo M, Kasmani MY, et al. 2021. A reservoir of stem-like $CD8^+$ T cells in the tumor-draining lymph node preserves the ongoing antitumor immune response. *Sci Immunol* **6:** eabg7836. doi:10.1126/sciimmunol.abg7836

Coppieters KT, Boettler T, von Herrath M. 2012. Virus infections in type 1 diabetes. *Cold Spring Harb Perspect Med* **2:** a007682. doi:10.1101/cshperspect.a007682

Costanzo A, Clarke D, Holt M, Sharma S, Nagy K, Tan X, Kain L, Abe B, Luce S, Boitard C, et al. 2024. Repositioning the early pathology of type 1 diabetes to the extraislet vasculature. *J Immunol* **212:** 1094–1104. doi:10.4049/jimmunol.2300769

Couper JJ, Harrison LC, Aldis JJ, Colman PG, Honeyman MC, Ferrante A. 1998. Igg subclass antibodies to glutamic acid decarboxylase and risk for progression to clinical insulin-dependent diabetes. *Hum Immunol* **59:** 493–499. doi:10.1016/S0198-8859(98)00040-8

Crawford SA, Wiles TA, Wenzlau JM, Powell RL, Barbour G, Dang M, Groegler J, Barra JM, Burnette KS, Hohenstein AC, et al. 2022. Cathepsin D drives the formation of hybrid insulin peptides relevant to the pathogenesis of type 1 diabetes. *Diabetes* **71:** 2793–2803. doi:10.2337/db22-0303

Creusot RJ, Postigo-Fernandez J, Teteloshvili N. 2018. Altered function of antigen-presenting cells in type 1 diabetes: a challenge for antigen-specific immunotherapy? *Diabetes* **67:** 1481–1494. doi:10.2337/db17-1564

Cui C, Wang J, Fagerberg E, Chen PM, Connolly KA, Damo M, Cheung JF, Mao T, Askari AS, Chen S, et al. 2021. Neoantigen-driven B cell and CD4 T follicular helper cell collaboration promotes anti-tumor CD8 T cell responses. *Cell* **184:** 6101–6118.e13. doi:10.1016/j.cell.2021.11.007

Culina S, Lalanne AI, Afonso G, Cerosaletti K, Pinto S, Sebastiani G, Kuranda K, Nigi L, Eugster A, Østerbye T, et al. 2018. Islet-reactive CD8$^+$ T cell frequencies in the pancreas, but not in blood, distinguish type 1 diabetic patients from healthy donors. *Sci Immunol* **3:** eaao4013. doi:10.1126/sciimmunol.aao4013

De George DJ, Ge T, Krishnamurthy B, Kay TWH, Thomas HE. 2023. Inflammation versus regulation: how interferon-γ contributes to type 1 diabetes pathogenesis. *Front Cell Dev Biol* **11:** 1205590. doi:10.3389/fcell.2023.1205590

Delong T, Wiles TA, Baker RL, Bradley B, Barbour G, Reisdorph R, Armstrong M, Powell RL, Reisdorph N, Kumar N, et al. 2016. Pathogenic CD4 T cells in type 1 diabetes recognize epitopes formed by peptide fusion. *Science* **351:** 711–714. doi:10.1126/science.aad2791

Denton AE, Wesselingh R, Gras S, Guillonneau C, Olson MR, Mintern JD, Zeng W, Jackson DC, Rossjohn J, Hodgkin PD, et al. 2011. Affinity thresholds for naive CD8$^+$ CTL activation by peptides and engineered influenza A viruses. *J Immunol* **187:** 5733–5744. doi:10.4049/jimmunol.1003937

DiLisio JE, Haskins K. 2021. Induction of antigen-specific tolerance in autoimmune diabetes with nanoparticles containing hybrid insulin peptides. *Biomedicines* **9:** 240. doi:10.3390/biomedicines9030240

DiLorenzo TP, Lieberman SM, Takaki T, Honda S, Chapman HD, Santamaria P, Serreze DV, Nathenson SG. 2002. During the early prediabetic period in NOD mice, the pathogenic CD8$^+$ T-cell population comprises multiple antigenic specificities. *Clin Immunol* **105:** 332–341. doi:10.1006/clim.2002.5298

Dong Y, Wang T, Wu H. 2024. Tertiary lymphoid structures in autoimmune diseases. *Front Immunol* **14:** 1322035. doi:10.3389/fimmu.2023.1322035

Dozio N, Belloni C, Girardi AM, Genovese S, Sodoyez JC, Bottazzo GF, Pozza G, Bosi E. 1994. Heterogeneous IgG subclass distribution of islet cell antibodies. *J Autoimmun* **7:** 45–53. doi:10.1006/jaut.1994.1004

Dubois-LaForgue D, Carel JC, Bougnères PF, Guillet JG, Boitard C. 1999. T-cell response to proinsulin and insulin in type 1 and pretype 1 diabetes. *J Clin Immunol* **19:** 127–134. doi:10.1023/A:1020558601175

Duckworth BC, Lafouresse F, Wimmer VC, Broomfield BJ, Dalit L, Alexandre YO, Sheikh AA, Qin RZ, Alvarado C, Mielke LA, et al. 2021. Effector and stem-like memory cell fates are imprinted in distinct lymph node niches directed by CXCR3 ligands. *Nat Immunol* **22:** 434–448. doi:10.1038/s41590-021-00878-5

Dwyer CJ, Ward NC, Pugliese A, Malek TR. 2016. Promoting immune regulation in type 1 diabetes using low-dose interleukin-2. *Curr Diab Rep* **16:** 46. doi:10.1007/s11892-016-0739-1

Eisenbarth SC. 2019. Dendritic cell subsets in T cell programming: location dictates function. *Nat Rev Immunol* **19:** 89–103. doi:10.1038/s41577-018-0088-1

Escobar G, Mangani D, Anderson AC. 2020. T cell factor 1: a master regulator of the T cell response in disease. *Sci Immunol* **5:** eabb9726. doi:10.1126/sciimmunol.abb9726

Eshima K, Mora C, Wong FS, Green EA, Grewal IS, Flavell RA. 2003. A crucial role of CD4 T cells as a functional source of CD154 in the initiation of insulin-dependent diabetes mellitus in the non-obese diabetic mouse. *Int Immunol* **15:** 351–357. doi:10.1093/intimm/dxg035

Espinosa-Carrasco G, Le Saout C, Fontanaud P, Stratmann T, Mollard P, Schaeffer M, Hernandez J. 2018. CD4$^+$ T helper cells play a key role in maintaining diabetogenic CD8$^+$ T cell function in the pancreas. *Front Immunol* **8:** 2001. doi:10.3389/fimmu.2017.02001

Espinosa-Carrasco G, Chiu E, Scrivo A, Zumbo P, Dave A, Betel D, Kang SW, Jang HJ, Hellmann MD, Burt BM, et al. 2024. Intratumoral immune triads are required for immunotherapy-mediated elimination of solid tumors. *Cancer Cell* **42:** 1202–1216.e8. doi:10.1016/j.ccell.2024.05.025

Fasolino M, Schwartz GW, Patil AR, Mongia A, Golson ML, Wang YJ, Morgan A, Liu C, Schug J, Liu J, et al. 2022. Single-cell multi-omics analysis of human pancreatic islets reveals novel cellular states in type 1 diabetes. *Nat Metab* **4:** 284–299. doi:10.1038/s42255-022-00531-x

Ferraro A, Socci C, Stabilini A, Valle A, Monti P, Piemonti L, Nano R, Olek S, Maffi P, Scavini M, et al. 2011. Expansion of Th17 cells and functional defects in T regulatory cells are key features of the pancreatic lymph nodes in patients with type 1 diabetes. *Diabetes* **60:** 2903–2913. doi:10.2337/db11-0090

Ferreira RC, Simons HZ, Thompson WS, Cutler AJ, Dopico XC, Smyth DJ, Mashar M, Schuilenburg H, Walker NM, Dunger DB, et al. 2015. IL-21 production by CD4$^+$ effector T cells and frequency of circulating follicular helper T cells are increased in type 1 diabetes patients. *Diabetologia* **58:** 781–790. doi:10.1007/s00125-015-3509-8

Ferris ST, Carrero JA, Mohan JF, Calderon B, Murphy KM, Unanue ER. 2014. A minor subset of Batf3-dependent antigen-presenting cells in islets of Langerhans is essential for the development of autoimmune diabetes. *Immunity* **41:** 657–669. doi:10.1016/j.immuni.2014.09.012

Ferris ST, Carrero JA, Unanue ER. 2016. Antigen presentation events during the initiation of autoimmune diabetes in the NOD mouse. *J Autoimmun* **71:** 19–25. doi:10.1016/j.jaut.2016.03.007

Feuerer M, Shen Y, Littman DR, Benoist C, Mathis D. 2009. How punctual ablation of regulatory T cells unleashes an autoimmune lesion within the pancreatic islets. *Immunity* **31:** 654–664. doi:10.1016/j.immuni.2009.08.023

Firdessa Fite R, Bechi Genzano C, Mallone R, Creusot RJ. 2023. Epitope-based precision immunotherapy of type 1 diabetes. *Hum Vaccin Immunother* **19:** 2154098. doi:10.1080/21645515.2022.2154098

Gagnerault MC, Luan JJ, Lotton C, Lepault F. 2002. Pancreatic lymph nodes are required for priming of β cell reactive T cells in NOD mice. *J Exp Med* **196:** 369–377. doi:10.1084/jem.20011353

Gamble DR, Kinsley ML, FitzGerald MG, Bolton R, Taylor KW. 1969. Viral antibodies in diabetes mellitus. *Br Med J* **3:** 627–630. doi:10.1136/bmj.3.5671.627

Garg G, Tyler JR, Yang JH, Cutler AJ, Downes K, Pekalski M, Bell GL, Nutland S, Peakman M, Todd JA, et al. 2012. Type 1 diabetes-associated *IL2RA* variation lowers IL-2 signaling and contributes to diminished CD4$^+$CD25$^+$ regulatory T cell function. *J Immunol* **188:** 4644–4653. doi:10.4049/jimmunol.1100272

Gearty SV, Dündar F, Zumbo P, Espinosa-Carrasco G, Shakiba M, Sanchez-Rivera FJ, Socci ND, Trivedi P, Lowe SW,

Lauer P, et al. 2022. An autoimmune stem-like CD8 T cell population drives type 1 diabetes. *Nature* **602:** 156–161. doi:10.1038/s41586-021-04248-x

Gioia L, Holt M, Costanzo A, Sharma S, Abe B, Kain L, Nakayama M, Wan X, Su A, Mathews C, et al. 2019. Position β57 of I-A^{g7} controls early anti-insulin responses in NOD mice, linking an MHC susceptibility allele to type 1 diabetes onset. *Sci Immunol* **4:** eaaw6329. doi:10.1126/sciimmunol.aaw6329

Gounari F, Khazaie K. 2022. TCF-1: a maverick in T cell development and function. *Nat Immunol* **23:** 671–678. doi:10.1038/s41590-022-01194-2

Grebinoski S, Zhang Q, Cillo AR, Manne S, Xiao H, Brunazzi EA, Tabib T, Cardello C, Lian CG, Murphy GF, et al. 2022. Autoreactive $CD8^+$ T cells are restrained by an exhaustion-like program that is maintained by LAG3. *Nat Immunol* **23:** 868–877. doi:10.1038/s41590-022-01210-5

Guleria I, Gubbels Bupp M, Dada S, Fife B, Tang Q, Ansari MJ, Trikudanathan S, Vadivel N, Fiorina P, Yagita H, et al. 2007. Mechanisms of PDL1-mediated regulation of autoimmune diabetes. *Clin Immunol* **125:** 16–25. doi:10.1016/j.clim.2007.05.013

Hamilton-Williams EE, Palmer SE, Charlton B, Slattery RM. 2003. β cell MHC class I is a late requirement for diabetes. *Proc Natl Acad Sci* **100:** 6688–6693. doi:10.1073/pnas.1131954100

Hannelius U, Beam CA, Ludvigsson J. 2020. Efficacy of GAD-alum immunotherapy associated with HLA-DR3-DQ2 in recently diagnosed type 1 diabetes. *Diabetologia* **63:** 2177–2181. doi:10.1007/s00125-020-05227-z

Haskins K, McDuffie M. 1990. Acceleration of diabetes in young NOD mice with a $CD4^+$ islet-specific T cell clone. *Science* **249:** 1433–1436. doi:10.1126/science.2205920

Hawa MI, Fava D, Medici F, Deng YJ, Notkins AL, De Mattia G, Leslie RD. 2000. Antibodies to IA-2 and GAD65 in type 1 and type 2 diabetes: isotype restriction and polyclonality. *Diabetes Care* **23:** 228–233. doi:10.2337/diacare.23.2.228

He R, Hou S, Liu C, Zhang A, Bai Q, Han M, Yang Y, Wei G, Shen T, Yang X, et al. 2016. Follicular CXCR5-expressing $CD8^+$ T cells curtail chronic viral infection. *Nature* **537:** 412–428. doi:10.1038/nature19317

Herold KC, Bundy BN, Long SA, Bluestone JA, DiMeglio LA, Dufort MJ, Gitelman SE, Gottlieb PA, Krischer JP, Linsley PS, et al. 2019. An anti-CD3 antibody, teplizumab, in relatives at risk for type 1 diabetes. *N Engl J Med* **381:** 603–613. doi:10.1056/NEJMoa1902226

Herold KC, Delong T, Perdigoto AL, Biru N, Brusko TM, Walker LSK. 2024. The immunology of type 1 diabetes. *Nat Rev Immunol* **24:** 435–451. doi:10.1038/s41577-023-00985-4

Höglund P, Mintern J, Waltzinger C, Heath W, Benoist C, Mathis D. 1999. Initiation of autoimmune diabetes by developmentally regulated presentation of islet cell antigens in the pancreatic lymph nodes. *J Exp Med* **189:** 331–339. doi:10.1084/jem.189.2.331

Hoppu S, Ronkainen MS, Kimpimäki T, Simell S, Korhonen S, Ilonen J, Simell O, Knip M. 2004. Insulin autoantibody isotypes during the prediabetic process in young children with increased genetic risk of type 1 diabetes. *Pediatr Res* **55:** 236–242. doi:10.1203/01.PDR.0000100905.41131.3F

Hu H, Zakharov PN, Peterson OJ, Unanue ER. 2020. Cytocidal macrophages in symbiosis with CD4 and CD8 T cells cause acute diabetes following checkpoint blockade of PD-1 in NOD mice. *Proc Natl Acad Sci* **117:** 31319–31330. doi:10.1073/pnas.2019743117

Im SJ, Hashimoto M, Gerner MY, Lee J, Kissick HT, Burger MC, Shan Q, Hale JS, Lee J, Nasti TH, et al. 2016. Defining $CD8^+$ T cells that provide the proliferative burst after PD-1 therapy. *Nature* **537:** 417–421. doi:10.1038/nature19330

Ito Y, Ashenberg O, Pyrdol J, Luoma AM, Rozenblatt-Rosen O, Hofree M, Christian E, Ferrari de Andrade L, Tay RE, Teyton L, et al. 2018. Rapid CLIP dissociation from MHC II promotes an unusual antigen presentation pathway in autoimmunity. *J Exp Med* **215:** 2617–2635. doi:10.1084/jem.20180300

James EA, Mallone R, Kent SC, DiLorenzo TP. 2020. T-cell epitopes and neo-epitopes in type 1 diabetes: a comprehensive update and reappraisal. *Diabetes* **69:** 1311–1335. doi:10.2337/dbi19-0022

Jamison BL, Neef T, Goodspeed A, Bradley B, Baker RL, Miller SD, Haskins K. 2019. Nanoparticles containing an insulin-ChgA hybrid peptide protect from transfer of autoimmune diabetes by shifting the balance between effector T cells and regulatory T cells. *J Immunol* **203:** 48–57. doi:10.4049/jimmunol.1900127

Jansen CS, Prokhnevska N, Master VA, Sanda MG, Carlisle JW, Bilen MA, Cardenas M, Wilkinson S, Lake R, Sowalsky AG, et al. 2019. An intra-tumoral niche maintains and differentiates stem-like CD8 T cells. *Nature* **576:** 465–470. doi:10.1038/s41586-019-1836-5

Jung M, Lee J, Seo HY, Lim JS, Kim EK. 2015. Cathepsin inhibition-induced lysosomal dysfunction enhances pancreatic β-cell apoptosis in high glucose. *PLoS ONE* **10:** e0116972. doi:10.1371/journal.pone.0116972

Kasmani MY, Ciecko AE, Brown AK, Petrova G, Gorski J, Chen YG, Cui W. 2022. Autoreactive CD8 T cells in NOD mice exhibit phenotypic heterogeneity but restricted TCR gene usage. *Life Sci Alliance* **5:** e202201503. doi:10.26508/lsa.202201503

Katz JD, Wang B, Haskins K, Benoist C, Mathis D. 1993. Following a diabetogenic T cell from genesis through pathogenesis. *Cell* **74:** 1089–1100. doi:10.1016/0092-8674(93)90730-E

Kendall PL, Yu G, Woodward EJ, Thomas JW. 2007. Tertiary lymphoid structures in the pancreas promote selection of B lymphocytes in autoimmune diabetes. *J Immunol* **178:** 5643–5651. doi:10.4049/jimmunol.178.9.5643

Kenefeck R, Wang CJ, Kapadi T, Wardzinski L, Attridge K, Clough LE, Heuts F, Kogimtzis A, Patel S, Rosenthal M, et al. 2015. Follicular helper T cell signature in type 1 diabetes. *J Clin Invest* **125:** 292–303. doi:10.1172/JCI76238

Khan O, Giles JR, McDonald S, Manne S, Ngiow SF, Patel KP, Werner MT, Huang AC, Alexander KA, Wu JE, et al. 2019. TOX transcriptionally and epigenetically programs $CD8^+$ T cell exhaustion. *Nature* **571:** 211–218. doi:10.1038/s41586-019-1325-x

King CG, Koehli S, Hausmann B, Schmaler M, Zehn D, Palmer E. 2012. T cell affinity regulates asymmetric division, effector cell differentiation, and tissue pathology. *Immunity* **37:** 709–720. doi:10.1016/j.immuni.2012.06.021

Knip M, Simell O. 2012. Environmental triggers of type 1 diabetes. *Cold Spring Harb Perspect Med* **2:** a007690. doi:10.1101/cshperspect.a007690

Kornete M, Mason ES, Girouard J, Lafferty EI, Qureshi S, Piccirillo CA. 2015. Th1-Like ICOS$^+$ Foxp3$^+$ Treg cells preferentially express CXCR3 and home to β-islets during pre-diabetes in BDC2.5 NOD mice. *PLoS ONE* **10:** e0126311. doi:10.1371/journal.pone.0126311

Korpos É, Kadri N, Loismann S, Findeisen CR, Arfuso F, Burke GW, Richardson SJ, Morgan NG, Bogdani M, Pugliese A, et al. 2021. Identification and characterisation of tertiary lymphoid organs in human type 1 diabetes. *Diabetologia* **64:** 1626–1641. doi:10.1007/s00125-021-05453-z

Kratchmarov R, Djeddi S, Dunlap G, He W, Jia X, Burk CM, Ryan T, McGill A, Allegretti JR, Kataru RP, et al. 2024. TCF1-LEF1 co-expression identifies a multipotent progenitor cell (TH2-MPP) across human allergic diseases. *Nat Immunol* **25:** 902–915. doi:10.1038/s41590-024-01803-2

Lasch S, Müller P, Bayer M, Pfeilschifter JM, Luster AD, Hintermann E, Christen U. 2015. Anti-CD3/anti-CXCL10 antibody combination therapy induces a persistent remission of type 1 diabetes in two mouse models. *Diabetes* **64:** 4198–4211. doi:10.2337/db15-0479

Lee KU, Amano K, Yoon JW. 1988. Evidence for initial involvement of macrophage in development of insulitis in NOD mice. *Diabetes* **37:** 989–991. doi:10.2337/diab.37.7.989

Leong YA, Chen Y, Ong HS, Wu D, Man K, Deleage C, Minnich M, Meckiff BJ, Wei Y, Hou Z, et al. 2016. CXCR5$^+$ follicular cytotoxic T cells control viral infection in B cell follicles. *Nat Immunol* **17:** 1187–1196. doi:10.1038/ni.3543

Levisetti MG, Suri A, Frederick K, Unanue ER. 2004. Absence of lymph nodes in *NOD* mice treated with lymphotoxin-β receptor immunoglobulin protects from diabetes. *Diabetes* **53:** 3115–3119. doi:10.2337/diabetes.53.12.3115

Li MO, Rudensky AY. 2016. T cell receptor signalling in the control of regulatory T cell differentiation and function. *Nat Rev Immunol* **16:** 220–233. doi:10.1038/nri.2016.26

Li Y, Liu Y, Chu CQ. 2015. Th17 cells in type 1 diabetes: role in the pathogenesis and regulation by gut microbiome. *Mediators Inflamm* **2015:** 638470. doi:10.1155/2015/638470

Li Y, Ramírez-Suástegui C, Harris R, Castañeda-Castro FE, Ascui G, Pérez-Jeldres T, Diaz A, Morong C, Giles DA, Chai J, et al. 2024. Stem-like T cells are associated with the pathogenesis of ulcerative colitis in humans. *Nat Immunol* **25:** 1231–1244. doi:10.1038/s41590-024-01860-7

Lieberman SM, Evans AM, Han B, Takaki T, Vinnitskaya Y, Caldwell JA, Serreze DV, Shabanowitz J, Hunt DF, Nathenson SG, et al. 2003. Identification of the β cell antigen targeted by a prevalent population of pathogenic CD8$^+$ T cells in autoimmune diabetes. *Proc Natl Acad Sci* **100:** 8384–8388. doi:10.1073/pnas.0932778100

Lin MY, Welsh RM. 1998. Stability and diversity of T cell receptor repertoire usage during lymphocytic choriomeningitis virus infection of mice. *J Exp Med* **188:** 1993–2005. doi:10.1084/jem.188.11.1993

Lohmann T, Hawa M, Leslie RD, Lane R, Picard J, Londei M. 2000. Immune reactivity to glutamic acid decarboxylase 65 in Stiffman syndrome and type 1 diabetes mellitus. *Lancet* **356:** 31–35. doi:10.1016/S0140-6736(00)02431-4

Long SA, Cerosaletti K, Bollyky PL, Tatum M, Shilling H, Zhang S, Zhang ZY, Pihoker C, Sanda S, Greenbaum C, et al. 2010. Defects in IL-2R signaling contribute to diminished maintenance of FOXP3 expression in CD4$^+$CD25$^+$ regulatory T-cells of type 1 diabetic subjects. *Diabetes* **59:** 407–415. doi:10.2337/db09-0694

Long SA, Thorpe J, DeBerg HA, Gersuk V, Eddy J, Harris KM, Ehlers M, Herold KC, Nepom GT, Linsley PS. 2016. Partial exhaustion of CD8 T cells and clinical response to teplizumab in new-onset type 1 diabetes. *Sci Immunol* **1:** eaai7793. doi:10.1126/sciimmunol.aai7793

Mallone R, Martinuzzi E, Blancou P, Novelli G, Afonso G, Dolz M, Bruno G, Chaillous L, Chatenoud L, Bach JM, et al. 2007. CD8$^+$ T-cell responses identify β-cell autoimmunity in human type 1 diabetes. *Diabetes* **56:** 613–621. doi:10.2337/db06-1419

Mannering SI, Rubin AF, Wang R, Bhattacharjee P. 2021. Identifying new hybrid insulin peptides (HIPs) in type 1 diabetes. *Front Immunol* **12:** 667870. doi:10.3389/fimmu.2021.667870

Martin AP, Marinkovic T, Canasto-Chibuque C, Latif R, Unkeless JC, Davies TF, Takahama Y, Furtado GC, Lira SA. 2009. CCR7 deficiency in NOD mice leads to thyroiditis and primary hypothyroidism. *J Immunol* **183:** 3073–3080. doi:10.4049/jimmunol.0900275

McClymont SA, Putnam AL, Lee MR, Esensten JH, Liu W, Hulme MA, Hoffmüller U, Baron U, Olek S, Bluestone JA, et al. 2011. Plasticity of human regulatory T cells in healthy subjects and patients with type 1 diabetes. *J Immunol* **186:** 3918–3926. doi:10.4049/jimmunol.1003099

McGuire HM, Walters S, Vogelzang A, Lee CM, Webster KE, Sprent J, Christ D, Grey S, King C. 2011a. Interleukin-21 is critically required in autoimmune and allogeneic responses to islet tissue in murine models. *Diabetes* **60:** 867–875. doi:10.2337/db10-1157

McGuire HM, Vogelzang A, Ma CS, Hughes WE, Silveira PA, Tangye SG, Christ D, Fulcher D, Falcone M, King C. 2011b. A subset of interleukin-21$^+$ chemokine receptor CCR9$^+$ T helper cells target accessory organs of the digestive system in autoimmunity. *Immunity* **34:** 602–615. doi:10.1016/j.immuni.2011.01.021

McKinney EF, Lee JC, Jayne DR, Lyons PA, Smith KG. 2015. T-cell exhaustion, co-stimulation and clinical outcome in autoimmunity and infection. *Nature* **523:** 612–616. doi:10.1038/nature14468

Miller BJ, Appel MC, O'Neil JJ, Wicker LS. 1988. Both the Lyt-2$^+$ and L3T4$^+$ T cell subsets are required for the transfer of diabetes in nonobese diabetic mice. *J Immunol* **140:** 52–58. doi:10.4049/jimmunol.140.1.52

Millward A, Hussain MJ, Peakman M, Pyke DA, Leslie RD, Vergani D. 1988. Characterization of islet cell antibody in insulin dependent diabetes: evidence for IgG1 subclass restriction and polyclonality. *Clin Exp Immunol* **71:** 353–356.

Mitchell AM, Alkanani AA, McDaniel KA, Pyle L, Waugh K, Steck AK, Nakayama M, Yu L, Gottlieb PA, Rewers MJ, et al. 2021. T-cell responses to hybrid insulin peptides prior to type 1 diabetes development. *Proc Natl Acad Sci* **118:** e2019129118. doi:10.1073/pnas.2019129118

Mitchell JS, Spanier JA, Dwyer AJ, Knutson TP, Alkhatib MH, Qian G, Weno ME, Chen Y, Shaheen ZR, Tucker CG, et al. 2024. CD4+ T cells reactive to a hybrid peptide from insulin-chromogranin A adopt a distinct effector fate and are pathogenic in autoimmune diabetes. *Immunity* **57:** 2399–2415.e8. doi:10.1016/j.immuni.2024.07.024

Mitchison NA, O'Malley C. 1987. Three-cell-type clusters of T cells with antigen-presenting cells best explain the epitope linkage and noncognate requirements of the in vivo cytolytic response. *Eur J Immunol* **17:** 1579–1583. doi:10.1002/eji.1830171109

Mollah ZU, Graham KL, Krishnamurthy B, Trivedi P, Brodnicki TC, Trapani JA, Kay TW, Thomas HE. 2012. Granzyme B is dispensable in the development of diabetes in non-obese diabetic mice. *PLoS ONE* **7:** e40357. doi:10.1371/journal.pone.0040357

Morris MA, McDuffie M, Nadler JL, Ley K. 2011. Prevention, but not cure, of autoimmune diabetes in a NOD.*scid* transfer model by FTY720 despite effective modulation of blood T cells. *Autoimmunity* **44:** 115–128. doi:10.3109/08916934.2010.499885

Nakayama M, Abiru N, Moriyama H, Babaya N, Liu E, Miao D, Yu L, Wegmann DR, Hutton JC, Elliott JF, et al. 2005. Prime role for an insulin epitope in the development of type 1 diabetes in NOD mice. *Nature* **435:** 220–223. doi:10.1038/nature03523

O'Flaherty E, Kaye J. 2003. TOX defines a conserved subfamily of HMG-box proteins. *BMC Genomics* **4:** 13. doi:10.1186/1471-2164-4-13

Ozga AJ, Moalli F, Abe J, Swoger J, Sharpe J, Zehn D, Kreutzfeldt M, Merkler D, Ripoll J, Stein JV. 2016. pMHC affinity controls duration of CD8+ T cell–DC interactions and imprints timing of effector differentiation versus expansion. *J Exp Med* **213:** 2811–2829. doi:10.1084/jem.20160206

Paley MA, Kroy DC, Odorizzi PM, Johnnidis JB, Dolfi DV, Barnett BE, Bikoff EK, Robertson EJ, Lauer GM, Reiner SL, et al. 2012. Progenitor and terminal subsets of CD8+ T cells cooperate to contain chronic viral infection. *Science* **338:** 1220–1225. doi:10.1126/science.1229620

Parras D, Solé P, Delong T, Santamaría P, Serra P. 2021. Recognition of multiple hybrid insulin peptides by a single highly diabetogenic T-cell receptor. *Front Immunol* **12:** 737428. doi:10.3389/fimmu.2021.737428

Patil AR, Schug J, Naji A, Kaestner KH, Faryabi RB, Vahedi G. 2023. Single-cell expression profiling of islets generated by the Human Pancreas Analysis Program. *Nat Metab* **5:** 713–715. doi:10.1038/s42255-023-00806-x

Patil AR, Schug J, Liu C, Lahori D, Descamps HC, Naji A; Human Pancreas Analysis Consortium; Kaestner KH, Faryabi RB, Vahedi G. 2024. Modeling type 1 diabetes progression using machine learning and single-cell transcriptomic measurements in human islets. *Cell Rep Med* **5:** 101535. doi:10.1016/j.xcrm.2024.101535

Peng Y, Xiao L, Rong H, Ou Z, Cai T, Liu N, Li B, Zhang L, Wu F, Lan T, et al. 2021. Single-cell profiling of tumor-infiltrating TCF1/TCF7+ T cells reveals a T lymphocyte subset associated with tertiary lymphoid structures/organs and a superior prognosis in oral cancer. *Oral Oncol* **119:** 105348. doi:10.1016/j.oraloncology.2021.105348

Philip M, Schietinger A. 2022. CD8+ T cell differentiation and dysfunction in cancer. *Nat Rev Immunol* **22:** 209–223. doi:10.1038/s41577-021-00574-3

Phillips JM, Parish NM, Raine T, Bland C, Sawyer Y, De La Peña H, Cooke A. 2009. Type 1 diabetes development requires both CD4+ and CD8+ T cells and can be reversed by non-depleting antibodies targeting both T cell populations. *Rev Diab Stud* **6:** 97–103. doi:10.1900/RDS.2009.6.97

Postigo-Fernandez J, Farber DL, Creusot RJ. 2019. Phenotypic alterations in pancreatic lymph node stromal cells from human donors with type 1 diabetes and NOD mice. *Diabetologia* **62:** 2040–2051. doi:10.1007/s00125-019-04984-w

Prasad S, Neef T, Xu D, Podojil JR, Getts DR, Shea LD, Miller SD. 2018. Tolerogenic Ag-PLG nanoparticles induce Tregs to suppress activated diabetogenic CD4 and CD8 T cells. *J Autoimmun* **89:** 112–124. doi:10.1016/j.jaut.2017.12.010

Probst HC, Tschannen K, Gallimore A, Martinic M, Basler M, Dumrese T, Jones E, van den Broek MF. 2003. Immunodominance of an antiviral cytotoxic T cell response is shaped by the kinetics of viral protein expression. *J Immunol* **171:** 5415–5422. doi:10.4049/jimmunol.171.10.5415

Pugliese A. 2017. Autoreactive T cells in type 1 diabetes. *J Clin Invest* **127:** 2881–2891. doi:10.1172/JCI94549

Purcell AW, Sechi S, DiLorenzo TP. 2019. The evolving landscape of autoantigen discovery and characterization in type 1 diabetes. *Diabetes* **68:** 879–886. doi:10.2337/dbi18-0066

Quesada-Masachs E, Zilberman S, Rajendran S, Chu T, McArdle S, Kiosses WB, Lee JM, Yesildag B, Benkahla MA, Pawlowska A, et al. 2022. Upregulation of HLA class II in pancreatic β cells from organ donors with type 1 diabetes. *Diabetologia* **65:** 387–401. doi:10.1007/s00125-021-05619-9

Redondo MJ, Steck AK, Pugliese A. 2018. Genetics of type 1 diabetes. *Pediatr Diabetes* **19:** 346–353. doi:10.1111/pedi.12597

Rich SS, Weitkamp LR, Barbosa J. 1984. Genetic heterogeneity of insulin-dependent (type 1) diabetes mellitus: evidence from a study of extended haplotypes. *Am J Hum Genet* **36:** 1015–1023.

Richard AC, Lun ATL, Lau WWY, Göttgens B, Marioni JC, Griffiths GM. 2018. T cell cytolytic capacity is independent of initial stimulation strength. *Nat Immunol* **19:** 849–858. doi:10.1038/s41590-018-0160-9

Ridge JP, Di Rosa F, Matzinger P. 1998. A conditioned dendritic cell can be a temporal bridge between a CD4+ T-helper and a T-killer cell. *Nature* **393:** 474–478. doi:10.1038/30989

Robertson CC, Inshaw JRJ, Onengut-Gumuscu S, Chen WM, Santa Cruz DF, Yang H, Cutler AJ, Crouch DJM, Farber E, Bridges SL, et al. 2021. Fine-mapping, trans-ancestral and genomic analyses identify causal variants, cells, genes and drug targets for type 1 diabetes. *Nat Genet* **53:** 962–971. doi:10.1038/s41588-021-00880-5

Rosenzwajg M, Salet R, Lorenzon R, Tchitchek N, Roux A, Bernard C, Carel JC, Storey C, Polak M, Beltrand J, et al. 2020. Low-dose IL-2 in children with recently diagnosed type 1 diabetes: a phase I/II randomised, double-blind, placebo-controlled, dose-finding study. *Diabetologia* **63:** 1808–1821. doi:10.1007/s00125-020-05200-w

Russell MA, Redick SD, Blodgett DM, Richardson SJ, Leete P, Krogvold L, Dahl-Jørgensen K, Bottino R, Brissova M, Spaeth JM, et al. 2019. HLA class II antigen processing and presentation pathway components demonstrated by transcriptome and protein analyses of islet β-cells from donors with type 1 diabetes. *Diabetes* **68:** 988–1001. doi:10.2337/db18-0686

Sade-Feldman M, Yizhak K, Bjorgaard SL, Ray JP, de Boer CG, Jenkins RW, Lieb DJ, Chen JH, Frederick DT, Barzily-Rokni M, et al. 2018. Defining T cell states associated with response to checkpoint immunotherapy in melanoma. *Cell* **175:** 998–1013.e20. doi:10.1016/j.cell.2018.10.038

Salomon B, Lenschow DJ, Rhee L, Ashourian N, Singh B, Sharpe A, Bluestone JA. 2000. B7/CD28 costimulation is essential for the homeostasis of the $CD4^+CD25^+$ immunoregulatory T cells that control autoimmune diabetes. *Immunity* **12:** 431–440. doi:10.1016/S1074-7613(00)80195-8

Samassa F, Mallone R. 2022. Self-antigens, benign autoimmunity and type 1 diabetes: a β-cell and T-cell perspective. *Curr Opin Endocrinol Diabetes Obes* **29:** 370–378. doi:10.1097/MED.0000000000000735

Sandor AM, Jacobelli J, Friedman RS. 2019. Immune cell trafficking to the islets during type 1 diabetes. *Clin Exp Immunol* **198:** 314–325. doi:10.1111/cei.13353

Sato Y, Jain A, Ohtsuki S, Okuyama H, Sturmlechner I, Takashima Y, Le KC, Bois MC, Berry GJ, Warrington KJ, et al. 2023. Stem-like $CD4^+$ T cells in perivascular tertiary lymphoid structures sustain autoimmune vasculitis. *Sci Transl Med* **15:** eadh0380. doi:10.1126/scitranslmed.adh0380

Schnell A, Huang L, Singer M, Singaraju A, Barilla RM, Regan BML, Bollhagen A, Thakore PI, Dionne D, Delorey TM, et al. 2021. Stem-like intestinal Th17 cells give rise to pathogenic effector T cells during autoimmunity. *Cell* **184:** 6281–6298.e23. doi:10.1016/j.cell.2021.11.018

Schober K, Voit F, Grassmann S, Müller TR, Eggert J, Jarosch S, Weißbrich B, Hoffmann P, Borkner L, Nio E, et al. 2020. Reverse TCR repertoire evolution toward dominant low-affinity clones during chronic CMV infection. *Nat Immunol* **21:** 434–441. doi:10.1038/s41590-020-0628-2

Schoenberger SP, Toes RE, van der Voort EI, Offringa R, Melief CJ. 1998. T-cell help for cytotoxic T lymphocytes is mediated by CD40–CD40L interactions. *Nature* **393:** 480–483. doi:10.1038/31002

Schuster C, Jonas F, Zhao F, Kissler S. 2018. Peripherally induced regulatory T cells contribute to the control of autoimmune diabetes in the NOD mouse model. *Eur J Immunol* **48:** 1211–1216. doi:10.1002/eji.201847498

Scott AC, Dündar F, Zumbo P, Chandran SS, Klebanoff CA, Shakiba M, Trivedi P, Menocal L, Appleby H, Camara S, et al. 2019. TOX is a critical regulator of tumour-specific T cell differentiation. *Nature* **571:** 270–274. doi:10.1038/s41586-019-1324-y

Selck C, Jhala G, De George DJ, Kwong CJ, Christensen MK, Pappas EG, Liu X, Ge T, Trivedi P, Kallies A, et al. 2024. Extraislet expression of islet antigen boosts T cell exhaustion to partially prevent autoimmune diabetes. *Proc Natl Acad Sci* **121:** e2315419121. doi:10.1073/pnas.2315419121

Seo H, Chen J, González-Avalos E, Samaniego-Castruita D, Das A, Wang YH, López-Moyado IF, Georges RO, Zhang W, Onodera A, et al. 2019. TOX and TOX2 transcription factors cooperate with NR4A transcription factors to impose $CD8^+$ T cell exhaustion. *Proc Natl Acad Sci* **116:** 12410–12415. doi:10.1073/pnas.1905675116

Shakiba M, Zumbo P, Espinosa-Carrasco G, Menocal L, Dündar F, Carson SE, Bruno EM, Sanchez-Rivera FJ, Lowe SW, Camara S, et al. 2022. TCR signal strength defines distinct mechanisms of T cell dysfunction and cancer evasion. *J Exp Med* **219:** e20201966. doi:10.1084/jem.20201966

Sharma S, Tan X, Boyer J, Clarke D, Costanzo A, Abe B, Kain L, Holt M, Armstrong A, Rihanek M, et al. 2023. Measuring anti-islet autoimmunity in mouse and human by profiling peripheral blood antigen-specific CD4 T cells. *Sci Transl Med* **15:** eade3614. doi:10.1126/scitranslmed.ade3614

Shevach EM, Thornton AM. 2014. Ttregs, pTregs, and iTregs: similarities and differences. *Immunol Rev* **259:** 88–102. doi:10.1111/imr.12160

Shizuru JA, Taylor-Edwards C, Banks BA, Gregory AK, Fathman CG. 1988. Immunotherapy of the nonobese diabetic mouse: treatment with an antibody to T-helper lymphocytes. *Science* **240:** 659–662. doi:10.1126/science.2966437

Siddiqui I, Schaeuble K, Chennupati V, Fuertes Marraco SA, Calderon-Copete S, Pais Ferreira D, Carmona SJ, Scarpellino L, Gfeller D, Pradervand S, et al. 2019. Intratumoral $Tcf1^+PD\text{-}1^+CD8^+$ T cells with stem-like properties promote tumor control in response to vaccination and checkpoint blockade immunotherapy. *Immunity* **50:** 195–211.e10. doi:10.1016/j.immuni.2018.12.021

Sim MJW, Lu J, Spencer M, Hopkins F, Tran E, Rosenberg SA, Long EO, Sun PD. 2020. High-affinity oligoclonal TCRs define effective adoptive T cell therapy targeting mutant KRAS-G12D. *Proc Natl Acad Sci* **117:** 12826–12835. doi:10.1073/pnas.1921964117

Sims EK, Bundy BN, Stier K, Serti E, Lim N, Long SA, Geyer SM, Moran A, Greenbaum CJ, Evans-Molina C, et al. 2021. Teplizumab improves and stabilizes β cell function in antibody-positive high-risk individuals. *Sci Transl Med* **13:** eabc8980. doi:10.1126/scitranslmed.abc8980

Singh N, Hocking AM, Buckner JH. 2023. Immune-related adverse events after immune check point inhibitors: understanding the intersection with autoimmunity. *Immunol Rev* **318:** 81–88. doi:10.1111/imr.13247

Skokos D, Shakhar G, Varma R, Waite JC, Cameron TO, Lindquist RL, Schwickert T, Nussenzweig MC, Dustin ML. 2007. Peptide-MHC potency governs dynamic interactions between T cells and dendritic cells in lymph nodes. *Nat Immunol* **8:** 835–844. doi:10.1038/ni1490

Spanier JA, Sahli NL, Wilson JC, Martinov T, Dileepan T, Burrack AL, Finger EB, Blazar BR, Michels AW, Moran A, et al. 2017. Increased effector memory insulin-specific $CD4^+$ T cells correlate with insulin autoantibodies in patients with recent-onset type 1 diabetes. *Diabetes* **66:** 3051–3060. doi:10.2337/db17-0666

Spanier JA, Fung V, Wardell CM, Alkhatib MH, Chen Y, Swanson LA, Dwyer AJ, Weno ME, Silva N, Mitchell JS, et al. 2023. Tregs with an MHC class II peptide-specific chimeric antigen receptor prevent autoimmune diabetes in mice. *J Clin Invest* **133:** e168601. doi:10.1172/JCI168601

Spolski R, Kashyap M, Robinson C, Yu Z, Leonard WJ. 2008. IL-21 signaling is critical for the development of type I diabetes in the NOD mouse. *Proc Natl Acad Sci* **105:** 14028–14033. doi:10.1073/pnas.0804358105

Sprouse ML, Scavuzzo MA, Blum S, Shevchenko I, Lee T, Makedonas G, Borowiak M, Bettini ML, Bettini M. 2018. High self-reactivity drives T-bet and potentiates Treg function in tissue-specific autoimmunity. *JCI Insight* **3:** e97322. doi:10.1172/jci.insight.97322

Stadinski BD, Cleveland SB, Brehm MA, Greiner DL, Huseby PG, Huseby ES. 2023. I-A^{g7} β56/57 polymorphisms regulate non-cognate negative selection to CD4$^+$ T cell orchestrators of type 1 diabetes. *Nat Immunol* **24:** 652–663. doi:10.1038/s41590-023-01441-0

Stone JD, Chervin AS, Kranz DM. 2009. T-cell receptor binding affinities and kinetics: impact on T-cell activity and specificity. *Immunology* **126:** 165–176. doi:10.1111/j.1365-2567.2008.03015.x

Suri A, Walters JJ, Gross ML, Unanue ER. 2005. Natural peptides selected by diabetogenic DQ8 and murine I-A (g7) molecules show common sequence specificity. *J Clin Invest* **115:** 2268–2276. doi:10.1172/JCI25350

Tan TG, Mathis D, Benoist C. 2016. Singular role for T-BET$^+$CXCR3$^+$ regulatory T cells in protection from autoimmune diabetes. *Proc Natl Acad Sci* **113:** 14103–14108. doi:10.1073/pnas.1616710113

Thomas HE, Parker JL, Schreiber RD, Kay TW. 1998. IFN-γ action on pancreatic β cells causes class I MHC upregulation but not diabetes. *J Clin Invest* **102:** 1249–1257. doi:10.1172/JCI2899

Thomas HE, Trapani JA, Kay TWH. 2010. The role of perforin and granzymes in diabetes. *Cell Death Differ* **17:** 577–585. doi:10.1038/cdd.2009.165

Thornton CA, Mulqueen RM, Torkenczy KA, Nishida A, Lowenstein EG, Fields AJ, Steemers FJ, Zhang W, McConnell HL, Woltjer RL, et al. 2021. Spatially mapped single-cell chromatin accessibility. *Nat Commun* **12:** 1274. doi:10.1038/s41467-021-21515-7

Trivedi P, Graham KL, Krishnamurthy B, Fynch S, Slattery RM, Kay TW, Thomas HE. 2016. Perforin facilitates β cell killing and regulates autoreactive CD8$^+$ T-cell responses to antigen in mouse models of type 1 diabetes. *Immunol Cell Biol* **94:** 334–341. doi:10.1038/icb.2015.89

Uenishi GI, Repic M, Yam JY, Landuyt A, Saikumar-Lakshmi P, Guo T, Zarin P, Sassone-Corsi M, Chicoine A, Kellogg H, et al. 2024. GNTI-122: an autologous antigen-specific engineered Treg cell therapy for type 1 diabetes. *JCI Insight* **9:** e171844. doi:10.1172/jci.insight.171844

Ueno T, Tomiyama H, Fujiwara M, Oka S, Takiguchi M. 2004. Functionally impaired HIV-specific CD8 T cells show high affinity TCR-ligand interactions. *J Immunol* **173:** 5451–5457. doi:10.4049/jimmunol.173.9.5451

Unanue ER. 2014. Antigen presentation in the autoimmune diabetes of the NOD mouse. *Annu Rev Immunol* **32:** 579–608. doi:10.1146/annurev-immunol-032712-095941

Utzschneider DT, Charmoy M, Chennupati V, Pousse L, Ferreira DP, Calderon-Copete S, Danilo M, Alfei F, Hofmann M, Wieland D, et al. 2016. T cell factor 1-expressing memory-like CD8$^+$ T cells sustain the immune response to chronic viral infections. *Immunity* **45:** 415–427. doi:10.1016/j.immuni.2016.07.021

Vecchione A, Jofra T, Gerosa J, Shankwitz K, Di Fonte R, Galvani G, Ippolito E, Cicalese MP, Schultz AR, Seay HR, et al. 2021. Reduced follicular regulatory T cells in spleen and pancreatic lymph nodes of patients with type 1 diabetes. *Diabetes* **70:** 2892–2902. doi:10.2337/db21-0091

Viisanen T, Ihantola EL, Näntö-Salonen K, Hyöty H, Nurminen N, Selvenius J, Juutilainen A, Moilanen L, Pihlajamäki J, Veijola R, et al. 2017. Circulating CXCR5$^+$ PD-1$^+$ICOS$^+$ follicular T helper cells are increased close to the diagnosis of type 1 diabetes in children with multiple autoantibodies. *Diabetes* **66:** 437–447. doi:10.2337/db16-0714

von Herrath M, Bain SC, Bode B, Clausen JO, Coppieters K, Gaysina L, Gumprecht J, Hansen TK, Mathieu C, Morales C, et al. 2021. Anti-interleukin-21 antibody and liraglutide for the preservation of β-cell function in adults with recent-onset type 1 diabetes: a randomised, double-blind, placebo-controlled, phase 2 trial. *Lancet Diabetes Endocrinol* **9:** 212–224. doi:10.1016/S2213-8587(21)00019-X

Walker LS, von Herrath M. 2016. CD4 T cell differentiation in type 1 diabetes. *Clin Exp Immunol* **183:** 16–29. doi:10.1111/cei.12672

Wan X, Thomas JW, Unanue ER. 2016. Class-switched anti-insulin antibodies originate from unconventional antigen presentation in multiple lymphoid sites. *J Exp Med* **213:** 967–978. doi:10.1084/jem.20151869

Wan X, Zinselmeyer BH, Zakharov PN, Vomund AN, Taniguchi R, Santambrogio L, Anderson MS, Lichti CF, Unanue ER. 2018. Pancreatic islets communicate with lymphoid tissues via exocytosis of insulin peptides. *Nature* **560:** 107–111. doi:10.1038/s41586-018-0341-6

Wang B, Gonzalez A, Benoist C, Mathis D. 1996. The role of CD8$^+$ T cells in the initiation of insulin-dependent diabetes mellitus. *Eur J Immunol* **26:** 1762–1769. doi:10.1002/eji.1830260815

Wang J, Yoshida T, Nakaki F, Hiai H, Okazaki T, Honjo T. 2005. Establishment of NOD-*Pdcd1*$^{-/-}$ mice as an efficient animal model of type I diabetes. *Proc Natl Acad Sci* **102:** 11823–11828. doi:10.1073/pnas.0505497102

Watts D, Janßen M, Jaykar M, Palmucci F, Weigelt M, Petzold C, Hommel A, Sparwasser T, Bonifacio E, Kretschmer K. 2021. Transient depletion of Foxp3$^+$ regulatory T cells selectively promotes aggressive β cell autoimmunity in genetically susceptible DEREG mice. *Front Immunol* **12:** 720133. doi:10.3389/fimmu.2021.720133

Wenzlau JM, DiLisio JE, Barbour G, Dang M, Hohenstein AC, Nakayama M, Delong T, Baker RL, Haskins K. 2022. Insulin B-chain hybrid peptides are agonists for T cells reactive to insulin B:9–23 in autoimmune diabetes. *Front Immunol* **13:** 926650. doi:10.3389/fimmu.2022.926650

Wesley JD, Pagni PP, Bergholdt R, Kreiner FF, von Herrath M. 2022. Induction of antigenic immune tolerance to delay type 1 diabetes—challenges for clinical translation. *Curr Opin Endocrinol Diabetes Obes* **29:** 379–385. doi:10.1097/MED.0000000000000742

Wiedeman AE, Muir VS, Rosasco MG, DeBerg HA, Presnell S, Haas B, Dufort MJ, Speake C, Greenbaum CJ, Serti E, et al. 2020. Autoreactive CD8+ T cell exhaustion distinguishes subjects with slow type 1 diabetes progression. *J Clin Invest* **130:** 480–490. doi:10.1172/JCI126595

Wiles TA, Delong T, Baker RL, Bradley B, Barbour G, Powell RL, Reisdorph N, Haskins K. 2017. An insulin-IAPP hybrid peptide is an endogenous antigen for CD4 T cells in the non-obese diabetic mouse. *J Autoimmun* **78:** 11–18. doi:10.1016/j.jaut.2016.10.007

Wiles TA, Powell R, Michel R, Beard KS, Hohenstein A, Bradley B, Reisdorph N, Haskins K, Delong T. 2019. Identification of hybrid insulin peptides (HIPs) in mouse and human islets by mass spectrometry. *J Proteome Res* **18:** 814–825. doi:10.1021/acs.jproteome.8b00875

Wiles TA, Saba LM, Delong T. 2021a. Peptide–spectrum match validation with internal standards (P–VIS): internally controlled validation of mass spectrometry-based peptide identifications. *J Proteome Res* **20:** 236–249. doi:10.1021/acs.jproteome.0c00355

Wiles TA, Hohenstein A, Landry LG, Dang M, Powell R, Guyer P, James EA, Nakayama M, Haskins K, Delong T, et al. 2021b. Characterization of human CD4 T cells specific for a C-peptide/C-peptide hybrid insulin peptide. *Front Immunol* **12:** 668680. doi:10.3389/fimmu.2021.668680

Wong FS, Karttunen J, Dumont C, Wen L, Visintin I, Pilip IM, Shastri N, Pamer EG, Janeway CA Jr. 1999. Identification of an MHC class I–restricted autoantigen in type 1 diabetes by screening an organ-specific cDNA library. *Nat Med* **5:** 1026–1031. doi:10.1038/12465

Wong J, Mathis D, Benoist C. 2007. TCR-based lineage tracing: no evidence for conversion of conventional into regulatory T cells in response to a natural self-antigen in pancreatic islets. *J Exp Med* **204:** 2039–2045. doi:10.1084/jem.20070822

Writing Committee for the Type 1 Diabetes TrialNet Oral Insulin Study Group; Krischer JP, Schatz DA, Bundy B, Skyler JS, Greenbaum CJ. 2017. Effect of oral insulin on prevention of diabetes in relatives of patients with type 1 diabetes: a randomized clinical trial. *JAMA* **318:** 1891–1902. doi:10.1001/jama.2017.17070

Wu T, Ji Y, Moseman EA, Xu HC, Manglani M, Kirby M, Anderson SM, Handon R, Kenyon E, Elkahloun A, et al. 2016. The TCF1-Bcl6 axis counteracts type I interferon to repress exhaustion and maintain T cell stemness. *Sci Immunol* **1:** eaai8593. doi:10.1126/sciimmunol.aai8593

Wu R, Veličkovič M, Burnum-Johnson KE. 2024. From single-cell to spatial multi-omics: unveiling molecular mechanisms in dynamic and heterogeneous systems. *Curr Opin Biotechnol* **89:** 103174. doi:10.1016/j.copbio.2024.103174

Xia Y, Sandor K, Pai JA, Daniel B, Raju S, Wu R, Hsiung S, Qi Y, Yangdon T, Okamoto M, et al. 2022. BCL6-dependent TCF-1+ progenitor cells maintain effector and helper CD4+ T cell responses to persistent antigen. *Immunity* **55:** 1200–1215.e6. doi:10.1016/j.immuni.2022.05.003

Yang SJ, Singh AK, Drow T, Tappen T, Honaker Y, Barahmand-Pour-Whitman F, Linsley PS, Cerosaletti K, Mauk K, Xiang Y, et al. 2022. Pancreatic islet-specific engineered Tregs exhibit robust antigen-specific and bystander immune suppression in type 1 diabetes models. *Sci Transl Med* **14:** eabn1716. doi:10.1126/scitranslmed.abn1716

Yao C, Sun HW, Lacey NE, Ji Y, Moseman EA, Shih HY, Heuston EF, Kirby M, Anderson S, Cheng J, et al. 2019. Single-cell RNA-seq reveals TOX as a key regulator of CD8+ T cell persistence in chronic infection. *Nat Immunol* **20:** 890–901. doi:10.1038/s41590-019-0403-4

Yeung WC, Rawlinson WD, Craig ME. 2011. Enterovirus infection and type 1 diabetes mellitus: systematic review and meta-analysis of observational molecular studies. *BMJ* **342:** d35. doi:10.1136/bmj.d35

Yi JS, Du M, Zajac AJ. 2009. A vital role for interleukin-21 in the control of a chronic viral infection. *Science* **324:** 1572–1576. doi:10.1126/science.1175194

Zakharov PN, Hu H, Wan X, Unanue ER. 2020. Single-cell RNA sequencing of murine islets shows high cellular complexity at all stages of autoimmune diabetes. *J Exp Med* **217:** e20192362. doi:10.1084/jem.20192362

Zander R, Kasmani MY, Chen Y, Topchyan P, Shen J, Zheng S, Burns R, Ingram J, Cui C, Joshi N, et al. 2022. Tfh-cell-derived interleukin 21 sustains effector CD8+ T cell responses during chronic viral infection. *Immunity* **55:** 475–493.e5. doi:10.1016/j.immuni.2022.01.018

Zehn D, Lee SY, Bevan MJ. 2009. Complete but curtailed T-cell response to very low-affinity antigen. *Nature* **458:** 211–214. doi:10.1038/nature07657

Zhang JY, Hamey F, Trzupek D, Mickunas M, Lee M, Godfrey L, Yang JHM, Pekalski ML, Kennet J, Waldron-Lynch F, et al. 2022. Low-dose IL-2 reduces IL-21+ T cell frequency and induces anti-inflammatory gene expression in type 1 diabetes. *Nat Commun* **13:** 7324. doi:10.1038/s41467-022-34162-3

Zhao Y, Scott NA, Quah HS, Krishnamurthy B, Bond F, Loudovaris T, Mannering SI, Kay TW, Thomas HE. 2015. Mouse pancreatic β cells express MHC class II and stimulate CD4+ T cells to proliferate. *Eur J Immunol* **45:** 2494–2503. doi:10.1002/eji.201445378

Zhao X, Shan Q, Xue HH. 2022. TCF1 in T cell immunity: a broadened frontier. *Nat Rev Immunol* **22:** 147–157. doi:10.1038/s41577-021-00563-6

Zhou L, Chong MM, Littman DR. 2009a. Plasticity of CD4+ T cell lineage differentiation. *Immunity* **30:** 646–655. doi:10.1016/j.immuni.2009.05.001

Zhou X, Bailey-Bucktrout SL, Jeker LT, Penaranda C, Martínez-Llordella M, Ashby M, Nakayama M, Rosenthal W, Bluestone JA. 2009b. Instability of the transcription factor Foxp3 leads to the generation of pathogenic memory T cells in vivo. *Nat Immunol* **10:** 1000–1007. doi:10.1038/ni.1774

Zhu J. 2018. T helper cell differentiation, heterogeneity, and plasticity. *Cold Spring Harb Perspect Biol* **10:** a030338. doi:10.1101/cshperspect.a030338

Zou D, Yin Z, Yi SG, Wang G, Guo Y, Xiao X, Li S, Zhang X, Gonzalez NM, Minze LJ, et al. 2024. CD4+ T cell immunity is dependent on an intrinsic stem-like program. *Nat Immunol* **25:** 66–76. doi:10.1038/s41590-023-01682-z

Genetics and Epigenetics of Type 1 Diabetes Self-Reactive T Cells

Tae Gun Kang and Benjamin Youngblood

Department of Immunology, St. Jude Children's Research Hospital, Memphis, Tennessee 38105, USA

Correspondence: benjamin.youngblood@stjude.org; taegun.kang@stjude.org

Type 1 diabetes (T1D) serves as an exemplar of chronic autoimmune disease characterized by insulin deficiency due to pancreatic β-cell destruction, leading to hyperglycemia and progressive organ failure. Until recently, therapeutic efforts to mitigate the root cause of disease have been limited by the challenges in studying mechanisms involved in immune tolerance in humans. The current clinical advances, and existing challenges, highlight a need to incorporate new insights into mechanisms into correlative studies that assess immune tolerance in the setting of delayed β-cell destruction. Among several factors known to promote T1D, autoreactive T cells play a critical role in initiating and sustaining disease through their direct recognition and destruction of β cells. Emerging research defining the genetic and epigenetic etiology of long-lived β-cell-specific T cells is providing new insight into mechanisms that promote lifelong disease and future opportunities for targeted therapeutic intervention. This article will provide an overview of recent progress toward understanding the development of autoreactive T cells and epigenetic mechanisms stabilizing their developmental state during T1D pathogenesis.

Type 1 diabetes (T1D) is demarcated by a progressive destruction of insulin-producing pancreatic β cells in the islets of Langerhans, and when untreated, results in increased blood glucose levels (hyperglycemia), that can ultimately cause failure of multiple organs. Such pathogenesis is the cause of one of the most severe childhood autoimmune diseases. While daily insulin injection delays secondary infirmities, T1D patients remain at high risk of serious complications, including cardiovascular mortality (DiMeglio et al. 2018). New interventions are, therefore, urgently required to prevent new-onset disease and treat individuals with established T1D.

The etiology of T1D has been largely linked to genetic, epigenetic, and environmental factors that enable the immune system to break tolerance and target pancreatic islets. T1D can be diagnosed by the emergence of autoantibodies arising many months or years before detectable pathology. Disease progression is broadly demarcated by the initial detection of two or more autoantibodies followed by a stage of the disease where autoantibodies are detected in conjunction with β-cell destruction (Herold et al. 2024). During the progression of T1D, these antibodies are not thought to be causing factors for T1D but serve as a robust diagnostic biomarker of the forthcom-

Cite this article as *Cold Spring Harb Perspect Med* doi: 10.1101/cshperspect.a041586

ing disease (Katsarou et al. 2017). Unlike the role of B cells and their autoantibodies in pathology of T1D, the emergence of autoreactive T cells is considered not only a correlate of disease but a major causal mechanism by targeting a broad repertoire of epitopes on pancreatic β cells leading to their direct lysis. Thus far, the majority of studies investigating the development of β-cell-specific T cells have focused on genetic factors derived genome-wide association studies (GWASs) and have identified human leukocyte antigen (HLA) alleles, which encode molecules that enable the presentation of the antigen recognized by T cells, or genes that support T-cell activation (Pugliese 2017; Bender et al. 2021). The observed association of specific HLA variants suggests that changes in peptide binding and signal transduction after interaction with the T-cell receptor allow for autoreactive T cells to escape thymic selection. However, it is unclear how these T cells can sustain a chronic immune response for very long periods of time without becoming terminally differentiated. Recent studies focused on defining the differentiation state of autoreactive T cells in T1D patients have begun to uncover the incredible longevity of these cells.

HETEROGENEOUS AUTOREACTIVE T-CELL SUBSETS IN T1D

The continuous cycling of naive T cells through secondary lymphoid organs helps ensure they encounter their cognate antigen by their congregating with professional antigen-presenting cells in a centralized location. Upon recognizing their cognate antigen, such as occurs during an acute viral infection, antigen-specific CD8 T cells can differentiate into functional effector T cells that subsequently traffic to the source of antigen. After clearance of infected cells, the majority of the effector T cells die, leaving a small subset of T cells that further differentiate into a quiescent pool of memory T cells. These memory T cells can populate lymphoid and nonlymphoid tissues, providing heightened surveillance and reactivation potential to guard against subsequent reinfections. In contrast to an acute antigen setting, chronic infections establish a source of antigen that cannot be easily eliminated, and, thus, T cells are persistently stimulated. This chronic activation of T cells often drives their development into a differentiation state that has limited effector function and proliferative potential, commonly referred to as T-cell exhaustion (Fig. 1A; Lugli et al. 2020; Lan et al. 2023). Although T-cell exhaustion was initially described with chronic viral infections, the core gene regulatory programs governing exhaustion can be observed across many disease settings, including cancer, establishing T-cell exhaustion as a general feature associated with robust chronic antigen exposure (Blank et al. 2019). However, despite having access to a chronic source of antigen, autoreactive T cells appear to escape this tolerance mechanism and can sustain their cytotoxic effector functions (Bluestone et al. 2015). This sustained effector response suggests that the T cells indeed have chronic access to the source antigen, but also can maintain their quantity. This stem and effector duality among the autoreactive T-cell pool thus raises questions regarding cellular and anatomical heterogeneity.

Addressing the issue of β-cell-specific T-cell functional persistence, several groups have leveraged known tolerance-inducing mechanisms as a therapeutic strategy to stably suppress the effector response. It is well established that activation of T cells through the T-cell receptor in the absence of costimulation induces a nonfunctional tolerized state described as anergy (Schwartz 2003; Crespo et al. 2013). Based on this concept, clinical approaches have been developed to broadly tolerize autoreactive T cells through the administration of a non-Fc-binding anti-CD3 antibody (teplizumab). Results from teplizumab studies have documented transient success with a significant increase in C-peptide levels (indicators of endogenous insulin production) (Ramos et al. 2023) and have created a framework for better understanding the heterogeneity issue described above. Specifically, it was noted that CD8 T cells in responder patients treated with teplizumab became enriched with a phenotype resembling exhausted T cells with higher expression of EOMES and KLRG1 as well as increased inhibitory receptor expression including TIGIT compared to CD8 T cells in nonresponders (Fig. 1B; Long et al. 2016). Addition-

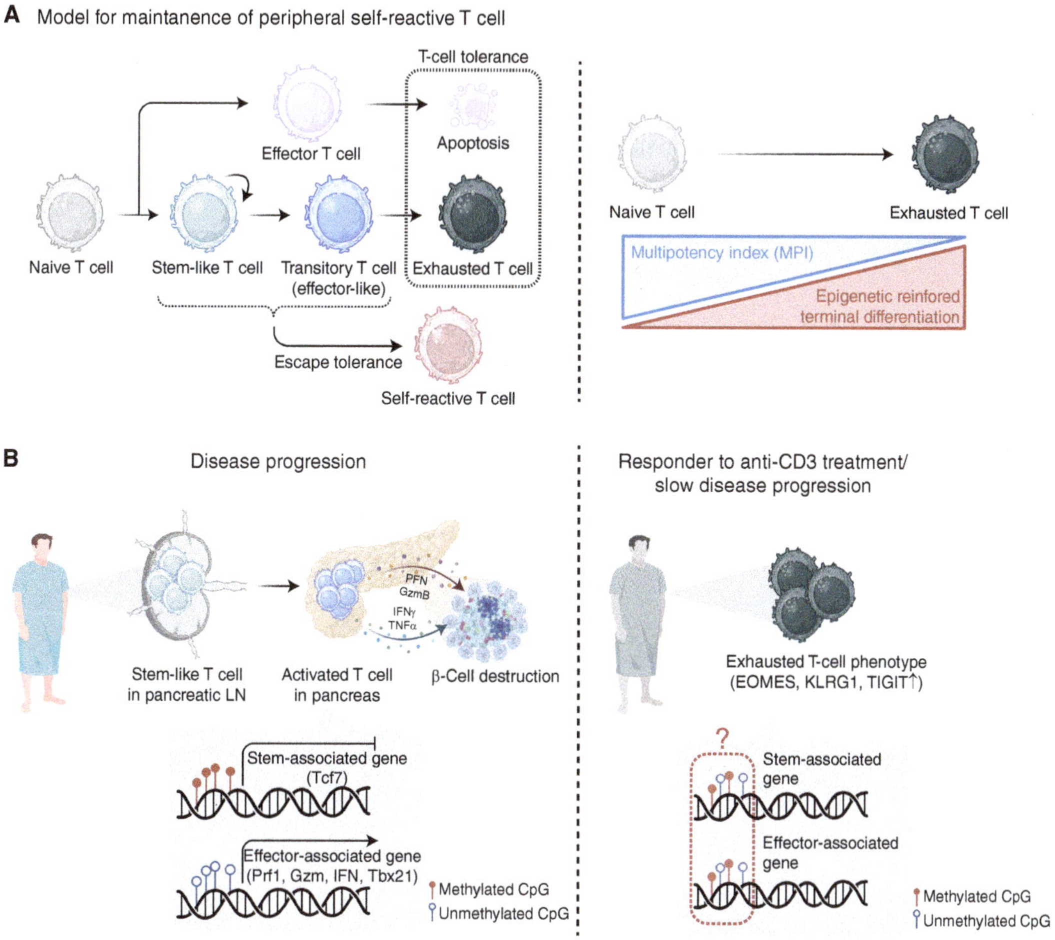

Figure 1. The generation of stem-like T cells and their potential impact on T1D disease. (*A*, *Left*) Naive antigen-specific CD8 T cells are activated and clonally expand in response to antigen presentation. During the early stage of the immune response, the expanded population bifurcates into effector and stem-like T cells. During sustained antigen exposure, effector T cells undergo apoptosis, whereas a stem-like T-cell subset continues to self-renew and can differentiate into transitory and exhausted T cells. Both apoptosis of effector T cells and terminal differentiation of stem-like T cells can be considered a form of T-cell tolerance to prevent hyperimmune responses. Some self-reactive T cells may escape these forms of tolerance during T-cell differentiation, resulting in long-lived autoimmune diseases. (*Right*) Schematic depiction of DNA methylation-based T-cell multipotency index (MPI). Epigenetic programs, including DNA methylation, are utilized during CD8 T-cell differentiation, to reinforce cell fate decisions such as T-cell exhaustion. Epigenetic modifications serve as a biomarker defining a T cell's developmental potential that can be used to assess therapeutic strategies for inducing tolerance. (*B*) Type 1 diabetes (T1D) has been associated with a stem-like T-cell phenotype and an epigenetic program that has accessibility among both stem-associated transcription factors and effector loci. Conversely, in murine models of T1D, β-cell-specific T cells that infiltrate the pancreas possess a terminal phenotype and epigenetic program. Clinical approaches have been developed to tolerize self-reactive T cells by treatment with the anti-CD3 antibody teplizumab. Responders to teplizumab exhibit an exhausted T-cell phenotype. It remains to be determined whether anti-CD3 antibody treatment can induce a stable epigenetic program that reinforces tolerization after therapy.

al analysis of teplizumab-treated patients documented greater circulation of central memory CD8 T cells in responders. The specific impact of teplizumab on the self-renewing stem-like T-cell population remains to be further characterized. However, it was noted that gene expression programs associated with T-cell activation among the pool of Tcm CD8 T cells in responders were repressed. This repressed state was also associated with increased expression of *IL-10* and *KLRC1*, and a reduction in pathogenic cytokines such as *IL-17A*. These observations suggest that teplizumab treatment may induce a tolerance-like program among Tcm cells (Tooley et al. 2016). This work has served as a proof of the principle that tolerance-inducing strategies may effectively induce long-term protection against disease progression if all of the long-lived autoreactive T cells can be anatomically accessed by the therapeutic antibody.

Further investigation of islet-specific T-cell phenotypes revealed that they are also detectable in individuals that have limited or slow development of diabetes. However, as opposed to having an activated transitional memory phenotype with a high proliferative potential, the autoreactive T cells in patients with slow disease progression exhibited an exhausted phenotype that included high EOMES expression as well as expression of multiple inhibitory receptors such as 2B4, PD-1, TIGIT, and CD160 (Wiedeman et al. 2020). Compared to healthy donors, most β-cell-specific autoreactive T cells from slow progressors exhibited a less-differentiated memory T-cell phenotype (Skowera et al. 2015). Consistent with the human studies, characterization of islet-specific CD8 T cells from nonobese diabetic (NOD) mice, a model possessing many genetic and immunological features of the human condition (Anderson and Bluestone 2005), identified T cells with an effector-memory phenotype within the islets that could emigrate to peripheral tissue (Chee et al. 2014). Collectively, these human and murine studies demonstrate that the phenotype of CD8 T cells is associated with T1D disease progression, and help define the population of T cells that need to be targeted by tolerance-inducing therapies to prevent or slow disease progression for long periods of time.

Recent efforts to determine how the pool of T cells recognizing a chronic source of antigen can be sustained have identified a stem-like CD8 T-cell subset expressing the transcription factor TCF-1 as a long-lived resource for generating effector progeny in settings of chronic infection (Utzschneider et al. 2016). This subset harbors critical gene expression programs that enable the cells to self-renew in the presence of antigen, resulting in the maintenance of functional T cells, and has been linked to the proliferative burst and ultimately the therapeutic efficacy arising from immune checkpoint blockade (Im et al. 2016; Gebhardt et al. 2023). While this stem-like population is beneficial in settings of tumor immunotherapy, it has the potential to limit tolerance-inducing therapies in the context of autoimmunity. Recent reports have revealed that such β-cell-specific CD8 T cells indeed acquire stem-associated gene expression programs in T1D patients (Abdelsamed et al. 2020). This observation raised the possibility that disease could be sustained by a self-renewing population of pathogenic T cells. Additionally, it was found using the NOD mouse model that β-cell-specific T cells indeed acquire a stem-like gene expression program among cells in the pancreatic draining lymph node (pLN) (Abdelsamed et al. 2020). This discovery was further extended by studies using the murine NOD model showing that the pool of β-cell-specific T cells could be preserved during serial transplantation into disease-free recipients. Importantly, this T-cell adoptive transfer model propagated disease into the new animals (Gearty et al. 2022). A parallel study confirmed that a stem-like T-cell population of autoreactive T cells populate the pLN in NOD mice, but the autoreactive T cells that traffic to the intraislets acquire an activated/exhaustion phenotype. While the phenotype suggested that the T cells in the intraislets were becoming exhausted, it was noted that they did not show an accumulation of reactive oxygen species (ROS), a hallmark of T-cell dysfunction often observed in tumor microenvironments (Scharping et al. 2016), and the cells maintained an ability to produce effector cytokines at a similar level to the autoreactive T cells from the pLN. A broader longitudinal analysis of the T cells in the

NOD mouse model of T1D documented a dramatic shift in the T-cell phenotype over time. At 4 weeks of age, it was shown that the manifestation of disease coincided with the enrichment of cytotoxic effector CD8 T cells. However, at a later stage of the disease (16 wk), the frequency of cytotoxic T cells decreased, and a stem-like population of CD8 T cells expressing *Tcf7* (a major transcription factor of stem-like CD8 T cells) was detected (Zakharov et al. 2020). The significance of this stem-like population of T cells has become increasingly appreciated over the last 10 years as it has been shown to serve as a resource for sustaining an effector response in various chronic antigen settings. This stem-like T-cell population likely plays a similar role in sustaining the effector T-cell population during T1D, suggesting that a greater understanding of its cellular origin and molecular features could provide key insights into the longevity of T1D disease and potential therapeutic interventions.

EPIGENETIC CHARACTERISTICS OF T CELLS IN T1D

To better understand the mechanism that enables T cells to sustain their effector potential for long periods of time and over many rounds of cell division, investigators have turned their attention to epigenetic modifications. Such covalent alterations to the genome include histone modifications and DNA methylation, that ultimately program the chromatin density, and thus enable or restrict specific regions of the genome for transcriptional activity. These mechanisms enable heritable changes to gene regulation and have been shown to play a critical role in reinforcing memory T-cell subset specification (Gray et al. 2017; Youngblood et al. 2017; Pace et al. 2018) and exhaustion (Ghoneim et al. 2017; Prinzing et al. 2021). Among the major epigenetic modifications, the role of DNA methylation in T1D has been the most extensively studied. As a first pass to assessing the epigenetics of T1D, the genome-wide DNA methylation profiles of CD4 T cells from 15 adult patients with latent autoimmune diabetes were measured. Overall, the total DNA methylation level among CD4 T cells was significantly higher in patients compared to healthy donor groups. Consistent with increased DNA methylation levels, expression of DNMT3B was also increased in the patients. Additionally, the expression of FOXP3, a major transcription factor of regulatory T cells, was decreased in patients, which was associated with specific hypermethylation of its promoter region (Li et al. 2011). Another study also reported hypermethylation of the *FOXP3* gene promoter along with decreased CTLA4 levels from peripheral blood mononuclear cells of patients with fulminant T1D. The authors of this study further reported that *FOXP3* promoter hypermethylation blocked interferon regulatory factor 7 binding to this region of the DNA and resulted in a reduction in *FOXP3* transcription (Wang et al. 2013). These results collectively indicated that alteration of DNA methylation status could contribute to the onset or progression of T1D pathogenesis by regulating the expression of autoimmune-related genes in CD4 T cells.

Similar to DNA methylation, several groups have examined the relationship between histone modifications of CD4 T cells and the development of T1D. As a metric for transcriptional repression, histone lysine 9 dimethylation (H3K9me2), was investigated from lymphocytes and monocytes of T1D patients and healthy groups (Padeken et al. 2022). Notably, a significant difference in H3K9me2 level between T1D and healthy groups was found in lymphocytes but not in monocytes. Specifically, the level of H3K9me2 at the *CTLA4* locus was increased in T1D patients. Ingenuity pathway analysis of the H3K9me2 profiles revealed that this modification was especially altered at genes associated with autoimmune and inflammation pathways including TGF-β, NF-κB, and TLR signaling (Miao et al. 2008). In another study investigating the total level of histone 3 lysine 9 methylation (H3K9me) in CD4 T cells, it was reported that individuals with latent autoimmune diabetes exhibited reduced global H3K9me levels in CD4 T cells compared to healthy individuals. Consistent with the decreased level of Histone 3, these patients exhibited diminished expression of SUV39H2, histone methyltransferase, and increased expression of histone demethylase KDM4C, resulting in a reduction of detectable global unmethylated H3 lysine 9 (Liu and Li 2017). While it is not clear whether histone modification is directly contributing to the progression of T1D, alterations in histone modification have been observed in patients of T1D. It might be important to elucidate the detailed causal relationship between histone modification and the progression of T1D through further studies.

In contrast to the large body of work investigating epigenetic modifications among CD4 T cells, until recently there has been very limited emphasis on epigenetic regulation of CD8 T cells in T1D. Early efforts to investigate epigenetic mechanisms involved in effector and memory CD8 T-cell differentiation documented DNA methylation, histone modifications, and chromatic accessibility profiles associated with effector and memory stages of an immune response to an acute viral infection in mice and humans (Russ et al. 2014; Sen et al. 2016; Akondy et al. 2017; Youngblood et al. 2017; Satpathy et al. 2019; Lan et al. 2023). These collective studies have established the concept that epigenetic programs serve as a mechanism to reinforce acquired gene expression programs that are associated with specific CD8 T-cell developmental fates. This epigenetic memory concept has recently been interrogated in the setting of long-lived human autoreactive CD8 T-cell responses during T1D. Profiling the DNA methylome of β-cell-specific CD8 T cells isolated from T1D patients revealed that this pool of autoreactive T cells retained epigenetic programs associated with both naive and effector CD8 T-cell subsets. Furthermore, analysis of the epigenome at the single-cell level using an assay for transposase-accessible chromatin confirmed that some individual β-cell-specific autoreactive CD8 T cells contained transcriptionally permissive regions at both naive and effector-associated loci. Consistent with the epigenetic analysis of human autoreactive T cells, mouse β-cell-specific CD8 T cells isolated from lymphoid tissues away from the source of antigen also retained a stem-like epigenetic state harboring both naive and effector programs. However, mouse autoreactive CD8 T cells isolated from the pancreas exhibited epigenetic programs more closely resembling a terminally differentiated state. Collectively, this study provided a putative mechanism to explain how the stem-like state of T cells can sustain the autoreactive immune response and highlights the potential use of epigenetic analysis to track the status of self-reactive T cells (Fig. 1B; Abdelsamed et al. 2020). Confirmation of this mechanism in treated patient T cells isolated from draining lymph nodes and pancreatic islets awaits future investigation.

The above-described comprehensive characterization of epigenetic programs at well-defined differentiation states, not only provided new insight into the durability of autoreactive T cells, but also enabled the development of an epigenetic-based tool for predicting T-cell differentiation potential that is agnostic to a T cell's phenotype or antigenic history. This bioinformatic tool uses the DNA methylation status on its own to approximate a T cell's differentiation potential. The DNA methylation-based assessment places the differentiation potential of the cell between two points of reference, a naive T cell with full effector and memory potential at one end of the spectrum and a terminally differentiated T cell that has lost its effector potential at the other end of the spectrum. This tool, referred to as the T-Cell Multipotency Index, not only enables finer characterization of samples with unknown antigen exposure history, which is often the case for human samples, but it also further reinforces the concept that epigenetic mechanisms serve as checkpoints for stages of T-cell differentiation in response to acute and chronic sources of antigen. Thus, the development of the methylation-based T-cell multipotency index provides a novel approach for assessing the induction of T-cell terminal differentiation and may be used to assess the stability of therapeutic approaches that seek to establish long-term tolerance (Fig. 1B).

THERAPEUTIC STRATEGIES FOR T-CELL SUPPRESSION IN T1D

Current strategies to treat T1D are predominantly designed to target nonspecific mechanisms of immunosuppression. Thus, novel therapeutic strategies to induce antigen-specific immune tolerance are needed. As described above, several recent studies have revealed the relationship between T1D progression and the phenotype of CD8 T cells. Specifically, autoreactive CD8 T cell exhibiting a stem-like phenotype is coupled to sustained disease (Abdelsamed et al. 2020; Wiedeman et al. 2020; Gearty et al. 2022). To attenuate the developmental potential of β-cell-specific CD8 T cells, it has become conceptually clear that current and new efforts for tolerization therapy must target the self-renewing population of autoreactive CD8 T cells. Supporting the feasibility of such an approach, it was reported that patients receiving exogenous insulin become enriched with an exhausted phenotype among insulin-specific T cells (Wiedeman et al. 2020), suggesting heightened conversion of the stem-like T cells into exhausted antigen-specific T cells through excess antigenic stimulation. However, among high-risk T1D patients, including children, exogenous insulin administration did not delay or prevent T1D (Diabetes Prevention Trial-Type 1 Diabetes Study Group 2002; Skyler et al. 2005; Krischer et al. 2017). Similar results and consideration have been reported when patients were immunized with GAD65, one of the dominant circulating autoantibodies during the early stage of T1D, or T1D-associated peptides (Ludvigsson et al. 2017; Smith and Peakman 2018). In addition, exogenous antigen administration could expand preexisting effector T cells instead of inducing T-cell exhaustion. Here, it is important to consider that mechanisms of T-cell exhaustion have been largely borne out of studies from murine chronic virus and tumor models. Therefore, the tolerance-avoiding mechanisms of autoreactive T cells in T1D may arise from a yet-to-be-defined mechanism that is not used in canonical models of T-cell dysfunction. Thus, future efforts for peptide-based tolerization of self-reactive T cells may be further informed by directly assessing mechanisms of T-cell longevity in autoimmune models.

While lacking the antigen specificity of peptide-based tolerizing approaches, the use of anti-CD3 antibodies, teplizumab, and otelixizumab, have established that loss of β-cell function can be attenuated by broadly reducing T-cell effector functions (Sherry et al. 2011; Herold et al. 2013). Notably, this proof-of-principle study also established that broad tolerizing mechanisms can result in transient reactivation of chronic herpes viruses. Specifically, reactivation of Epstein–Barr virus (EBV) was observed after treatment with otelixizumab (Keymeulen et al. 2010; Kroll et al. 2013), which was subsequently controlled by the endogenous immune response. Immunological control of the EBV infection included virus-specific T cells that mounted an effector response and raises questions about the strength of stimulation needed to tolerize auto versus viral reactive T cells. In addition to anti-CD3 therapies, blocking costimulatory signals is being considered as an alternative immunomodulating approaches. Blockade of CD80 and CD86 via the cytotoxic T-lymphocyte-associated protein 4 (CTLA-4) for 2 years markedly prolonged β-cell function in new-onset T1D patients and was accompanied by increased numbers of T cells (Orban et al. 2011, 2014). However, in a clinical trial targeting the early stage of T1D, patients treated with anti-CTLA-4 continued to progress to T1D (Russell et al. 2023), indicating that blockade of CTLA4 alone may be insufficient to delay disease progression. Another targeted approach involves specifically depleting the pool of stem-like autoreactive CD8 T cells. High expression of the glucose transporter 1 (GLUT1) is a hallmark of circulating stem-like T cells, and can be targeted with the GLUT1 selective inhibitor, WZB117. This approach resulted in the inhibition of stem-like T-cell generation and expansion (Vignali et al. 2018), suggesting that the depletion of stem-like CD8 T cells by specific markers of these cells in T1D patients can be considered.

In the field of cancer immunotherapy, epigenetic reprogramming of CD8 T cells is now being considered to extend antitumor activity. Disruption of Dnmt3a in mouse and human antiviral and antitumor T cells prevents the acquisition of bona fide exhaustion DNA methylation programs and significantly improves the therapeutic utility of the T cells (Ghoneim et al. 2017; Prinzing et al. 2021). In addition, it was recently reported that disruption of the DNA demethylating enzyme, Tet2, in CAR-T cells results in substantial improvement in tumor control without resulting in leukemic transformation (Fraietta et al. 2018; Jain et al. 2023). These studies conceptually identify DNA methylation programming as a putative mechanism for inducing tolerance. While this mechanism is currently being exploited for the purpose of sustaining an immune response, the opposite may also be possible. To determine whether β-cell-specific CD8 T cells can be targeted for epigenetic mechanisms of exhaustion, we recently characterized mouse and human β-cell-specific T cells in circulation (human), within the draining lymph node and within the pancreas (mouse) (Abdelsamed et al. 2020). Results from this study indicated that β-cell-specific T cells away from the source of antigen were able to maintain a stem-like epigenetic state (Fig. 1B). To further, investigate the impact these epigenetic programs have on transcriptional permissiveness, we assessed the genome-wide chromatin accessibility of β-cell-specific T cells. Specifically, we performed single-cell ATAC-seq to determine whether the stem and effector epigenetic state observed from the bulk DNA methylation profiles arose from two discreet subsets of cells, or whether a single cell could possess both programs. Notably, analysis of the chromatin for single β-cell-specific T cells from individuals with T1D indeed demonstrated that the cells possessed a stem-like epigenetic state that consisted of both naive and effector chromatin profiles. The existence of this hybrid chromatin state further supports the concept that the pathology can be sustained by a long-lived population of autoreactive T cells that retain effector potential. Based on this discovery, future work is needed to define mechanisms for inducing tolerance among T cells that have differentiated into a stem-like developmental state.

While the engineering approaches described above that target-specific T-cell subsets for epigenetic reprogramming have yet to be developed for T1D, recent efforts have tested the use of nonspecific epigenetic reprogramming strategies. Treatment of NOD mice with 5-Aza-2′-Deoxycotidie (DAC), a cytosine analog that inhibits the activity of DNA methyltransferase, has recently been reported to induce Foxp3 expression in CD4 T cell through demethylation of a CpG island in the first intron of the *Foxp3* gene. These cells exhibited enhanced immunosuppressive function compared to controls, indicating that inhibition of DNA methylation can prevent the development of T1D in the NOD model (Zheng et al. 2009). Recent studies have also documented the association between histone deacetylases (HDACs) and T1D progression. The expression of HDAC1 has been reported to increase in islets from T1D patients, while the expression of HDAC2 and HDAC3 is decreased (Lundh et al. 2012). Oral administration of the HDAC inhibitor, valproic acid (VPA), for 3 weeks in patients has been reported to improve glucose homeostasis through stimulating the proliferation and function of islet β cells by reducing the apoptosis of β cells (Khan and Jena 2016). While the pleiotropic effector of nonspecifically targeting epigenetic mechanisms to control gene expression programs among T cells within the pancreas remains a challenge, these studies have paved the way for future targeted approaches.

CONCLUDING REMARKS

In summary, investigation into the origin, maintenance, and anatomical partitioning of stem-like T cells during T1D has provided mechanistic insight into the longevity of autoreactive CD8 T cells and the overall duration of disease. The use of new omics technologies to investigate T-cell heterogeneity has greatly advanced fundamental investigation of autoreactive T-cell development in humans and murine model systems and enabled in-depth correlates of response to tolerization-focused therapies. These conceptual and technical breakthroughs have led to the discovery that epigenetic mechanisms reinforcing a stem-like T-cell population are associated with T1D pathogenesis, and new therapeutic approaches will need to consider a mechanism for inducing an epigenetic signature of T-cell tolerance. Moreover, as approaches for establishing long-term T-cell tolerance emerge for T1D, such strategies may be applied to other autoimmune diseases that arise from the development and maintenance of self-reactive T cells.

ACKNOWLEDGMENTS

Studies were supported by the Center for Translational Immunology and Immunotherapy

(CeTI²) at St. Jude. In addition, this work was supported by the National Institutes of Health (NIH) (R01AI114442 and R01CA237311 to B.Y.), Stand Up To Cancer (SU2C to B.Y.), ASSISI Foundation funding (to B.Y.), and the American Lebanese Syrian Associated Charities (ALSAC to B.Y.). This work does not represent the opinion of the NIH.

REFERENCES

Abdelsamed HA, Zebley CC, Nguyen H, Rutishauser RL, Fan Y, Ghoneim HE, Crawford JC, Alfei F, Alli S, Ribeiro SP, et al. 2020. β-Cell-specific CD8⁺ T cells maintain stem cell memory-associated epigenetic programs during type 1 diabetes. *Nat Immunol* **21:** 578–587. doi:10.1038/s41590-020-0633-5

Akondy RS, Fitch M, Edupuganti S, Yang S, Kissick HT, Li KW, Youngblood BA, Abdelsamed HA, McGuire DJ, Cohen KW, et al. 2017. Origin and differentiation of human memory CD8 T cells after vaccination. *Nature* **552:** 362–367. doi:10.1038/nature24633

Anderson MS, Bluestone JA. 2005. The NOD mouse: a model of immune dysregulation. *Annu Rev Immunol* **23:** 447–485. doi:10.1146/annurev.immunol.23.021704.115643

Bender C, Rajendran S, Von Herrath MG. 2021. New insights into the role of autoreactive CD8 T cells and cytokines in human type 1 diabetes. *Front Endocrinol* **11:** 606434. doi:10.3389/fendo.2020.606434

Blank CU, Haining WN, Held W, Hogan PG, Kallies A, Lugli E, Lynn RC, Philip M, Rao A, Restifo NP, et al. 2019. Defining 'T cell exhaustion'. *Nat Rev Immunol* **19:** 665–674. doi:10.1038/s41577-019-0221-9

Bluestone JA, Bour-Jordan H, Cheng M, Anderson M. 2015. T cells in the control of organ-specific autoimmunity. *J Clin Invest* **125:** 2250–2260. doi:10.1172/JCI78089

Chee J, Ko HJ, Skowera A, Jhala G, Catterall T, Graham KL, Sutherland RM, Thomas HE, Lew AM, Peakman M, et al. 2014. Effector-memory T cells develop in islets and report islet pathology in type 1 diabetes. *J Immunol* **192:** 572–580. doi:10.4049/jimmunol.1302100

Crespo J, Sun H, Welling TH, Tian Z, Zou W. 2013. T cell anergy, exhaustion, senescence, and stemness in the tumor microenvironment. *Curr Opin Immunol* **25:** 214–221. doi:10.1016/j.coi.2012.12.003

Diabetes Prevention Trial-Type 1 Diabetes Study Group. 2002. Effects of insulin in relatives of patients with type 1 diabetes mellitus. *N Engl J Med* **346:** 1685–1691. doi:10.1056/NEJMoa012350

DiMeglio LA, Evans-Molina C, Oram RA. 2018. Type 1 diabetes. *Lancet* **391:** 2449–2462. doi:10.1016/S0140-6736(18)31320-5

Fraietta JA, Nobles CL, Sammons MA, Lundh S, Carty SA, Reich TJ, Cogdill AP, Morrissette JJ, DeNizio JE, Reddy S, et al. 2018. Disruption of TET2 promotes the therapeutic efficacy of CD19-targeted T cells. *Nature* **558:** 307–312. doi:10.1038/s41586-018-0178-z

Gearty SV, Dündar F, Zumbo P, Espinosa-Carrasco G, Shakiba M, Sanchez-Rivera FJ, Socci ND, Trivedi P, Lowe SW, Lauer P, et al. 2022. An autoimmune stem-like CD8 T cell population drives type 1 diabetes. *Nature* **602:** 156–161. doi:10.1038/s41586-021-04248-x

Gebhardt T, Park SL, Parish IA. 2023. Stem-like exhausted and memory CD8⁺ T cells in cancer. *Nat Rev Cancer* **23:** 780–798. doi:10.1038/s41568-023-00615-0

Ghoneim HE, Fan Y, Moustaki A, Abdelsamed HA, Dash P, Dogra P, Carter R, Awad W, Neale G, Thomas PG, et al. 2017. De novo epigenetic programs inhibit PD-1 blockade-mediated T cell rejuvenation. *Cell* **170:** 142–157.e19. doi:10.1016/j.cell.2017.06.007

Gray SM, Amezquita RA, Guan T, Kleinstein SH, Kaech SM. 2017. Polycomb repressive complex 2-mediated chromatin repression guides effector CD8⁺ T cell terminal differentiation and loss of multipotency. *Immunity* **46:** 596–608. doi:10.1016/j.immuni.2017.03.012

Herold KC, Gitelman SE, Ehlers MR, Gottlieb PA, Greenbaum CJ, Hagopian W, Boyle KD, Keyes-Elstein L, Aggarwal S, Phippard D, et al. 2013. Teplizumab (anti-CD3 mAb) treatment preserves C-peptide responses in patients with new-onset type 1 diabetes in a randomized controlled trial: metabolic and immunologic features at baseline identify a subgroup of responders. *Diabetes* **62:** 3766–3774. doi:10.2337/db13-0345

Herold KC, Delong T, Perdigoto AL, Biru N, Brusko TM, Walker LS. 2024. The immunology of type 1 diabetes. *Nat Rev Immunol* **24:** 435–451. doi:10.1038/s41577-023-00985-4

Im SJ, Hashimoto M, Gerner MY, Lee J, Kissick HT, Burger MC, Shan Q, Hale JS, Lee J, Nasti TH, et al. 2016. Defining CD8⁺ T cells that provide the proliferative burst after PD-1 therapy. *Nature* **537:** 417–421. doi:10.1038/nature19330

Jain N, Zhao Z, Feucht J, Koche R, Iyer A, Dobrin A, Mansilla-Soto J, Yang J, Zhan Y, Lopez M, et al. 2023. TET2 guards against unchecked BATF3-induced CAR T cell expansion. *Nature* **615:** 315–322. doi:10.1038/s41586-022-05692-z

Katsarou A, Gudbjörnsdottir S, Rawshani A, Dabelea D, Bonifacio E, Anderson BJ, Jacobsen LM, Schatz DA, Lernmark Å. 2017. Type 1 diabetes mellitus. *Nat Rev Dis Primers* **3:** 1–17. doi:10.1038/nrdp.2017.16

Keymeulen B, Candon S, Fafi-Kremer S, Ziegler A, Leruez-Ville M, Mathieu C, Vandemeulebroucke E, Walter M, Crenier L, Thervet E, et al. 2010. Transient Epstein-Barr virus reactivation in CD3 monoclonal antibody-treated patients. *Blood* **115:** 1145–1155. doi:10.1182/blood-2009-02-204875

Khan S, Jena G. 2016. Valproic acid improves glucose homeostasis by increasing β-cell proliferation, function, and reducing its apoptosis through HDAC inhibition in juvenile diabetic rat. *J Biochem Mol Toxicol* **30:** 438–446. doi:10.1002/jbt.21807

Krischer JP, Schatz DA, Bundy B, Skyler JS, Greenbaum CJ. 2017. Effect of oral insulin on prevention of diabetes in relatives of patients with type 1 diabetes: a randomized clinical trial. *J Am Med Assoc* **318:** 1891–1902. doi:10.1001/jama.2017.17070

Kroll JL, Beam C, Li S, Viscidi R, Dighero B, Cho A, Boulware D, Pescovitz M, Weinberg A; Type 1 Diabetes TrialNet Anti CD-20 Study Group. 2013. Reactivation of latent viruses in individuals receiving rituximab for new onset type 1 diabetes. *J Clin Virol* **57:** 115–119. doi:10.1016/j.jcv.2013.01.016

Lan X, Zebley CC, Youngblood B. 2023. Cellular and molecular waypoints along the path of T cell exhaustion. *Sci Immunol* **8:** eadg3868. doi:10.1126/sciimmunol.adg3868

Li Y, Zhao M, Hou C, Liang G, Yang L, Tan Y, Wang Z, Yin H, Zhou Z, Lu Q. 2011. Abnormal DNA methylation in $CD4^+$ T cells from people with latent autoimmune diabetes in adults. *Diabetes Res Clin Pract* **94:** 242–248. doi:10.1016/j.diabres.2011.07.027

Liu XY, Li H. 2017. Reduced histone H3 lysine 9 methylation contributes to the pathogenesis of latent autoimmune diabetes in adults via regulation of SUV39H2 and KDM4C. *J Diabetes Res* **2017:** 8365762. doi:10.1155/2017/8365762

Long SA, Thorpe J, DeBerg HA, Gersuk V, Eddy JA, Harris KM, Ehlers M, Herold KC, Nepom GT, Linsley PS. 2016. Partial exhaustion of CD8 T cells and clinical response to teplizumab in new-onset type 1 diabetes. *Sci Immunol* **1:** eaai7793. doi:10.1126/sciimmunol.aai7793

Ludvigsson J, Wahlberg J, Casas R. 2017. Intralymphatic injection of autoantigen in type 1 diabetes. *N Engl J Med* **376:** 697–699. doi:10.1056/NEJMc1616343

Lugli E, Galletti G, Boi SK, Youngblood BA. 2020. Stem, effector, and hybrid states of memory $CD8^+$ T cells. *Trends Immunol* **41:** 17–28. doi:10.1016/j.it.2019.11.004

Lundh M, Christensen D, Damgaard Nielsen M, Richardson S, Dahllöf M, Skovgaard T, Berthelsen J, Dinarello C, Stevenazzi A, Mascagni P, et al. 2012. Histone deacetylases 1 and 3 but not 2 mediate cytokine-induced β cell apoptosis in INS-1 cells and dispersed primary islets from rats and are differentially regulated in the islets of type 1 diabetic children. *Diabetologia* **55:** 2421–2431. doi:10.1007/s00125-012-2615-0

Miao F, Smith DD, Zhang L, Min A, Feng W, Natarajan R. 2008. Lymphocytes from patients with type 1 diabetes display a distinct profile of chromatin histone H3 lysine 9 dimethylation: an epigenetic study in diabetes. *Diabetes* **57:** 3189–3198. doi:10.2337/db08-0645

Orban T, Bundy B, Becker DJ, DiMeglio LA, Gitelman SE, Goland R, Gottlieb PA, Greenbaum CJ, Marks JB, Monzavi R, et al. 2011. Co-stimulation modulation with abatacept in patients with recent-onset type 1 diabetes: a randomised, double-blind, placebo-controlled trial. *Lancet* **378:** 412–419. doi:10.1016/S0140-6736(11)60886-6

Orban T, Bundy B, Becker DJ, DiMeglio LA, Gitelman SE, Goland R, Gottlieb PA, Greenbaum CJ, Marks JB, Monzavi R, et al. 2014. Costimulation modulation with abatacept in patients with recent-onset type 1 diabetes: follow-up 1 year after cessation of treatment. *Diabetes Care* **37:** 1069–1075. doi:10.2337/dc13-0604

Pace L, Goudot C, Zueva E, Gueguen P, Burgdorf N, Waterfall JJ, Quivy JP, Almouzni G, Amigorena S. 2018. The epigenetic control of stemness in $CD8^+$ T cell fate commitment. *Science* **359:** 177–186. doi:10.1126/science.aah6499

Padeken J, Methot SP, Gasser SM. 2022. Establishment of H3K9-methylated heterochromatin and its functions in tissue differentiation and maintenance. *Nat Rev Mol Cell Biol* **23:** 623–640. doi:10.1038/s41580-022-00483-w

Prinzing B, Zebley CC, Petersen CT, Fan Y, Anido AA, Yi Z, Nguyen P, Houke H, Bell M, Haydar D, et al. 2021. Deleting DNMT3A in CAR T cells prevents exhaustion and enhances antitumor activity. *Sci Transl Med* **13:** eabh0272. doi:10.1126/scitranslmed.abh0272

Pugliese A. 2017. Autoreactive T cells in type 1 diabetes. *J Clin Invest* **127:** 2881–2891. doi:10.1172/JCI94549

Ramos EL, Dayan CM, Chatenoud L, Sumnik Z, Simmons KM, Szypowska A, Gitelman SE, Knecht LA, Niemoeller E, Tian W, et al. 2023. Teplizumab and β-cell function in newly diagnosed type 1 diabetes. *N Engl J Med* **389:** 2151–2161. doi:10.1056/NEJMoa2308743

Russ BE, Olshanksy M, Smallwood HS, Li J, Denton AE, Prier JE, Stock AT, Croom HA, Cullen JG, Nguyen ML, et al. 2014. Distinct epigenetic signatures delineate transcriptional programs during virus-specific $CD8^+$ T cell differentiation. *Immunity* **41:** 853–865. doi:10.1016/j.immuni.2014.11.001

Russell WE, Bundy BN, Anderson MS, Cooney LA, Gitelman SE, Goland RS, Gottlieb PA, Greenbaum CJ, Haller MJ, et al. 2023. Abatacept for delay of type 1 diabetes progression in stage 1 relatives at risk: a randomized, double-masked, controlled trial. *Diabetes Care* **46:** 1005–1013. doi:10.2337/dc22-2200

Satpathy AT, Granja JM, Yost KE, Qi Y, Meschi F, McDermott GP, Olsen BN, Mumbach MR, Pierce SE, Corces MR, et al. 2019. Massively parallel single-cell chromatin landscapes of human immune cell development and intratumoral T cell exhaustion. *Nat Biotechnol* **37:** 925–936. doi:10.1038/s41587-019-0206-z

Scharping NE, Menk AV, Moreci RS, Whetstone RD, Dadey RE, Watkins SC, Ferris RL, Delgoffe GM. 2016. The tumor microenvironment represses T cell mitochondrial biogenesis to drive intratumoral T cell metabolic insufficiency and dysfunction. *Immunity* **45:** 374–388. doi:10.1016/j.immuni.2016.07.009

Schwartz RH. 2003. T cell anergy. *Annu Rev Immunol* **21:** 305–334. doi:10.1146/annurev.immunol.21.120601.141110

Sen DR, Kaminski J, Barnitz RA, Kurachi M, Gerdemann U, Yates KB, Tsao HW, Godec J, LaFleur MW, Brown FD, et al. 2016. The epigenetic landscape of T cell exhaustion. *Science* **354:** 1165–1169. doi:10.1126/science.aae0491

Sherry N, Hagopian W, Ludvigsson J, Jain SM, Wahlen J, Ferry RJ, Bode B, Aronoff S, Holland C, Carlin D, et al. 2011. Teplizumab for treatment of type 1 diabetes (Protégé study): 1-year results from a randomised, placebo-controlled trial. *Lancet* **378:** 487–497. doi:10.1016/S0140-6736(11)60931-8

Skowera A, Ladell K, McLaren JE, Dolton G, Matthews KK, Gostick E, Kronenberg-Versteeg D, Eichmann M, Knight RR, Heck S, et al. 2015. β-Cell-specific CD8 T cell phenotype in type 1 diabetes reflects chronic autoantigen exposure. *Diabetes* **64:** 916–925. doi:10.2337/db14-0332

Skyler JS, Krischer JP, Wolfsdorf J, Cowie C, Palmer JP, Greenbaum C, Cuthbertson D, Rafkin-Mervis LE, Chase HP, Leschek E. 2005. Effects of oral insulin in relatives of patients with type 1 diabetes: the diabetes prevention trial-type 1. *Diabetes Care* **28:** 1068–1076. doi:10.2337/diacare.28.7.1630

Smith EL, Peakman M. 2018. Peptide immunotherapy for type 1 diabetes—clinical advances. *Front Immunol* **9:** 392. doi:10.3389/fimmu.2018.00392

Tooley JE, Vudattu N, Choi J, Cotsapas C, Devine L, Raddassi K, Ehlers MR, McNamara JG, Harris KM, Kanaparthi S, et al. 2016. Changes in T-cell subsets identify responders to FcR-nonbinding anti-CD3 mAb (teplizumab) in patients with type 1 diabetes. *Eur J Immunol* **46:** 230–241. doi:10.1002/eji.201545708

Utzschneider DT, Charmoy M, Chennupati V, Pousse L, Ferreira DP, Calderon-Copete S, Danilo M, Alfei F, Hofmann M, Wieland D, et al. 2016. T cell factor 1-expressing memory-like $CD8^+$ T cells sustain the immune response to chronic viral infections. *Immunity* **45:** 415–427. doi:10.1016/j.immuni.2016.07.021

Vignali D, Cantarelli E, Bordignon C, Canu A, Citro A, Annoni A, Piemonti L, Monti P. 2018. Detection and characterization of $CD8^+$ autoreactive memory stem T cells in patients with type 1 diabetes. *Diabetes* **67:** 936–945. doi:10.2337/db17-1390

Wang Z, Zheng Y, Hou C, Yang L, Li X, Lin J, Huang G, Lu Q, Wang CY, Zhou Z. 2013. DNA methylation impairs TLR9 induced Foxp3 expression by attenuating IRF-7 binding activity in fulminant type 1 diabetes. *J Autoimmun* **41:** 50–59. doi:10.1016/j.jaut.2013.01.009

Wiedeman AE, Muir VS, Rosasco MG, DeBerg HA, Presnell S, Haas B, Dufort MJ, Speake C, Greenbaum CJ, Serti E, et al. 2020. Autoreactive $CD8^+$ T cell exhaustion distinguishes subjects with slow type 1 diabetes progression. *J Clin Invest* **130:** 480–490. doi:10.1172/JCI126595

Youngblood B, Hale JS, Kissick HT, Ahn E, Xu X, Wieland A, Araki K, West EE, Ghoneim HE, Fan Y, et al. 2017. Effector CD8 T cells dedifferentiate into long-lived memory cells. *Nature* **552:** 404–409. doi:10.1038/nature25144

Zakharov PN, Hu H, Wan X, Unanue ER. 2020. Single-cell RNA sequencing of murine islets shows high cellular complexity at all stages of autoimmune diabetes. *J Exp Med* **217:** e20192362. doi:10.1084/jem.20192362

Zheng Q, Xu Y, Liu Y, Zhang B, Li X, Guo F, Zhao Y. 2009. Induction of Foxp3 demethylation increases regulatory $CD4^+CD25^+$ T cells and prevents the occurrence of diabetes in mice. *J Mol Med* **87:** 1191–1205. doi:10.1007/s00109-009-0530-8

Epitope Hierarchy in Type 1 Diabetes Pathogenesis

Thomas Delong[1] and Maki Nakayama[2,3,4]

[1]Department of Pharmaceutical Sciences, Skaggs School of Pharmacy and Pharmaceutical Sciences, University of Colorado Anschutz Medical Campus, Aurora, Colorado 80045, USA

[2]Barbara Davis Center for Childhood Diabetes, [3]Department of Pediatrics, [4]Department of Immunology and Microbiology, University of Colorado School of Medicine, Aurora, Colorado 80045, USA

Correspondence: Thomas.delong@cuanschutz.edu; maki.nakayama@cuanschutz.edu

Type 1 diabetes (T1D) is an autoimmune disease mediated by T cells destroying insulin-producing β cells. Identifying the antigenic epitopes targeted by autoreactive T cells is crucial for understanding pathogenesis, detecting biomarkers, and developing immunotherapies. This paper covers T-cell epitopes in T1D, focusing on pre-proinsulin and hybrid insulin peptides (HIPs) as major autoantigens. Substantial evidence highlights epitopes in the insulin B-chain and C-peptide as dominant targets for pathogenic CD4 and CD8 T cells infiltrating the islets. HIPs, formed by proinsulin fragments ligated to other peptides, constitute a novel class of epitopes detected in human and mouse islets. In addition, the paper also examines neoepitopes arising from posttranslational modifications, splice variants, and defective ribosomal products. A key challenge is differentiating genuinely pathogenic epitopes driving disease from nonpathogenic mimotopes. Identifying any essential, indispensable epitopes among this array could enable the development of antigen-specific immunotherapies targeting the root causative factors underlying T1D.

Type 1 diabetes (T1D) is an autoimmune disease characterized by the T-cell-mediated destruction of insulin-producing β cells in the pancreas (Herold et al. 2013; Atkinson et al. 2014; Pugliese 2017; Bluestone et al. 2021). Both CD4 and CD8 T cells play critical roles in orchestrating β-cell destruction through recognition of islet autoantigens presented on MHC class I and class II molecules, respectively. The identification of epitopes derived from β-cell proteins that are targeted by autoreactive T cells is critical for several reasons. First, defining the epitopes recognized provides insight into disease pathogenesis and the mechanisms triggering autoimmunity against specific β-cell components. Second, characterizing autoreactive T-cell epitope recognition enables immune monitoring in patients by detection of epitope-specific T cells as biomarkers. Third, knowledge of epitope specificities is necessary for developing antigen-specific immunotherapies that can modulate T-cell responses. Over the past decades, significant advances have been made leading to the detection of T-cell epitopes relevant to T1D pathogenesis. So far, several

Cite this article as *Cold Spring Harb Perspect Med* doi: 10.1101/cshperspect.a041594

proteins have been identified as the source antigenic epitopes based on the reactivity of patient T cells and autoantibodies. A recent comprehensive effort cataloged and analyzed T-cell epitopes derived from human proteins that are potentially relevant to T1D, using a combination of PubMed and Immune Epitope Database (IEDB) searches (Pugliese 2017). Here, the literature delineates a comprehensive collection, surpassing 100 unique HLA class I–restricted CD8$^+$ T-cell epitopes and exceeding 300 distinct HLA class II–restricted CD4$^+$ T-cell epitopes derived from these proteins (Fig. 1). Of those proteins, a total of seven—namely, pre-proinsulin (PPI), 65 kDa glutamic acid decarboxylase (GAD65), a tyrosine phosphatase-like protein (IA2), zinc transporter 8 (ZnT8), islet-specific glucose-6-phosphatase catalytic subunit-related protein (IGRP), S100 calcium-binding protein B (S100B), and chromogranin A (ChgA)—were identified as the source of epitopes for both CD4 and CD8 T cells. Additionally, neoepitopes, such as posttranslationally modified (Dunne et al. 2012) and alternately spliced (Juan-Mateu et al. 2016), as well as defective ribosomal products (DRiPs) (Kracht et al. 2017) have been identified as antigens recognized by autoreactive T cells. In the past decade, a significant focus has been placed on posttranslationally modified epitopes, which include hybridized, deamidated, citrullinated, as well as oxidized peptide epitopes. Major gaps remain in the current knowledge of islet antigens recognized in T1D. Only a limited number of epitopes has been defined using T cells isolated from target tissues like the pancreas and pancreatic lymph nodes. Furthermore, many reported epitopes lack robust evidence that they are naturally processed and presented as true targets for adaptive immune cells contributing to disease pathogenesis. Among the identified epitopes, PPI and hybrid peptides

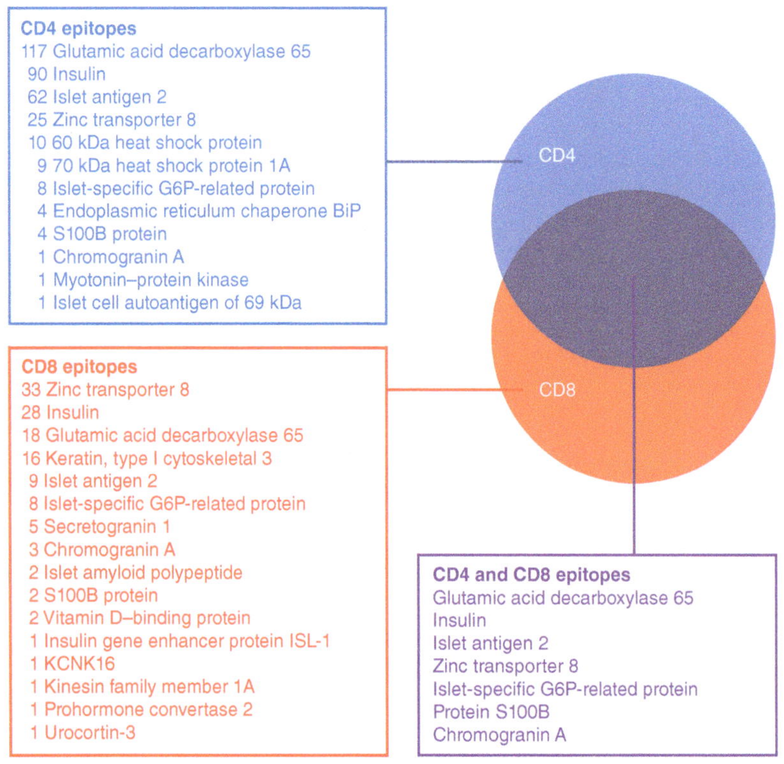

Figure 1. Autoantigens linked to type 1 diabetes (T1D). Various unmodified peptide epitopes have been identified as targets for CD4 and/or CD8 T cells in the pathogenesis of T1D. The numerical value preceding each protein's name indicates the count of distinct epitopes so far associated with T cells linked to T1D.

stand out with evidence implicating a disease-critical role. Here, we will review discoveries of these antigens and describe current challenges as well as requirements toward identifying antigens useful for the developments of biomarkers and immunotherapies.

ANTIGENS TARGETED BY ISLET-ASSOCIATED AUTOANTIBODIES

It is well established that autoantibodies directed against islet proteins are often detectable in individuals developing T1D. Such autoantibodies include those against proinsulin, GAD65, IA2, and ZnT8. These four autoantibodies have been used in clinics as well as clinical trials to diagnose or predict T1D development. More than 70% of individuals with two or more autoantibodies to these four islet proteins develop T1D within 10 years (Ziegler et al. 2013), and thus, the measurement of islet autoantibodies has been a hallmark not only to identify at-risk individuals but also to classify the stages of disease development (Insel et al. 2015). Currently, individuals who have developed two or more islet autoantibodies without showing symptoms of dysglycemia are defined as stage 1 in the disease progression. However, islet autoimmunity may have already been initiated before the detection of the currently used four autoantibodies, and it is important to detect the disease development as early as possible to accurately interpret clinical trial data and understand the trigger and initiation of T1D development. For this purpose, autoantibodies directed to other islet antigens have been explored. For instance, a pilot study assessing the detection of autoantibodies specifically targeting the extracellular domain of ZnT8 shows that these autoantibodies appear before insulin autoantibodies (Gu et al. 2021). Studies using larger sample sizes may demonstrate whether additional autoantibodies can further improve the prediction of T1D development at an earlier stage. The definition of stage 1 requires the detection of multiple islet autoantibodies, because a large portion of individuals developing only one out of the four islet autoantibodies does not progress to developing T1D. By improving the specificity and affinity for each autoantibody detection may allow using single autoantibody positivity to accurately identify individuals developing T1D. Indeed, it was suggested that affinity of autoantibodies is an important factor to reduce false positivity as high-affinity autoantibodies but not low-affinity autoantibodies are associated with T1D development (Achenbach et al. 2004; Mayr et al. 2007; Miao et al. 2015; Jia et al. 2021). Overall, autoantibody measurements have been advantageous for use as reliable biomarkers to determine the stages of T1D. Understanding the chronological order in which individual autoantibodies emerge in prediabetic individuals can also be beneficial for categorizing the disease phenotype and tracking its progression. This is supported by data from the TEDDY (The Environmental Determinants of Diabetes in the Young) study, in which a trend was reported that insulin autoantibodies appear first in individuals with the HLA-DR4-DQ8 haplotype, whereas GAD65 autoantibodies appear first in individuals with HLA-DR3-DQ2. In summary, the measurement of islet autoantibodies has been instrumental in identifying at-risk individuals and classifying the stages of T1D development, with potential implications for improving the prediction and understanding of disease progression.

HLA MOLECULES AND T-CELL ANTIGENS

The identification of T-cell antigens has lagged the detection of autoantibodies due to several factors. Traditional T-cell assays rely on live cell samples, which adds complexity to the process. In addition, the frequencies of autoreactive T cells in peripheral blood are exceedingly low, making their detection challenging. Furthermore, T-cell antigens used for assays may vary depending on the HLA molecules that each individual has. Nevertheless, given the pivotal role of T cells in destroying pancreatic β cells in the pathogenesis of T1D, numerous investigators have dedicated significant efforts to identifying epitopes that are targeted by T cells involved in the development of T1D. Many T-cell clones reactive to islet antigens have been established from T1D patients and animal models such as nonobese diabetic

(NOD) mice, which spontaneously develop autoimmune diabetes and share several characteristics with human T1D (Atkinson and Leiter 1999). Notably, NOD mice express an MHC class II molecule, I-A^{g7}, ortholog to the human T1D-risk HLA allele DQ8. These MHC class II molecules show a common characteristic: The absence of an aspartic acid residue at position 57 of their β-chains influences the configuration of their P9 peptide binding pockets. Consequently, I-A^{g7} and DQ8 favor the presentation of peptides containing negatively charged amino acids at their carboxy-terminal end (Corper et al. 2000; Lee et al. 2001; Suri et al. 2005). Furthermore, these preferences in peptides presented by specific HLA molecules influence the selection of T-cell receptors (TCRs), which are the ligands for peptide-MHC complexes, expressed by individual CD4 T cells. It was shown that TCRs expressed by CD4 T cells of NOD mice tend to have hydrophobic amino acids in the complementarity determining region 3 (CDR3) of β-chains, a characteristic of self-reactive TCRs, whereas TCR repertoires in those with a mutated I-A^{g7} having an aspartic acid at the β-chain position 57 abrogate this feature (Stadinski et al. 2023). Moreover, analyses on insulin-specific TCR repertoires established that carboxy-terminal amino acid residues of the insulin peptides anchoring into the I-A^{g7} or DQ8 peptide groove determine the preferred amino acid usage of TCRs at the CDR3-β segment (Yoshida et al. 2010; Gioia et al. 2019). Thus, peptide repertoires presented by T1D-risk MHC class II molecules show similar characteristics, ultimately determining TCR repertoires expressed by T cells involved in T1D pathogenesis.

The expression of HLA class I molecules in islets of organ donors with T1D is elevated, strongly implicating that CD8 T cells play a key role in β-cell destruction (Coppieters et al. 2012; Richardson et al. 2016). Although most CD8 T-cell epitopes identified to date are presented by HLA-A2 (Ouyang et al. 2006; Standifer et al. 2006; Mallone et al. 2007; Toma et al. 2009; Luce et al. 2011; Scotto et al. 2012; Culina et al. 2018; Gonzalez-Duque et al. 2018; Calviño-Sampedro et al. 2019), it is likely because the HLA-A2 epitopes have been extensively studied. Indeed, unbiased HLA restriction analyses of PPI-specific CD8 T cells showed that those in the islets of organ donors with T1D recognize their target epitopes presented by a number of different HLA class I molecules (Anderson et al. 2021). However, individuals with particular HLA class I alleles tend to have a higher frequency of PPI-specific CD8 T cells in the islets than those without (Anderson et al. 2021). Epitopes preferentially presented by particular HLA class I molecules may contribute to shaping pathogenic CD8 T-cell repertoires in the islets. In addition, it was shown that HLA-B molecules are up-regulated more dramatically upon cytokine exposure compared to HLA-A molecules (Carré et al. 2023). This finding may implicate that peptides exclusively presented in an inflammatory environment are preferentially presented by HLA-B and potentially HLA-C molecules, resulting in activating a subset of CD8 T cells restricted to these "minor" HLA molecules whose basal expression levels are low. It will be important to broadly search for such disease-specific CD8 epitopes, apart from specific HLA restriction.

THE ROLE OF PRE-PROINSULIN IN T1D

PPI, the precursor of both proinsulin and insulin, stands out as the most abundant protein selectively synthesized by β cells, garnering significant attention as a key target in the study of T cells implicated in the onset of T1D. A substantial portion of proteins produced in both human and mouse β cells is PPI and PPI-derived products (i.e., proinsulin and insulin) (Hutton 1989; Bollheimer et al. 1998; Boland et al. 2017). Notably, through immunopeptidome analyses, numerous peptides derived from PPI have been identified, elucidating their presence in the peptide repertoire presented by MHC class I and class II molecules, as revealed by mass spectrometry (Skowera et al. 2008; Gonzalez-Duque et al. 2018; Wan et al. 2020). This underscores the pivotal role of PPI peptides in engaging T cells in the immune response. Furthermore, genetic evidence supports PPI as a T-cell antigen involved in T1D pathogenesis. The insulin variable number of tandem repeats (VNTRs) gene element, located in the PPI promoter region, has been identified as a genetic region associated with T1D development (Pugliese et al. 1997; Vafiadis et al. 1997). Individuals with protective insulin VNTR class III alleles express higher levels of PPI mRNA, resulting in fewer T cells stained with proinsulin tetramers in the peripheral blood compared to those with susceptible class I alleles, who have high levels of proinsulin-specific T cells (Durinovic-Belló et al. 2010). Thus, accumulated evidence suggests that T cells specific to PPI are involved in T1D development.

Since the 1990s, numerous CD4 and CD8 T-cell clones have been isolated from pancreatic islets and immune organs of NOD mice. A significant portion of these T cells were reactive to proinsulin peptides (Wegmann et al. 1994; Wong et al. 1999; Chen et al. 2001; Haskins 2005; Mohan et al. 2013; Lamont et al. 2014). The majority of insulin-reactive CD4 T-cell clones were reactive to an insulin B-chain peptide (insulin B:9–23) (Daniel et al. 1995), and therefore reactivity to peptides within this region has been extensively studied as epitopes involved in T1D development in the NOD mouse model. Interestingly, a portion of this peptide, insulin B:15–23, has also been identified as a target for CD8 T cells in the islets of NOD mice (Wong et al. 1999). The insulin B:9–23-reactive CD4 T-cell clones abolish the response when an amino acid at position 16 is exchanged from tyrosine to alanine (Alleva et al. 2002). Importantly, NOD mice having this mutation do not have immune cell infiltration in the islets and are completely protected from diabetes development, demonstrating that peptides in the B:9–23 region serve as essential targets for provoking autoimmunity to β cells (French et al. 1997; Jaeckel et al. 2004; Nakayama et al. 2005, 2007). Further studies have shown that the presence of anti-insulin responses is required for the development of T-cell responses to IGRP, but vice versa is not true (Krishnamurthy et al. 2006). Additionally, insulin tolerance induced during the neonatal stage is sufficient to suppress diabetes development throughout life (Jhala et al. 2016). These studies elucidate that there is a hierarchical order of antigens recognized by β-cell-specific T cells over the course of developing disease, and activation of anti-insulin autoimmunity occurs at the initial stage.

Insulin B:9–23-reactive T cells are currently classified into two subsets: One specific to an insulin B-chain 13–21 segment (insulin B:13–21) and reactive to insulin processed in antigen-presenting cells, and the other specific to only a segment insulin B-chain 12–20 (insulin B:12–20) but not reacting to native insulin (Mohan et al. 2010, 2011). Of conceptual importance, the latter subset responds to islet-derived dendritic cells but not thymic dendritic or epithelial cells, suggesting a failure of eliminating or regulating these cells (Mohan et al. 2011). Indeed, B:12–20-specific T cells are a dominant population in the islets of NOD mice, particularly in young animals, and induce diabetes when transferred into immunocompromised NOD mice, thus contributing considerably to anti-islet autoimmunity (Mohan et al. 2010, 2011; Gioia et al. 2019). Truncated B-chain peptides, including insulin B:9–23 and insulin B:11–23, are predominantly detected in crinosomes rather than insulin-containing granules. Crinosomes are vesicles that are formed in β cells when secretory granules containing insulin fuse with lysosomes. This fusion results in the degradation of excess or damaged insulin granules (Wan et al. 2018). These truncated peptides are released from β cells upon glucose stimulation, activating insulin B:12–20-specific T cells in the lymphoid tissues (Wan et al. 2018). Further studies have linked the expression of peptides presented by MHC class II molecules to T-cell responses against peptides contained in crinosomes (Wan et al. 2020). Peptides truncated from insulin B-chain and C-peptide are dominantly detected in MHC class II immunopeptidomes from islet cells expressing the I-A^{g7} MHC class II molecule in NOD mice. Furthermore, while not all peptides abundantly expressed by MHC class II molecules are antigenic, a carboxy-terminal insulin B-chain segment, including the B:12–20 region as well as a carboxy-terminal segment in C-peptide are recognized by T cells in the islets and pancreatic lymph nodes. Altogether, peptides derived from the insulin B-chain are generated in crinosomes of β cells and presented by the T1D-risk I-A^{g7} MHC class II molecule, and T cells specific to I-A^{g7}/insulin B:12–20 are activated and accumulate in the islets as well as in the draining lymph nodes. In separate studies, insulin B:9–23-specific T cells were classified based on their preferred specificity to insulin B:9–23 peptides with amino acid substitutions at the carboxyl terminus: One subset preferably responds to a peptide with a mutation R22E (termed Reg 3A), and the other to peptides with mutations E21G and R22E (termed Reg 3B) (Crawford et al. 2011; Gao et al. 2017; Smith et al. 2024). T cells stained with tetramers composed of these peptides are detected in the pancreas of NOD mice as well as in the peripheral blood of T1D patients, suggesting the participation of these T cells in islet autoimmunity (Crawford et al. 2011; Pauken et al. 2013; Yang et al. 2014; Nakayama et al. 2015). Both peptides have a mutation from arginine (R) to glutamic acid (E) at position 22 of the insulin B-chain, forcing the insulin B:14–22 segment to bind to the I-A^{g7} molecule pockets 1–9, whereas the latter has an additional mutation from glutamic acid (E) to glycine (G) at position 21. The E21G mutation removes a side chain from the surface structure exposed to a TCR molecule, which determines TCR repertoires that preferably recognize this peptide (Gao et al. 2017; Wang et al. 2019). This series of structural analyses raises an intriguing hypothesis that insulin B-chain peptides with posttranslational modifications (PTMs) at the carboxyl terminus may be biological epitopes activating the T cells stained with these tetramers. While peptide hybridization reactions, as discussed below, have the potential to introduce such modifications to the B-chain, there is currently no evidence validating the formation of such modified B-chain epitopes in β cells. Currently, it is unknown whether the two types of insulin-specific T-cell subsets defined by the separate studies described above designate the same T-cell populations; there seem to be at least some overlaps. Identification of biologically occurring posttranslationally modified epitopes may lead us to understand how T cells specific to the insulin B-chain peptide and potentially their derivatives are activated, differentiated, and involved in the T1D pathogenesis.

While PPI amino acid sequences are identical between people with and without T1D, insulin peptides do not provoke T-cell activation in most people protected from autoimmunity against β cells. As discussed above, factors such as expression levels in the thymus, truncation into peptides suitable for MHC presentation, and MHC-binding affinity may determine whether PPI peptides become antigens eliciting T-cell activations in individuals. Peptide modifications may also be an important determinant, and all these factors ultimately shape T-cell phenotypes and functions. Studies showed that phenotypes of T cells stained with insulin tetramers are mixtures of Th1-like, Foxp3-positive regulatory, and anergic T cells (Pauken et al. 2013; Baker et al. 2018; Spence et al. 2018; Gioia et al. 2019). Age and types of insulin recognition (i.e., B:12–20 or B:13–21; alternatively, Reg 3A or Reg 3B) are not correlated with phenotypes and clonotype selection in the thymus (Gioia et al. 2019; Smith et al. 2024). Instead, TCR affinity to the insulin peptide/MHC complex determined T-cell deletion in the thymus mediated by the autoimmune regulator (Smith et al. 2024). A recent study analyzing T cells in NOD islets revealed a positive correlation between TCR signaling intensity, presumably reflecting reactivity to islets, and effector functions (Kong et al. 2022). Thus, TCR affinity to peptide/MHC complexes may be crucial in determining T-cell fate and functions. Biological epitopes targeted by individual insulin B:9–23-specific T cells, even within the same subsets classified based on their recognition patterns of the insulin peptides, may vary. Therefore, identifying the epitopes that genuinely elicit T-cell activation in the pancreas is important for precisely evaluating TCR affinity and its association with T-cell functions.

In 2015, antigen specificity of CD4 T cells in the islets of organ donors with T1D was reported first (Pathiraja et al. 2015), and subsequently, two separate studies using islet samples from donors recovered through collaborative efforts by organ donor networks such as the Network for Pancreatic Organ Donors with Diabetes (nPOD) have been published (Babon et al. 2016; Michels et al. 2017). One team analyzed the antigen specificity of 50 CD4 and CD8 T-cell lines established from nine organ donors who had T1D for 2–20 years (Babon et al. 2016). These enormous efforts led to the discoveries that one-third of T-cell lines were reactive to islet antigens, indicating that T-cell repertoires in the islets of established T1D donors contain T cells recognizing a variety of antigens, including proinsulin (Babon et al. 2016). The pioneering study analyzing more than 50 CD4 T-cell clones from a donor who had T1D for 3 years identified CD4 T cells in the islets responding to epitopes contained in C-peptide presented by HLA-DQ8 or DQ8/DQ2 transdimer molecules (Pathiraja et al. 2015). The other study has further demonstrated that C-peptide-specific CD4 T cells are detected in the blood of recent-onset T1D patients and precisely mapped epitopes in C-peptide, the majority of which are presented by T1D-risk HLA-DQ molecules (So et al. 2018). The other team also found CD4 T cells expressing TCRs reactive to C-peptide presented by DQ2 or DQ8/DQ2 transdimers from the islets of different donors (Michels et al. 2017; Landry et al. 2021), and thus peptide-MHC complexes composed of C-peptide and T1D risk HLA-DQ molecules are common targets for CD4 T cells in the islets of T1D individuals. This evidence provides an underlying rationale that immunotherapies targeting proinsulin may be more effective than those targeting only insulin, which does not contain C-peptide (Roep et al. 2013). In addition to C-peptide-reactive T cells, CD4 T cells reacting to the insulin B:9–23 peptide presented by HLA-DQ8 were identified in islets samples of T1D organ donors (Michels et al. 2017), recapitulating the finding from the NOD mouse model in human T1D. Furthermore, a recent study comprehensively analyzing 166 TCRs expressed by CD4 T cells in the islets or pancreas of six T1D donors identified 14 TCR clonotypes reactive to epitopes spread out in the mature proinsulin protein presented by various HLA molecules, in which half of the TCR clonotypes are restricted with HLA-DQ (Landry et al. 2021). Of importance, 12 out of the 14 TCRs responded to islet lysates, confirming the specificity to β cells. In summary, islets of individuals with T1D contain CD4 T cells targeting various proinsulin-derived peptides, including insulin B:9–23 and those within C-peptide presented by T1D-risk HLA-DQ molecules. It will be important to determine frequencies of T cells specific to these epitopes in the islets as well as draining lymph nodes, intensity of responsiveness to the cognate epitopes, and phenotypes of T cells targeting these epitopes in each stage of T1D development to understand how proinsulin-specific CD4 T cells are involved in the T1D pathogenesis.

Well-evidenced PPI-specific CD8 epitopes in human T1D were first identified using CD8 T-cell clones established from peripheral blood samples of T1D patients: One, a PPI 15–24 peptide (PPI:15–24) presented by HLA-A2, and the other, a PPI 3–11 peptide presented by HLA-A24 (Skowera et al. 2008; Kronenberg et al. 2012). These studies demonstrate two crucial pieces of evidence: (1) the epitopes are naturally processed and presented in human β cells; and (2) CD8 T cells reacting to the epitope can kill β cells. Subsequently, the presence of PPI:15–24/HLA-A2-specific CD8 T cells in the islets of T1D organ donors was confirmed (Coppieters et al. 2012; Anderson et al. 2021; Rodriguez-Calvo et al. 2021), further reinforcing the conclusion that the PPI:15–24 peptide is a major antigen targeted by CD8 T cells to destroy β cells and may be used for immunotherapies to treat T1D patients having HLA-A2. Recently, TCRs expressed by CD8 T cells in the islets or pancreas of organ donors with and without T1D were comprehensively analyzed for the response to PPI peptides (Anderson et al. 2021). All of the seven T1D donors investigated had at least one PPI-specific TCRs derived from CD8 T cells in the pancreas, whereas only one of four nondiabetic control donors had an insulin B-chain-reactive TCR. In addition, the insulin-specific TCR found in the nondiabetic donor required high peptide concentrations—in the millimolar range—to be stimulated, and thus it was an extremely low-affinity TCR. On the other hand, TCRs found from T1D donors were activated by their cognate peptides at nanomolar to low micromolar concentrations, suggesting that CD8 T cells expressing high-affinity TCRs infiltrate the islets over the course of T1D development. While only a limited number of TCRs specific to each PPI epitope has been identified, there is a trend that high-affinity but not low-affinity TCRs targeting the same epitopes share similar motifs. Approximately a quarter of the TCRs identified from the pancreas of

T1D organ donors are found in other individuals, and a portion of these shared TCRs was predominantly detected in the peripheral blood of T1D patients compared to nondiabetic individuals (Mitchell et al. 2023). Accumulating additional islet-specific TCR sequence information, especially from high-affinity TCRs, could enhance the prediction of antigen specificity of individual TCRs (Nakayama and Michels 2021).

THE ROLE OF HYBRID INSULIN PEPTIDES IN T1D

ChgA has emerged as an epitope that is targeted by autoreactive CD4 T cells in both NOD mice (Stadinski et al. 2010) and human patients with T1D (Gottlieb et al. 2014). In early investigations, the peptide WE14, a naturally occurring cleavage product of ChgA with unknown biological function, was identified as an epitope recognized by various diabetes-triggering CD4 T-cell clones in NOD mice. These T-cell clones, which encompass BDC-2.5, BDC-10.1, and BDC-9.46, were established from lymph nodes or spleens of separate diabetic NOD mice, suggesting a broad significance of ChgA in the pathogenesis of NOD mice (Haskins 2005). In human disease, recent-onset patients with T1D showed significantly elevated T-cell responses in their peripheral blood mononuclear cells (PBMCs) to WE14 through IFN-γ ELISPOT assays, which distinguished the patients from nondiabetic control subjects (Gottlieb et al. 2014). This indicated that WE14 is a target of autoreactive T cells in early–stage 3 patients with T1D, which is the final stage at which the disease becomes symptomatic (Faustman et al. 1990). Notably, studies on NOD mice deficient in ChgA showed protection from disease onset (Baker et al. 2016), placing ChgA on par with insulin as a potentially critical autoantigen. However, unlike insulin, ChgA is expressed in various cell types and can also be found in secretory vesicles of neurons and endocrine cells, including chromaffin cells in the adrenal medulla, paraganglia, and enterochromaffin-like cells (Helman et al. 1988). The expression of ChgA in unaffected tissues of NOD mice suggested that the primary epitope for autoreactive T cells is a modified form of ChgA exclusive to β cells. Subsequent studies led to the identification of a hybrid insulin peptide (HIP) that was recognized by these diabetes-triggering CD4 T-cell clones (Delong et al. 2016). This peptide contains a distinct fragment of C-peptide linked through a peptide bond to the amino terminus of WE14. The designation of this epitope is 2.5HIP, as it is recognized by the prototypic CD4 T-cell clone BDC-2.5 at low nanomolar concentrations (Table 1). Significantly, BDC-2.5 and other 2.5HIP-reactive CD4 T-cell clones also respond to the nonligated ChgA peptide WE14. However, for this T-cell stimulation to occur, nonphysiological concentrations of WE14—in the micromolar range concentrations—were needed. HIPs contain amino acid sequences not encoded in the genome, offering a plausible explanation for how HIP-reactive T cells may bypass the negative selection process in the thymus. Here, the lack of the distinct β-cell peptide processing machinery, responsible for generating substantial levels of essential HIP-precursor peptides like WE14 or C-peptide, makes it unlikely that significant levels of these HIPs form in medullary thymic epithelial cells, which are pivotal in T-cell development and selection within the thymus. Mass spectrometric analyses on murine islet extracts verified the presence of 2.5HIP as well as other HIPs. These HIPs include 6.9HIP, which forms between the same C-peptide fragment and a natural cleavage product of islet amyloid polypeptide (Delong et al. 2016; Wiles et al. 2017, 2019). This HIP is recognized by the diabetes-triggering T-cell clones BDC-6.9 and BDC-9.3. More recently, the diabetes-triggering CD4 TCR NY4.1 was shown to respond to various HIP sequences (Parras et al. 2021). However, the presence of only one of these HIPs (HIP11) in murine islets was validated through mass spectrometric analyses (Wiles et al. 2019). Notably, HIP11 is composed of the amino terminus of intact C-peptide that is linked to the same C-peptide fragment forming 2.5HIP and 6.9HIP (Table 1). Disease-relevance of the above-mentioned HIPs has been demonstrated in immunodeficient NOD.scid mice, each expressing only a monoclonal T-cell population (retrogenic mice) derived from 17 distinct TCRs against various autoantigens (Burton et al. 2008). Here, it was shown that only a small subset of five

Table 1. Hybrid insulin peptides (HIPs) are T-cell epitopes in type 1 diabetes (T1D)

Identifier	Amino terminal	Carboxy terminal	T-cell clones
Nonobese diabetic (NOD) mice			
2.5HIP	...DLQTLAL	WSRMDQL... (WE14)	BDC-2.5, BDC-10.1, BDC-9.46
6.9HIP	...DLQTLAL	NAARDPN... (IAPP2)	BDC-6.9, BDC-9.3
HIP11	...DLQTLAL	EVEDPQV... (C-Peptide)	NY4.1
Human type 1 diabetes (T1D) (residual islets)			
HIP4	...QVELGGG	GIVEQCC... (A-Chain)	
HIP5	...QVELGGG	TPIESHQ... (IAPP1)	
HIP6	...QVELGGG	NAVEVLK... (IAPP2)	
HIP8	...QVELGGG	SSPETLI... (NPY)	
HIP11	...SLQPLAL	EAEDPQV... (PPI)	GSE.8E3
Human T1D (peripheral blood mononuclear cells [PBMCs])			
HIP4	...QVELGGG	GIVEQCC... (A-Chain)	
HIP11	...SLQPLAL	EAEDPQV... (C-Peptide)	E2
HIP12	...SLQPLAL	GIVEQCC... (A-Chain)	
HIP16	...SLQPLAL	SSPETLI... (NPY)	

HIPs form in β cells through peptide bonding between proinsulin fragments on the amino-terminal side and various β-cell peptides in the carboxy-terminal side. Table shows amino- and carboxy-terminal amino acid sequences of HIPs that have been identified as targets for diabetes-triggering T cells in NOD mice, as well as T cells or TCRs identified in PBMCs of recent-onset T1D patients, or residual islets of T1D organ donors. The presence of a limited number of HIPs—namely, 2.5HIP, 6.9HIP, and HIP11—has been validated in NOD islets. In human islets, the presence of HIP11 has been confirmed by mass spectrometry.

autoantigen-specific TCRs could initiate islet infiltration and β-cell destruction independently. The pathogenic TCRs included those from the HIP-reactive T-cell clones BDC-2.5, BDC-10.1, NY4.1, and BDC-6.9 (Table 1), as well as insulin B:9–23-specific T-cell clones. The remaining TCRs, specific to other epitopes associated with T1D—namely, GAD65, IA2, and phogrin (IA2-β)—did not induce disease onset in these retrogenic mice. This highlights the important fact that autoreactivity does not inherently imply pathogenicity and supports the roles of insulin and HIPs as potentially critical epitopes for β-cell destruction. Furthermore, efforts to induce antigen-specific tolerance in NOD mice with poly(lactic-co-glycolic acid) nanoparticles (NPs) loaded with 2.5HIP significantly extended the survival of islet grafts in mice (Neef et al. 2021). The protection observed in mice treated with 2.5HIP NPs was attributed to two factors: The simultaneous induction of anergy in 2.5HIP-specific effector T cells and the expansion of $Foxp3^{+}$ regulatory T cells specific for the same antigen. The findings also indicate a significant impairment in the effector function of CD4 and CD8 T cells specific to other β-cell epitopes that infiltrated the graft. This further supports a key role of this ChgA-bearing epitope in NOD mice as a target for the T-cell-mediated destruction of β cells.

In human disease, a study using IFN-γ ELISPOT analyses revealed the presence of HIP-reactive T cells in PBMCs of recent-onset patients with T1D (Baker et al. 2019). Here, different samples, each containing a unique HIP, yielded significantly elevated levels of proinflammatory T-cell responses, when compared to samples lacking HIPs. This distinguished patients from nondiabetic control subjects, in which the significant elevation of HIP-reactive T cells was not observed. In this study, a total of four HIPs triggered such significantly elevated T-cell responses (Table 1). However, it is important to note that the presence of only one of these HIPs has so far been validated through mass spectrometric analyses on pancreatic islets of nondiabetic organ donors (Wiles et al. 2021). This HIP is the human equivalent of HIP11, which is targeted by the diabetes-triggering CD4 TCR NY4.1 derived from NOD mice (Table 1; Parras et al. 2021). A HIP11-reactive CD4 T-cell clone (E2) was also isolated from the peripheral blood of a recent-onset T1D patients. This T-cell clone responds to HIP11 in the low nanomolar range (Baker et al. 2019). In a separate study, a HIP11-reactive TCR was also identified in residual pancreatic islets of an organ donor with T1D (Wiles et al. 2021). Furthermore, CD4 T-cell clones infiltrating human islets, isolated from the residual islets of a T1D patient, demonstrated recognition of HIPs when presented, leading to IFN-γ secretion upon peptide stimulation. Notably, two distinct T-cell clones specifically recognized a HIP that formed between a C-peptide fragment linked to a natural cleavage product of islet amyloid polypeptide (IAPP) (GQVELGGG-NAVEVLK) (Delong et al. 2016). In another study, several islet infiltrating $CD4^+$ T-cell lines grown from T1D organ donors were also found to recognize this HIP. This study also identified a T-cell clone responding to a HIP containing the same C-peptide fragment, linked to the amino terminus of the insulin A-chain (GQVELGGG-GIVEQCC) (Babon et al. 2016). Furthermore, a CD4 T-cell line from a 20-year-old male with 7 years of T1D also secreted IFN-γ in response to a HIP formed by the fusion of proinsulin C-peptide to neuropeptide Y (GQVELGGG-SSPETLI). However, it is again important to note that the presence of these HIPs in pancreatic islets from nondiabetic organ donors has not been confirmed.

The formation of several disease-relevant HIPs, specifically 2.5HIP, 6.9HIP, and HIP11, has been attributed to the reverse proteolytic activity of the aspartic protease cathepsin D (CatD) (Crawford et al. 2022). Immunogold electron microscopy was used to investigate the subcellular localization of 6.9HIP, revealing its presence within insulin secretory granules and crinophagic bodies in NOD islets (Wenzlau et al. 2024). Crinophagic bodies, formed by the fusion of lysosomes and insulin granules, play a crucial role in sequestering and isolating indigestible waste materials resulting from autophagic processes. The presence of CatD within insulin granules, further supported by mass spectrometric analyses of highly purified insulin granule preparations (Brunner et al. 2007), challenges the traditional view of CatD as a lysosomal enzyme and highlights the importance of these specialized secretory vesicles in the generation of autoantigens in T1D. In addition to CatD-mediated HIP formation, another mechanism involving an aspartic anhydride intermediate of a C-peptide fragment has been shown to contribute to the formation of HIPs and their isomers (isoHIPs) (Crawford et al. 2023). This process occurs spontaneously in an acidic environment and leads to the formation of peptide bonds at aspartic acid residues or isopeptide bonds at the side chain of aspartic acid residues. Although these HIPs have been detected in both human and murine islets, their relevance to T1D pathogenesis remains to be established. These findings shed new light on the intracellular processes that contribute to the development of autoimmunity and open new avenues for exploring the mechanisms underlying the pathogenesis of T1D. Further research into the factors regulating HIP formation within insulin granules and the potential impact of these autoantigens on β-cell function and immune recognition may provide valuable insights for the development of novel therapeutic strategies. By understanding the complex interplay between the formation of HIPs, their subcellular localization, and the role of crinophagic bodies in cellular homeostasis, we can gain a more comprehensive understanding of the pathogenic mechanisms driving T1D and identify potential targets for intervention.

THE ROLE OF ADDITIONAL NEOEPITOPES IN T1D

Neoepitopes can emerge due to various factors, such as PTMs, alternate splicing or DRiP formation. This field has been of great interest in the past decade, and evidence supporting the involvement of neoepitopes in the pathogenesis of T1D has accumulated. The resulting neoepitopes may not be present in the healthy state and could provide a priming target for autoimmune diseases. However, it is important to note that the mere presence of neoepitopes does not automatically lead to an autoimmune response. For example, the presence of several HIPs, which are a form of PTM, can be confidently validated not only in islets of NOD mice, but also in islets of BALB/c mice, which do not develop autoimmune diabetes (Wiles et al. 2019). Furthermore, the presence of various HIPs in pancreatic islets obtained from nondiabetic organ donors has also been validated through mass spectrometric analyses (Wiles et al. 2019, 2021; Crawford et al. 2023).

Enzymatic PTMs

In general, PTMs of proteins represent important mechanisms for regulating protein structure and function in normal physiology. However, such modifications may provide epitopes that accelerate or initiate the destruction of target tissue through autoimmune mechanisms. This may especially be plausible for modifications that do not occur at significant yields within the thymus, allowing autoreactive T cells to evade the negative selection process. In addition to HIPs, there is evidence for several PTMs that may contribute to the development of T1D. When tolerance to these modified self-epitopes fails, the result can be the activation and clonal expansion of pathogenic autoimmune cells. One type of PTMs is formed through the process of deamidation, which involves the conversion of the amino acid glutamine to its deamidated counterpart glutamic acid. This reaction may be catalyzed by members of the transglutaminase family, with tissue transglutaminase 2 (TG2) being a prominent member (van Lummel et al. 2014; Callebaut et al. 2021). The expression and activity of TG2 can be influenced by factors like cytokines and oxidative stress. In the context of autoimmunity, TG2 has been implicated in generating deamidated neoepitopes, such as deamidated gluten epitopes that provide critical epitopes in celiac disease (Mothes 2007; Qiao et al. 2012). In T1D, TG2-catalyzed deamidation has been observed in islet proteins, emphasizing its role in generating modified antigens. Studies in NOD mice and humans have identified deamidated neoepitopes, particularly in proinsulin (Wan et al. 2020). Another type of PTMs linked to autoimmunity are citrullinations, which are catalyzed by the protein arginine deiminase (PAD) family of enzymes through a calcium-dependent process that converts the guanidine group of arginine to a ureido group. Multiple PADs are expressed in humans with varying sequence specificities, and their activity is influenced by calcium levels, linking citrullination to inflammatory processes affecting intracellular and extracellular calcium levels. Citrullination has been implicated in autoimmune diseases such as systemic lupus erythematosus (Ciesielski et al. 2022), celiac disease (Caio et al. 2019), and T1D (Yang et al. 2021), but it is most strongly associated with rheumatoid arthritis (Nava-Quiroz et al. 2023). In T1D, citrullinated targets include GRP78, GAD65, IA-2, IGRP, IAPP, and glucokinase, which has been linked to impaired β-cell function (Yang et al. 2022b). Studies reveal that citrullination (Ireland and Unanue 2011, 2012) can also occur within autophagy vesicles of antigen-presenting cells, particularly macrophages and dendritic cells.

Nonenzymatic PTMs

In addition to enzymatically introduced PTMs, there are various modifications that lead to protein modifications nonenzymatically. This includes HIP-formation, which was shown to not only occur in β cells through a CatD-mediated transpeptidation reaction (Crawford et al. 2022), but also through a spontaneous reaction involving an aspartic anhydride intermediate (Crawford et al. 2023). Another reaction that may occur spontaneously is the deamidation of glutamine or asparagine residues, leading to the formation of glutamic or aspartic acid residues. The acidic environments of insulin secretory granules or crinophagic bodies can facilitate the spontaneous deamidation through an acid catalyzed reaction mechanism (Callebaut et al. 2021). Oxidation reactions can also occur spontaneously. In β cells, the oxidizing environment of the endoplasmic reticulum (ER) contributes to the folding of proinsulin and the oxidative formation of its disulfide bonds (Vakilian et al. 2019). When disulfide bonds are incorrectly formed or if there are mispairings between cysteine residues, protein disulfide isomerases can act to reduce these disulfide bonds and assist in rearranging them to achieve the correct pairing (Wang and Wang 2023). This process of disulfide bond reduction and isomerization helps prevent the accumulation of misfolded or unfolded proteins in the ER. Indeed, the insulin A-chain containing an atypical disulfide bridge was identified as a cognate epitope for a T-cell clone isolated from a T1D patient. In this epitope, the insulin A-chain contains an atypical disulfide bridge. PTM introduced by reactive oxidants represents another mechanism for the generation of neoepitopes. It was shown that most individuals with T1D (Strollo et al. 2015) or children at risk of diabetes (Strollo et al. 2017) have autoantibodies to oxidative posttranslationally modified insulin. Hence, antibodies to oxidized forms of insulin were detected in several patients who were negative to the standard islet autoantibodies (Strollo et al. 2015, 2019). Various patients also showed a coherent autoimmune reaction to oxidized insulin, involving concurrent activation of CD4 and CD8 T cells alongside the presence of autoantibodies (Strollo et al. 2023). Protein carbonylation represents another PTM that can occur in tissue proteins when exposed to oxidative stress (Yang et al. 2022a). Proteomic analyses of islets from prediabetic NOD mice revealed the presence of several carbonylated proteins, including prolyl-4-hydroxylase β (P4Hb), which is responsible for proinsulin folding and trafficking. Increased carbonylation of P4Hb was also found in human islets exposed to oxidative stress or inflammatory cytokines, associated with impaired insulin secretion and elevated proinsulin/insulin ratios. Carbonyl modification of P4Hb likely impairs its role in proinsulin folding, causing misfolded proinsulin accumulation and autoimmunity. These findings suggest the carbonylation of P4Hb and resulting proinsulin misfolding may be an important event in T1D autoimmunity and β-cell dysfunction.

RNA Splice Variants and Defective Ribosomal Products (DRiPs)

Splice variants refer to different versions of a gene transcript that are generated through alternative splicing of precursor messenger RNA (pre-mRNA). These variants can generate novel sequences that can act as neoepitopes not subject to normal tolerance mechanisms (Guyer et al. 2023). For example, a splice variant of cyclin I, a protein implicated in cell cycle regulation, was discovered within the HLA class I peptidome (Guyer et al. 2023). This neoepitope was recognized by CD4 T cells in the peripheral blood of T1D patients. Furthermore, a partially overlapping peptide of this neoepitope was also recognized by CD8 T cells of T1D patients, suggesting a linked recognition. Another source for neoepitopes arises from errors in insulin mRNA translation. Leaky ribosome scanning and stress-induced effects on translation are proposed as mechanisms driving the production of such DRiPs (Kracht et al. 2017; Anderson et al. 2021; Thomaidou et al. 2021). It was discovered that an alternative open reading frame in human PPI mRNA encodes a highly immunogenic peptide. T cells responsive to the amino-terminal peptide of this aberrant translation product were detected in the pancreas of T1D patients. Furthermore, CD8 T cells reactive to this peptide were found in the islets of T1D donors (Anderson et al. 2021), and CD8 T-cell clones specific for this epitope were shown to kill human β cells in vitro, confirming the peptide is naturally processed and presented (Kracht et al. 2017). Single-nucleotide polymorphisms in the alternative reading frame determined epitope variants that correlated with T1D risk. The findings reveal DRiPs of insulin mRNA translation act as neoepitopes targeted in T1D pathogenesis. It has been proposed that such translational errors create neoepitopes that break immune tolerance and trigger cytotoxic responses against β cells in T1D.

PERSPECTIVES AND CONCLUSIONS

Accumulating efforts have yielded the identification of numerous T-cell epitopes (James et al. 2020; Amdare et al. 2021). This progress highlights two crucial points. First, it raises the question of which epitopes genuinely activate the T cells involved in T1D pathogenesis. Second, among these pathogenic epitopes, it prompts the inquiry of which antigenic targets are indispensable drivers of T1D development.

Pathogenic Epitopes versus Nonpathogenic Mimotopes

A single TCR can interact with hundreds of thousands of distinct epitopes presented by appropriate MHC molecules (Wooldridge et al. 2012). For example, the NOD-derived TCR NY4.1 has been demonstrated to recognize numerous HIP sequences presented by I-A^{g7} (Parras et al. 2021). However, among these HIPs, the presence of only HIP11 has been confirmed through mass spectrometric analyses on murine islets. This indicates that the remaining HIPs, which contained amino acid sequences partially overlapping with HIP11, were mimicking the sequence of HIP11 but play no role in disease. In human disease, a study using IFN-γ ELISPOT analyses revealed the presence of HIP11-reactive T cells in peripheral blood mononuclear cells (PBMCs) of patients with recent-onset T1D (E2, see Table 1; Baker et al. 2019). Conversely, a TCR identified in the residual islets of a T1D donor showed dual reactivity to HIP11 and native C-peptide (GSE.8E3, see Table 1; Wiles et al. 2021). The presence of both C-peptide and HIP11 has been validated by mass spectrometry on human islets. Despite HIP11 eliciting a strong response at lower peptide concentrations compared to C-peptide, the GSE.8E3 TCR responds to islet lysate fractions containing C-peptide rather than those containing HIP11, raising the question of which epitope acts as the disease-driving antigen for this TCR. Differentiating such "pathogenic" epitopes that elicit T-cell activations in vivo from potentially nonpathogenic mimotopes that are recognized by T cells but not actual targets in the pancreas will be important to understand T1D pathogenesis and use them for therapies. For this, evidence from both T cells and β cells will be crucial. Here, we propose three criteria to define pathogenic epitopes involved in T1D pathogenesis.

1. Evidence for the presence of epitopes in β cells. The presence of epitopes in β cells must be confirmed through mass spectrometric analyses. Immunopeptidomics evidence demonstrating presentations of epitopes by MHC molecules is ideal. While some epitopes such as PPI:15–24 are detected in primary β cells regardless of donor types (i.e., donors with and without T1D) (Gonzalez-Duque et al. 2018), some epitopes may be produced only in β cells of T1D donors or require specific β-cell manipulations that mimic the disease environment, such as inducing ER stress, exposing them to an inflammatory microenvironment, or even subjecting them to proper viral infection, to generate and process antigens into epitopes recognized by TCRs.
2. Evidence for the presence of epitope-reactive T cells in the pancreas or draining lymph nodes of individuals developing T1D. The mere presence of T cells in the islets of individuals with T1D does not guarantee their relevance to T1D development. Confirming that the T cells in question react to β cells or islet extracts is essential. While self-reactive T cells are present in individuals who do not develop T1D, frequencies and phenotypes of islet-reactive T cells in the pancreas and draining lymph nodes but not peripheral blood distinguish T1D patients from nondiabetic controls (Nakayama et al. 2015; Skowera et al. 2015; Gonzalez-Duque et al. 2018; Bender et al. 2020). Therefore, studying T cells in the target organs is crucial (James et al. 2020). Additionally, as high-affinity islet autoantibodies can predict disease development more accurately than low-affinity ones (Steck et al. 2016; Jia et al. 2021; Triolo et al. 2022), TCR affinity or response levels to epitopes may be a critical factor to discriminate pathogenic epitopes from nonpathogenic mimotopes. Of note, T cells expressing high-affinity TCRs for islet antigens have been detected in the pancreas of organ donors with T1D but not those without (Anderson et al. 2021).
3. Evidence of the indispensability of epitopes for T cells to respond to β cells or β-cell extracts. T cells may cross-react to multiple epitopes. Therefore, validating which epitope(s) expressed by β cells stimulate given TCRs is important. For instance, could the response to β cells by T cells be suppressed by autoantibodies specific to a given peptide-MHC complex? Alternatively, can T cells expressing a cognate TCR migrate to native islets but not to those devoid of epitope expression in animal models? These investigations will confirm epitopes that are genuinely recognized by T cells to be activated.

TCRs expressed by T cells can recognize antigens only when presented as epitopes by MHC molecules. This fundamental concept suggests that antigen-specific T-cell activation requires either T cells expressing high-affinity TCRs interacting with a limited number of proper peptide-MHC complexes, or β cells or antigen-presenting cells expressing numerous peptide-MHC molecules recognized by a substantial number of TCRs on T cells. Alternatively, self-reactive T cells may be activated through lower TCR signaling intensity compared to conventional T cells. Establishing connections between epitope production, processing, presentation, and TCR affinity, avidity, and signaling is crucial for identifying genuinely pathogenic epitopes.

Essential versus Nonessential Epitopes

A critical question remains: Are there epitopes essential for T cells to provoke islet autoimmunity, and if so, what are they? Studies in NOD mice indicate a hierarchy of antigens to which T cells respond in T1D development (Nakayama et al. 2005; Krishnamurthy et al. 2006). While there may be multiple epitopes critical for T1D development, identifying a set of such essential epitopes could inform the developing antigen-specific immunotherapies. Distinguishing essential epitopes from those contributing to but not essential for T1D development is pivotal for devising effective immunotherapies. Nonessential epitopes tend to be targeted by T cells in the pancreas in which β-cell destruction has already occurred, and, therefore, investigators are keen to identify antigen specificity at early stages of T1D development, especially those initiating islet autoimmunity. However, not only T1D patients but also nondiabetic individuals have T cells specific to islet antigens, so-called "benign islet autoimmunity" (von Herrath and Bonifacio 2021; Samassa and Mallone 2022). This concept suggests that the "initiation" of anti-islet immune responses may be occurring under physiological conditions in individuals not developing T1D. Islet-specific T cells in the peripheral blood of nondiabetic individuals tend to be naive or anergic, whereas those of T1D patients contain more effector and memory types of T cells. However, in the pancreas, individuals with T1D have higher numbers of ZnT8-specific T cells than those without (Culina et al. 2018). Moreover, PPI-specific T cells accumulate in the islets of T1D individuals, whereas those in nondiabetic controls stay in the exocrine tissue of the pancreas (Bender et al. 2020). Importantly, response levels of PPI-specific TCRs in the pancreas of T1D individuals are orders of magnitude higher when compared to those of nondiabetic individuals (Anderson et al. 2021). This series of studies indicate that different sets of islet-specific T-cell repertoires, presumably T cells expressing higher affinity TCRs, are activated and recruited to the pancreas to cause "pathogenic" islet autoimmunity, or different epitopes may provoke activation of T cells that were naive or regulated in the benign islet autoimmunity phase (Fig. 2). This "change of gear" may manifest through T cells targeting the same epitopes as those involved in benign autoimmunity but expressing higher affinity TCRs, or it could be provoked by T cells targeting different epitopes. Furthermore, T cells not only specific to an epitope in the benign autoimmunity stage but also cross-reactive to different epitopes, such as neoepitopes generated exclusively in diseased β cells, may drive the gear change. Among the identified pathogenic epitopes, it will be crucial to distinguish essential epitopes from nonessential ones. Ultimately, understanding at which stage—initiation or "gear change"—T cells specific to a given epitope become activated and drive islet autoimmunity is paramount for selecting proper antigens for immunotherapies. For instance, antigens such as PPI:15–24, which is abundantly expressed by β cells positive for HLA-A2, would be an appropriate target to direct therapeutic reagents/cells to the microenvironment in the pancreatic islets of individuals with HLA-A2. Alternatively, 2.5HIP has been shown to be a major target for effector T cells in the islets of NOD mice. An NP therapy that modulates 2.5HIP-specific T-cell functions suppresses syngeneic graft rejection transplanted in diabetic NOD mice (Jamison et al. 2022). Insights into the temporal dynamics of epitope production, spreading and the hierarchy of pathogenic epitopes involved in T1D pathogenesis will provide

 Cite this article as *Cold Spring Harb Perspect Med* doi: 10.1101/cshperspect.a041594

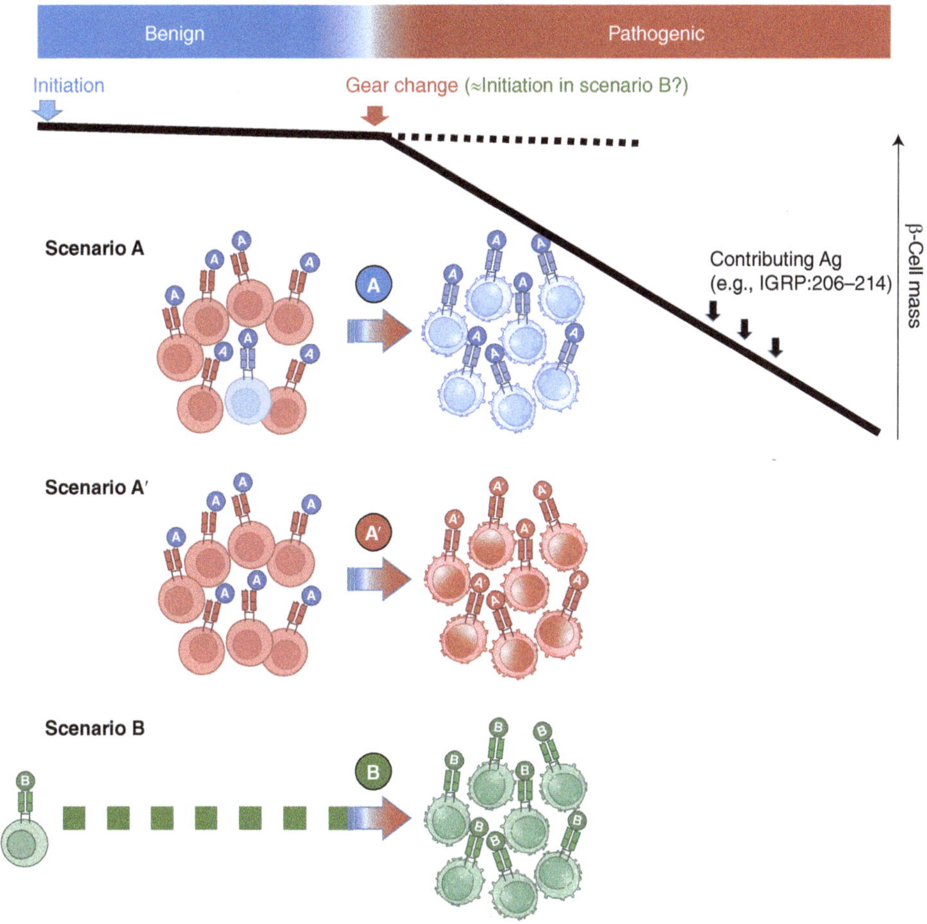

Figure 2. Classification of antigen-specific T cells in the development of type 1 diabetes (T1D). Three possible models for T cells that are essential for T1D development are illustrated. Scenario (*A*): The majority of T cells recognizing epitope "A" are low-affinity (represented by red T cells) and regulated within benign autoimmunity. T cells recognizing "A" with high affinity (represented by blue T cells) become activated, leading the progress to the pathogenic phase. Scenario (*A*′) An epitope "A′," which is a modification of "A," serves as a high-affinity antigen for T cells that recognize "A" with low affinity. When "A′" is produced in sick β cells and presented to T cells, the A/A′-cross-reactive T cells (represented by red T cells) are regulated in the benign phase but become activated upon exposure to the modified epitope "A,′" triggering the disease progression to the pathogenic phase. In both scenarios, the epitopes "A" and "A′" play roles in inducing progression to pathogenic autoimmunity. Scenario (*B*): T cells recognizing epitope "B" (represented by green T cells) are naive and do not participate in benign autoimmunity. Upon exposure to "B," these T cells become activated and initiate the development of T1D. (Figure created with BioRender.com.)

rationales for using proper antigens for T1D immunotherapies.

CLOSING REMARKS

Evidence from both β cells and T cells will permit the identification of pathogenic epitopes, particularly those that initiate or change the mode of the disease process. This will ultimately enable us to determine the timing, location, and mechanisms by which essential epitopes are generated and prime autoreactive T cells, culminating in islet autoimmunity. Elucidating these insights holds promise for interventional opportunities to halt the destructive autoimmune cascade before clinical onset of T1D. Unraveling the hierarchy and dynamics of pathogenic epitope spreading is vital to developing strategies that can preemptively or therapeutically target the root causative factors driving disease pathogenesis.

ACKNOWLEDGMENTS

This work was supported by the National Institutes of Diabetes and Digestive and Kidney Diseases (R01DK119529, R01DK099317, R01DK032083, and R01DK133457).

REFERENCES

Achenbach P, Koczwara K, Knopff A, Naserke H, Ziegler AG, Bonifacio E. 2004. Mature high-affinity immune responses to (pro)insulin anticipate the autoimmune cascade that leads to type 1 diabetes. *J Clin Invest* **114:** 589–597. doi:10.1172/JCI200421307

Alleva DG, Gaur A, Jin L, Wegmann D, Gottlieb PA, Pahuja A, Johnson EB, Motheral T, Putnam A, Crowe PD, et al. 2002. Immunological characterization and therapeutic activity of an altered-peptide ligand, NBI-6024, based on the immunodominant type 1 diabetes autoantigen insulin B-chain (9–23) peptide. *Diabetes* **51:** 2126–2134. doi:10.2337/diabetes.51.7.2126

Amdare N, Purcell AW, DiLorenzo TP. 2021. Noncontiguous T cell epitopes in autoimmune diabetes: from mice to men and back again. *J Biol Chem* **297:** 100827. doi:10.1016/j.jbc.2021.100827

Anderson AM, Landry LG, Alkanani AA, Pyle L, Powers AC, Atkinson MA, Mathews CE, Roep BO, Michels AW, Nakayama M. 2021. Human islet T cells are highly reactive to preproinsulin in type 1 diabetes. *Proc Natl Acad Sci* **118:** e2107208118. doi:10.1073/pnas.2107208118

Atkinson MA, Leiter EH. 1999. The NOD mouse model of type 1 diabetes: as good as it gets? *Nat Med* **5:** 601–604. doi:10.1038/9442

Atkinson MA, Eisenbarth GS, Michels AW. 2014. Type 1 diabetes. *Lancet* **383:** 69–82. doi:10.1016/S0140-6736(13)60591-7

Babon JA, DeNicola ME, Blodgett DM, Crèvecoeur I, Buttrick TS, Maehr R, Bottino R, Naji A, Kaddis J, Elyaman W, et al. 2016. Analysis of self-antigen specificity of islet-infiltrating T cells from human donors with type 1 diabetes. *Nat Med* **22:** 1482–1487. doi:10.1038/nm.4203

Baker RL, Bradley B, Wiles TA, Lindsay RS, Barbour G, Delong T, Friedman RS, Haskins K. 2016. Cutting edge: nonobese diabetic mice deficient in chromogranin A are protected from autoimmune diabetes. *J Immunol* **196:** 39–43. doi:10.4049/jimmunol.1501190

Baker RL, Jamison BL, Wiles TA, Lindsay RS, Barbour G, Bradley B, Delong T, Friedman RS, Nakayama M, Haskins K. 2018. CD4 T cells reactive to hybrid insulin peptides are indicators of disease activity in the NOD mouse. *Diabetes* **67:** 1836–1846. doi:10.2337/db18-0200

Baker RL, Rihanek M, Hohenstein AC, Nakayama M, Michels A, Gottlieb PA, Haskins K, Delong T. 2019. Hybrid insulin peptides are autoantigens in type 1 diabetes. *Diabetes* **68:** 1830–1840. doi:10.2337/db19-0128

Bender C, Rodriguez-Calvo T, Amirian N, Coppieters KT, von Herrath MG. 2020. The healthy exocrine pancreas contains preproinsulin-specific CD8 T cells that attack islets in type 1 diabetes. *Sci Adv* **6:** eabc5586. doi:10.1126/sciadv.abc5586

Bluestone JA, Buckner JH, Herold KC. 2021. Immunotherapy: building a bridge to a cure for type 1 diabetes. *Science* **373:** 510–516. doi:10.1126/science.abh1654

Boland BB, Rhodes CJ, Grimsby JS. 2017. The dynamic plasticity of insulin production in β-cells. *Mol Metab* **6:** 958–973. doi:10.1016/j.molmet.2017.04.010

Bollheimer LC, Skelly RH, Chester MW, McGarry JD, Rhodes CJ. 1998. Chronic exposure to free fatty acid reduces pancreatic β cell insulin content by increasing basal insulin secretion that is not compensated for by a corresponding increase in proinsulin biosynthesis translation. *J Clin Invest* **101:** 1094–1101. doi:10.1172/JCI420

Brunner Y, Iezzi M, Foti M, Fukuda M, Hochstrasser DF, Wollheim CB, Sanchez J-C. 2007. Proteomics analysis of insulin secretory granules. *Mol Cell Proteomics* **6:** 1007–1017. doi:10.1074/mcp.M600443-MCP200

Burton AR, Vincent E, Arnold PY, Lennon GP, Smeltzer M, Li CS, Haskins K, Hutton J, Tisch RM, Sercarz EE, et al. 2008. On the pathogenicity of autoantigen-specific T-cell receptors. *Diabetes* **57:** 1321–1330. doi:10.2337/db07-1129

Caio G, Volta U, Sapone A, Leffler DA, De Giorgio R, Catassi C, Fasano A. 2019. Celiac disease: a comprehensive current review. *BMC Med* **17:** 142. doi:10.1186/s12916-019-1380-z

Callebaut A, Derua R, Vig S, Delong T, Mathieu C, Overbergh L. 2021. Identification of deamidated peptides in cytokine-exposed MIN6 cells through LC-MS/MS using a shortened digestion time and inspection of MS2 spectra. *J Proteome Res* **20:** 1405–1414. doi:10.1021/acs.jproteome.0c00801

Calviño-Sampedro C, Gomez-Tourino I, Cordero OJ, Reche PA, Gómez-Perosanz M, Sánchez-Trincado JL, Rodríguez M, Sueiro AM, Viñuela JE, Calviño RV. 2019. Naturally presented HLA class I–restricted epitopes from the neurotrophic factor S100-β are targets of the autoimmune response in type 1 diabetes. *FASEB J* **33:** 6390–6401. doi:10.1096/fj.201802270R

Carré A, Zhou Z, Perez-Hernandez J, Samassa F, Lekka C, Manganaro A, Oshima M, Liao H, Parker R, Nicastri A, et al. 2023. Interferon-α promotes neo-antigen formation and preferential HLA-B-restricted antigen presentation in pancreatic β-cells. bioRxiv doi:10.1101/2023.09.15.557918

Chen W, Bergerot I, Elliott JF, Harrison LC, Abiru N, Eisenbarth GS, Delovitch TL. 2001. Evidence that a peptide spanning the B-C junction of proinsulin is an early autoantigen epitope in the pathogenesis of type 1 diabetes. *J Immunol* **167:** 4926–4935. doi:10.4049/jimmunol.167.9.4926

Ciesielski O, Biesiekierska M, Panthu B, Soszyński M, Pirola L, Balcerczyk A. 2022. Citrullination in the pathology of inflammatory and autoimmune disorders: recent advances and future perspectives. *Cell Mol Life Sci* **79:** 94. doi:10.1007/s00018-022-04126-3

Coppieters KT, Dotta F, Amirian N, Campbell PD, Kay TW, Atkinson MA, Roep BO, von Herrath MG. 2012. Demonstration of islet-autoreactive CD8 T cells in insulitic lesions from recent onset and long-term type 1 diabetes patients. *J Exp Med* **209:** 51–60. doi:10.1084/jem.2011 1187

Corper AL, Stratmann T, Apostolopoulos V, Scott CA, Garcia KC, Kang AS, Wilson IA, Teyton L. 2000. A structural framework for deciphering the link between I-Ag^7 and autoimmune diabetes. *Science* **288:** 505–511. doi:10 .1126/science.288.5465.505

Crawford F, Stadinski B, Jin N, Michels A, Nakayama M, Pratt P, Marrack P, Eisenbarth G, Kappler JW. 2011. Specificity and detection of insulin-reactive CD4$^+$ T cells in type 1 diabetes in the nonobese diabetic (NOD) mouse. *Proc Natl Acad Sci* **108:** 16729–16734. doi:10.1073/pnas .1113954108

Crawford SA, Wiles TA, Wenzlau JM, Powell RL, Barbour G, Dang M, Groegler J, Barra JM, Burnette KS, Hohenstein AC, et al. 2022. Cathepsin D drives the formation of hybrid insulin peptides relevant to the pathogenesis of type 1 diabetes. *Diabetes* **71:** 2793–2803. doi:10.2337/db22-0303

Crawford SA, Groegler J, Dang M, Michel C, Powell RL, Hohenstein AC, Reyes K, Haskins K, Wiles TA, Delong T. 2023. Hybrid insulin peptide isomers spontaneously form in pancreatic β-cells from an aspartic anhydride intermediate. *J Biol Chem* **299:** 105264. doi:10.1016/j.jbc .2023.105264

Culina S, Lalanne AI, Afonso G, Cerosaletti K, Pinto S, Sebastiani G, Kuranda K, Nigi L, Eugster A, Østerbye T, et al. 2018. Islet-reactive CD8$^+$ T cell frequencies in the pancreas, but not in blood, distinguish type 1 diabetic patients from healthy donors. *Sci Immunol* **3:** eaao4013. doi:10 .1126/sciimmunol.aao4013

Daniel D, Gill RG, Schloot N, Wegmann D. 1995. Epitope specificity, cytokine production profile and diabetogenic activity of insulin-specific T cell clones isolated from NOD mice. *Eur J Immunol* **25:** 1056–1062. doi:10.1002/ eji.1830250430

Delong T, Wiles TA, Baker RL, Bradley B, Barbour G, Reisdorph R, Armstrong M, Powell RL, Reisdorph N, Kumar N, et al. 2016. Pathogenic CD4 T cells in type 1 diabetes recognize epitopes formed by peptide fusion. *Science* **351:** 711–714. doi:10.1126/science.aad2791

Dunne JL, Overbergh L, Purcell AW, Mathieu C. 2012. Posttranslational modifications of proteins in type 1 diabetes: the next step in finding the cure? *Diabetes* **61:** 1907–1914. doi:10.2337/db11-1675

Durinovic-Belló I, Wu RP, Gersuk VH, Sanda S, Shilling HG, Nepom GT. 2010. Insulin gene VNTR genotype associates with frequency and phenotype of the autoimmune response to proinsulin. *Genes Immun* **11:** 188–193. doi:10 .1038/gene.2009.108

Faustman D, Eisenbarth G, Breitmeyer J. 1990. Analysis of T lymphocyte subsets in all stages of diabetes. *J Autoimmun* **3:** 111–116. doi:10.1016/S0896-8411(09)90019-1

French MB, Allison J, Cram DS, Thomas HE, Dempsey-Collier M, Silva A, Georgiou HM, Kay TW, Harrison LC, Lew AM. 1997. Transgenic expression of mouse proinsulin II prevents diabetes in nonobese diabetic mice. *Diabetes* **46:** 34–39. doi:10.2337/diab.46.1.34

Gao H, Li C, Ramesh B, Hu N. 2017. Cloning, purification and characterization of novel Cu-containing nitrite reductase from the *Bacillus firmus* GY-49. *World J Microbiol Biotechnol* **34:** 10. doi:10.1007/s11274-017-2383-6

Gioia L, Holt M, Costanzo A, Sharma S, Abe B, Kain L, Nakayama M, Wan X, Su A, Mathews C, et al. 2019. Position β57 of I-A^{g7} controls early anti-insulin responses in NOD mice, linking an MHC susceptibility allele to type 1 diabetes onset. *Sci Immunol* **4:** eaaw6329. doi:10.1126/ sciimmunol.aaw6329

Gonzalez-Duque S, Azoury ME, Colli ML, Afonso G, Turatsinze JV, Nigi L, Lalanne AI, Sebastiani G, Carré A, Pinto S, et al. 2018. Conventional and neo-antigenic peptides presented by β cells are targeted by circulating naïve CD8$^+$ T cells in type 1 diabetic and healthy donors. *Cell Metab* **28:** 946–960.e6. doi:10.1016/j.cmet.2018.07.007

Gottlieb PA, Delong T, Baker RL, Fitzgerald-Miller L, Wagner R, Cook G, Rewers MR, Michels A, Haskins K. 2014. Chromogranin A is a T cell antigen in human type 1 diabetes. *J Autoimmun* **50:** 38–41. doi:10.1016/j.jaut.2013 .10.003

Gu Y, Merriman C, Guo Z, Jia X, Wenzlau J, Li H, Li H, Rewers M, Yu L, Fu D. 2021. Novel autoantibodies to the β-cell surface epitopes of ZnT8 in patients progressing to type-1 diabetes. *J Autoimmun* **122:** 102677. doi:10.1016/j .jaut.2021.102677

Guyer P, Arribas-Layton D, Manganaro A, Speake C, Lord S, Eizirik DL, Kent SC, Mallone R, James EA. 2023. Recognition of mRNA splice variant and secretory granule epitopes by CD4$^+$ T cells in type 1 diabetes. *Diabetes* **72:** 85–96. doi:10.2337/db22-0191

Haskins K. 2005. Pathogenic T-cell clones in autoimmune diabetes: more lessons from the NOD mouse. *Adv Immunol* **87:** 123–162. doi:10.1016/S0065-2776(05)87004-X

Helman LJ, Ahn TG, Levine MA, Allison A, Cohen PS, Cooper MJ, Cohn DV, Israel MA. 1988. Molecular cloning and primary structure of human chromogranin A (secretory protein I) cDNA. *J Biol Chem* **263:** 11559–11563. doi:10.1016/S0021-9258(18)37995-X

Herold KC, Vignali DA, Cooke A, Bluestone JA. 2013. Type 1 diabetes: translating mechanistic observations into effective clinical outcomes. *Nat Rev Immun* **13:** 243–256. doi:10.1038/nri3422

Hutton JC. 1989. The insulin secretory granule. *Diabetologia* **32:** 271–281. doi:10.1007/BF00265542

Insel RA, Dunne JL, Atkinson MA, Chiang JL, Dabelea D, Gottlieb PA, Greenbaum CJ, Herold KC, Krischer JP, Lernmark Å, et al. 2015. Staging presymptomatic type 1 diabetes: a scientific statement of JDRF, the Endocrine Society, and the American Diabetes Association. *Diabetes Care* **38:** 1964–1974. doi:10.2337/dc15-1419

Ireland JM, Unanue ER. 2011. Autophagy in antigen-presenting cells results in presentation of citrullinated peptides to CD4 T cells. *J Exp Med* **208:** 2625–2632. doi:10 .1084/jem.20110640

Ireland JM, Unanue ER. 2012. Processing of proteins in autophagy vesicles of antigen-presenting cells generates citrullinated peptides recognized by the immune system. *Autophagy* **8:** 429–430. doi:10.4161/auto.19261

Jaeckel E, Lipes MA, von Boehmer H. 2004. Recessive tolerance to preproinsulin 2 reduces but does not abolish type 1 diabetes. *Nat Immunol* **5:** 1028–1035. doi:10.1038/ni1120

James EA, Mallone R, Kent SC, DiLorenzo TP. 2020. T-cell epitopes and neo-epitopes in type 1 diabetes: a comprehensive update and reappraisal. *Diabetes* **69:** 1311–1335. doi:10.2337/dbi19-0022

Jamison BL, DiLisio JE, Beard KS, Neef T, Bradley B, Goodman J, Gill RG, Miller SD, Baker RL, Haskins K. 2022. Tolerogenic delivery of a hybrid insulin peptide markedly prolongs islet graft survival in the NOD mouse. *Diabetes* **71:** 483–496. doi:10.2337/db20-1170

Jhala G, Chee J, Trivedi PM, Selck C, Gurzov EN, Graham KL, Thomas HE, Kay TW, Krishnamurthy B. 2016. Perinatal tolerance to proinsulin is sufficient to prevent autoimmune diabetes. *JCI insight* **1:** e86065. doi:10.1172/jci.insight.86065

Jia X, He L, Miao D, Waugh K, Rasmussen CG, Dong F, Steck AK, Rewers M, Yu L. 2021. High-affinity ZnT8 autoantibodies by electrochemiluminescence assay improve risk prediction for type 1 diabetes. *J Clin Endocrinol Metab* **106:** 3455–3463. doi:10.1210/clinem/dgab575

Juan-Mateu J, Villate O, Eizirik DL. 2016. Mechanisms in endocrinology: alternative splicing: the new frontier in diabetes research. *Eur J Endocrinol* **174:** R225–R238. doi:10.1530/EJE-15-0916

Kong Y, Jing Y, Allard D, Scavuzzo MA, Sprouse ML, Borowiak M, Bettini ML, Bettini M. 2022. A dormant T-cell population with autoimmune potential shows low self-reactivity and infiltrates islets in type 1 diabetes. *Eur J Immunol* **52:** 1158–1170. doi:10.1002/eji.202149690

Kracht MJ, van Lummel M, Nikolic T, Joosten AM, Laban S, van der Slik AR, van Veelen PA, Carlotti F, de Koning EJ, Hoeben RC, et al. 2017. Autoimmunity against a defective ribosomal insulin gene product in type 1 diabetes. *Nat Med* **23:** 501–507. doi:10.1038/nm.4289

Krishnamurthy B, Dudek NL, McKenzie MD, Purcell AW, Brooks AG, Gellert S, Colman PG, Harrison LC, Lew AM, Thomas HE, et al. 2006. Responses against islet antigens in NOD mice are prevented by tolerance to proinsulin but not IGRP. *J Clin Invest* **116:** 3258–3265. doi:10.1172/JCI29602

Kronenberg D, Knight RR, Estorninho M, Ellis RJ, Kester MG, de Ru A, Eichmann M, Huang GC, Powrie J, Dayan CM, et al. 2012. Circulating preproinsulin signal peptide-specific CD8 T cells restricted by the susceptibility molecule HLA-A24 are expanded at onset of type 1 diabetes and kill β-cells. *Diabetes* **61:** 1752–1759. doi:10.2337/db11-1520

Lamont D, Mukherjee G, Kumar PR, Samanta D, McPhee CG, Kay TW, Almo SC, DiLorenzo TP, Serreze DV. 2014. Compensatory mechanisms allow undersized anchor-deficient class I MHC ligands to mediate pathogenic autoreactive T cell responses. *J Immunol* **193:** 2135–2146. doi:10.4049/jimmunol.1400997

Landry LG, Anderson AM, Russ HA, Yu L, Kent SC, Atkinson MA, Mathews CE, Michels AW, Nakayama M. 2021. Proinsulin-reactive CD4 T cells in the islets of type 1 diabetes organ donors. *Front Endocrinol* **12:** 622647. doi:10.3389/fendo.2021.622647

Lee KH, Wucherpfennig KW, Wiley DC. 2001. Structure of a human insulin peptide-HLA-DQ8 complex and susceptibility to type 1 diabetes. *Nat Immunol* **2:** 501–507. doi:10.1038/88694

Luce S, Lemonnier F, Briand JP, Coste J, Lahlou N, Muller S, Larger E, Rocha B, Mallone R, Boitard C. 2011. Single insulin-specific $CD8^+$ T cells show characteristic gene expression profiles in human type 1 diabetes. *Diabetes* **60:** 3289–3299. doi:10.2337/db11-0270

Mallone R, Martinuzzi E, Blancou P, Novelli G, Afonso G, Dolz M, Bruno G, Chaillous L, Chatenoud L, Bach JM, et al. 2007. $CD8^+$ T-cell responses identify β-cell autoimmunity in human type 1 diabetes. *Diabetes* **56:** 613–621. doi:10.2337/db06-1419

Mayr A, Schlosser M, Grober N, Kenk H, Ziegler AG, Bonifacio E, Achenbach P. 2007. GAD autoantibody affinity and epitope specificity identify distinct immunization profiles in children at risk for type 1 diabetes. *Diabetes* **56:** 1527–1533. doi:10.2337/db06-1715

Miao D, Steck AK, Zhang L, Guyer KM, Jiang L, Armstrong T, Muller SM, Krischer J, Rewers M, Yu L. 2015. Electrochemiluminescence assays for insulin and glutamic acid decarboxylase autoantibodies improve prediction of type 1 diabetes risk. *Diabetes Technol Ther* **17:** 119–127. doi:10.1089/dia.2014.0186

Michels AW, Landry LG, McDaniel KA, Yu L, Campbell-Thompson M, Kwok WW, Jones KL, Gottlieb PA, Kappler JW, Tang Q, et al. 2017. Islet-derived CD4 T cells targeting proinsulin in human autoimmune diabetes. *Diabetes* **66:** 722–734. doi:10.2337/db16-1025

Mitchell AM, Baschal EE, McDaniel KA, Fleury T, Choi H, Pyle L, Yu L, Rewers MJ, Nakayama M, Michels AW. 2023. Tracking DNA-based antigen-specific T cell receptors during progression to type 1 diabetes. *Sci Adv* **9:** eadj6975. doi:10.1126/sciadv.adj6975

Mohan JF, Levisetti MG, Calderon B, Herzog JW, Petzold SJ, Unanue ER. 2010. Unique autoreactive T cells recognize insulin peptides generated within the islets of Langerhans in autoimmune diabetes. *Nat Immunol* **11:** 350–354. doi:10.1038/ni.1850

Mohan JF, Petzold SJ, Unanue ER. 2011. Register shifting of an insulin peptide-MHC complex allows diabetogenic T cells to escape thymic deletion. *J Exp Med* **208:** 2375–2383. doi:10.1084/jem.20111502

Mohan JF, Calderon B, Anderson MS, Unanue ER. 2013. Pathogenic $CD4^+$ T cells recognizing an unstable peptide of insulin are directly recruited into islets bypassing local lymph nodes. *J Exp Med* **210:** 2403–2414. doi:10.1084/jem.20130582

Mothes T. 2007. Deamidated gliadin peptides as targets for celiac disease-specific antibodies. *Adv Clin Chem* **44:** 35–63. doi:10.1016/S0065-2423(07)44002-1

Nakayama M, Michels AW. 2021. Using the T cell receptor as a biomarker in type 1 diabetes. *Front Immunol* **12:** 777788. doi:10.3389/fimmu.2021.777788

Nakayama M, Abiru N, Moriyama H, Babaya N, Liu E, Miao D, Yu L, Wegmann DR, Hutton JC, Elliott JF, et al. 2005. Prime role for an insulin epitope in the development of type 1 diabetes in NOD mice. *Nature* **435:** 220–223. doi:10.1038/nature03523

Nakayama M, Beilke JN, Jasinski JM, Kobayashi M, Miao D, Li M, Coulombe MG, Liu E, Elliott JF, Gill RG, et al. 2007. Priming and effector dependence on insulin B:9–23 peptide in NOD islet autoimmunity. *J Clin Invest* **117:** 1835–1843. doi:10.1172/JCI31368

Nakayama M, McDaniel K, Fitzgerald-Miller L, Kiekhaefer C, Snell-Bergeon JK, Davidson HW, Rewers M, Yu L, Gottlieb P, Kappler JW, et al. 2015. Regulatory vs. inflammatory cytokine T-cell responses to mutated insulin peptides in healthy and type 1 diabetic subjects. *Proc Natl Acad Sci* **112:** 4429–4434. doi:10.1073/pnas.1502967112

Nava-Quiroz KJ, López-Flores LA, Pérez-Rubio G, Rojas-Serrano J, Falfán-Valencia R. 2023. Peptidyl arginine deiminases in chronic diseases: a focus on rheumatoid arthritis and interstitial lung disease. *Cells* **12:** 2829. doi:10.3390/cells12242829

Neef T, Ifergan I, Beddow S, Penaloza-MacMaster P, Haskins K, Shea LD, Podojil JR, Miller SD. 2021. Tolerance induced by antigen-loaded PLG nanoparticles affects the phenotype and trafficking of transgenic $CD4^+$ and $CD8^+$ T cells. *Cells* **10:** 3445. doi:10.3390/cells10123445

Ouyang Q, Standifer NE, Qin H, Gottlieb P, Verchere CB, Nepom GT, Tan R, Panagiotopoulos C. 2006. Recognition of HLA class I-restricted β-cell epitopes in type 1 diabetes. *Diabetes* **55:** 3068–3074. doi:10.2337/db06-0065

Parras D, Solé P, Delong T, Santamaría P, Serra P. 2021. Recognition of multiple hybrid insulin peptides by a single highly diabetogenic T-cell receptor. *Front Immunol* **12:** 737428. doi:10.3389/fimmu.2021.737428

Pathiraja V, Kuehlich JP, Campbell PD, Krishnamurthy B, Loudovaris T, Coates PT, Brodnicki TC, O'Connell PJ, Kedzierska K, Rodda C, et al. 2015. Proinsulin-specific, HLA-DQ8, and HLA-DQ8-transdimer-restricted $CD4^+$ T cells infiltrate islets in type 1 diabetes. *Diabetes* **64:** 172–182. doi:10.2337/db14-0858

Pauken KE, Linehan JL, Spanier JA, Sahli NL, Kalekar LA, Binstadt BA, Moon JJ, Mueller DL, Jenkins MK, Fife BT. 2013. Cutting edge: type 1 diabetes occurs despite robust anergy among endogenous insulin-specific CD4 T cells in NOD mice. *J Immunol* **191:** 4913–4917. doi:10.4049/jimmunol.1301927

Pugliese A. 2017. Autoreactive T cells in type 1 diabetes. *J Clin Invest* **127:** 2881–2891. doi:10.1172/JCI94549

Pugliese A, Zeller M, Fernandez A Jr, Zalcberg LJ, Bartlett RJ, Ricordi C, Pietropaolo M, Eisenbarth GS, Bennett ST, Patel DD. 1997. The insulin gene is transcribed in the human thymus and transcription levels correlated with allelic variation at the INS VNTR-IDDM2 susceptibility locus for type 1 diabetes. *Nat Genet* **15:** 293–297. doi:10.1038/ng0397-293

Qiao SW, Iversen R, Ráki M, Sollid LM. 2012. The adaptive immune response in celiac disease. *Semin Immunopathol* **34:** 523–540. doi:10.1007/s00281-012-0314-z

Richardson SJ, Rodriguez-Calvo T, Gerling IC, Mathews CE, Kaddis JS, Russell MA, Zeissler M, Leete P, Krogvold L, Dahl-Jørgensen K, et al. 2016. Islet cell hyperexpression of HLA class I antigens: a defining feature in type 1 diabetes. *Diabetologia* **59:** 2448–2458. doi:10.1007/s00125-016-4067-4

Rodriguez-Calvo T, Krogvold L, Amirian N, Dahl-Jørgensen K, von Herrath M. 2021. One in ten $CD8^+$ cells in the pancreas of living individuals with recent-onset type 1 diabetes recognizes the preproinsulin epitope PPI_{15-24}. *Diabetes* **70:** 752–758. doi:10.2337/db20-0908

Roep BO, Solvason N, Gottlieb PA, Abreu JRF, Harrison LC, Eisenbarth GS, Yu L, Leviten M, Hagopian WA, Buse JB, et al. 2013. Plasmid-encoded proinsulin preserves C-peptide while specifically reducing proinsulin-specific $CD8^+$ T cells in type 1 diabetes. *Sci Transl Med* **5:** a182.

Samassa F, Mallone R. 2022. Self-antigens, benign autoimmunity and type 1 diabetes: a β-cell and T-cell perspective. *Curr Opin Endocrinol Diabetes Obes* **29:** 370–378. doi:10.1097/MED.0000000000000735

Scotto M, Afonso G, Larger E, Raverdy C, Lemonnier FA, Carel JC, Dubois-Laforgue D, Baz B, Levy D, Gautier JF, et al. 2012. Zinc transporter (ZnT)8(186–194) is an immunodominant $CD8^+$ T cell epitope in HLA-$A2^+$ type 1 diabetic patients. *Diabetologia* **55:** 2026–2031. doi:10.1007/s00125-012-2543-z

Skowera A, Ellis RJ, Varela-Calviño R, Arif S, Huang GC, Van-Krinks C, Zaremba A, Rackham C, Allen JS, Tree TI, et al. 2008. CTLs are targeted to kill β cells in patients with type 1 diabetes through recognition of a glucose-regulated preproinsulin epitope. *J Clin Invest* **118:** 3390–3402. doi:10.1172/JCI35449

Skowera A, Ladell K, McLaren JE, Dolton G, Matthews KK, Gostick E, Kronenberg-Versteeg D, Eichmann M, Knight RR, Heck S, et al. 2015. β-cell-specific CD8 T cell phenotype in type 1 diabetes reflects chronic autoantigen exposure. *Diabetes* **64:** 916–925. doi:10.2337/db14-0332

Smith JA, Yuen BTK, Purtha W, Balolong JM, Phipps JD, Crawford F, Bluestone JA, Kappler JW, Anderson MS. 2024. Aire mediates tolerance to insulin through thymic trimming of high-affinity T cell clones. *Proc Natl Acad Sci* **121:** e2320268121. doi:10.1073/pnas.2320268121

So M, Elso CM, Tresoldi E, Pakusch M, Pathiraja V, Wentworth JM, Harrison LC, Krishnamurthy B, Thomas HE, Rodda C, et al. 2018. Proinsulin C-peptide is an autoantigen in people with type 1 diabetes. *Proc Natl Acad Sci* **115:** 10732–10737. doi:10.1073/pnas.1809208115

Spence A, Purtha W, Tam J, Dong S, Kim Y, Ju CH, Sterling T, Nakayama M, Robinson WH, Bluestone JA, et al. 2018. Revealing the specificity of regulatory T cells in murine autoimmune diabetes. *Proc Natl Acad Sci* **115:** 5265–5270. doi:10.1073/pnas.1715590115

Stadinski BD, Delong T, Reisdorph N, Reisdorph R, Powell RL, Armstrong M, Piganelli JD, Barbour G, Bradley B, Crawford F, et al. 2010. Chromogranin A is an autoantigen in type 1 diabetes. *Nat Immunol* **11:** 225–231. doi:10.1038/ni.1844

Stadinski BD, Cleveland SB, Brehm MA, Greiner DL, Huseby PG, Huseby ES. 2023. I-A^{g7} β56/57 polymorphisms regulate non-cognate negative selection to $CD4^+$ T cell orchestrators of type 1 diabetes. *Nat Immunol* **24:** 652–663. doi:10.1038/s41590-023-01441-0

Standifer NE, Ouyang Q, Panagiotopoulos C, Verchere CB, Tan R, Greenbaum CJ, Pihoker C, Nepom GT. 2006. Identification of Novel HLA-A*0201-restricted epitopes in recent-onset type 1 diabetic subjects and antibody-positive relatives. *Diabetes* **55:** 3061–3067. doi:10.2337/db06-0066

Steck AK, Fouts A, Miao D, Zhao Z, Dong F, Sosenko J, Gottlieb P, Rewers MJ, Yu L. 2016. ECL-IAA and ECL-

GADA can identify high-risk single autoantibody-positive relatives in the TrialNet Pathway to Prevention Study. *Diabetes Technol Ther* **18:** 410–414. doi:10.1089/dia.2015.0316

Strollo R, Vinci C, Arshad MH, Perrett D, Tiberti C, Chiarelli F, Napoli N, Pozzilli P, Nissim A. 2015. Antibodies to post-translationally modified insulin in type 1 diabetes. *Diabetologia* **58:** 2851–2860. doi:10.1007/s00125-015-3746-x

Strollo R, Vinci C, Napoli N, Pozzilli P, Ludvigsson J, Nissim A. 2017. Antibodies to post-translationally modified insulin as a novel biomarker for prediction of type 1 diabetes in children. *Diabetologia* **60:** 1467–1474. doi:10.1007/s00125-017-4296-1

Strollo R, Vinci C, Napoli N, Fioriti E, Maddaloni E, Åkerman L, Casas R, Pozzilli P, Ludvigsson J, Nissim A. 2019. Antibodies to oxidized insulin improve prediction of type 1 diabetes in children with positive standard islet autoantibodies. *Diabetes Metab Res Rev* **35:** e3132. doi:10.1002/dmrr.3132

Strollo R, Vinci C, Man YKS, Bruzzaniti S, Piemonte E, Alhamar G, Briganti SI, Malandrucco I, Tramontana F, Fanali C, et al. 2023. Autoantibody and T cell responses to oxidative post-translationally modified insulin neoantigenic peptides in type 1 diabetes. *Diabetologia* **66:** 132–146. doi:10.1007/s00125-022-05812-4

Suri A, Walters JJ, Gross ML, Unanue ER. 2005. Natural peptides selected by diabetogenic DQ8 and murine I-A (g7) molecules show common sequence specificity. *J Clin Invest* **115:** 2268–2276. doi:10.1172/JCI25350

Thomaidou S, Slieker RC, van der Slik AR, Boom J, Mulder F, Munoz-Garcia A, 't Hart LM, Koeleman B, Carlotti F, Hoeben RC, et al. 2021. Long RNA sequencing and ribosome profiling of inflamed β-cells reveal an extensive translatome landscape. *Diabetes* **70:** 2299–2312. doi:10.2337/db20-1122

Toma A, Laïka T, Haddouk S, Luce S, Briand JP, Camoin L, Connan F, Lambert M, Caillat-Zucman S, Carel JC, et al. 2009. Recognition of human proinsulin leader sequence by class I–restricted T-cells in HLA-A*0201 transgenic mice and in human type 1 diabetes. *Diabetes* **58:** 394–402. doi:10.2337/db08-0599

Triolo TM, Pyle L, Broncucia H, Armstrong T, Yu L, Gottlieb PA, Steck AK. 2022. Association of high-affinity autoantibodies with type 1 diabetes high-risk HLA haplotypes. *J Clin Endocrinol Metab* **107:** e1510–e1517. doi:10.1210/clinem/dgab853

Vafiadis P, Bennett ST, Todd JA, Nadeau J, Grabs R, Goodyer CG, Wickramasinghe S, Colle E, Polychronakos C. 1997. Insulin expression in human thymus is modulated by INS VNTR alleles at the IDDM2 locus. *Nat Genet* **15:** 289–292. doi:10.1038/ng0397-289

Vakilian M, Tahamtani Y, Ghaedi K. 2019. A review on insulin trafficking and exocytosis. *Gene* **706:** 52–61. doi:10.1016/j.gene.2019.04.063

van Lummel M, Duinkerken G, van Veelen PA, de Ru A, Cordfunke R, Zaldumbide A, Gomez-Touriño I, Arif S, Peakman M, Drijfhout JW, et al. 2014. Posttranslational modification of HLA-DQ binding islet autoantigens in type 1 diabetes. *Diabetes* **63:** 237–247. doi:10.2337/db12-1214

von Herrath M, Bonifacio E. 2021. How benign autoimmunity becomes detrimental in type 1 diabetes. *Proc Natl Acad Sci* **118:** e2116508118. doi:10.1073/pnas.2116508118

Wan X, Zinselmeyer BH, Zakharov PN, Vomund AN, Taniguchi R, Santambrogio L, Anderson MS, Lichti CF, Unanue ER. 2018. Pancreatic islets communicate with lymphoid tissues via exocytosis of insulin peptides. *Nature* **560:** 107–111. doi:10.1038/s41586-018-0341-6

Wan X, Vomund AN, Peterson OJ, Chervonsky AV, Lichti CF, Unanue ER. 2020. The MHC-II peptidome of pancreatic islets identifies key features of autoimmune peptides. *Nat Immunol* **21:** 455–463. doi:10.1038/s41590-020-0623-7

Wang L, Wang CC. 2023. Oxidative protein folding fidelity and redoxtasis in the endoplasmic reticulum. *Trends Biochem Sci* **48:** 40–52. doi:10.1016/j.tibs.2022.06.011

Wang Y, Sosinowski T, Novikov A, Crawford F, White J, Jin N, Liu Z, Zou J, Neau D, Davidson HW, et al. 2019. How Carboxy-terminal additions to insulin B-chain fragments create superagonists for T cells in mouse and human type 1 diabetes. *Sci Immunol* **4:** eaav7517. doi:10.1126/sciimmunol.aav7517

Wegmann DR, Norbury-Glaser M, Daniel D. 1994. Insulin-specific T cells are a predominant component of islet infiltrates in pre-diabetic NOD mice. *Eur J Immunol* **24:** 1853–1857. doi:10.1002/eji.1830240820

Wenzlau JM, Peterson OJ, Vomund AN, DiLisio JE, Hohenstein A, Haskins K, Wan X. 2024. Mapping of a hybrid insulin peptide in the inflamed islet β-cells from NOD mice. *Front Immunol* **15:** 1348131. doi:10.3389/fimmu.2024.1348131

Wiles TA, Delong T, Baker RL, Bradley B, Barbour G, Powell RL, Reisdorph N, Haskins K. 2017. An insulin-IAPP hybrid peptide is an endogenous antigen for CD4 T cells in the non-obese diabetic mouse. *J Autoimmun* **78:** 11–18. doi:10.1016/j.jaut.2016.10.007

Wiles TA, Powell R, Michel R, Beard KS, Hohenstein A, Bradley B, Reisdorph N, Haskins K, Delong T. 2019. Identification of hybrid insulin peptides (HIPs) in mouse and human islets by mass spectrometry. *J Proteome Res* **18:** 814–825. doi:10.1021/acs.jproteome.8b00875

Wiles TA, Hohenstein A, Landry LG, Dang M, Powell R, Guyer P, James EA, Nakayama M, Haskins K, Delong T, et al. 2021. Characterization of human CD4 T cells specific for a C-peptide/C-peptide hybrid insulin peptide. *Front Immunol* **12:** 668680. doi:10.3389/fimmu.2021.668680

Wong FS, Karttunen J, Dumont C, Wen L, Visintin I, Pilip IM, Shastri N, Pamer EG, Janeway CA Jr. 1999. Identification of an MHC class I–restricted autoantigen in type 1 diabetes by screening an organ-specific cDNA library. *Nat Med* **5:** 1026–1031. doi:10.1038/12465

Wooldridge L, Ekeruche-Makinde J, van den Berg HA, Skowera A, Miles JJ, Tan MP, Dolton G, Clement M, Llewellyn-Lacey S, Price DA, et al. 2012. A single autoimmune T cell receptor recognizes more than a million different peptides. *J Biol Chem* **287:** 1168–1177. doi:10.1074/jbc.M111.289488

Yang J, Chow IT, Sosinowski T, Torres-Chinn N, Greenbaum CJ, James EA, Kappler JW, Davidson HW, Kwok WW. 2014. Autoreactive T cells specific for insulin B:11–23 recognize a low-affinity peptide register in human subjects with autoimmune diabetes. *Proc Natl Acad Sci* **111:** 14840–14845. doi:10.1073/pnas.1416864111

Yang ML, Sodré FMC, Mamula MJ, Overbergh L. 2021. Citrullination and PAD enzyme biology in type 1 diabetes—regulators of inflammation, autoimmunity, and pathology. *Front Immunol* **12:** 678953. doi:10.3389/fimmu.2021.678953

Yang ML, Connolly SE, Gee RJ, Lam TT, Kanyo J, Peng J, Guyer P, Syed F, Tse HM, Clarke SG, et al. 2022a. Carbonyl posttranslational modification associated with early-onset type 1 diabetes autoimmunity. *Diabetes* **71:** 1979–1993. doi:10.2337/db21-0989

Yang ML, Horstman S, Gee R, Guyer P, Lam TT, Kanyo J, Perdigoto AL, Speake C, Greenbaum CJ, Callebaut A, et al. 2022b. Citrullination of glucokinase is linked to autoimmune diabetes. *Nat Commun* **13:** 1870. doi:10.1038/s41467-022-29512-0

Yoshida K, Corper AL, Herro R, Jabri B, Wilson IA, Teyton L. 2010. The diabetogenic mouse MHC class II molecule I-Ag7 is endowed with a switch that modulates TCR affinity. *J Clin Invest* **120:** 1578–1590. doi:10.1172/JCI41502

Ziegler AG, Rewers M, Simell O, Simell T, Lempainen J, Steck A, Winkler C, Ilonen J, Veijola R, Knip M, et al. 2013. Seroconversion to multiple islet autoantibodies and risk of progression to diabetes in children. *JAMA* **309:** 2473–2479. doi:10.1001/jama.2013.6285

Integrating Omics into Functional Biomarkers of Type 1 Diabetes

S. Alice Long[1] and Peter S. Linsley[2]

[1]Center for Translational Immunology; [2]Center for Systems Immunology, Benaroya Research Institute, Seattle, Washington 98101, USA

Correspondence: along@benaroyaresearch.org; plinsley@benaroyaresearch.org

Biomarkers are critical to the staging and diagnosis of type 1 diabetes (T1D). Functional biomarkers offer insights into T1D immunopathogenesis and are often revealed using "omics" approaches that integrate multiple measures to identify involved pathways and functions. Application of the omics biomarker discovery may enable personalized medicine approaches to circumvent the more recently appreciated heterogeneity of T1D progression and treatment. Use of omics to define functional biomarkers is still in its early years, yet findings to date emphasize the role of cytokine signaling and adaptive immunity in biomarkers of progression and response to therapy. Here, we share examples of the use of omics to define functional biomarkers focusing on two signatures, T-cell exhaustion and T-cell help, which have been associated with outcomes in both the natural history and treatment contexts.

We live in an era defined by the intersection of three powerful trends in medicine. One trend is the evolution of personalized medicine, which seeks to match the right drugs to the right patients at the right doses and times. Personalized medicine has been most successful where a therapeutic agent is clearly linked to the genetic basis or cause of the disease. So far, personalized medicine has been less successful with genetically complex diseases like type 1 diabetes (T1D), which is caused by the autoimmune destruction of pancreatic β cells. Another powerful trend in the current era is the explosive growth of the identification and use of biomarkers for a host of different purposes during the disease process, including risk of disease, diagnosis, prognosis and course, as well as prediction, safety, and response of therapeutic intervention. Yet a third trend is the development over the past two decades of multiple "omics" technologies, which make simultaneous parallel measurements on tens of thousands of individual analytes (e.g., proteins, DNA, RNA, metabolites, etc.). These measurements are then analyzed using powerful statistical techniques to provide unbiased insights into disease mechanisms, drug targets, and biomarkers. While progress in these three trends has perhaps been less rapid than initially hoped, they have established themselves in the mainstream and there remains a great deal of excitement about their potential (Quezada et al. 2017; Chen et al. 2023; Lim et al. 2024).

In this review, we highlight recent developments that illustrate the value and future

Cite this article as *Cold Spring Harb Perspect Med* doi: 10.1101/cshperspect.a041602

prospects of omics technologies for discovering and applying functional immune biomarkers in T1D to better understand disease mechanisms and guide precision medicine. As examples, we focus on exhausted CD8 T cells induced by T-cell reduction therapies and alterations in helper T cells induced by T-cell costimulation blockade.

BIOMARKERS IN T1D

A biomarker is defined by the U.S. Food and Drug Administration (FDA) as "a defined characteristic that is measured as an indicator of normal biological processes, pathogenic processes, or biological responses to an exposure or intervention, including therapeutic interventions" (FDA-NIH Biomarker Working Group 2016). Biomarker measurements may be functional or physiological, biochemical, or molecular in nature (IPCS INCHEM 1993). There are multiple types of biomarkers, including those to assess disease susceptibility or risk, diagnosis, prognosis and course, prediction, and the safety and response of therapeutic intervention (Table 1). Several recent reviews have covered biomarkers for disease susceptibility, diagnosis, prognosis, and course of T1D (Brenu et al. 2023; Fyvie and Gillespie 2023; Sarkar et al. 2023), so we will focus here on emerging biomarkers of prediction and response to therapy aided by omics technologies.

A pharmacodynamic (PD) biomarker that "indicates biologic activity of a medical product or environmental agent" (FDA-NIH Biomarker Working Group 2016) is one type of measure indicating response to therapy. During drug development, PD biomarkers are used to measure drug activity for dose selection or to ensure that a drug is acting as predicted. The relevance of PD biomarkers for T1D therapy is indicated by analysis of samples from multiple clinical studies in T1D including studies with rituximab (Linsley et al. 2018a), abatacept (Linsley et al. 2019b), and teplizumab (Linsley et al. 2021b). Overall, these analyses showed evidence for nonuniform PD activity, with better response to therapy occurring in subjects with higher PD activity as discussed below.

Individual variation in drug response can be partly exploited in the context of drug development (Polasek et al. 2018). However, the clinical study of many different doses in many different patients is impractical and expensive, so drug developers generally use a more practical one-dose-fits-all model. In addition, regulatory agencies usually require safe and effective doses for a population, not the best dose for each individual patient. Moreover, since clinical trials usually have tight inclusion criteria and focus on relatively homogenous populations, increased inter-individual variation in optimal dosing is to be expected when trial results are extrapolated to larger populations after approval.

Another factor affecting the linkage between drug PD activity and therapeutic benefit in T1D is the common practice of treating younger patients using dosing primarily determined in adults. Typically, drugs, including biologics such as monoclonal antibodies and fusion proteins (Liu et al. 2019), are approved with more extensive dosing information available for adults than children. Approved doses are oftentimes "weight tiered," and it may be unclear how best to extrapolate doses determined in adults to children. Thus, while desirable, the concept of "precision dosing" (Polasek et al. 2018) is difficult to

Table 1. Examples of biomarkers in type 1 diabetes (T1D)

Biomarker type	Example	Stage of development
Susceptibility or risk	AAb number	In clinical use
Diagnosis and course	HbA1c, C-peptide	In clinical use
Susceptibility or risk	PRS	Development and validation
Prediction	Insufficient data	Discovery
Safety and response to therapy	Insufficient data	Discovery

(PRS) Polygenic risk score, (AAb) autoantibody.

achieve in practice, especially in a disease such as T1D, which affects children.

One way to achieve more optimal dosing is to use treat-to-target (T2T) strategies (Garber 2014). T2T is a medical strategy that sets a goal of altering target disease activity values to reach targeted values for each individual patient. Activity values may be derived from measurements made with biomarkers, laboratory tests, or clinical examination. If target values are not reached, types or doses of medications may be adjusted according to a predefined protocol. The process may be iterated until the target values are achieved. T2T strategies have been explored in investigations of medications and dosing in T1D (Mathieu et al. 2016; Russell-Jones et al. 2023), T2D (Mathieu et al. 2023; Philis-Tsimikas et al. 2023), and other autoimmune disease (van Vollenhoven 2019; Garcia et al. 2022; Parra Sánchez et al. 2022). While T2T strategies typically use disease biomarkers, a potentially powerful approach for the future would be to incorporate PD biomarkers that are functional in nature and capable of measuring drug responses across time and age (Kearns and Artman 2015) that may inform when to initiate treatment, repeat dosing, or change therapies.

APPLICATION OF OMICS IN T1D

Since the sequencing of the human genome, developments in several technologies have facilitated the simultaneous and parallel measurement of biological molecules at genome-wide scales (National Research Council (US) Committee on a Framework for Developing a New Taxonomy of Disease 2011; Dzau et al. 2017). The vast amounts of data obtained using these technologies have enabled unbiased examination of biological processes at a previously unobtainable scale and have provided numerous candidate biomarkers. Collectively, the scientific technologies associated with measuring such biological molecules in a high-throughput way are termed "omics" (National Guideline Centre (UK) 2018). The technologies used in these studies include "proteomics, transcriptomics, genomics, metabolomics, lipidomics, and epigenomics, which correspond to global analyses of proteins, RNA, genes, metabolites, lipids, and methylated DNA or modified histone proteins in chromosomes, respectively" (National Guideline Centre (UK) 2018). In oncology, the use of omics for biomarker discovery has advanced to such a degree that there now are multiple commercially available transcriptomic-based tests for prognosis, prediction of metastasis probability, and treatment recommendations for several cancer types (Tsakiroglou et al. 2023). While there also has been considerable effort with omics-based studies in T1D (Fig. 1), in contrast to cancer, none of these studies have yet progressed to the extent of generating commercial products in widespread use.

Some T1D studies have used genomics data to reveal risk and prognostic biomarkers, useful as measures of susceptibility but not rate of progression. The decreased costs of generating genomics data and the increased availability of genetic data have facilitated the development of polygenic scores that aggregate risk variants from multiple loci into a single genetic or polygenic risk score (GRS or PRS, respectively). The current status of GRS studies was recently reviewed (Luckett et al. 2023). GRSs are being tested in several studies of disease risk in the general population (Sims et al. 2022). A factor limiting the use of GRS is that most early studies of T1D genetics have been conducted in European ancestry populations (Luckett et al. 2023). European-based GRSs are a powerful tool that will be improved upon with future large case-control studies from non-European populations, which will increase the accuracy of GRSs across diverse ancestries (Luckett et al. 2023).

There is a long history of transcriptomic studies in T1D, with studies dating back decades, largely focusing on the ability to predict or determine risk for T1D (Maas et al. 2002; Liu et al. 2006). Most transcriptomic studies in humans have focused on peripheral blood, which has the advantage of being easily accessed but the disadvantage of being collected distal to the primary site of disease (the pancreas). The majority of early transcriptomic studies with peripheral blood were investigator-driven and involved small cohorts and have not led to consensus diagnostic T1D signatures. However, there are several more recent studies involving larger and

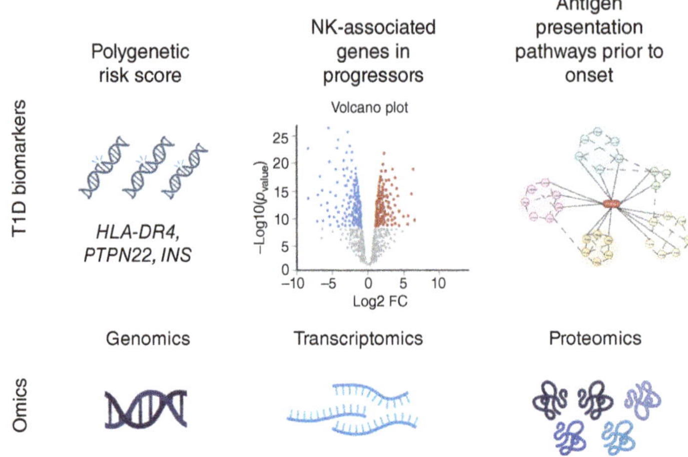

Figure 1. Examples of omics integration into functional biomarkers in type 1 diabetes (T1D). Omics technologies have been used to define functional biomarkers in many genetic diseases. Application to complex diseases like T1D is in its early stages, with some examples shown.

more highly powered cohorts that may overcome some of the limitations of earlier studies that focus on predicting disease progression and onset even when limited to peripheral blood samples. Measurement of β-cell death using cell-free DNA (cfDNA) in sera is a new and evolving field. Elevations of cfDNA levels can be measured in the periphery in the transplant setting (Ventura-Aguiar et al. 2022; Foda et al. 2023). Another approach being investigated is to measure changes in methylation patterns (methylone) (Spector et al. 2023). Methylation changes in cfDNA in T1D have been reported (Voss et al. 2021; Abdel-Karim et al. 2024; Drawshy et al. 2024), but these have not yet been robustly distinguished from chronic inflammation. Yet another evolving omics field in T1D is the microbiome. Early studies have suggested a role for the microbiome in T1D, glycemic control, and disease-related complications (van Heck et al. 2022).

The Environmental Determinants of Diabetes in the Young (TEDDY) consortium is a prospective cohort study aimed at determining the genetic and environmental interactions causing T1D (TEDDY Study Group 2008). A recent transcriptomic study with the TEDDY cohort analyzed longitudinal blood transcriptomes of 2013 samples from 400 individuals before the development of both T1D and islet autoimmunity (Xhonneux et al. 2021). These investigators identified age-associated changes in gene expression in healthy infancy and age-independent changes tracking with progression to islet autoimmunity and T1D. A model developed from these data to predict individual risk of T1D onset and the association of a natural killer (NK) cell signature with progression was validated with an independent cohort.

Another approach to transcriptomic studies was demonstrated by a meta-analysis of multiple previously published investigator-generated transcriptomic data sets (Ochsner et al. 2022) with the aim of generating testable hypotheses around signaling pathway dysfunction in T1D. These investigators repurposed and combined 17 data sets from the Gene Expression Omnibus (GEO) database to interrogate gene expression differences between T1D and normoglycemic controls. Genes that were preferentially induced or repressed in T1D immune cells were identified and validated against community benchmarks. They then used these genes to infer and validate signaling node networks regulating the expression of these gene sets. They further developed use cases demonstrating how informed integration of these networks with complementary digital resources can be useful. The entire data matrix was made available for unrestricted access and reuse by the research community.

Proteomics research presents technological challenges that have led the field, in general, to lag behind transcriptomics research. Despite these limitations, the TEDDY consortium recently described a proteomics study that perhaps came closer to developing usable progression biomarkers than any transcriptomic study to date (Nakayasu et al. 2023). This study used untargeted proteomics of 2252 samples from 184 individuals to identify 376 proteins regulated even before autoimmunity. Additionally, they found that extracellular matrix and antigen presentation proteins were differentially regulated in individuals who progressed to T1D compared with those that remained in autoimmunity. Using targeted proteomics measurements, the investigators identified 167 proteins in 6426 samples from 990 individuals and validated 83 of these biomarkers. Machine learning analysis of these biomarkers accurately predicted whether individuals would remain in autoimmunity or develop T1D 6 months before autoantibody appearance.

BIOLOGY LEARNED FROM OMICS STUDIES IN T1D

Omics data can provide prognostic and response biomarker signatures from which biological function is beginning to be inferred. These biological findings from single omics data can then be verified using more focused and functional techniques. In this manner, some early clues about the immunopathogenesis of T1D have been revealed using omics in an unbiased manner (Fig. 2). For example, a signature enriched for B-cell-specific transcripts is present upon autoantibody conversion indicative of initiation of autoimmunity (Xhonneux et al. 2021). In a reciprocal manner, B-cell signatures have also been associated with kidney transplant tolerance (Newell et al. 2010). Further studies are required to better understand the functional role of B cells in these settings. Concomitant with this T1D B-cell signature are features that are associated with the rate of disease progression. NK and memory CD4 T-cell signatures increased preferentially in HLA DR4 individuals who developed autoantibodies to insulin first and early in life. By comparison, an early TNF-enriched monocyte signature marked HLA DR3 individuals who developed early autoantibodies to GADA first. Single-cell studies measuring a more limited number of features confirmed changes in cytokine signaling, B-cell subsets, and NK function with disease progression (for review, see Long and Buckner 2022) offering evidence for genetics, cytokine-, and cell-specific influence on T1D

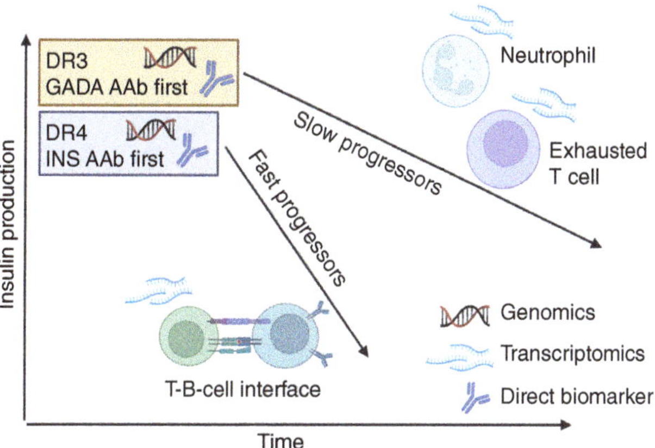

Figure 2. Examples of omics used to predict outcome in type 1 diabetes (T1D). Stable (boxes) and dynamic (arrows) features are associated with slow or fast loss of insulin production over time. Shown are examples of functional biomarkers identified using omics. INS and GADA AAb (autoantibody) first refer to the initial AAb in islet autoimmunity.

severity. In a related example, higher levels of a neutrophil transcriptomic signature and lower levels of a B-cell transcriptomic signature were associated with slower progression in two complementary studies comparing a large number of placebo subjects from clinical trials (Dufort et al. 2019; Suomi et al. 2023). Together these individual studies demonstrate the potential of omics discovery combined with focused studies, to identify immune biomarkers that predict the rate of disease progression.

Exploratory omics studies of T1D-associated T-cell receptor (TCR) sequences have also underscored the integral role of T cells in T1D pathogenesis. The TCR is comprised most commonly of an α and β chain that both contain regions of high sequence variability (complementarity determining regions or CDRs). Sequence differences within the most variable of these regions (CDR3) can serve as biomarkers for T-cell clonality and have been most commonly studied across TCR β chains (Jacobsen et al. 2017). TCRs may be unique to one individual (private) or shared across multiple individuals, either in the general population or with T1D (public). Since public TCRs are found in a larger segment of the population, they are more suitable for therapeutic targets and biomarker studies. More than 30 public TCRs have been identified to date in the pancreas and peripheral blood of individuals with T1D. Shared TCR β chains from these public TCRs are increased in individuals with earlier disease onset T1D (Mitchell et al. 2022, 2023), offering candidate genomic biomarkers of disease progression with the caveat that these initial studies were performed in genetically similar cohorts.

Beyond these advances with TCR β-chain sequencing, much remains to be determined about TCR biology and its application as a predictive or prognostic biomarker. The specificities of most sequenced public TCRs remain undefined, many of which may also be useful for biomarker studies. The usefulness of TCR α chains is also poorly understood with the exception of recent studies that provide insight into common islet reactivity of shared TCR sequences (Linsley et al. 2021a, 2023). In another study, TCRs reactive to preproinsulin, a precursor of secreted insulin, were found at a higher proportion in T1D as compared to HLA-matched healthy controls (Anderson et al. 2021). Thus, while in its infancy, TCR genomics is beginning to offer clues about the specificity of a finite number of shared T1D-associated TCR sequences and, with additional studies and deeper sampling, has the potential to be used to predict early disease onset and severity.

Omics studies of PD biomarkers in the context of immunotherapy offer clues as to how and why a treatment may work better in one individual than another and the underlying immunopathology, but this variability has also limited the discovery of robust biomarkers common to all T1D individuals. A recent review of treatment PD biomarkers (Linsley et al. 2021b) emphasized the potential use of PD biomarkers in personalized medicine. In general, the signature and timing of PD biomarkers are specific to the treatment. However, when looking across treatments, collectively, PD biomarkers of better response indicate a role for cytokine and cell-type-specific inflammation with adaptive cells playing a prominent role. Yet, a challenge of these studies is that few associations with response have been validated given the requirement to perform additional clinical trials. Two notable exceptions are signatures of T-cell exhaustion and T-cell help that are associated with response in multiple contexts discussed here in detail.

EXHAUSTED CD8 T CELLS AS A FUNCTIONAL BIOMARKER OF BETTER OUTCOME IN T1D

Common features across autoimmune diseases may limit disease progression, consistent with a finite number of mechanisms of immune tolerance. Epigenetic and transcriptional signatures define exhausted CD8 T cells (Tex) (Blank et al. 2019). In a hallmark study across multiple diseases, a gene signature with features of Tex was associated with slower autoimmune disease progression (McKinney et al. 2010, 2015). This finding laid the conceptual foundation for the discovery of signatures of Tex associated with better outcomes in T1D.

CD8 T-cell exhaustion is a unique lineage that develops in a setting of chronic antigen stimulation such as cancer and chronic viral infection, and more recently appreciated in autoimmunity (McLane et al. 2019). In T1D, a whole blood transcriptomic signature with features of Tex was increased in responders to anti-CD3 therapy (Long et al. 2016). This increase was confirmed in additional trials using the T1D Tex-associated EOMES, TIGIT, and KLRG1 cellular phenotype (Herold et al. 2019; Mathieu et al. 2024). Given that Tex were not originally characterized in T1D, follow-up studies were performed to confirm the tolerance-promoting function of these cells. The CD8 T-cell signature was marked by transcription factors and inhibitory receptors common to Tex. Progressive loss of proinflammatory cytokine production is a feature of Tex and this hyporesponsiveness was augmented following therapy (Sims et al. 2021) and in vitro upon inhibitory receptor ligation (Long et al. 2016). Thus, across multiple studies, transcriptomics facilitated the discovery and functional definition of Tex in the context of anti-CD3 treatment in T1D.

Tex association with better outcome in T1D is not restricted to anti-CD3 therapy. Higher levels of a whole blood and CD8 T-cell transcriptional signature of Tex following treatment with LFA3-Ig, a fusion protein that binds CD2, also associated with better response to therapy (Diggins et al. 2021). As in the anti-CD3 studies, the LFA3-Ig Tex-associated signature was confirmed to mark hyporesponsive cells expressing multiple inhibitory receptors indicative of Tex. Beyond the therapeutic setting, higher frequencies of CD8 Tex were associated with slower progression (McKinney et al. 2010, 2015; Wiedeman et al. 2020) and autoreactive T cells have been shown to be restrained by increased exhaustion-associated inhibitory receptors (Wiedeman et al. 2020; Grebinoski et al. 2022). While not as well understood, CD4 T cells expressing multiple inhibitory receptors are also increased with T-cell therapy (Rigby et al. 2015; Jacobsen et al. 2023), although their function has not been well defined. Taken together, these omics and functional studies suggest that higher levels of T1D-associated Tex are linked to better response to T-cell reduction therapies in T1D.

FOLLICULAR HELPER T CELLS AS A FUNCTIONAL BIOMARKER OF WORSE OUTCOME IN T1D

Follicular helper T (TfH) cells are a specialized subset of CD4 T cells that are essential for providing help to B cells (Song and Craft 2024). A peripheral blood counterpart of TfH, termed circulating TfH (cTfH), are found in the peripheral blood and share many features of TfH making them a tractable biomarker in T1D. cTfH, defined by a transcriptional signature and cytometry, were increased in at-risk and T1D subjects as compared to healthy controls (Shao et al. 2020), and higher levels of activated cTfH associated with faster disease progression (Habib et al. 2019; Long and Buckner 2022). The primary role of TfH is to interact with B cells and aberrations in B cells are also associated with faster disease progression (Smith et al. 2020). Thus, the TfH B-cell axis may be critical in driving more severe disease. CTLA4Ig treatment blocks the TfH B cells interaction, and TpH levels at the time of treatment were found to predict beneficial response to therapy in recent-onset T1D individuals (Edner et al. 2020). In contrast, the expansion of B cells following therapy marks poor response to CTLA4Ig (Linsley et al. 2019b). This is consistent with TfH being increased early in the disease and associated with more severe autoimmunity in general (Walker 2022). Thus, TfH cells have a unique signature that associates with worse outcome in T1D and autoimmunity more broadly.

CD8 Tex and TfH have opposing associations with outcome in T1D, yet they share several features (Fig. 3). Both Tex and TfH development are multistage processes (Walker 2022). These processes lead to appreciable heterogeneity with the potential for multiple factors to influence Tex and TfH-cell subsets over the course of T1D. Beyond T1D, both cell subsets have been associated with outcome in cancer. However, in contrast to autoimmunity, TfH are beneficial in cancer (Cui et al. 2023) while increased Tex are associated with worse tumor clearance (McLane et al. 2019). This dichotomy in Tex and Tfh function in T1D is also exemplified with cancer therapy. Many cancers can be successfully treated with

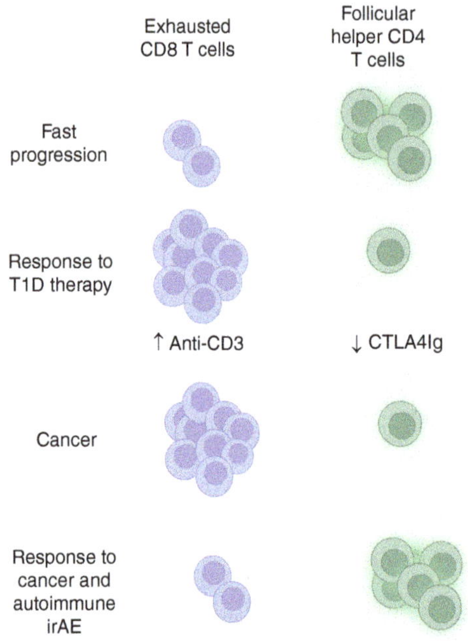

Figure 3. Multipronged identification of T-cell subsets associated with dichotomous type 1 diabetes (T1D) outcome. Reciprocal levels of exhausted T cells and follicular helper T cells, discovered using transcriptomics and cytometry, are associated with outcome in T1D natural progression, response to therapy, and immune response adverse event (irAE) in cancer therapy.

inhibitory checkpoint blockade (ICB) thought to deplete or antagonize Tex. However, autoimmunity may occur as an immune-related adverse event (irAE) of ICB treatment, sometimes including T1D (Dougan and Pietropaolo 2020) and TfH (Lechner et al. 2023). Thus, multipronged evidence supports the interpretation that CD8 Tex and CD4 TfH are associated with outcome in T1D, cancer, and irAEs, but in a reciprocal manner. With additional validation, changes in the abundance of these cell types may serve as biomarkers of disease progression and response.

CONCLUDING REMARKS

Direct autoantibody and serum biomarkers linked to insulin production are the foundation of disease staging of T1D (Insel et al. 2015). This staging ultimately led to the first FDA-approved therapy for the prevention of T1D (Hirsch 2023). Functional biomarkers differ from direct biomarkers in that they provide insight into the immunopathology of T1D. Translation of functional biomarkers is in its infancy, but it holds promise to determine who will progress more quickly and who will respond to what treatment. Functional biomarkers identified to date in T1D have primarily been transcriptional. However, new single-cell technologies using a range of omics and improved computational analyses are already beginning to expand the number and type of functional biomarkers in T1D including new multimodal approaches. These approaches will be further advanced with the integration of current and future large data sets and the use of artificial intelligence (AI)-driven analyses. Given the speed of advances in omics techniques and analyses and increased collaborative efforts in the field of T1D, the hope is that omics will enable personalized medicine for complex diseases like T1D in the near future.

REFERENCES

Abdel-Karim TR, Hodges JS, Herold KC, Pruett TL, Ramanathan KV, Hering BJ, Dunn TB, Kirchner VA, Beilman GJ, Bellin MD. 2024. Peri-transplant inflammation and long-term diabetes outcomes were not impacted by either etanercept or α-1-antitrypsin treatment in islet autotransplant recipients. *Transpl Int* **37:** 12320. doi:10.3389/ti.2024.12320

Anderson AM, Landry LG, Alkanani AA, Pyle L, Powers AC, Atkinson MA, Mathews CE, Roep BO, Michels AW, Nakayama M. 2021. Human islet T cells are highly reactive to preproinsulin in type 1 diabetes. *Proc Natl Acad Sci* **118:** e2107208118. doi:10.1073/pnas.2107208118

Blank CU, Haining WN, Held W, Hogan PG, Kallies A, Lugli E, Lynn RC, Philip M, Rao A, Restifo NP, et al. 2019. Defining "T cell exhaustion." *Nat Rev Immunol* **19:** 665–674. doi:10.1038/s41577-019-0221-9

Brenu EW, Harris M, Hamilton-Williams EE. 2023. Circulating biomarkers during progression to type 1 diabetes: a systematic review. *Front Endocrinol (Lausanne)* **14:** 1117076. doi:10.3389/fendo.2023.1117076

Chen C, Wang J, Pan D, Wang X, Xu Y, Yan J, Wang L, Yang X, Yang M, Liu GP. 2023. Applications of multi-omics analysis in human diseases. *MedComm (2020)* **4:** e315. doi:10.1002/mco2.315

Cui C, Craft J, Joshi NS. 2023. T follicular helper cells in cancer, tertiary lymphoid structures, and beyond. *Semin Immunol* **69:** 101797. doi:10.1016/j.smim.2023.101797

Diggins KE, Serti E, Muir VS, Rosasco MG, Lu T, Balmas E, Nepom GT, Long SA, Linsley PS. 2021. Exhausted-like $CD8^+$ T cell phenotypes linked to C-peptide preservation in alefacept-treated T1D subjects. *JCI Insight* **6:** e142680. doi:10.1172/jci.insight.142680

Dougan M, Pietropaolo M. 2020. Time to dissect the autoimmune etiology of cancer antibody immunotherapy. *J Clin Invest* **130:** 51–61. doi:10.1172/JCI131194

Drawshy Z, Neiman D, Fridlich O, Peretz A, Magenheim J, Rozo AV, Doliba NM, Stoffers DA, Kaestner KH, Schatz DA, et al. 2024. DNA methylation-based assessment of cell composition in human pancreas and islets. *Diabetes* **73:** 554–564. doi:10.2337/db23-0704

Dufort MJ, Greenbaum CJ, Speake C, Linsley PS. 2019. Cell type-specific immune phenotypes predict loss of insulin secretion in new-onset type 1 diabetes. *JCI Insight* **4:** e125556. doi:10.1172/jci.insight.125556

Dzau VJ, Ginsburg GS, Chopra A, Goldman D, Green ED, Leonard DGB, McClellan MB, Plump A, Terry SF, Yamamoto KR. 2017. Realizing the full potential of precision medicine in health and health care. In *Vital directions for health & health care: an initiative of the National Academy of Medicine* (ed. National Academy of Medicine; Finkelman EM, McGinnis JM, McClellan MB, et al.), pp. 249–268. National Academies Press, Washington, DC.

Edner NM, Heuts F, Thomas N, Wang CJ, Petersone L, Kenefeck R, Kogimtzis A, Ovcinnikovs V, Ross EM, Ntavli E, et al. 2020. Follicular helper T cell profiles predict response to costimulation blockade in type 1 diabetes. *Nat Immunol* **21:** 1244–1255. doi:10.1038/s41590-020-0744-z

FDA-NIH Biomarker Working Group. 2016. *BEST (Biomarkers, EndpointS, and other Tools) resource.* Food and Drug Administration (US), Bethesda, MD, National Institutes of Health (US), Silver Spring, MD.

Foda ZH, Annapragada AV, Boyapati K, Bruhm DC, Vulpescu NA, Medina JE, Mathios D, Cristiano S, Niknafs N, Luu HT, et al. 2023. Detecting liver cancer using cell-free DNA fragmentomes. *Cancer Discov* **13:** 616–631. doi:10.1158/2159-8290.CD-22-0659

Fyvie MJ, Gillespie KM. 2023. The importance of biomarker development for monitoring type 1 diabetes progression rate and therapeutic responsiveness. *Front Immunol* **14:** 1158278. doi:10.3389/fimmu.2023.1158278

Garber AJ. 2014. Treat-to-target trials: uses, interpretation and review of concepts. *Diabetes Obes Metab* **16:** 193–205. doi:10.1111/dom.12129

Garcia NM, Cohen NA, Rubin DT. 2022. Treat-to-target and sequencing therapies in Crohn's disease. *United European Gastroenterol J* **10:** 1121–1128. doi:10.1002/ueg2.12336

Grebinoski S, Zhang Q, Cillo AR, Manne S, Xiao H, Brunazzi EA, Tabib T, Cardello C, Lian CG, Murphy GF, et al. 2022. Autoreactive CD8$^+$ T cells are restrained by an exhaustion-like program that is maintained by LAG3. *Nat Immunol* **23:** 868–877. doi:10.1038/s41590-022-01210-5

Habib T, Long SA, Samuels PL, Brahmandam A, Tatum M, Funk A, Hocking AM, Cerosaletti K, Mason MT, Whalen E, et al. 2019. Dynamic immune phenotypes of B and T helper cells mark distinct stages of T1D progression. *Diabetes* **68:** 1240–1250. doi:10.2337/db18-1081

Herold KC, Bundy BN, Long SA, Bluestone JA, DiMeglio LA, Dufort MJ, Gitelman SE, Gottlieb PA, Krischer JP, Linsley PS, et al. 2019. An anti-CD3 antibody, teplizumab, in relatives at risk for type 1 diabetes. *N Engl J Med* **381:** 603–613. doi:10.1056/NEJMoa1902226

Hirsch JS. 2023. FDA approves teplizumab: a milestone in type 1 diabetes. *Lancet Diabetes Endocrinol* **11:** 18. doi:10.1016/S2213-8587(22)00351-5

Insel RA, Dunne JL, Atkinson MA, Chiang JL, Dabelea D, Gottlieb PA, Greenbaum CJ, Herold KC, Krischer JP, Lernmark A, et al. 2015. Staging presymptomatic type 1 diabetes: a scientific statement of JDRF, the Endocrine Society, and the American Diabetes Association. *Diabetes Care* **38:** 1964–1974. doi:10.2337/dc15-1419

IPCS INCHEM. 1993. *Biomarkers and risk assessment: concepts and principles (Environmental Health Criteria 155).* World Health Organization, Geneva, Switzerland

Jacobsen LM, Posgai A, Seay HR, Haller MJ, Brusko TM. 2017. T cell receptor profiling in type 1 diabetes. *Curr Diab Rep* **17:** 118. doi:10.1007/s11892-017-0946-4

Jacobsen LM, Diggins K, Blanchfield L, McNichols J, Perry DJ, Brant J, Dong X, Bacher R, Gersuk VH, Schatz DA, et al. 2023. Responders to low-dose ATG induce CD4$^+$ T cell exhaustion in type 1 diabetes. *JCI Insight* **8:** e161812. doi:10.1172/jci.insight.161812

Kearns GL, Artman M. 2015. Functional biomarkers: an approach to bridge pharmacokinetics and pharmacodynamics in pediatric clinical trials. *Curr Pharm Des* **21:** 5636–5642. doi:10.2174/1381612821666150901105337

Lechner MG, Zhou Z, Hoang AT, Huang N, Ortega J, Scott LN, Chen HC, Patel AY, Yakhshi-Tafti R, Kim K, et al. 2023. Clonally expanded, thyrotoxic effector CD8$^+$ T cells driven by IL-21 contribute to checkpoint inhibitor thyroiditis. *Sci Transl Med* **15:** eadg0675. doi:10.1126/scitranslmed.adg0675

Lim J, Park C, Kim M, Kim H, Kim J, Lee DS. 2024. Advances in single-cell omics and multiomics for high-resolution molecular profiling. *Exp Mol Med* **56:** 515–526. doi:10.1038/s12276-024-01186-2

Linsley PS, Greenbaum CJ, Rosasco M, Presnell S, Herold KC, Dufort MJ. 2019a. Elevated T cell levels in peripheral blood predict poor clinical response following rituximab treatment in new-onset type 1 diabetes. *Genes Immun* **20:** 293–307. doi:10.1038/s41435-018-0032-1

Linsley PS, Greenbaum CJ, Speake C, Long SA, Dufort MJ. 2019b. B lymphocyte alterations accompany Abatacept resistance in new-onset type 1 diabetes. *JCI Insight* **4:** e126136. doi:10.1172/jci.insight.126136

Linsley PS, Barahmand-Pour-Whitman F, Balmas E, DeBerg HA, Flynn KJ, Hu AK, Rosasco MG, Chen J, O'Rourke C, Serti E, et al. 2021a. Autoreactive T cell receptors with shared germline-like α chains in type 1 diabetes. *JCI Insight* **6:** e151349. doi:10.1172/jci.insight.151349

Linsley PS, Greenbaum CJ, Nepom GT. 2021b. Uncovering pathways to personalized therapies in type 1 diabetes. *Diabetes* **70:** 831–841. doi:10.2337/db20-1185

Linsley P, Nakayama M, Balmas E, Chen J, Pour F, Bansal S, Serti E, Speake C, Pugliese A, Cerosaletti K. 2023. Self-reactive germline-like TCR α chains shared between blood and pancreas. *Res Sq* doi:10.21203/rs.3.rs-3446917/v1

Liu Z, Maas K, Aune TM. 2006. Identification of gene expression signatures in autoimmune disease without the influence of familial resemblance. *Hum Mol Genet* **15:** 501–509. doi:10.1093/hmg/ddi466

Liu XI, Dallmann A, Wang YM, Green DJ, Burnham JM, Chiang B, Wu P, Sheng M, Lu K, van den Anker JN, et al. 2019. Monoclonal antibodies and Fc-fusion proteins for pediatric use: dosing, immunogenicity, and modeling and simulation in data submitted to the US Food and Drug Administration. *J Clin Pharmacol* **59:** 1130–1143. doi:10.1002/jcph.1406

Long SA, Buckner JH. 2022. Clinical and experimental treatment of type 1 diabetes. *Clin Exp Immunol* **210:** 105–113. doi:10.1093/cei/uxac077

Long SA, Thorpe J, DeBerg HA, Gersuk V, Eddy J, Harris KM, Ehlers M, Herold KC, Nepom GT, Linsley PS. 2016. Partial exhaustion of CD8 T cells and clinical response to teplizumab in new-onset type 1 diabetes. *Sci Immunol* **1:** 1–9. doi:10.1126/sciimmunol.aai7793

Luckett AM, Weedon MN, Hawkes G, Leslie RD, Oram RA, Grant SFA. 2023. Utility of genetic risk scores in type 1 diabetes. *Diabetologia* **66:** 1589–1600. doi:10.1007/s00125-023-05955-y

Maas K, Chan S, Parker J, Slater A, Moore J, Olsen N, Aune TM. 2002. Cutting edge: molecular portrait of human autoimmune disease. *J Immunol* **169:** 5–9. doi:10.4049/jimmunol.169.1.5

Mathieu C, Zinman B, Hemmingsson JU, Woo V, Colman P, Christiansen E, Linder M, Bode B. 2016. Efficacy and safety of liraglutide added to insulin treatment in type 1 diabetes: the adjunct one treat-to-target randomized trial. *Diabetes Care* **39:** 1702–1710. doi:10.2337/dc16-0691

Mathieu C, Ásbjörnsdóttir B, Bajaj HS, Lane W, Matos A, Murthy S, Stachlewska K, Rosenstock J. 2023. Switching to once-weekly insulin icodec versus once-daily insulin glargine U100 in individuals with basal-bolus insulin-treated type 2 diabetes (ONWARDS 4): a phase 3a, randomised, open-label, multicentre, treat-to-target, non-inferiority trial. *Lancet* **401:** 1929–1940. doi:10.1016/S0140-6736(23)00520-2

Mathieu C, Wiedeman A, Cerosaletti K, Long SA, Serti E, Cooney L, Vermeiren J, Caluwaerts S, Van Huynegem K, Steidler L, et al. 2024. A first-in-human, open-label Phase 1b and a randomised, double-blind Phase 2a clinical trial in recent-onset type 1 diabetes with AG019 as monotherapy and in combination with teplizumab. *Diabetologia* **67:** 27–41. doi:10.1007/s00125-023-06014-2

McKinney EF, Lyons PA, Carr EJ, Hollis JL, Jayne DR, Willcocks LC, Koukoulaki M, Brazma A, Jovanovic V, Kemeny DM, et al. 2010. A CD8$^+$ T cell transcription signature predicts prognosis in autoimmune disease. *Nat Med* **16:** 586–591. doi:10.1038/nm.2130

McKinney EF, Lee JC, Jayne DR, Lyons PA, Smith KG. 2015. T-cell exhaustion, co-stimulation and clinical outcome in autoimmunity and infection. *Nature* **523:** 612–616. doi:10.1038/nature14468

McLane LM, Abdel-Hakeem MS, Wherry EJ. 2019. CD8 T cell exhaustion during chronic viral infection and cancer. *Annu Rev Immunol* **37:** 457–495. doi:10.1146/annurev-immunol-041015-055318

Mitchell AM, Baschal EE, McDaniel KA, Simmons KM, Pyle L, Waugh K, Steck AK, Yu L, Gottlieb PA, Rewers MJ, et al. 2022. Temporal development of T cell receptor repertoires during childhood in health and disease. *JCI Insight* **7:** e161885. doi:10.1172/jci.insight.161885

Mitchell AM, Baschal EE, McDaniel KA, Fleury T, Choi H, Pyle L, Yu L, Rewers MJ, Nakayama M, Michels AW. 2023. Tracking DNA-based antigen-specific T cell receptors during progression to type 1 diabetes. *Sci Adv* **9:** eadj6975. doi:10.1126/sciadv.adj6975

Nakayasu ES, Bramer LM, Ansong C, Schepmoes AA, Fillmore TL, Gritsenko MA, Clauss TR, Gao Y, Piehowski PD, Stanfill BA, et al. 2023. Plasma protein biomarkers predict the development of persistent autoantibodies and type 1 diabetes 6 months prior to the onset of autoimmunity. *Cell Rep Med* **4:** 101093. doi:10.1016/j.xcrm.2023.101093

National Guideline Centre (UK). 2018. Treat-to-target: rheumatoid arthritis in adults: diagnosis and management. In *NICE evidence reviews collection*. National Institute for Health and Care Excellence (NICE), London.

National Research Council (US) Committee on a Framework for Developing a New Taxonomy of Disease. 2011. *Toward precision medicine: building a knowledge network for biomedical research and a new taxonomy of disease*. National Academies Press, Washington, DC.

Newell KA, Asare A, Kirk AD, Gisler TD, Bourcier K, Suthanthiran M, Burlingham WJ, Marks WH, Sanz I, Lechler RI, et al. 2010. Identification of a B cell signature associated with renal transplant tolerance in humans. *J Clin Invest* **120:** 1836–1847. doi:10.1172/JCI39933

Ochsner SA, Pillich RT, Rawool D, Grethe JS, McKenna NJ. 2022. Transcriptional regulatory networks of circulating immune cells in type 1 diabetes: a community knowledge base. *iScience* **25:** 104581. doi:10.1016/j.isci.2022.104581

Parra Sánchez AR, Voskuyl AE, van Vollenhoven RF. 2022. Treat-to-target in systemic lupus erythematosus: advancing towards its implementation. *Nat Rev Rheumatol* **18:** 146–157. doi:10.1038/s41584-021-00739-3

Philis-Tsimikas A, Asong M, Franek E, Jia T, Rosenstock J, Stachlewska K, Watada H, Kellerer M. 2023. Switching to once-weekly insulin icodec versus once-daily insulin degludec in individuals with basal insulin-treated type 2 diabetes (ONWARDS 2): a phase 3a, randomised, open label, multicentre, treat-to-target trial. *Lancet Diabetes Endocrinol* **11:** 414–425. doi:10.1016/S2213-8587(23)00093-1

Polasek TM, Shakib S, Rostami-Hodjegan A. 2018. Precision dosing in clinical medicine: present and future. *Expert Rev Clin Pharmacol* **11:** 743–746. doi:10.1080/17512433.2018.1501271

Quezada H, Guzmán-Ortiz AL, Díaz-Sánchez H, Valle-Rios R, Aguirre-Hernández J. 2017. Omics-based biomarkers: current status and potential use in the clinic. *Bol Med Hosp Infant Mex* **74:** 219–226. doi:10.1016/j.bmhimx.2017.03.003

Rigby MR, Harris KM, Pinckney A, DiMeglio LA, Rendell MS, Felner EI, Dostou JM, Gitelman SE, Griffin KJ, Tsalikian E, et al. 2015. Alefacept provides sustained clinical and immunological effects in new-onset type 1 diabetes patients. *J Clin Invest* **125:** 3285–3296. doi:10.1172/JCI81722

Russell-Jones D, Babazono T, Cailleteau R, Engberg S, Irace C, Kjaersgaard MIS, Mathieu C, Rosenstock J, Woo V, Klonoff DC. 2023. Once-weekly insulin icodec versus once-daily insulin degludec as part of a basal-bolus regimen in individuals with type 1 diabetes (ONWARDS 6): a phase 3a, randomised, open-label, treat-to-target trial. *Lancet* **402:** 1636–1647. doi:10.1016/S0140-6736(23)02179-7

Sarkar S, Elliott EC, Henry HR, Ludovico ID, Melchior JT, Frazer-Abel A, Webb-Robertson BJ, Davidson WS, Holers VM, Rewers MJ, et al. 2023. Systematic review of type 1 diabetes biomarkers reveals regulation in circulating proteins related to complement, lipid metabolism, and immune response. *Clin Proteomics* **20:** 38. doi:10.1186/s12014-023-09429-6

Shao F, Zheng P, Yu D, Zhou Z, Jia L. 2020. Follicular helper T cells in type 1 diabetes. *FASEB J* **34:** 30–40. doi:10.1096/fj.201901637R

Sims EK, Bundy BN, Stier K, Serti E, Lim N, Long SA, Geyer SM, Moran A, Greenbaum CJ, Evans-Molina C, et al. 2021. Teplizumab improves and stabilizes β cell function in antibody-positive high-risk individuals. *Sci Transl Med* **13:** eabc8980. doi:10.1126/scitranslmed.abc8980

Sims EK, Besser REJ, Dayan C, Geno Rasmussen C, Greenbaum C, Griffin KJ, Hagopian W, Knip M, Long AE, Martin F, et al. 2022. Screening for type 1 diabetes in the general population: a status report and perspective. *Diabetes* **71:** 610–623. doi:10.2337/dbi20-0054

Smith MJ, Cambier JC, Gottlieb PA. 2020. Endotypes in T1D: B lymphocytes and early onset. *Curr Opin Endocrinol Diabetes Obes* **27:** 225–230. doi:10.1097/MED.0000000000000547

Song W, Craft J. 2024. T follicular helper cell heterogeneity. *Annu Rev Immunol* **42:** 127–152. doi:10.1146/annurev-immunol-090222-102834

Spector BL, Harrell L, Sante D, Wyckoff GJ, Willig L. 2023. The methylome and cell-free DNA: current applications in medicine and pediatric disease. *Pediatr Res* **94:** 89–95. doi:10.1038/s41390-022-02448-3

Suomi T, Starskaia I, Kalim UU, Rasool O, Jaakkola MK, Grönroos T, Välikangas T, Brorsson C, Mazzoni G, Bruggraber S, et al. 2023. Gene expression signature predicts rate of type 1 diabetes progression. *EBioMedicine* **92:** 104625. doi:10.1016/j.ebiom.2023.104625

TEDDY Study Group. 2008. The Environmental Determinants of Diabetes in the Young (TEDDY) study. *Ann NY Acad Sci* **1150:** 1–13. doi:10.1196/annals.1447.062

Tsakiroglou M, Evans A, Pirmohamed M. 2023. Leveraging transcriptomics for precision diagnosis: lessons learned from cancer and sepsis. *Front Genet* **14:** 1100352. doi:10.3389/fgene.2023.1100352

van Heck JIP, Gacesa R, Stienstra R, Fu J, Zhernakova A, Harmsen HJM, Weersma RK, Joosten LAB, Tack CJ. 2022. The gut microbiome composition is altered in long-standing type 1 diabetes and associates with glycemic control and disease-related complications. *Diabetes Care* **45:** 2084–2094. doi:10.2337/dc21-2225

van Vollenhoven R. 2019. Treat-to-target in rheumatoid arthritis—are we there yet? *Nat Rev Rheumatol* **15:** 180–186. doi:10.1038/s41584-019-0170-5

Ventura-Aguiar P, Ramirez-Bajo MJ, Rovira J, Bañón-Maneus E, Hierro N, Lazo M, Cuatrecasas M, Garcia-Criado MA, Liang N, Swenerton RK, et al. 2022. Donor-derived cell-free DNA shows high sensitivity for the diagnosis of pancreas graft rejection in simultaneous pancreas-kidney transplantation. *Transplantation* **106:** 1690–1697. doi:10.1097/TP.0000000000004088

Voss MG, Cuthbertson DD, Cleves MM, Xu P, Evans-Molina C, Palmer JP, Redondo MJ, Steck AK, Lundgren M, Larsson H, et al. 2021. Time to peak glucose and peak C-peptide during the progression to type 1 diabetes in the diabetes prevention trial and TrialNet cohorts. *Diabetes Care* **44:** 2329–2336. doi:10.2337/dc21-0226

Walker LSK. 2022. The link between circulating follicular helper T cells and autoimmunity. *Nat Rev Immunol* **22:** 567–575. doi:10.1038/s41577-022-00693-5

Wiedeman AE, Muir VS, Rosasco MG, DeBerg HA, Presnell S, Haas B, Dufort MJ, Speake C, Greenbaum CJ, Serti E, et al. 2020. Autoreactive $CD8^+$ T cell exhaustion distinguishes subjects with slow type 1 diabetes progression. *J Clin Invest* **130:** 480–490. doi:10.1172/JCI126595

Xhonneux LP, Knight O, Lernmark A, Bonifacio E, Hagopian WA, Rewers MJ, She JX, Toppari J, Parikh H, Smith KGC, et al. 2021. Transcriptional networks in at-risk individuals identify signatures of type 1 diabetes progression. *Sci Transl Med* **13:** eabd5666. doi:10.1126/scitranslmed.abd5666

Checkpoint Inhibitor-Induced Autoimmune Diabetes: An Autoinflammatory Disease

Zoe Quandt,[1] Ana Perdigoto,[2,3] Mark S. Anderson,[1] and Kevan C. Herold[4]

[1]Department of Internal Medicine and Diabetes Center, University of California San Francisco, San Francisco, California 94115, USA

[2]Department of Internal Medicine, Yale University, New Haven, Connecticut 06510, USA

[3]Veterans Administration Hospital, West Haven, Connecticut 06516, USA

[4]Departments of Immunobiology and Internal Medicine, Yale University, New Haven, Connecticut 06510, USA

Correspondence: kevan.herold@yale.edu

Immunomodulatory agents targeting immune checkpoints are now the state-of-the-art for the treatment of many cancers, but at the same time have led to autoimmune side effects, including autoimmune diabetes: immune checkpoint inhibitor-induced diabetes (CPI-DM). Emerging research shows the importance of preexisting autoimmune disease risk that has been identified through genetics, and autoantibodies. Key associated clinical findings also include increased levels of lipase before diagnosis suggesting that the inflammatory process in the pancreas extends beyond the islets of Langerhans. There is selectivity for the blockade of programmed cell death protein 1 (PD-1)/programmed death-ligand 1 (PD-L1) for this adverse event, consistent with the role of this checkpoint in maintaining tolerance to autoimmune diabetes.

Over the last decade, there have been major advances in cancer-immune therapy with now widespread use of immune checkpoint inhibitors (CPIs) to treat certain cancers. Treatment with these drugs, which most often block the T-cell inhibitory receptors CTLA-4 and programmed cell death protein 1 (PD-1), and their ligands can also trigger autoimmunity in certain subjects with a wide spectrum of different autoimmune manifestations being described (Postow et al. 2018). Although somewhat infrequent, it is now recognized that some patients develop an autoimmune disease that shares many features with spontaneous type 1 diabetes (T1D). This emerging condition we term checkpoint inhibitor-induced diabetes (CPI-DM) is a new opportunity to understand the triggers for T1D and also how tolerance to the pancreatic islets is maintained. Here, we discuss key features of the disease and recent insights into how autoimmune diabetes emerges in these patients.

INTRODUCTION TO IMMUNE CHECKPOINT INHIBITORS

The immune system is charged with both identifying and eradicating foreign and malignant entities, such as bacteria and cancer cells, but also with maintaining self-tolerance. Among multiple approaches, malignant cells coopt mech-

Cite this article as *Cold Spring Harb Perspect Med* doi: 10.1101/cshperspect.a041603

anisms used for self-tolerance to evade the immune response. The ability to reinvigorate the immune system to fight cancer was initially discovered by William Coley, when he injected streptococcal cultures into a soft tissue sarcoma and induced an 8-year remission (Starnes 1992; Bucktrout et al. 2018). Following this experiment, work with immunomodulation to treat cancer was sidelined until the last few decades. The current pivotal treatments arose from immunomodulation at three different immune checkpoints, CTLA-4, PD-1/programmed death-ligand 1 (PD-L1), and LAG3, which effect T-cell activation. The blockade of these checkpoints leads to enhanced immune activation to target malignant cells, but also allows for adverse events termed immune-related adverse events (irAEs). IrAEs, which have been termed the "Achille's heal" of immunotherapy (June et al. 2017), can effect almost every organ and can limit the use of CPIs but also may portend improved response (Young et al. 2018). These irAEs offer an opportunity to study corollary conventional autoimmune disease but are also critical to improving the efficacy of CPI therapy.

IMMUNE CHECKPOINT INHIBITOR-INDUCED DIABETES DEFINITION

CPI-DM is infrequent, occurring in 0.2%–1.9% of individuals exposed to CPI (Quandt et al. 2021). CPI-DM lacks a consensus definition that leads to differences in clinical manifestations between case reports, case series, and reviews. There is also potential heterogeneity within CPI-DM such that a simple definition is not adequate. There are nonetheless key features that are consistent across reports. The unambiguous CPI-DM cases are characterized by insulinopenia, as documented by either presentation in DKA or very low C-peptide (a measure of endogenous insulin production), with an ongoing requirement for insulin following exposure to CPI therapy for cancer. Herein is one such complexity: This extreme insulinopenia may represent one end of the spectrum of the irAE, and CPI-DM definitions that are limited to patients with undetectable C-peptide may lack nuance and exclude the opportunity for intervention if patients are initially identified while still producing insulin. Patients with C-peptide levels that are both inappropriate for the degree of concurrent hyperglycemia and persistently low but detectable may also represent diabetes that is induced or exacerbated by CPIs. There are of course additional causes of hyperglycemia that are contextually related to CPI therapy but may not represent a targeted β-cell-immune attack. There are some patients who may have a history of well-controlled/mild type 2 (non-autoimmune) diabetes (T2D) whose metabolic condition precipitously deteriorates leading to an insulin requirement. Finally, most hyperglycemia that occurs in patients on CPI is due to concurrent steroid use (Mulla et al. 2023), which should not be considered a direct effect of CPI therapy. Treatment with glucocorticoids at the time of cancer therapies may also worsen preexisting T2D but insulin deficiency is not absolute and the direct association with CPI therapy is not certain.

In summary, there should be clear evidence of marked hyperglycemia resulting from the reduction in insulin production following CPI therapy to diagnose CPI-DM, and while the presence of T1D autoantibodies supports the diagnosis, they are not always present. As has already been done in T1D, further work is required to define possible endotypes within CPI-DM that might account for differences in the degree of insulinopenia and the presence of T1D autoantibodies.

EPIDEMIOLOGY AND NATURAL HISTORY

Aside from a handful of cases (Stamatouli et al. 2018; Wright et al. 2018), CPI-DM occurs following exposure to PD-1 or PD-L1 inhibitors alone or in combination with CTLA-4 inhibitors or other therapies. There is a suggestion that, like other irAEs, the rates may be higher in those exposed to combination CPI rather than monotherapy (Grimmelmann et al. 2021; Quandt et al. 2022). Although CPI-DM occurs across many cancer types, the majority of diagnosed patients suffer from metastatic melanoma. However, this is likely a consequence of PD-1/PD-L1 inhibitors having first been approved for the treatment of this disease resulting in many more patients being treated for melanoma (Marsiglio et al. 2023). It is unknown whether any particular cancer type has a greater predisposition to CPI-DM than others.

The time from CPI initiation to diagnosis with CPI-DM can vary widely. The reported median times range from 10 to 29 weeks (Stamatouli et al. 2018; Grimmelmann et al. 2021; Marsiglio et al. 2023; Wu et al. 2023a,b; Zhang et al. 2023) with the largest compilation of cases reporting 12 weeks (Wu et al. 2023b). CPI-DM in particular can be a delayed irAE; CPI-DM has been observed 6 months or even longer after cessation of CPI therapy (Stamatouli et al. 2018; Hatayama et al. 2022; Marsiglio et al. 2023) or only occurs after monotherapy is changed to combination therapy. The clinical onset of disease is often quite acute and the frequency of DKA in CPI-DM is higher compared to spontaneous T1D (Tittel et al. 2021; Qiu et al. 2022). In one study, white patients developed CPI-DM faster than Asian patients (40 vs. 110 days; Qiu et al. 2022), but, as detailed below, there are many phenotypic differences in CPI-DM in these populations.

In CPI-DM, there are frequently signs of non-islet pancreatic dysfunction, including elevated levels of enzymes, exocrine pancreatic insufficiency, and pancreatic volume loss, before the discovery of hyperglycemia. Multiple cohorts have reported increases in lipase that occur before (peaked at 1 week to 1 month; Grimmelmann et al. 2021; Wu et al. 2023a) or at CPI-DM diagnosis (Stamatouli et al. 2018). A recent retrospective, multicenter case series detected lipase elevation in 48% of patients (Wu et al. 2023a). Interestingly, baseline, pretreatment pancreatic volumes were lower in CPI-DM patients compared to CPI-treated controls in this study. Like a CPI-induced pancreatitis cohort, there was an ~40% decline in pancreatic volume from pretreatment to 6 months after DM diagnosis. This decline was not detected in patients with asymptomatic CPI-induced lipase elevation or control CPI-treated patients. These findings are consistent with pancreatic exocrine involvement in the pathogenesis of CPI-DM at least in some patients. Furthermore, patients who develop CPI-DM may have pancreatic changes at baseline that predispose them to develop diabetes, such as a prior injury or lower pancreatic reserve. Pancreatic volume has been shown to be decreased in people at risk for T1D (defined as single autoantibody positive) and T1D, even at T1D onset, compared to normal controls (Campbell-Thompson et al. 2012; Williams et al. 2012; Virostko et al. 2019), suggesting a parallel change in both forms of autoimmune diabetes.

Patients with CPI-DM are also more likely to have prior thyroid irAEs or preexisting autoimmune thyroid disease (Stamatouli et al. 2018; Grimmelmann et al. 2021; Zhang et al. 2021). Cohort studies have reported thyroid irAEs in 33%–64% (Stamatouli et al. 2018; Zhang et al. 2021; Marsiglio et al. 2023; Wu et al. 2023a). It is not clear that there is overlapping risk with other irAEs or the risk for subsequent irAEs.

Case series, meta-analyses of case reports, and cohort studies have found a frequency of islet-specific autoantibodies ranging from 18% to 54% (Zhang et al. 2021, 2023) with larger cohorts describing autoantibody prevalence of 40%–50% (Stamatouli et al. 2018; Wu et al. 2023b). The majority of CPI-DM patients who have a T1D autoantibody tend to have only a single positive autoantibody, the most common of which is anti-GAD65. This is in contrast to spontaneous T1D in which two or more positive autoantibodies (which also include anti-insulin, anti-ZnT8, anti-IA2) are frequently found at diagnosis but occur in <25% of patients with CPI-DM. Furthermore, high-affinity anti-GAD antibodies are more specific for progression to T1D than conventional anti-GAD antibodies, but as of yet, these high-affinity autoantibodies have not been assessed in patients with CPI-DM (Bender et al. 2014; Krause et al. 2014). In some studies, patients with CPI-DM with autoantibodies had a more rapid time to diagnosis than those without autoantibodies (Stamatouli et al. 2018; Qiu et al. 2022). Patients with positive autoantibodies at diagnosis are also more likely to present in DKA (Qiu et al. 2022), suggesting more complete β-cell failure. T1D autoantibodies are not routinely checked before or during CPI treatments, but there is a suggestion that their presence before CPI exposure identifies patients at increased for CPI-DM (Quandt et al. 2023). The features and frequencies of these autoantibodies are similar to thyroid irAEs in which there is a lower prevalence of autoantibodies than spontaneous disease. The frequency of autoantibodies in CPI-DM may vary by patient cohort: In one study, white people with CPI-DM had a higher prevalence of autoantibodies than Asian patients (Qiu et al. 2022). These variations in particular suggest that there are potential endotypes of CPI-DM and studies will need to account for these differences moving forward.

Together, the combination of this risk profile identifies patients at higher risk for islet autoimmunity and can be considered a group that may benefit from closer surveillance, although additional prospective studies are needed to determine the value of monitoring strategies. Considerations may include T1D autoantibody-positive patients, family history of T1D, autoimmune thyroid disease (whether CPI-induced or preexisting), and/or lipase elevations while on treatment. Other features, such as HLA or other genetic typing (described below) and changes in pancreatic volume require further investigations. The need for early identification is to consider, in the future, interventions that may prevent the complete loss of insulin production without affecting antitumor immunity.

A key clinical question is whether the appearance of this irAE has prognostic value for the anticancer response. This has been suggested for CPI-DM and also for other irAEs (Faje et al. 2018; Stamatouli et al. 2018; Muniz et al. 2022) but the sample sizes do not easily allow for direct comparison to cancer subjects that do not develop CPI-DM or adjustment for survival bias.

MECHANISMS OF CPI-DM

Genetic Determinants

Certain HLA alleles contribute the strongest genetic risk to spontaneous T1D and, in particular, HLA-DR4, a haplotype associated with spontaneous T1D, is enriched in CPI-DM patients. HLA-DR4 was found in 76% of our series of 27 patients, and other series have identified T1D susceptibility HLA alleles (DR3 and/or DR4) in 59% of patients (Wu et al. 2023b). Although a high frequency of HLA-DR4 was found in a single center case series from China (DRB1*0901-DQA1*03-DQB1*0303 (DR9) and DRB1*0405-DQA1*03-DQB1*0401 (Qiu et al. 2022; Liu et al. 2023), the overall frequency of the T1D susceptibility alleles is less than in spontaneous disease (HLA-DR3 and/or 4 can be found in >90% of patients with T1D) (Wu et al. 2023a). Interestingly, HLA haplotypes known to be protective of T1D appear to be decreased in CPI-DM, but likewise, the effects of these alleles are not completely understood (Wu et al. 2023a).

We recently completed whole exome sequencing of tumors from (13) patients with CPI-DM and identified a missense mutation (Pro191Leu) in NLRC5 in 9 of the 13 tumors. This mutation was subsequently found to be a germline mutation detectable in DNA extracted from peripheral blood mononuclear cells (Caulfield et al. 2023). This was significantly greater than in the general population or patients with the same cancers treated with the same drugs. NLRC5 is a regulator of class I–dependent immune responses analogous to the class II transactivator (CIITA). It interacts with major histocompatibility complex (MHC) promoter factors and thereby controls the loading of peptides onto the MHC molecules. It is not predicted to affect the function of NLRC5, but further studies are underway to determine how it may affect class I MHC loading and antigen presentation. Together with HLA-DR4, NLRC5 may serve as a useful marker for identifying individuals at increased risk for CPI-DM but prospective studies are needed.

Cellular Mechanisms

The data noted above suggest that inflammation of the whole pancreas is involved in CPI-DM. Multiple studies have shown evidence of exocrine pancreas inflammation with lipase and/or amylase elevation and reduced pancreatic volume in patients with CPI-DM (Stamatouli et al. 2018; Marchand et al. 2019; Grimmelmann et al. 2021; Perdigoto et al. 2022). We have little knowledge of the immune and islet cell changes occurring in the pancreas of patients with CPI-DM. T-cell infiltrate was detected in the pancreatic islets of a patient with CPI-DM, but very few β cells were identified in the tissue (Yoneda et al. 2019). Within these islets, $CD4^+$ T cells and $CD8^+$ T cells were noted in a peri-islet distribution in a patient with CPI-DM as well as expression of IFN-γ and TNF-α (Perdigoto et al. 2022). Additionally, checkpoint molecules such as PD-L1 and IDO were expressed on β cells. PD-L1 expression has been shown to be inducible in human islets in response to IFN-α and IFN-γ and expressed in β cells of patients with T1D (Colli et al. 2018; Osum et al. 2018).

Due to the limited availability of tissue from patients with CPI-DM, studies of CPI-DM in the nonobese diabetic (NOD) mouse have provided insights into cellular mechanisms and have suggested potential treatment approaches. NOD mice spontaneously develop autoimmune diabetes beginning at 12 weeks of age, but in younger mice, anti-PD-1 or PD-L1 mAb treatment can rapidly precipitate disease (Lenschow et al. 1995; Ansari et al. 2003). Anti-CTLA-4 agents will only precipitate diabetes in the NOD mouse if given in the neonatal period (Lenschow et al. 1995; Lühder et al. 1998). Hu et al. (2020) investigated immune mediators of CPI-DM in anti-PD-1-treated NOD mice and identified a central role for exhausted $CD8^+$ T cells expressing IFN-γ in CPI-DM. Activated T cells led to the recruitment of monocyte-derived macrophages that in turn became activated in response to IFN-γ and showed cytocidal activity against β cells. We compared transcriptional differences in β cells and islet-infiltrating immune cells in NOD mice treated with anti-PD-L1 versus anti-CTLA-4 mAbs before the onset of hyperglycemia. While both anti-CTLA-4 and anti-PD-L1 mAbs caused cellular infiltrates, single-cell RNA sequencing identified differences in the infiltrating immune cells and β cells in these NOD mice. We found that anti-PD-L1 resulted in infiltration of IFN-γ-expressing $CD8^+$ T cells with a cytotoxic phenotype (Perdigoto et al. 2022). We also identified changes in macrophages consistent with activation in response to IFN-γ (Perdigoto et al. 2022).

Gene expression changes in β cells that were unique to anti-PD-L1 treatment and primarily mediated by IFN-γ and TNF-α were also identified. Upon anti-PD-L1 treatment, there was a novel β-cell cluster with features of dedifferentiation that may occur in response to inflammatory stressors and contribute to the loss of functional β cells in CPI-DM. Neutralizing IFN-γ and TNF-α in vivo in anti-PD-L1-treated NOD mice prevented the development of diabetes pointing to the central role of these inflammatory mediators in this process. A similar approach was employed by Collier et al. (2023) who used single-cell RNA sequencing and T-cell receptor (TCR) sequencing to compare anti-PD-L1 mAb-induced diabetes to spontaneous diabetes in the NOD mouse. Collier et al. (2023) found increased terminally exhausted/effector-like $CD8^+$ T cells, T-bet^{hi} $CD4^+$ FoxP3-T cells, and reduced memory $CD4^+$ $FoxP3^-$ and $CD8^+$ T cells in anti-PD-1-treated NOD mice compared to spontaneous diabetes.

The role of antigen-specific T cells in CPI-DM remains unclear. The fact that CPI-DM can occur with CPI treatment of multiple cancers suggests that a tumor-defined antigen is not the target of the adaptive immune response. Ge et al. (2022) identified increased IGRP-specific $CD8^+$ T cells in the peripheral lymphoid organs of NOD mice treated with anti-PD-L1. Similarly, Collier et al. (2023) detected increased IGRP-specific $CD8^+$ T cells in the pancreatic lymph node and peripheral blood of anti-PD1-treated NOD mice, even higher than in spontaneously diabetic NOD mice. To more broadly investigate the diabetogenic T-cell repertoire, beyond known diabetic antigens, the authors used TCR sequencing to identify shared T-cell clones in the periphery (pancreatic lymph nodes and blood) and the pancreas. They found that anti-PD1 resulted in increased TCR sharing between the pancreas and the periphery and that $CD8^+$ T cells with shared clonotypes had an increased proportion of terminally exhausted/effector-like T cells. These data suggest that diabetogenic $CD8^+$ T cells are increased in the pancreatic lymph nodes and blood of CPI-DM in mice and that infiltration into the pancreas is mechanistically important for the development of CPI-DM. Further studies in human CPI-DM are needed.

Selectivity for One CPI versus Another

Ipilimumab (anti-CTLA-4 monoclonal antibody; mAb) was approved for clinical use in 2011 but the first cases of CPI-DM were not reported until nivolumab was introduced a few years later. CPI-DM has been described in a few patients with cancers treated with ipilimumab treatment alone

(Wright et al. 2018), but the majority of cases have occurred with the combination of drugs or anti-PD-1 or anti-PD-L1 mAb alone.

As noted, anti-PD-L1 or anti-PD-1 mAbs can rapidly and uniformly induce diabetes in young prediabetic NOD mice, while anti-CTLA-4 mAbs will induce diabetes only if given in the neonatal period (Ansari et al. 2003). Blockade or knockout of PD-1 or PD-L1 in NOD mice results in accelerated development of diabetes and PD-L1 overexpression inhibits the development of diabetes (Ansari et al. 2003; Wang et al. 2005; Keir et al. 2006; El Khatib et al. 2015). Thus, the strong association for selectivity of PD-1 blockade for CPI-DM is bolstered by data in the NOD mouse. Furthermore, either anti-PD-1 or anti-PD-L1 antibodies, but not anti-CTLA-4 mAb can break tolerance that is induced by anti-CD3 mAb, which collectively suggests that the PD-1/L1 costimulatory pathway is involved in the maintenance of tolerance to β cells.

Mouse β cells express PD-L1 as diabetes progresses and immune cells infiltrate the islet (Rui et al. 2017; Osum et al. 2018). Fife et al. described how PD-1 blockade alleviated the stop signal that was induced with TCR stimulation and limits the expansion of autoreactive T cells (Guleria et al. 2007; Fife et al. 2009). In addition, studies from our laboratory and others have shown that PD-L1 but not CD80 or CD86 is induced on human β cells when they are cultured with IFN-γ together with chemokines such as CXCL10 that can recruit effector T cells to the pancreas.

Studies by Kier et al. (2006) using bone marrow chimeras to express PD-L1 or PD-L2 on nonlymphoid hematopoietic immune cells showed that expression on these cells alone was not sufficient to protect from diabetes that could be rapidly transferred with T cells from a wild-type (WT) NOD mouse. Furthermore, PD-L1 expression on islet cells protected against diabetes after transplantation of syngeneic islets into PD-L1/L2 knockout (KO) diabetic recipients but the effect of the ligand on islet cells themselves was less clear when the islets were transplanted into WT diabetic recipients (Fig. 1). These studies together suggest that PD-L1 expression on nonlymphoid cells is needed for peripheral tolerance but also indicate that PD-L1 expression alone on β cells may not be sufficient alone to prevent diabetes that recurs in islet transplants when PD-L1/L2 is available on other cells and the repertoire is activated.

In the pancreas of a patient who died with PD-1-induced CPI-DM, we identified increased PD-L1 expression on β cells. Further bolstering a strong link of PD-1 dysfunction to T1D predilection is a recent case report of a child with a homozygous frameshift mutation of PD-1 who developed autoimmune diabetes at 3 years of age (Ogishi et al. 2021). Together, these data suggest

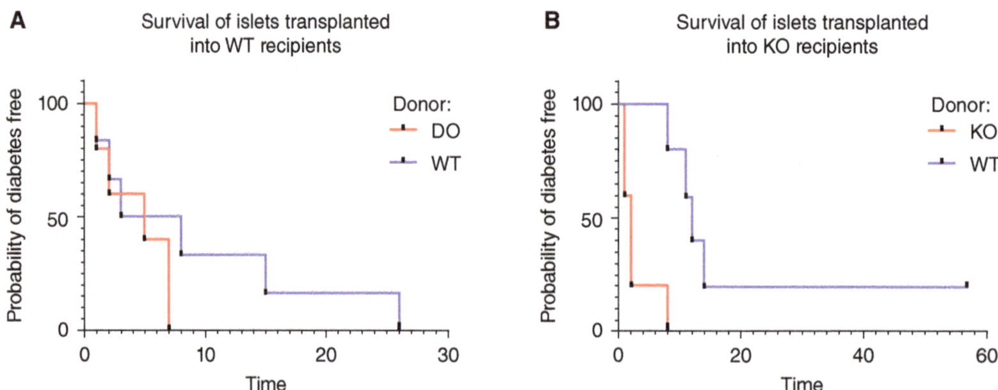

Figure 1. Survival of programmed death-ligand 1/2 (PD-L1/L2) knockout (KO) or wild-type (WT) islets once transplanted into WT (*A*) or KO (*B*) nonobese diabetic (NOD) mice. There is a significant hastening of the killing of the KO islets when they are transplanted into the KO recipients (median survival 2 vs. 12 days, $P = 0.005$). (Figure based on data from Keir et al. 2006.)

that PD-L1 expression on β cells is important for the maintenance of tolerance to these cells.

The availability of ligand expression may also be responsible for the control of autoimmunity and the differential effects of the anticheckpoint mAbs. In contrast to PD-L1, which is expressed on β cells, CTLA-4 ligands (CD80/CD86) are not detected on β cells but are found on antigen-presenting cells such as $CD14^+$ or $CD16^+$ cells. These infiltrating antigen-presenting cells represent a small proportion of cells within the islet and therefore, the availability of ligands that can engage inhibitory ligands like CTLA-4 is limited and most likely to occur with interactions between immune cells. However, the relationship between ligand expression on the tissue cells and proclivity to CPI-AEs is not certain. In a patient with a gain-of-function mutation of STAT1, which would be expected to enhance PD-L1 expression on β cells, autoimmune diabetes developed at a young age. We have not identified PD-L1 expression on colonic epithelial cells but other groups have reported its expression on these cells (Mann et al. 2023; J Mann, pers. comm.). Finally, it is unlikely that differential effects on regulatory T cells explain the differences as both PD-1 and CTLA-4 are expressed on Tregs.

Collectively, these experimental observations from different settings suggest that blockade of PD-1 or blockade or loss of PD-L1 is sufficient to trigger autoimmune killing of β cells when on a permissive genetic background that may include, in mice, NOD genotype, and in humans, HLA-DR4, NLRC5 polymorphism, or potentially other contributory loci. A polymorphism in the PD-1 gene has been associated with the development of spontaneous T1D (Nielsen et al. 2003). However, expression of PD-L1 alone is not sufficient to maintain tolerance since under inflammatory conditions, with available IFN-γ or other interferons, PD-L1 expression may be induced on β cells but is not sufficient to prevent islet-directed immunity.

CPI-DM MONITORING, DIAGNOSIS, AND TREATMENT

Guidelines for screening and monitoring for CPI-DM have not been codified, but the following suggestions are based on the above studies (Fig. 2). Genetic screening (e.g., for HLA-DR4, NLRC5 mutations) may identify those who are most likely to develop the disease, but it is important to recognize that a high percentage of patients do not have these genetic risk markers. Monitoring PD-1/L1 and combination therapy–treated patients with lipase as well as blood glucose levels should be done initially with every cycle (for 12 cycles) and then every 3–6 weeks (Brahmer et al. 2018). If glucocorticoids are used, an HbA1c before steroid initiation may help to understand the etiology of impaired metabolic control. The utility of monitoring pancreatic volumes in the detection of CPI-DM has not been formally evaluated.

In patients who develop CPI-DM, we recommend initiating insulin therapy as would be done with patients with T1D. It may initially be difficult to differentiate CPI-DM from other causes of diabetes such as worsening T2D or potentially steroid-induced diabetes and in such cases, insulin should be initiated until further diagnostic clarity is obtained. In case of severe symptomatic hyperglycemia or DKA, pausing the CPI therapy may be done to treat the severe hyperglycemia, but once frank hyperglycemia has developed it is unlikely that it can be reversed. HbA1c targets should be individualized and, given these patients are often older and with active malignancies, relaxed target levels may be appropriate, with the goal of avoiding DKA, symptomatic hyperglycemia, and hypoglycemia. Because C-peptide decline has been shown to be rapid and permanent in CPI-DM, we recommend follow-up C-peptide and glucose levels to verify the CPI-DM diagnosis, the need for continuous insulin treatment, and the risk for DKA in case the patient has a ketosis-prone or glucotoxic phenotype of diabetes rather than CPI-DM (Tsang et al. 2019; Wu et al. 2023a).

Given that CPI-DM is permanent in almost all cases, insulin therapy will need to be continued either through a basal bolus regimen or an insulin pump. Of note, there have been some reports of stopping insulin therapy in patients diagnosed with CPI-DM, but those patients were not insulinopenic (Hansen et al. 2016; Trinh et al. 2019) even at CPI-DM diagnosis. In

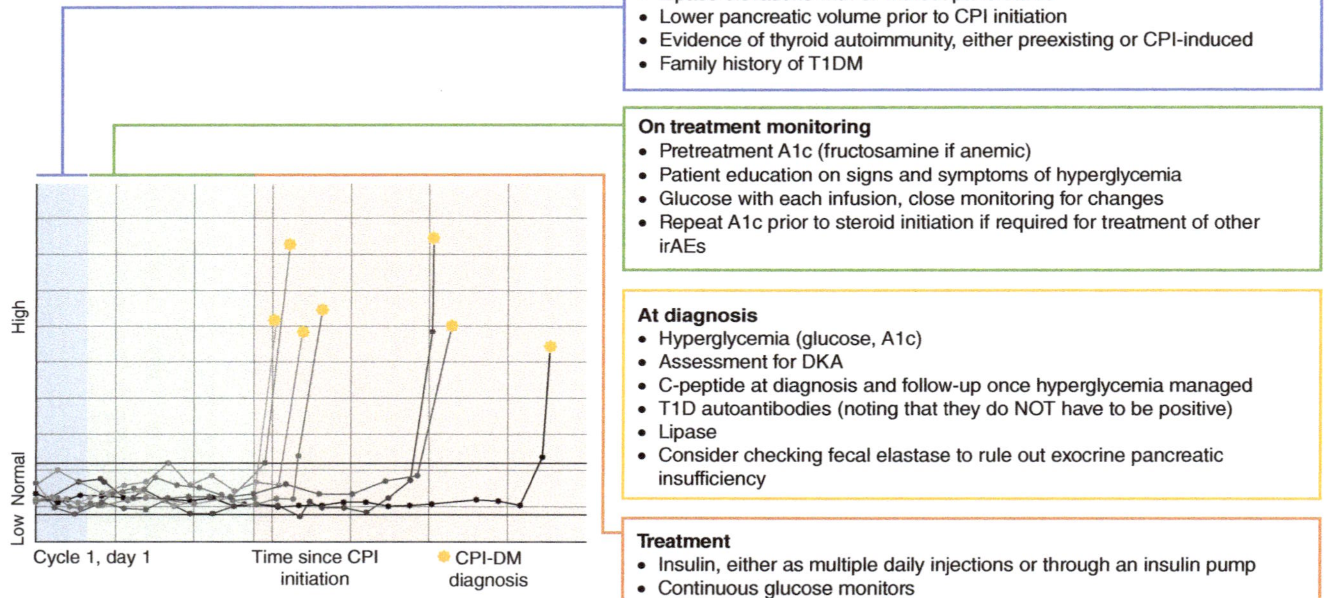

Figure 2. Schematic of the natural history of checkpoint inhibitor-induced diabetes (CPI-DM) development. The *left* panel shows the random glucose in patients as they start immune checkpoint inhibitor (CPI) therapy. As can be seen, the onset of significant hyperglycemia is most often acute, without preceding mild increases in glucose. The *right* panel summarizes risk factors, monitoring recommendations, diagnostic workup, and treatment considerations.

Cite this article as *Cold Spring Harb Perspect Med* doi: 10.1101/cshperspect.a041603

our clinical experience, glucose control is labile in patients with CPI-DM. Given their low C-peptide levels, patients are prone to hypoglycemia and continuous glucose monitoring should be considered in these patients. Glucose monitoring systems have been shown in a small study to potentially be effective in the management of CPI-DM to prevent severe hyperglycemia as well as hypoglycemia just as they are in T1D (Rodríguez De Vera-Gómez et al. 2022).

FUTURE OPPORTUNITIES FOR TREATMENT AND PREVENTION

To be useful as a treatment, an agent would need to be able to arrest the mechanisms of CPI-DM without blocking the antitumor effects of the CPI. Preclinical and clinical studies that have identified a role of cytokine signaling (particularly TNF and IFN-γ) in inducing PD-L1 on β cells and in the development of CPI-DM suggest that blockade of these pathways may be exploited for therapeutic purposes. Our preclinical studies suggested the neutralization of IFN-γ and TNF with antibodies may prevent the induction of diabetes with CPI in NOD mice (Perdigoto et al. 2022). One case report described improvement of diabetes in a patient treated with infliximab for oligoarthritis. The patient in that case report had been on steroids and was not insulinopenic leaving questions as to the efficacy of this TNF inhibitor in other cases of CPI-DM (Trinh et al. 2019).

JAK inhibitors, which are small molecule therapies that suppress cytokine production in T-cell-mediated inflammatory pathways are another potential pharmacologic class in CPI-DM. JAK inhibitors, particularly tofacitinib, which is a JAK1/JAK2/JAK3 inhibitor, have been successfully used to treat other CPI-induced irAEs (CPI-induced colitis, arthritis, and myocarditis; Esfahani et al. 2020; Liu and Jiang 2021; Murray et al. 2021; Sasson et al. 2021). Recently, a preclinical study by Ge et al. (2022) suggests they may be useful for the treatment of CPI diabetes. Ge et al. (2022) demonstrated that inhibition of the JAK1/JAK2 pathway with a pharmacological inhibitor could both prevent diabetes when given to NOD mice before or after anti-PD-L1 treatment as well as reverse hyperglycemia following checkpoint inhibitor treatment. The authors went on to show that JAK1/JAK2 inhibition prevented diabetes by reducing T-cell proliferation and T-cell infiltration into the islet as well as reducing islet-specific T cells in the peripheral lymphoid organs. A JAK inhibitor (baricitinib, a JAK1/JAK2 inhibitor) has been used to successfully preserve β-cell function in T1D in humans and to reverse conventional diabetes in NOD mouse models in the absence of checkpoint inhibition (Trivedi et al. 2017; Chaimowitz et al. 2020; Ge et al. 2020; Waibel et al. 2023). The efficacy of this agent, which affects IFN-γ and TNF, further highlights the importance of the IFN-γ and TNF cytokines in CPI-DM.

For these agents to be deployable in the irAE setting, they must not impede antitumor immunity. In the preclinical models described, Ge and colleagues use of JAK1/JAK2 inhibition to prevent diabetes did not affect the efficacy of CPI therapy for a transplantable tumor model. As mentioned, infliximab and JAK inhibitors (among other immunomodulators including CTLA-4 Ig) have been used as nonsteroidal approaches for other irAEs through ongoing trials, but preliminary evidence supports their use (Verheijden et al. 2023).

In contrast to other irAEs, glucocorticoids have no known efficacy in CPI-DM and could worsen hyperglycemia. Further work is needed to elucidate the efficacy of these agents in CPI-DM in clinical settings. This will need to include efficacy to prevent CPI-DM without impeding antitumor immunity and should focus on highly targeted therapies that might include islet-specific immunosuppression.

CONCLUSIONS

The emergence and recognition of CPI-DM as a complication of cancer immune therapy has created a new area for research on autoimmune diabetes that may not only identify their pathogenesis in the setting of checkpoint blockade but also for understanding tolerance to β cells and mechanisms that may underlie spontaneous disease. The predilection of triggering of CPI-DM by PD-1 blockade over CTLA-4 blockade suggests that maintenance of the PD-1 pathway is an active process in many adult patients. The role of genetic factors in enabling these CPIs to precipitate disease is an ongoing area of investigation. The finding that not all patients have conventional autoantibodies may suggest that antigens other than those that are recognized in spontaneous disease drive the disease but the scope of the inflammatory response that is associated with the disease, which may also involve the exocrine pancreas, suggests a broader inflammatory response.

The observations from preclinical models and the limited data from human studies have suggested strategies that may be useful to prevent or treat the disease. If new antigens are involved, new targets for immune therapies may be suggested. Like T1D, the timing of any intervention to prevent or attenuate CPI-DM is critical for efficacy. If there is very minimal endogenous insulin production, it will be much less likely for these interventions to be effective since there is no evidence for reversal once β-cell function is lost. Finally, the implication of the work in this uncommon form of autoimmune diabetes is an effective strategy for preventing spontaneous disease using PD-1 agonists—an active area of drug development (Tuttle et al. 2023).

ACKNOWLEDGMENTS

Z.Q. was supported by the NIH NIDDK DiabDocs K12DK133995 and a Larry L Hillblom Foundation Start Up Grant. A.P. was supported by the NIH NCI grant 1K08CA282972 and the Yale SPORE in Skin Cancer Career Enhancement Program Award. M.S.A. was supported by the JDRF Northern California Center of Excellence, Helmsley Charitable Trust, and Chan-Zuckerberg Biohub. K.C.H. was supported by the NIH NIDDK and NCI grants DK057846, DK045735, and CA2277473 and funding from the Parker Institute for Cancer Immunotherapy.

REFERENCES

Ansari MJI, Salama AD, Chitnis T, Smith RN, Yagita H, Akiba H, Yamazaki T, Azuma M, Iwai H, Khoury SJ, et al. 2003. The programmed death-1 (PD-1) pathway regulates autoimmune diabetes in nonobese diabetic (NOD) mice. *J Exp Med* **198:** 63–69. doi:10.1084/jem.20022125

Bender C, Schlosser M, Christen U, Ziegler AG, Achenbach P. 2014. GAD autoantibody affinity in schoolchildren from the general population. *Diabetologia* **57:** 1911–1918. doi:10.1007/s00125-014-3294-9

Brahmer JR, Lacchetti C, Schneider BJ, Atkins MB, Brassil KJ, Caterino JM, Chau I, Ernstoff MS, Gardner JM, Ginex P, et al. 2018. Management of immune-related adverse events in patients treated with immune checkpoint inhibitor therapy: American Society of Clinical Oncology Clinical Practice guideline. *J Clin Oncol* **36:** 1714–1768. doi:10.1200/JCO.2017.77.6385

Bucktrout SL, Bluestone JA, Ramsdell F. 2018. Recent advances in immunotherapies: from infection and autoimmunity, to cancer, and back again. *Genome Med* **10:** 79. doi:10.1186/s13073-018-0588-4

Campbell-Thompson M, Wasserfall C, Montgomery EL, Atkinson MA, Kaddis JS. 2012. Pancreas organ weight in individuals with disease-associated autoantibodies at risk for type 1 diabetes. *J Am Med Assoc* **308:** 2337–2339. doi:10.1001/jama.2012.15008

Caulfield JI, Aizenbud L, Perdigoto AL, Meffre E, Jilaveanu L, Michalek DA, Rich SS, Aizenbud Y, Adeniran A, Herold KC, et al. 2023. Germline genetic variants are associated with development of insulin-dependent diabetes in cancer patients treated with immune checkpoint inhibitors. *J Immunother Cancer* **11:** e006570. doi:10.1136/jitc-2022-006570

Chaimowitz NS, Ebenezer SJ, Hanson IC, Anderson M, Forbes LR. 2020. STAT1 gain of function, type 1 diabetes, and reversal with JAK inhibition. *N Engl J Med* **383:** 1494–1496. doi:10.1056/NEJMc2022226

Colli ML, Hill JLE, Marroqui L, Chaffey J, Dos Santos RS, Leete P, Coomans de Brachene A, Paula FMM, Op de Beeck A, Castela A, et al. 2018. PDL1 is expressed in the islets of people with type 1 diabetes and is up-regulated by interferons-α and-γ via IRF1 induction. *EBioMedicine* **36:** 367–375. doi:10.1016/j.ebiom.2018.09.040

Collier JL, Pauken KE, Lee CAA, Patterson DG, Markson SC, Conway TS, Fung ME, France JA, Mucciarone KN, Lian CG, et al. 2023. Single-cell profiling reveals unique features of diabetogenic T cells in anti-PD-1-induced type 1 diabetes mice. *J Exp Med* **220:** e20221920. doi:10.1084/jem.20221920

El Khatib MM, Sakuma T, Tonne JM, Mohamed MS, Holditch SJ, Lu B, Kudva YC, Ikeda Y. 2015. β-Cell-targeted blockage of PD1 and CTLA4 pathways prevents development of autoimmune diabetes and acute allogeneic islets rejection. *Gene Ther* **22:** 430–438. doi:10.1038/gt.2015.18

Esfahani K, Hudson M, Batist G. 2020. Tofacitinib for refractory immune-related colitis from PD-1 therapy. *N Engl J Med* **382:** 2374–2375. doi:10.1056/NEJMc2002527

Faje AT, Lawrence D, Flaherty K, Freedman C, Fadden R, Rubin K, Cohen J, Sullivan RJ. 2018. High-dose glucocorticoids for the treatment of ipilimumab-induced hypophysitis is associated with reduced survival in patients with melanoma. *Cancer* **124:** 3706–3714. doi:10.1002/cncr.31629

Fife BT, Pauken KE, Eagar TN, Obu T, Wu J, Tang Q, Azuma M, Krummel MF, Bluestone JA. 2009. Interactions between PD-1 and PD-L1 promote tolerance by blocking the TCR-induced stop signal. *Nat Immunol* **10:** 1185–1192. doi:10.1038/ni.1790

Ge T, Jhala G, Fynch S, Akazawa S, Litwak S, Pappas EG, Catterall T, Vakil I, Long AJ, Olson LM, et al. 2020. The JAK1 selective inhibitor ABT 317 blocks signaling through interferon-γ and common γ chain cytokine receptors to reverse autoimmune diabetes in NOD mice. *Front Immunol* **11:** 588543. doi:10.3389/fimmu.2020.588543

Ge T, Phung AL, Jhala G, Trivedi P, Principe N, De George DJ, Pappas EG, Litwak S, Sanz-Villanueva L, Catterall T, et al. 2022. Diabetes induced by checkpoint inhibition in nonobese diabetic mice can be prevented or reversed by a JAK1/JAK2 inhibitor. *Clin Transl Immunology* **11:** e1425. doi:10.1002/cti2.1425

Grimmelmann I, Momma M, Zimmer L, Hassel JC, Heinzerling L, Pföhler C, Loquai C, Ruini C, Utikal J, Thoms KM, et al. 2021. Lipase elevation and type 1 diabetes mellitus related to immune checkpoint inhibitor therapy—a multicentre study of 90 patients from the German Dermatooncology Group. *Eur J Cancer* **149:** 1–10. doi:10.1016/j.ejca.2021.02.017

Guleria I, Gubbels Bupp M, Dada S, Fife B, Tang Q, Ansari MJ, Trikudanathan S, Vadivel N, Fiorina P, Yagita H, et al. 2007. Mechanisms of PDL1-mediated regulation of autoimmune diabetes. *Clin Immunol* **125:** 16–25. doi:10.1016/j.clim.2007.05.013

Hansen E, Sahasrabudhe D, Sievert L. 2016. A case report of insulin-dependent diabetes as immune-related toxicity of pembrolizumab: presentation, management and outcome. *Cancer Immunol Immunother* **65:** 765–767. doi:10.1007/s00262-016-1835-4

Hatayama S, Kodama S, Kawana Y, Otake S, Sato D, Horiuchi T, Takahashi K, Kaneko K, Imai J, Katagiri H. 2022. Two cases with fulminant type 1 diabetes that developed long after cessation of immune checkpoint inhibitor treatment. *J Diabetes Investig* **13:** 1458–1460. doi:10.1111/jdi.13807

Hu H, Zakharov PN, Peterson OJ, Unanue ER. 2020. Cytocidal macrophages in symbiosis with CD4 and CD8 T cells cause acute diabetes following checkpoint blockade of PD-1 in NOD mice. *Proc Natl Acad Sci* **117:** 31319–31330. doi:10.1073/pnas.2019743117

June CH, Warshauer JT, Bluestone JA. 2017. Is autoimmunity the Achilles' heel of cancer immunotherapy? *Nat Med* **23:** 540–547. doi:10.1038/nm.4321

Keir ME, Liang SC, Guleria I, Latchman YE, Qipo A, Albacker LA, Koulmanda M, Freeman GJ, Sayegh MH, Sharpe AH. 2006. Tissue expression of PD-L1 mediates peripheral T cell tolerance. *J Exp Med* **203:** 883–895. doi:10.1084/jem.20051776

Krause S, Landherr U, Agardh CD, Hausmann S, Link K, Hansen JM, Lynch KF, Powell M, Furmaniak J, Rees-Smith B, et al. 2014. GAD autoantibody affinity in adult patients with latent autoimmune diabetes, the study participants of a GAD65 vaccination trial. *Diabetes Care* **37:** 1675–1680. doi:10.2337/dc13-1719

Lenschow DJ, Ho SC, Sattar H, Rhee L, Gray G, Nabavi N, Herold KC, Bluestone JA. 1995. Differential effects of anti-B7-1 and anti-B7-2 monoclonal antibody treatment on the development of diabetes in the nonobese diabetic mouse. *J Exp Med* **181:** 1145–1155. doi:10.1084/jem.181.3.1145

Liu Y, Jiang L. 2021. Tofacitinib for treatment in immune-mediated myocarditis: the first reported cases. *J Oncol Pharm Pract* **27:** 739–746. doi:10.1177/1078155220947141

Liu YC, Liu H, Zhao SL, Chen K, Jin P. 2023. Clinical and HLA genotype analysis of immune checkpoint inhibitor-associated diabetes mellitus: a single-center case series from China. *Front Immunol* **14:** 1164120. doi:10.3389/fimmu.2023.1164120

Lühder F, Höglund P, Allison JP, Benoist C, Mathis D. 1998. Cytotoxic T lymphocyte-associated antigen 4 (CTLA-4) regulates the unfolding of autoimmune diabetes. *J Exp Med* **187:** 427–432. doi:10.1084/jem.187.3.427

Mann JE, Lucca L, Austin MR, Merkin RD, Robert ME, Al Bawardy B, Raddassi K, Aizenbud L, Joshi NS, Hafler DA, et al. 2023. ScRNA-seq defines dynamic T-cell subsets in longitudinal colon and peripheral blood samples in immune checkpoint inhibitor-induced colitis. *J Immunother Cancer* **11:** e007358. doi:10.1136/jitc-2023-007358

Marchand L, Thivolet A, Dalle S, Chikh K, Reffet S, Vouillarmet J, Fabien N, Cugnet-Anceau C, Thivolet C. 2019. Diabetes mellitus induced by PD-1 and PD-L1 inhibitors: description of pancreatic endocrine and exocrine phenotype. *Acta Diabetol* **56:** 441–448. doi:10.1007/s00592-018-1234-8

Marsiglio J, McPherson JP, Kovacsovics-Bankowski M, Jeter J, Vaklavas C, Swami U, Grossmann D, Erickson-Wayman A, Soares HP, Kerrigan K, et al. 2023. A single center case series of immune checkpoint inhibitor-induced type 1 diabetes mellitus, patterns of disease onset and long-term clinical outcome. *Front Immunol* **14:** 1229823. doi:10.3389/fimmu.2023.1229823

Mulla K, Farag S, Moore B, Matharu S, Young K, Larkin J, Popat S, Morganstein DL. 2023. Hyperglycaemia following immune checkpoint inhibitor therapy—incidence, aetiology and assessment. *Diabet Med* **40:** e15053. doi:10.1111/dme.15053

Muniz TP, Araujo DV, Savage KJ, Cheng T, Saha M, Song X, Gill S, Monzon JG, Grenier D, Genta S, et al. 2022. CANDIED: a pan-Canadian cohort of immune checkpoint inhibitor-induced insulin-dependent diabetes mellitus. *Cancers (Basel)* **14:** 89. doi:10.3390/cancers14010089

Murray K, Floudas A, Murray C, Fabre A, Crown J, Fearon U, Veale D. 2021. First use of tofacitinib to treat an immune checkpoint inhibitor-induced arthritis. *BMJ Case Rep* **14:** e238851. doi:10.1136/bcr-2020-238851

Nielsen C, Hansen D, Husby S, Jacobsen BB, Lillevang ST. 2003. Association of a putative regulatory polymorphism in the *PD-1* gene with susceptibility to type 1 diabetes. *Tissue Antigens* **62:** 492–497. doi:10.1046/j.1399-0039.2003.00136.x

Ogishi M, Yang R, Aytekin C, Langlais D, Bourgey M, Khan T, Ali FA, Rahman M, Delmonte OM, Chrabieh M, et al. 2021. Inherited PD-1 deficiency underlies tuberculosis and autoimmunity in a child. *Nat Med* **27:** 1646–1654. doi:10.1038/s41591-021-01388-5

Osum KC, Burrack AL, Martinov T, Sahli NL, Mitchell JS, Tucker CG, Pauken KE, Papas K, Appakalai B, Spanier JA, et al. 2018. Interferon-γ drives programmed death-ligand 1 expression on islet β cells to limit T cell function during autoimmune diabetes. *Sci Rep* **8:** 8295. doi:10.1038/s41598-018-26471-9

Perdigoto AL, Deng S, Du KC, Kuchroo M, Burkhardt DB, Tong A, Israel G, Robert ME, Weisberg SP, Kirkiles-Smith N, et al. 2022. Immune cells and their inflammatory mediators modify β cells and cause checkpoint inhibitor-induced diabetes. *JCI Insight* **7:** e156330. doi:10.1172/jci.insight.156330

Postow MA, Sidlow R, Hellmann MD. 2018. Immune-related adverse events associated with immune checkpoint blockade. *N Engl J Med* **378:** 158–168. doi:10.1056/NEJMra1703481

Qiu J, Luo S, Yin W, Guo K, Xiang Y, Li X, Liu Z, Zhou Z. 2022. Characterization of immune checkpoint inhibitor-associated fulminant type 1 diabetes associated with autoantibody status and ethnic origin. *Front Immunol* **13:** 968798. doi:10.3389/fimmu.2022.968798

Quandt Z, Young A, Perdigoto AL, Herold KC, Anderson MS. 2021. Autoimmune endocrinopathies: an emerging complication of immune checkpoint inhibitors. *Annu Rev Med* **72:** 313–330. doi:10.1146/annurev-med-050219-034237

Quandt ZE, Hill V, Dib JE, Burian J, Tessler S, Naqash AR, Anderson MS, Othus M, Sharon E. 2022. Immune checkpoint inhibitor-induced diabetes mellitus across NCI trials. *J Clin Oncol* **40:** 2668. doi:10.1200/JCO.2022.40.16_suppl.2668

Quandt Z, Liang S, Lucas A, Thompson M, Saha A, Hammer C, Herold K, Young A, Spencer C, Anderson M. 2023. Risk evaluation of immune checkpoint inhibitor diabetes through islet autoantibodies and HLA types in a large, real-world cohort. *J Immunother Cancer* **11:** A1366.

Rodríguez De Vera-Gómez P, Piñar-Gutiérrez A, Guerrero-Vázquez R, Bellido V, Morales-Portillo C, Sancho-Márquez MP, Espejo-García P, Gros-Herguido N, López-Gallardo G, Martínez-Brocca MA, et al. 2022. Flash glucose monitoring and diabetes mellitus induced by immune checkpoint inhibitors: an approach to clinical practice. *J Diabetes Res* **2022:** 1–16. doi:10.1155/2022/4508633

Rui J, Deng S, Arazi A, Perdigoto AL, Liu Z, Herold KC. 2017. β Cells that resist immunological attack develop during progression of autoimmune diabetes in NOD mice. *Cell Metab* **25:** 727–738. doi:10.1016/j.cmet.2017.01.005

Sasson SC, Slevin SM, Cheung VTF, Nassiri I, Olsson-Brown A, Fryer E, Ferreira RC, Trzupek D, Gupta T, Al-Hillawi L, et al. 2021. Interferon-γ-producing $CD8^+$ tissue resident memory T cells are a targetable hallmark of immune checkpoint inhibitor-colitis. *Gastroenterology* **161:** 1229–1244.e9. doi:10.1053/j.gastro.2021.06.025

Stamatouli AM, Quandt Z, Perdigoto AL, Clark PL, Kluger H, Weiss SA, Gettinger S, Sznol M, Young A, Rushakoff R, et al. 2018. Collateral damage: insulin-dependent diabetes induced with checkpoint inhibitors. *Diabetes* **67:** 1471–1480. doi:10.2337/dbi18-0002

Starnes CO. 1992. Coley's toxins in perspective. *Nature* **357:** 11–12. doi:10.1038/357011a0

Tittel SR, Laubner K, Schmid SM, Kress S, Merger S, Karges W, Wosch FJ, Altmeier M, Pavel M, Holl RW. 2021. Immune-checkpoint inhibitor-associated diabetes compared to other diabetes types—a prospective, matched control study. *J Diabetes* **13:** 1007–1014. doi:10.1111/1753-0407.13215

Trinh B, Donath MY, Laubli H. 2019. Successful treatment of immune checkpoint inhibitor-induced diabetes with infliximab. *Diabetes Care* **42:** e153–e154. doi:10.2337/dc19-0908

Trivedi PM, Graham KL, Scott NA, Jenkins MR, Majaw S, Sutherland RM, Fynch S, Lew AM, Burns CJ, Krishnamurthy B, et al. 2017. Repurposed JAK1/JAK2 inhibitor reverses established autoimmune insulitis in NOD mice. *Diabetes* **66:** 1650–1660. doi:10.2337/db16-1250

Tsang VHM, McGrath RT, Clifton-Bligh RJ, Scolyer RA, Jakrot V, Guminski AD, Long GV, Menzies AM. 2019. Checkpoint inhibitor-associated autoimmune diabetes is distinct from type 1 diabetes. *J Clin Endocrinol Metab* **104:** 5499–5506. doi:10.1210/jc.2019-00423

Tuttle J, Drescher E, Simón-Campos JA, Emery P, Greenwald M, Kivitz A, Rha H, Yachi P, Kiley C, Nirula A. 2023. A phase 2 trial of peresolimab for adults with rheumatoid arthritis. *N Engl J Med* **388:** 1853–1862. doi:10.1056/NEJMoa2209856

Verheijden RJ, van Eijs MJM, May AM, van Wijk F, Suijkerbuijk KPM. 2023. Immunosuppression for immune-related adverse events during checkpoint inhibition: an intricate balance. *NPJ Precis Oncol* **7:** 41. doi:10.1038/s41698-023-00380-1

Virostko J, Williams J, Hilmes M, Bowman C, Wright JJ, Du L, Kang H, Russell WE, Powers AC, Moore DJ. 2019. Pancreas volume declines during the first year after diagnosis of type 1 diabetes and exhibits altered diffusion at disease onset. *Diabetes Care* **42:** 248–257. doi:10.2337/dc18-1507

Waibel M, Wentworth JM, So M, Couper JJ, Cameron FJ, MacIsaac RJ, Atlas G, Gorelik A, Litwak S, Sanz-Villanueva L, et al. 2023. Baricitinib and β-cell function in patients with new-onset type 1 diabetes. *N Engl J Med* **389:** 2140–2150. doi:10.1056/NEJMoa2306691

Wang J, Yoshida T, Nakaki F, Hiai H, Okazaki T, Honjo T. 2005. Establishment of NOD-Pdcd1$^{-/-}$ mice as an efficient animal model of type I diabetes. *Proc Natl Acad Sci* **102:** 11823–11828. doi:10.1073/pnas.0505497102

Williams AJ, Thrower SL, Sequeiros IM, Ward A, Bickerton AS, Triay JM, Callaway MP, Dayan CM. 2012. Pancreatic volume is reduced in adult patients with recently diagnosed type 1 diabetes. *J Clin Endocrinol Metab* **97:** E2109–E2113. doi:10.1210/jc.2012-1815

Wright JJ, Salem JE, Johnson DB, Lebrun-Vignes B, Stamatouli A, Thomas JW, Herold KC, Moslehi J, Powers AC. 2018. Increased reporting of immune checkpoint inhibitor-associated diabetes. *Diabetes Care* **41:** e150–e151. doi:10.2337/dc18-1465

Wu L, Carlino MS, Brown DA, Long GV, Clifton-Bligh R, Mellor R, Moore K, Sasson SC, Menzies AM, Tsang V, et al. 2023a. Checkpoint inhibitor associated autoimmune diabetes mellitus is characterised by C-peptide loss and pancreatic atrophy. *J Clin Endocrinol Metab* **109:** 1301–1307. doi:10.1210/clinem/dgad685

Wu L, Tsang V, Menzies AM, Sasson SC, Carlino MS, Brown DA, Clifton-Bligh R, Gunton JE. 2023b. Risk factors and characteristics of checkpoint inhibitor-associated autoimmune diabetes mellitus (CIADM): a systematic review and delineation from type 1 diabetes. *Diabetes Care* **46:** 1292–1299. doi:10.2337/dc22-2202

Yoneda S, Imagawa A, Hosokawa Y, Baden MY, Kimura T, Uno S, Fukui K, Goto K, Uemura M, Eguchi H, et al. 2019. T-Lymphocyte infiltration to islets in the pancreas of a patient who developed type 1 diabetes after administration of immune checkpoint inhibitors. *Diabetes Care* **42:** e116–e118. doi:10.2337/dc18-2518

Young A, Quandt Z, Bluestone JA. 2018. The balancing act between cancer immunity and autoimmunity in response to immunotherapy. *Cancer Immunol Res* **6:** 1445–1452. doi:10.1158/2326-6066.CIR-18-0487

Zhang AL, Wang F, Chang LS, McDonnell ME, Min L. 2021. Coexistence of immune checkpoint inhibitor-induced autoimmune diabetes and pancreatitis. *Front Endocrinol (Lausanne)* **12:** 620522. doi:10.3389/fendo.2021.620522

Zhang Z, Sharma R, Hamad L, Riebandt G, Attwood K. 2023. Incidence of diabetes mellitus in patients treated with immune checkpoint inhibitors (ICI) therapy—a comprehensive cancer center experience. *Diabetes Res Clin Pract* **202:** 110776. doi:10.1016/j.diabres.2023.110776

Rebalancing the Immune System to Treat Type 1 Diabetes

Yannick D. Muller,[1,2] Patrick Ho,[3] Jeffrey A. Bluestone,[3,4] and Qizhi Tang[3,5,6]

[1]Division of Immunology and Allergy, Department of Medicine, Lausanne University Hospital and University of Lausanne, 1005 Lausanne, Switzerland

[2]Center for Human Immunology Lausanne, Lausanne University Hospital and University of Lausanne, 1005 Lausanne, Switzerland

[3]Diabetes Center, University of California San Francisco, San Francisco, California 94143, USA

[4]Sonoma Biotherapeutics, South San Francisco, California 94080, USA

[5]Department of Surgery, Division of Transplantation, University of California San Francisco, San Francisco, California 94143, USA

[6]Gladstone UCSF Institute of Genome Immunology, San Francisco, California 94158, USA

Correspondence: Qizhi.Tang@ucsf.edu

In type 1 diabetes (T1D), the immune system mistakenly attacks the pancreatic islet β cells resulting in the loss of insulin secretion. Insulin-replacement therapy developed more than a century ago provided means to manage the symptoms of diabetes without addressing the root cause of the disease—the faulty immune system. A healthy immune system has built-in mechanisms to limit unwanted, excessive immune activation and prevents damages to self-tissues. These immune self-tolerance mechanisms are often impaired in autoimmune patients including those with T1Ds. Understanding how immune self-tolerance is broken in patients with T1D can inform the design of new curative therapies that correct the immune defects. In this paper, we will summarize the mechanisms of immune tolerance, review their relevance to T1Ds, and discuss novel therapeutic approaches to rebalance the immune system for the treatment of T1Ds.

In type 1 diabetes (T1D), the immune system mistakenly destroys the insulin-producing pancreatic islet β cells. Understanding how the immune system naturally avoids autoimmune diseases such as T1D may inform the development of novel therapeutics that treat the root causes of these diseases. In this paper, we will review how immune self-tolerance is normally established, summarize evidence of tolerance defects in T1D, and propose strategies for developing curative therapies for T1D by repairing these defects. Since T cells are the principal driver of T1D, we will focus our review on T-cell tolerance.

THE CONCEPT OF A BALANCED IMMUNE SYSTEM

To protect the body against invading pathogens, the immune system must be able to recognize a vast array of antigens and respond rapidly to

Cite this article as *Cold Spring Harb Perspect Med* doi: 10.1101/cshperspect.a041599

eliminate them. At the same time, the immune system must avoid "friendly fire" against the body's own tissue and innocuous environmental antigens originating from food, pollen, and the commensal microbiome. Multilayered and redundant mechanisms have evolved to provide counterbalances and prevent uncontrolled immune activation. First, most immature T cells with self-reactive receptors are deleted from the mature immune repertoire during development in the thymus through a process called central tolerance. In the thymus, a few self-reactive T cells escape deletion and are instructed to become regulatory T cells (Tregs) dedicated to suppressing unwanted immune responses. Mature T cells and Tregs populate the peripheral lymphoid organs where an array of peripheral tolerance mechanisms help to further safeguard immune self-tolerance.

Central Tolerance

During the first step of T-cell development, a repertoire of immature T cells with a vast array of distinct T-cell receptors (TCRs) are produced at random that permit recognition of the gamut of pathogens that an individual may encounter in a lifetime. However, many of the TCRs on the immature T cells also recognize molecules expressed by normal self-tissues. The T-cell development program has a built-in process for purging cells with self-reactivity to achieve the balance of maximizing protective immunity while avoiding autoimmune attacks.

T-cell development in humans begins in the fetus during midgestation in an environment normally devoid of invading pathogens. Ligands that trigger the TCRs of immature T cells at this stage are, therefore, expressed by normal self-tissue. This creates a window in time to distinguish between self- and foreign antigens. TCR-mediated signaling within this window induces programmed cell death, thus eliminating T cells with self-reactive TCRs. This process, referred to as negative selection, occurs in the thymus, an organ dedicated to producing T cells. Ubiquitously expressed and serum proteins are naturally present in the thymus, enabling deletion of T cells that are reactive to these self-antigens (Klein et al. 2014). However, the deletion of T cells reactive to tissue-restricted antigens, such as insulin made by the pancreatic β cells, relies on the protein autoimmune regulator (AIRE). AIRE drives the expression of peripheral tissue-restricted antigens in thymic medullary epithelial cells, thus purging the developing T-cell repertoire of TCRs reactive to tissue-restricted antigens (Anderson et al. 2002). Patients with mutation in AIRE develop a systemic autoimmune disease referred to as autoimmune polyglandular syndrome type 1 (APS-1), demonstrating the indispensable role of AIRE-mediated central tolerance (Husebye et al. 2018). Recently, a constellation of "mimetic cells" among medullary thymic epithelial cells has been reported (Bornstein et al. 2018; Miller et al. 2018; Bautista et al. 2021; Michelson et al. 2022). These cells mimic the gene expression and even the morphology of highly specialized cells in peripheral tissues, such as tuft cells of the mucosal barriers, the M cells of the gut, and keratinocytes of the skin. These cells transiently express AIRE and their development is partially AIRE dependent. Together with AIRE-expressing cells, they project peripheral self-antigens in the thymus so that the immature thymocytes reactive to these peripheral antigens can be deleted.

Another important function of central tolerance is the production of thymic Tregs (tTregs), a population of T cells dedicated to peripheral tolerance as discussed in the next section. Some immature thymocytes expressing TCRs with moderate affinity for self-antigens develop into Tregs (Owen et al. 2019b). TCR stimulation of developing CD4 single-positive thymocytes induces two tTreg precursors, $FoxP3^{low}CD25^{-}$ and $CD25^{+}FoxP3^{-}$, and subsequent interleukin (IL)-2 signaling in these precursor cells induces $CD25^{+}FoxP3^{+}$ Tregs (Lio and Hsieh 2008; Tai et al. 2013; Owen et al. 2019a). Importantly, continued self-antigen engagement by the TCR and IL-2 signaling secures Treg lineage commitment by programming the epigenetic landscape to ensure sustained expression of FoxP3 (Ohkura et al. 2012; Herppich et al. 2019). AIRE-expressing cells and mimetic medullary thymic epithelial cells play an important role in tTreg development by expressing peripheral tissue antigens (Malchow et al. 2016; Bluestone and Anderson

2020). Interestingly, Tregs developed from the FoxP3^{low}CD25^{-} precursor have a distinct TCR repertoire from those developed from the CD25^{+}FoxP3^{-}, pointing to differential reactivity to self-antigens (Owen et al. 2019a). tTreg development from either precursor depends on FoxP3. Genetic defects in the FoxP3 gene result in systemic autoimmune disease called polyendocrinopathy enteropathy X-linked syndrome (IPEX) in humans, corresponding to *scurfy* in mice (Bacchetta et al. 2006; Bluestone and Anderson 2020). Notably, a high percentage of IPEX patients suffer from T1D, suggesting a specialized function of Tregs in the prevention of autoimmune reaction against the pancreatic islets (Gambineri et al. 2003).

T cells generally do not recognize full-length protein antigens, but short peptide fragments instead. These peptides are presented to T cells by major histocompatibility complexes (MHCs), also referred to as human leukocyte antigens (HLAs) in humans. Among the 12 HLA genes in the human genome, HLA-A, B, C, E, F, G, DRA, DRB, DPA, DPB, DQA, and DQB, nine are highly polymorphic (all except HLA-E, F, and G). Thus, apart from identical twins, each individual inherits a unique array of HLA alleles from their parents. Different HLAs have differing abilities to bind and present peptides from self-antigens, which can impact thymic deletion of autoreactive cells and selection of Tregs. This forms the basis of the HLA linkage that characterizes many autoimmune diseases (Dendrou et al. 2018).

In summary, the major impact of central tolerance is to remove autoreactive T cells from the mature T-cell repertoire and seed the repertoire with Tregs to maintain tolerance in the periphery (i.e., beyond thymus). Factors that influence the processes of central tolerance, such as HLA and AIRE, can impact the efficiency of central tolerance and the risks of autoimmune diseases.

Peripheral Tolerance

Peripheral T-cell tolerance depends on both cell-intrinsic and extrinsic mechanisms that regulate T-cell activation. Several mechanisms of cell-intrinsic T-cell tolerance exist to restrain T-cell activation. Antigen-stimulated T cells express checkpoint coinhibitory receptors such as CTLA-4 and programmed cell death 1 (PD-1). CTLA-4 shares 30% amino acid homology with CD28 and competitively sequesters their shared ligands CD80 and CD86, thereby reducing CD28-mediated costimulatory signaling and limiting further T-cell activation (Krummel and Allison 1995; Walunas et al. 1996; Kim and Choi 2022). PD-1 is also up-regulated upon T-cell activation and facilitates the recruitment of phosphatases that extinguish TCR and CD28 signaling (Boussiotis 2016; Hui et al. 2017). The importance of these molecules in inhibiting T-cell responses is best shown by the efficacy of immune checkpoint inhibitors that interfere with these molecular brakes to unleash T-cell responses against tumors (Ribas and Wolchok 2018; Sharma et al. 2023). Up to 0.2%–1.9% of cancer patients develop T1D after receiving PD-1 blockade therapy, demonstrating that this pathway is also a gatekeeper of T-cell tolerance to pancreatic β cells (Quandt et al. 2021).

In addition to the inhibitory tolerance mechanisms described above, two other forms of cell-intrinsic tolerance have been described. Chronic antigen exposure induces a progressive state of exhaustion characterized by a decline in proliferative potential and a loss of cytokine secretion and cytotoxic functions (Kahan and Zajac 2019). Curiously, T-cell exhaustion is often observed among T cells in a tumor microenvironment, but not at sites of autoimmune tissue destruction (Gearty et al. 2022). Another form of T-cell tolerance, termed anergy, results from TCR signaling (signal 1) and NFAT translocation into the nucleus in the absence of engagement by costimulatory receptors (signal 2) such as CD28 (Macian 2005). It has been reported that this anergic state may be a precursor to the conversion of conventional T cells (Tconvs) into peripherally induced Tregs (pTregs) (Kalekar et al. 2016; Kuczma et al. 2021). This notion is corroborated by the report that activating mouse Tconv cells while intentionally blocking CD28 efficiently converts them into pTregs (Mikami et al. 2020). This process may naturally expand the specificities of the repertoire of tTregs to include antigens encountered in the periphery in the absence of infection or inflammation. tTregs and pTregs together are the main instigators of cell-extrinsic dominant tolerance, which is described in the next section.

The Role of Tregs

tTregs are exported from the thymus to exert their dominant immune suppressive action in the periphery. Together with pTregs, they are the essential guardians of immune self-tolerance (Sakaguchi et al. 2020; Dikiy and Rudensky 2023). A key feature of Treg function is "bystander suppression"—once activated by a specific antigen, Tregs exert suppressive effects on other immune cells (T cells, B cells, and innate immune cells) in an antigen-nonspecific fashion in the local tissue environment (Esensten et al. 2018; Ferreira et al. 2019). Another feature of Treg function is "infectious tolerance"—Tregs create an immunosuppressive milieu that promotes the conversion of other antigen-activated T cells in the local tissue to become pTregs, enabling the tolerogenic influence to linger beyond their own survival (Kendal and Waldmann 2010). These two features allow Tregs to maintain local immune tolerance dominantly and persistently. Additionally, Tregs have tissue-repair activities, either directly via secretion of growth factors such as amphiregulin or indirectly by promoting myeloid cells to adopt an anti-inflammatory and prohealing state (Fig. 1; Li et al. 2018; Ou et al. 2023).

The potency of Tregs largely lies in their versatility and adaptability, with the ability to deploy over a dozen different suppression mechanisms (Tang and Bluestone 2008; Dikiy and Rudensky 2023; Ou et al. 2023). In a steady-state condition without overt immune activation, Tregs maintain immune quiescence by depriving other T cells of IL-2, mediated by constitutive expression of the high-affinity receptor for IL-2 (Pandiyan et al. 2007; Sitrin et al. 2013). In addition, Tregs strip CD80 and CD86, costimulatory ligands for CD28, from dendritic cells by *trans*-endocytosis because of their high expression of CTLA-4

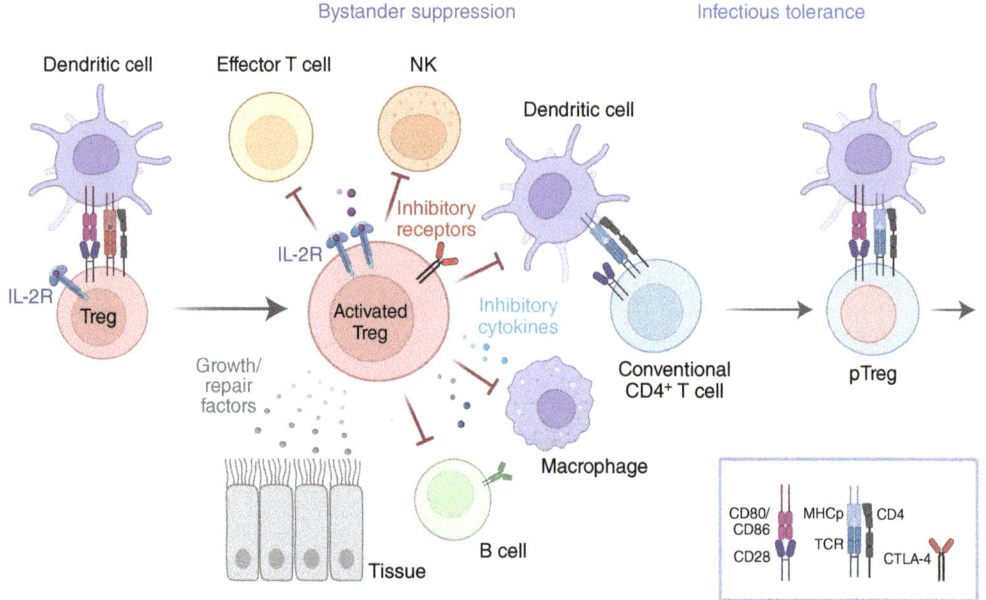

Figure 1. Mechanisms of regulatory T cells (Tregs) suppression. Antigen-activated Tregs dominantly suppress other immune cells in the vicinity via bystander suppression. Conventional $CD4^+$ T cells with distinct antigen specificity activated under the influence of Tregs can adopt a peripheral Treg (pTreg) cell fate and through infectious tolerance. (Figure generated with BioRender; biorender.com.)

(Qureshi et al. 2011), thus preventing T-cell activation and instead potentially promoting the development of pTregs. In the context of activated immune responses, Tregs are also activated to proliferate and express additional immunosuppressive molecules to prevent immune overactivation. Activated Tregs often adopt specialized phenotypes tailored to suppress specific types of immune response more effectively. For example, in a Th1-mediated immune response, expression of Th1 transcription factor T-bet enables Tregs to express the chemokine receptor CXCR3 and better traffic to sites of Th1 inflammation (Campbell and Koch 2011). Similar Treg "shadow" programs have also been described for Th2 and Th17 responses (Chaudhry et al. 2009; Zheng et al. 2009).

Most of the insights on the mechanisms of Treg function are derived from experiments in mice, and some similarities are found in human Tregs. For example, human Tregs also constitutively express high-affinity IL-2 receptor and CTLA-4 that can reduce the bioavailability of IL-2 and CD28 ligands, respectively. Additionally, activated human Tregs mediate bystander suppression using a variety of suppressive molecules (Sakaguchi et al. 2010) and confer infectious tolerance in vitro (Jonuleit et al. 2002; Stassen et al. 2004). Together, the localized, autonomous, polypharmaceutical functions of Tregs are difficult to replicate with conventional drugs, which underlies the enthusiasm for Treg-cell therapy for curbing unwanted immune responses (see below).

LOSS OF TOLERANCE IN TYPE 1 DIABETES

T1D is primarily a T lymphocyte–mediated autoimmune disease. The pathogenesis of T1D is still not fully understood, although genetic and environmental factors play critical roles in disease progression.

Genetic Factors

The most influential genetic contribution to T1D is from HLA genes on chromosome 6p21. Specific HLA allelic combinations increase the risk of developing T1D by over 40-fold. T1D risk alleles include the DRB1*0301-DQA1*0501-DQB1*0201 (DR3-DQ2.5) and DRB1*0401-DQA1*0301-DQB1*0302 (DR4-DQ8) haplotypes (Pociot et al. 2010; Wen et al. 2020). Interestingly, children expressing the DR4-DQ8 haplotype often develop anti-insulin autoantibodies and clinical disease early in life, while those expressing the DR3-DQ2.5 develop anti-GAD65 autoantibodies and clinical disease later in life (Krischer et al. 2015; Zhao et al. 2022). In stark contrast, the DRB1*15:01-DQB1*06:02 (DR15-DQ6) haplotype is robustly protective against T1D.

Specific HLA alleles may influence T1D risk by altering self-antigen presentation both during T-cell development in the thymus and antigen encounter in the periphery. For example, in non-T1D-associated HLA-DQ alleles, the aspartic acid residue at position 57 of the β-chain and the arginine residue at position 76 of the α-chain form a salt bridge that stabilizes the complex and influences peptide binding. T1D-associated DQ2.5 and DQ8 cannot form this salt bridge due to the absence of the β57 aspartic acid residue (Todd et al. 1987; Corper et al. 2000). This structural distinction may shape the repertoire of peptides presented by T1D-associated HLAs and impact thymic selection or peripheral activation of autoreactive T cells, thereby contributing to the susceptibility of T1D. Intriguingly, a recent study reported that nearly 10% of peptides presented by HLA-DQ8 have posttranslational modifications (PTMs), including hybrid insulin peptides (Tran et al. 2021). Presentation of posttranslationally modified neoantigens is one way to override immune self-tolerance because the absence of these PTMs during thymic selection preclude clonal TCR deletion or tTreg induction for these specificities.

The dominant protection of diabetes by the DR15-DQ6 haplotype is not completely understood. DR6 was shown to compete with coexpressed DQ8 in the presentation of islet autoantigens by antigen-presenting cells (van Lummel et al. 2019). However, it is not clear why presenting islet autoantigen by DR6 instead of DQ8 is protective. Individuals with the DR15-DQ6 haplotype paradoxically have higher frequencies of circulating islet-specific $CD4^+$ T cells and Tregs when compared to those with T1D-susceptible haplotypes (Wen et al. 2020). This finding suggests that the presence of robust Tregs may exert dominant control over autoreactive T cells to prevent islet destruction.

Beyond HLA distinctions, recent work in fine-grained genomic mapping of more than 60,000 T1D subjects identified 78 genetic loci associated with T1D (Robertson et al. 2021). Notably, the majority of the genes at these loci are expressed by immune cells, supporting the autoimmune etiology of T1D. The second-most correlative genetic locus for T1D contains the insulin gene itself. The specific region within the risk allele results in reduced expression of insulin in the thymus, thus making the deletion of insulin-specific T cells and/or the generation of insulin-specific tTregs less efficient.

Environmental Factors

The contribution of environmental factors is supported by the incomplete penetrance of T1D in monozygotic twins (Hyttinen et al. 2003). In the nonobese diabetic (NOD) murine model of autoimmune diabetes, manipulating the intestinal microbiota in a germ-free environment or using specific antibiotics dramatically shapes the risk of developing insulitis and diabetes (Silverman et al. 2017). The pancreatic lymph nodes (LNs) are key to initiating autoimmunity against pancreatic β cells in mice, as this is the site of initial expansion for small numbers of islet-specific T cells that escaped thymic deletion (Turley et al. 2003). In mice, drainage of the pancreas occurs in three LNs: the liver, celiac, and duodenal (Brown et al. 2023). The existence of a codrainage among the pancreas, gut, and liver may facilitate immune cross talk among these organs. For example, intestinal viral infections can promote pancreatic autoimmunity, food allergies, and celiac disease (Bouziat et al. 2017; Esterházy et al. 2019; Brown et al. 2023). An immune response to an infection may license antigen-presenting cells such as dendritic cells and B cells (e.g., via up-regulation of CD80 and CD86) to convert a homeostatically tolerogenic tissue environment to an immunogenic one. Indeed, the ongoing international The Environmental Determinants of Diabetes in the Young (TEDDY) study has found episodes of respiratory and gastrointestinal infections and the gut virome to be associated with the development of anti-islet autoantibodies (Rewers et al. 2018).

Treg Defects

While CD28-mediated costimulation is critical to initiate an immune response, it is also paradoxically essential to generate thymus-derived Tregs. In NOD mice, preventing CD28 ligation either by CTLA-4 Ig treatment or by deletion of the CD28 gene significantly reduced the number of Tregs and exacerbated diabetes (Salomon et al. 2000). CD28 costimulation is essential both for thymic development and peripheral homeostasis of Tregs (Tang et al. 2003; Tai et al. 2005). Interestingly, CD28 signaling also contributes to thymic deletion of self-reactive Tconv cells, although the intracellular domains required for tTreg differentiation and deletion appear to be distinct (Riley and June 2005; Watanabe et al. 2020).

A central hallmark of Tregs is the inability to produce IL-2, despite the requirement of IL-2 signaling to maintain FoxP3 expression and cell survival. Instead, Tregs constitutively express CD25, the α subunit of the trimeric IL-2 receptor complex (α [CD25], β [CD122], and γ [CD132]). This trimeric form of the IL-2 receptor has heightened affinity and responsiveness for IL-2 relative to the dimeric form lacking CD25 (Abbas et al. 2018). IL-2 is necessary for tTreg development, as well as pTreg induction, persistence, and survival (Setoguchi et al. 2005; Toomer and Malek 2018). In NOD mice, the paucity of IL-2 in chronically inflamed islets impairs the function of Tregs, preventing effective suppression of pancreatic β-cell destruction (Tang et al. 2008). In T1D patients, circulating Tregs also have an impaired response to IL-2 correlating with reduced phosphorylation of STAT5 (pSTAT5), a transcription factor essential for Treg lineage maintenance (Long et al. 2010, 2011; Garg et al. 2012). Intriguingly, NOD mice and some T1D patients have anti-IL-2 autoantibodies, which could limit the bioavailability of IL-2 and contribute to Treg impairment (Pérol et al. 2016). Lastly, a recent meta-analysis identified nine core genes whose expressions were altered under the influence of T1D-associated genetic loci. Many of these core genes, including FOXP3, CTLA-4, STAT1, and IL-10RA, were implicated in Treg development and function, suggesting an overall defect in Tregs as an underlying driver of the disease (Iakovliev et al. 2023).

Regulation-Resistant Effector T Cells

In addition to Treg impairment, experiments in mice show that autoreactive effector T cells can gain resistance to Treg control during the course of chronic activation (You et al. 2005; D'Alise et al. 2008). Analyses of human peripheral blood have also identified that T cells from T1D patients are more resistant to Treg suppression than T cells from normal donors (Lawson et al. 2008; Schneider et al. 2008). Inflammatory cytokines (e.g., IL-1, IL-6, IL-15, and IL-21) promote effector T cells resistance to Treg suppression in both mouse and human systems (Pasare and Medzhitov 2003; Peluso et al. 2007; Hmida et al. 2012; Schenten et al. 2014). In addition, the strength of TCR signaling and CD28 costimulation received by the effector T cells help them to overcome suppression by Tregs (Wohlfert and Clark 2007). In this regard, it is tempting to speculate that the neoantigen-specific effector T cells, such as posttranslationally modified peptides and hybrid insulin peptide (Wiles and Delong 2019; Nguyen et al. 2021), are likely to be more difficult to suppress because of their high-affinity TCRs due to a lack of negative selection against the neoantigens during thymic development (Fig. 2).

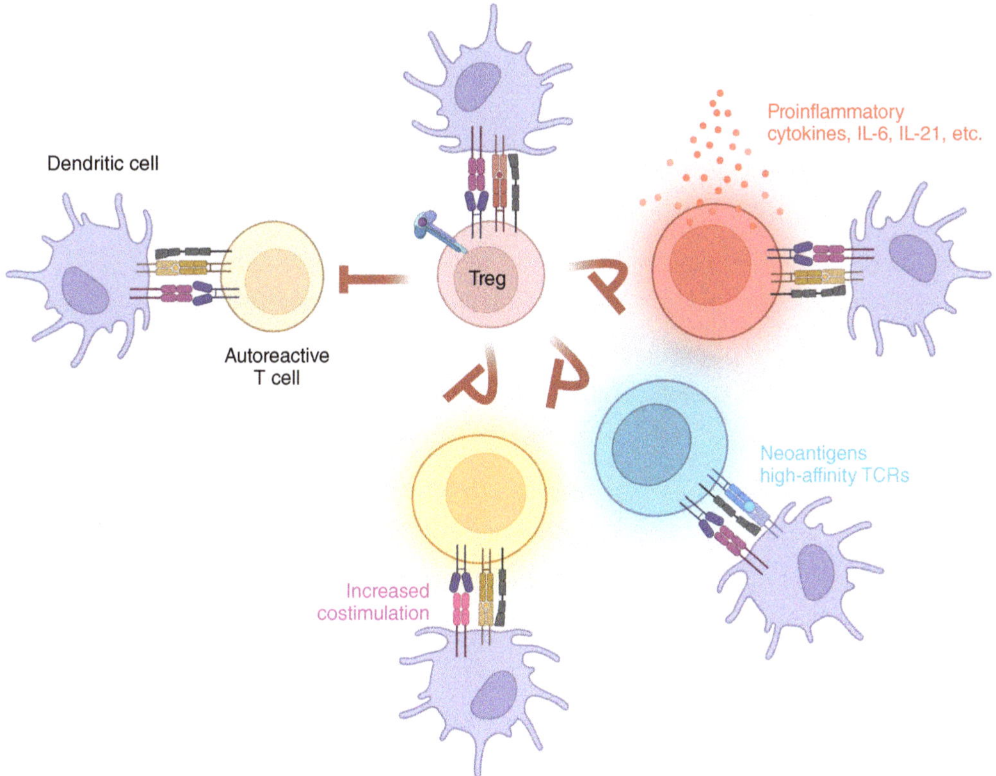

Figure 2. Mechanisms of regulatory T-cell (Treg) resistance. The presence of proinflammatory cytokine effector cells with high-affinity T-cell receptors (TCRs) such as those that react to neoantigens and high expression costimulation ligands on antigen-presenting cells can override Treg-mediated suppression. (Figure generated with BioRender; biorender.com.)

REBALANCING THE IMMUNE SYSTEM IN T1D

Purging the Effectors

T-Cell Depletion and Inactivation

Several approaches to disrupt islet-specific effector T cells have been explored, aiming to slow the autoimmune process and preserve pancreatic β cells. The most aggressive protocol consists of an autologous nonmyeloablative hematopoietic stem cell transplantation combining the administration of cyclophosphamide and high doses of antithymocyte globulin (ATG) for leukocyte depletion (Voltarelli et al. 2007). More than 50% of individuals experienced insulin independence, but only 32% remained insulin-independent after up to 48 months of follow-up (D'Addio et al. 2014). Considering the toxicity and side effects associated with this approach, others have tried to administer ATG alone, which failed to preserve islet function (Gitelman et al. 2016). ATG infusion induces profound T-cell depletion followed by incomplete recovery. Lymphopenia induces "spontaneous" T-cell proliferation and T-cell activation that may exacerbate autoimmune conditions. This consideration has prompted the evaluation of low-dose ATG for T1D. Initial study of low-dose ATG (2.5 mg/kg) combined with pegylated granulocyte colony stimulating factor (G-CSF) (ATG + G-CSF), used to mobilize hematopoietic stem cells, had early promising results at 1 and 2 years in new-onset T1D (Haller et al. 2015, 2018, 2019), but no statistically significant improvement in stimulated C-peptide when compared with placebo controls at 5 years (Lin et al. 2021). A follow-up study compared the effect of low-dose ATG alone or in combination with G-CSF in new-onset T1D and found low-dose ATG alone significantly improved C-peptide preservation over placebos at 1 and 2 years, whereas the additional of G-CSF did not provide therapeutic benefit (Haller et al. 2018, 2019). Mechanistic analyses of the peripheral blood of trial patients show milder depletion of T cells and relative preservation of Tregs in most patients, whereas effector T-cell exhaustion was associated with therapeutic response to low-dose ATG (Jacobsen et al. 2023). Ongoing efforts in Europe are aiming at determining the minimum effective low dose of ATG for the treatment of T1D (Wilhelm-Benartzi et al. 2021), whereas a U.S. group is evaluating efficacy of low-dose ATG in delaying T1D onset in at-risk autoantibody-positive individuals (Foster et al. 2024).

Alefacept, an LFA-3 IgG fusion molecule, demonstrated sustained C-peptide preservation after two courses of treatment in 30% of the new-onset T1D individuals (Rigby et al. 2013, 2015). LFA-3 is a ligand of T-cell costimulatory molecule CD2, which is highly expressed on memory and effector T cells but relatively low on naive T cells and Tregs. Thus, alefacept treatment favors deletion of effector cells while being relatively sparing of Tregs. Analyses of samples collected from subjects enrolled in the trial show the emergence of exhausted $CD57^{+}TIGIT^{+}KLRG1^{+}$ CD8 T cells in those who responded to the treatment (Diggins et al. 2021). In contrast, the presence of islet antigen-reactive TNF-α and GM-CSF-producing $CD4^{+}$ T cells in peripheral blood mononuclear cells (PBMCs) before treatment predicted a failure to respond to alefacept (Balmas et al. 2023).

The first biologic that has been approved by the US Food and Drug Administration (FDA) to delay T1D in children (8 yr or older) is teplizumab, an anti-CD3 monoclonal antibody engineered to avoid its binding to the FC receptors (FcRs) (Herold et al. 2019; Ramos et al. 2023a). Anti-CD3 antibodies typically form high-order clustering of the TCR-CD3 complex at the interface of T cells and FcR-expressing cells to activate T cells. By mutating the FcR-binding domain, teplizumab engages T cells bivalently, resulting in alternative signaling in T cells that specifically kills and anergizes CD8 and Th1 effector cells while sparing native cells and Tregs (Penaranda et al. 2011). Consequently, despite the ability to bind all T cells, FcR-nonbinding (FNB) anti-CD3 selectively disarms activated effector T cells. When administered at the peak of an immune response driven by clonal T-cell expansion, FNB anti-CD3 reduces T cells specific for the response-driving target antigens, leading to tissue-specific immune modulation in mouse models. This mode of action is reflected in the preclinical observation that short-term treatment with FNB anti-CD3 induces stable diabetes remission in NOD mice when administered at the time of diabetes onset, when more islet-specific autoreactive T cells are activated (Chatenoud et al. 1994). Similarly, while prophylactic treatment with FNB anti-CD3 delayed islet transplant rejection, treatment at the peak of the alloimmune response (i.e., 7–11 days after transplantation) induced long-term graft tolerance (Goto et al. 2013). In addition, there is evidence that the partial agonist signal induces cells with regulatory function in the draining LNs and gut in mice and $CD8^{+}$ T cells with signs of exhaustion in the peripheral blood of patients (Belghith et al. 2003; Esplugues et al. 2011; Penaranda et al. 2011; Waldron-Lynch et al. 2012). It is worth noting that mechanisms of action of teplizumab in T1D patients are more challenging to elucidate and likely to be variable in different subset of patients with distinct immunological features (Tooley et al. 2016).

B-Lymphocyte Depletion

T1D is not considered to be an antibody-mediated disease, notably because the disease can develop in patients with X-linked agammaglobulinemia bearing a complete or near-complete absence of antibodies (Martin et al. 2001). Yet, in the vast majority of T1D patients, several autoantibodies are produced against insulin, the insulinoma-associated tyrosine phosphatase-like protein (IA-2), the 65-kDa glutamic acid decarboxylase isoform (GAD65), or the zinc transporter 8 (ZnT8). Thus, the risk of developing T1D was evaluated in a large western cohort of children, and the number of autoantibodies at seroconversion (preceding the disease) predicted the risk of developing the disease later (Gorus et al. 2017; Anand et al. 2021). However, in NOD mice, depleting the IgM (mu) B cells resulted in protection from disease (Noorchashm et al. 1997). Transient B-cell depletion with rituximab delayed C-peptide decline in patients with new onset T1D (Pescovitz et al. 2009), although it did not prevent the reemergence of autoreactive B cells and anti-islet antibodies (Chamberlain et al. 2016). Thus, while autoantibodies are considered nonpathogenic, their presence indicates the involvement of B lymphocytes in the autoimmune response in other way. For example, B lymphocytes can serve as antigen-presenting cells in T1D (Noorchashm et al. 1999; Rivera et al. 2001). B-cell presentation of autoantigens may be enhanced as a subset of the cells express B-cell receptors specific for autoantigens that allow the cells to bind and internalize autoantigens and present immunogenic peptides in the context of MHC. In addition, B cells express a high level of costimulatory molecules that can increase the activation potential of the cells. Thus, like in many autoimmune diseases, most prominently multiple sclerosis (Carlson et al. 2024), the role of B cells goes beyond their autoantibody-producing activity.

Boosting Tregs

IL-2 and IL-2 Mutein Therapies

Considering the frequent association of polymorphisms in IL-2 and IL-2RA (i.e., CD25) with autoimmune diseases, and the essential role of IL-2 in Treg development, homeostasis, and function, there has been substantial interest in developing Treg-targeted low-dose IL-2 therapies to treat autoimmune diseases, including T1D. In the NOD model, expressing a mutant transgenic IL-2 receptor with reduced signaling in all T cells increases diabetes incidence, due to a selective impairment of Tregs (Dwyer et al. 2017). Conversely, IL-2 administration not only prevents but also reverses diabetes, notably by restoring the clonotypic expansion of activated islet-specific Tregs ($CD44^{high}CD62L^{low}$) (Tang et al. 2008; Grinberg-Bleyer et al. 2010; Mhanna et al. 2021). These preclinical results encouraged trials to evaluate low-dose IL-2 treatment in T1D patients. Results from several clinical trials thus far have shown good tolerability and a selective increase in the proportion of Tregs relative to effector T cells (Todd et al. 2016; Rosenzwajg et al. 2020; Lorenzon et al. 2024). In the phase 1/2 DF-IL2-Child cohort study involving 24 children with T1D (NCT01862120), the authors showed improved maintenance of induced C-peptide production at 1 year in the seven Treg high responders as compared with low responders further supporting the potential of Tregs in regulating autoimmunity in T1D (Rosenzwajg et al. 2020). The results of another efficacy trial are still pending (NCT02411253, completed, no results posted). Thus, IL-2 therapy for human autoimmune diseases is in early stage of development (Raeber et al. 2023).

In fact, in some clinical trials, the IL-2 therapy may have resulted in increased β-cell destruction (Long et al. 2012; Dong et al. 2021), since activated natural killer (NK) and CD8 cells can express high levels of CD25 effector cells and respond to the low dose IL-2 treatment (Rosenzwajg et al. 2015). Thus, alternative approaches are under development to refine the selectivity for Tregs. One strategy is to engineer IL-2 muteins to be more dependent on CD25 by increasing their affinity for CD25 and/or decreasing their affinity for CD122/CD132 (Peterson et al. 2018; Efe et al. 2024). Another strategy is to complex IL-2 with monoclonal antibodies that compete with the CD122/CD132 subunits (Webster et al. 2009; Létourneau et al. 2010). Certain antibodies, upon binding, modify the conformation of IL-2 via an allosteric effect. This modulates the affinity for CD25 and gives a competitive advantage for Tregs (Trotta et al. 2018). By complexing with antibodies, this approach also increases the half-life of IL-2 from minutes to hours. More recently, it has been shown that the stability of the cytokine/antibody complex can be enhanced by fusing both molecules as a single-chain protein that confers protection in mouse models of colitis and checkpoint inhibitor-induced diabetes (VanDyke et al. 2022). Yet another strategy engages the noncanonical IL-2-CD25-CCR7 chemokine receptor signaling pathway, which promotes the suppressive function of Tregs and ameliorates murine experimental autoimmune encephalomyelitis (Sun et al. 2023). Lastly, bispecific approaches are also being tested to target IL-2 and IL-2 muteins to sites of inflammation or to bind to other molecules selectively expressed on Tregs.

Adoptive Treg-Cell Therapy

In the NOD mouse, a single infusion of islet antigen-specific, TCR transgenic Tregs was orders of magnitude more effective at preventing diabetes than polyclonal Tregs (Tang et al. 2004; Tarbell et al. 2004). Similarly, the adoptive transfer of polyclonal islet-infiltrating Tregs naturally pre-enriched for islet antigen specificity, but not polyclonal Tregs isolated from pancreatic LNs or the spleen, prevented islet destruction (Spence et al. 2018). The infused islet antigen-specific Tregs trafficked to the pancreatic LN, where they become activated and prevent activation of effector T cells (Tang et al. 2006). The therapeutic Tregs also efficiently trafficked to inflamed islets and suppressed inflammation and cytotoxic effector T cells within a few days and prevented further influx of T cells and inflammatory monocytes (Mahne et al. 2015; Klementowicz et al. 2017). It is worth noting that not all islet antigen-specific Tregs have the same efficacy and Tregs that showed better protection were more activated in the pancreatic draining LNs (Tang et al. 2004).

The robust preclinical data of Treg therapy in diabetes protection inspired the translation of this therapy to T1D patients by developing a process to manufacture highly pure human Tregs (Earle et al. 2005; Liu et al. 2006; Putnam et al. 2009). Early phase safety studies showed that it was feasible to manufacture billions of autologous Tregs, with infusions well-tolerated by T1D patients (Marek-Trzonkowska et al. 2012; Bluestone et al. 2015). Moreover, by labeling the cells with deuterium during cell manufacturing, the fate of the infused autologous Tregs can be tracked. The infused Tregs peaked in the peripheral blood in the first 2 weeks and sharply declined in the next 10 weeks. In most patients, deuterium signal could be detected among circulating Tregs at 1 year after infusion, demonstrating that some of the infused Tregs were long-lived. Moreover, no deuterium signal was detected among Tconvs, suggesting that the Treg products maintained lineage identity after infusion. To investigate whether the reduction of infused Tregs in the first 3 months was due to lower IL-2 availability in vivo when compared to that in the in vitro culture medium, a follow-up study was conducted to assess the impact of low-dose IL-2 on Treg persistence after infusion. Low doses of IL-2 after Treg infusion indeed promoted Treg persistence but also led to the activation of NK, mucosal-associated invariant T, and clonal CD8$^+$ T cells (Dong et al. 2021). Thus, the decline of infused Tregs was likely due to IL-2 withdrawal and could be corrected by IL-2 supplementation. However, a phase 2 T-rex study in patients with new-onset T1D failed to demonstrate efficacy in preventing C-peptide decline by infusion of autologous polyclonal Tregs (NCT02691247; Bender et al. 2024). Together early clinical experiences show the feasibility and safety of Treg adoptive therapy in T1D, and also identify increasing Treg persistence and islet antigen-specificity as means to increase the efficacy of the therapy in future development.

Future Directions

In the past decade, many immunotherapies have been evaluated to restore tolerance in T1D and none have achieved durable restoration of tolerance. Natural immune self-tolerance is established via deletion of self-reactive cells and installation of dominant Tregs. This conceptual framework can guide the design of tolerance-promoting therapies in the future.

Inactivating Islet Antigen-Specific Effectors

The optimal approach to inactivating effector T cells should spare Tregs and be selective for islet antigen-specific effectors. Alefacept, low-dose ATG, and teplizumab are all relatively Treg sparing, which may explain the persistent preservation of C-peptide after a short course of the drugs. However, C-peptide declines in most participants after a delay of a few years, demonstrating reemergence of effectors. It is possible that repeated dosing may reinforce the favorable tipping of Treg versus effector balance to further extend the therapeutic benefit with these therapies. All these agents induce transient and partial decrease of T cells in circulation.

Particularly, the therapeutic actions of alefacept and ATG are mainly though antibody-dependent- and complement-dependent cytotoxicity (Mohty 2007; Binder et al. 2020). Deleting a large fraction of the T-cell compartment can promote homeostatic T-cell proliferation and activation of the remaining effector T cells, thereby antagonizing the therapeutic effects. Antigen-specific deletional approaches may avoid this problem. In this regard, multiple platform technologies are in active preclinical development. Polymeric nanoparticles and liposomes loaded with islet antigens can inactivate antigen-specific T cells in vivo and prevent diabetes (Tsai et al. 2010; Yeste et al. 2016; Jamison et al. 2019; Lewis et al. 2019; Bergot et al. 2020). A challenge to antigen-specific inactivation of effector cells is the multiple known and unknown specificities and heterogenous pathophysiology in a diverse patient population. Some of the antigen-targeting strategies also boost antigen-specific Tregs, which may induce dominant suppression of effectors without needed to deplete all of them.

Next-Generation Tregs for T1D

A direct way of increasing Tregs is adoptive Treg-cell therapy. As noted above, clinical Treg-cell therapy development thus far has pointed to the need to enhance Treg specificity for pancreatic islets and to improve Treg persistence after infusion. Treg specificity can be redirected using engineered TCRs or chimeric antigen receptors (CARs). Preclinical data suggest that the efficacy of islet antigen-specific Tregs is associated with stronger in vivo activation by islet antigens. Thus, targeting antigens that are presented in sufficient abundance with strongly reactive TCRs may help ensure therapeutic efficacy. A challenge for TCR engineering is the HLA-restricted nature of TCR-mediated antigen recognition. However, since T1D is strongly linked to HLA class II, a few carefully selected TCRs targeting antigen presented by T1D-associated HLAs (e.g., DQ8, DR4, etc.) would enable coverage across most T1D patients. An alternative approach would be to redirect the specificity against islet antigens using CARs, which can be designed to target any surface-bound antigen. Anti-insulin and anti-tetraspanin 7 CARs have been generated and shown to be functional in vitro, but lack efficacy in vivo (Tenspolde et al. 2019; Pieper et al. 2023). More recently, two groups reported that mouse Tregs engineered with a CAR specific for an MHC-II-presented insulin B chain–derived peptide effectively suppressed spontaneous diabetes, providing an important proof-of-concept of this strategy (Obarorakpor et al. 2023; Spanier et al. 2023).

Synthetic immunology may offer a solution to ensure the long-term survival of infused Tregs. IL-2 is essential for Treg homeostasis and lineage stability, but the pleotropic effect of IL-2 and the narrow therapeutic window between stimulating Tregs versus other IL-2-responsive cells make it difficult to use in vivo. The development of orthogonal IL-2 and orthogonal IL-2R systems may solve this challenge in the context of Treg-cell therapy (Sockolosky et al. 2018). Therapeutic Tregs can be engineered to express an orthogonal IL-2 receptor, and the recipients can be treated with the orthogonal IL-2 that only stimulate Tregs expressing the cognate receptor. This approach has been shown to selectively expand Tregs without activating CD8 T cells in a mouse model of graft-versus-host disease (Ramos et al. 2023b).

Lastly, while human Treg lineage instability has not been observed in clinical trials thus far, lineage-tracing murine models have revealed a natural susceptibility for Tregs to convert into exFoxP3 T cells that can acquire proinflammatory and/or cytotoxic functions. As strategies to engineer Tregs that specifically target and persist in pancreatic islets continue to mature, it will become increasingly necessary to ensure the stability of Treg identity in the cellular products. Given its central importance to Treg identity and function, one strategy is to overexpress FOXP3, an approach that has been shown to improve the stability, efficacy, and safety of human Tregs in preclinical models (McGovern et al. 2022; Henschel et al. 2023). As an additional precaution, kill switches may be engineered to further safeguard against the potential malignant transformation or proinflammatory conversion of engineered Treg therapeutics (Mohseni et al. 2020).

Combinational Therapy

Convincing preclinical and clinical evidence suggests that T1D arise from an imbalance of pathogenic effector T cells and protective Tregs. While inactivating effectors and promoting Tregs individually may offer long-term disease protection in some T1D patients as seen in preclinical models and in some clinical trials, a more reliable approach to restore immune self-tolerance may require combining the two modalities. A recent trial randomized children with recent onset of T1D into three groups of Treg therapy alone, Tregs and anti-CD20 mAb (rituximab), and untreated control and observed superior C-peptide preservation in the combination group during the 2-year follow-up. However, the study did not include an anti-CD20-only arm, so it is difficult to know whether the combination therapy was better than B-cell depletion alone (Zieliński et al. 2022). Considering the prolonger therapeutic benefit of targeting effector T cells with teplizumab therapy in T1D, it would be interesting to determine whether infusion of Tregs would further extend the protection by reinforcing dominant regulatory tolerance.

CONCLUSION

The discovery of insulin and its therapeutic application in 1921 completely changed the course of T1D, which was otherwise universally fatal. It must be acknowledged that insulin is effective in managing the symptoms of T1D, but it does not modify the pathophysiology of the disease. In 2022, more than 100 years after the discovery of insulin, the first disease-modifying therapy for T1D, teplizumab, was approved by the FDA. Research advances have provided a roadmap to restore immune tolerance in T1D, including an ever deeper understanding of T1D pathophysiology and an armamentarium of new technologies for generating small molecules, proteins, and cells with designed therapeutic properties. The pace of therapeutic development will undoubtedly quicken, so it is reasonable to stride toward the goal of developing tolerance-promoting curative therapies to eradicate T1D.

REFERENCES

Abbas AK, Trotta E, Simeonov DR, Marson A, Bluestone JA. 2018. Revisiting IL-2: biology and therapeutic prospects.

Sci Immunol **3:** eaat1482. doi:10.1126/sciimmunol.aat1482

Anand V, Li Y, Liu B, Ghalwash M, Koski E, Ng K, Dunne JL, Jönsson J, Winkler C, Knip M, et al. 2021. Islet autoimmunity and HLA markers of presymptomatic and clinical type 1 diabetes: joint analyses of prospective cohort studies in Finland, Germany, Sweden, and the U.S. *Diabetes Care* **44:** 2269–2276. doi:10.2337/dc20-1836

Anderson MS, Venanzi ES, Klein L, Chen Z, Berzins SP, Turley SJ, von Boehmer H, Bronson R, Dierich A, Benoist C, et al. 2002. Projection of an immunological self shadow within the thymus by the AIRE protein. *Science* **298:** 1395–1401. doi:10.1126/science.1075958

Bacchetta R, Passerini L, Gambineri E, Dai M, Allan SE, Perroni L, Dagna-Bricarelli F, Sartirana C, Matthes-Martin S, Lawitschka A, et al. 2006. Defective regulatory and effector T cell functions in patients with FOXP3 mutations. *J Clin Invest* **116:** 1713–1722. doi:10.1172/JCI25112

Balmas E, Chen J, Hu AK, DeBerg HA, Rosasco MG, Gersuk VH, Serti E, Speake C, Greenbaum CJ, Nepom GT, et al. 2023. Islet-autoreactive CD4$^+$ T cells are linked with response to alefacept in type 1 diabetes. *JCI Insight* **8:** e167881. doi:10.1172/jci.insight.167881

Bautista JL, Cramer NT, Miller CN, Chavez J, Berrios DI, Byrnes LE, Germino J, Ntranos V, Sneddon JB, Burt TD, et al. 2021. Single-cell transcriptional profiling of human thymic stroma uncovers novel cellular heterogeneity in the thymic medulla. *Nat Commun* **12:** 1096. doi:10.1038/s41467-021-21346-6

Belghith M, Bluestone JA, Barriot S, Mégret J, Bach JF, Chatenoud L. 2003. TGF-β-dependent mechanisms mediate restoration of self-tolerance induced by antibodies to CD3 in overt autoimmune diabetes. *Nat Med* **9:** 1202–1208. doi:10.1038/nm924

Bender C, Wiedeman AE, Hu A, Ylescupidez A, Sietsema WK, Herold KC, Griffin KJ, Gitelman SE, Long SA, T-Rex SG, et al. 2024. A phase 2 randomized trial with autologous polyclonal expanded regulatory T cells in children with new-onset type 1 diabetes. *Sci Transl Med* **16:** eadn2404. doi:10.1126/scitranslmed.adn2404

Bergot AS, Buckle I, Cikaluru S, Naranjo JL, Wright CM, Zheng G, Talekar M, Hamilton-Williams EE, Thomas R. 2020. Regulatory T cells induced by single-peptide liposome immunotherapy suppress islet-specific T cell responses to multiple antigens and protect from autoimmune diabetes. *J Immunol* **204:** 1787–1797. doi:10.4049/jimmunol.1901128

Binder C, Cvetkovski F, Sellberg F, Berg S, Paternina Visbal H, Sachs DH, Berglund E, Berglund D. 2020. CD2 immunobiology. *Front Immunol* **11:** 1090. doi:10.3389/fimmu.2020.01090

Bluestone JA, Anderson M. 2020. Tolerance in the age of immunotherapy. *N Engl J Med* **383:** 1156–1166. doi:10.1056/NEJMra1911109

Bluestone JA, Buckner JH, Fitch M, Gitelman SE, Gupta S, Hellerstein MK, Herold KC, Lares A, Lee MR, Li K, et al. 2015. Type 1 diabetes immunotherapy using polyclonal regulatory T cells. *Sci Transl Med* **7:** 315ra189. doi:10.1126/scitranslmed.aad4134

Bornstein C, Nevo S, Giladi A, Kadouri N, Pouzolles M, Gerbe F, David E, Machado A, Chuprin A, Tóth B, et al. 2018. Single-cell mapping of the thymic stroma identifies IL-25-producing tuft epithelial cells. *Nature* **559:** 622–626. doi:10.1038/s41586-018-0346-1

Boussiotis VA. 2016. Molecular and biochemical aspects of the PD-1 checkpoint pathway. *N Engl J Med* **375:** 1767–1778. doi:10.1056/NEJMra1514296

Bouziat R, Hinterleitner R, Brown JJ, Stencel-Baerenwald JE, Ikizler M, Mayassi T, Meisel M, Kim SM, Discepolo V, Pruijssers AJ, et al. 2017. Reovirus infection triggers inflammatory responses to dietary antigens and development of celiac disease. *Science* **356:** 44–50. doi:10.1126/science.aah5298

Brown H, Komnick MR, Brigleb PH, Dermody TS, Esterházy D. 2023. Lymph node sharing between pancreas, gut, and liver leads to immune crosstalk and regulation of pancreatic autoimmunity. *Immunity* **56:** 2070–2085.e11. doi:10.1016/j.immuni.2023.07.008

Campbell DJ, Koch MA. 2011. Phenotypical and functional specialization of FOXP3$^+$ regulatory T cells. *Nat Rev Immunol* **11:** 119–130. doi:10.1038/nri2916

Carlson AK, Amin M, Cohen JA. 2024. Drugs targeting CD20 in multiple sclerosis: pharmacology, efficacy, safety, and tolerability. *Drugs* **84:** 285–304. doi:10.1007/s40265-024-02011-w

Chamberlain N, Massad C, Oe T, Cantaert T, Herold KC, Meffre E. 2016. Rituximab does not reset defective early B cell tolerance checkpoints. *J Clin Invest* **126:** 282–287. doi:10.1172/JCI83840

Chatenoud L, Thervet E, Primo J, Bach JF. 1994. Anti-CD3 antibody induces long-term remission of overt autoimmunity in nonobese diabetic mice. *Proc Natl Acad Sci* **91:** 123–127. doi:10.1073/pnas.91.1.123

Chaudhry A, Rudra D, Treuting P, Samstein RM, Liang Y, Kas A, Rudensky AY. 2009. CD4$^+$ regulatory T cells control TH17 responses in a Stat3-dependent manner. *Science* **326:** 986–991. doi:10.1126/science.1172702

Corper AL, Stratmann T, Apostolopoulos V, Scott CA, Garcia KC, Kang AS, Wilson IA, Teyton L. 2000. A structural framework for deciphering the link between I-Ag7 and autoimmune diabetes. *Science* **288:** 505–511. doi:10.1126/science.288.5465.505

D'Addio F, Valderrama Vasquez A, Ben Nasr M, Franek E, Zhu D, Li L, Ning G, Snarski E, Fiorina P. 2014. Autologous nonmyeloablative hematopoietic stem cell transplantation in new-onset type 1 diabetes: a multicenter analysis. *Diabetes* **63:** 3041–3046. doi:10.2337/db14-0295

D'Alise AM, Auyeung V, Feuerer M, Nishio J, Fontenot J, Benoist C, Mathis D. 2008. The defect in T-cell regulation in NOD mice is an effect on the T-cell effectors. *Proc Natl Acad Sci* **105:** 19857–19862. doi:10.1073/pnas.0810713105

Dendrou CA, Petersen J, Rossjohn J, Fugger L. 2018. HLA variation and disease. *Nat Rev Immunol* **18:** 325–339. doi:10.1038/nri.2017.143

Diggins KE, Serti E, Muir V, Rosasco M, Lu T, Balmas E, Nepom G, Long SA, Linsley PS. 2021. Exhausted-like CD8$^+$ T cell phenotypes linked to C-peptide preservation in alefacept-treated T1D subjects. *JCI Insight* **6:** e142680. doi:10.1172/jci.insight.142680

Dikiy S, Rudensky AY. 2023. Principles of regulatory T cell function. *Immunity* **56:** 240–255. doi:10.1016/j.immuni.2023.01.004

Dong S, Hiam-Galvez KJ, Mowery CT, Herold KC, Gitelman SE, Esensten JH, Liu W, Lares AP, Leinbach AS, Lee M, et al. 2021. The effect of low-dose IL-2 and Treg adoptive cell therapy in patients with type 1 diabetes. *JCI Insight* **6:** e147474. doi:10.1172/jci.insight.147474

Dwyer CJ, Bayer AL, Fotino C, Yu L, Cabello-Kindelan C, Ward NC, Toomer KH, Chen Z, Malek TR. 2017. Altered homeostasis and development of regulatory T cell subsets represent an IL-2R-dependent risk for diabetes in NOD mice. *Sci Signal* **10:** eaam9563. doi:10.1126/scisignal.aam9563

Earle KE, Tang Q, Zhou X, Liu W, Zhu S, Bonyhadi ML, Bluestone JA. 2005. In vitro expanded human $CD4^+CD25^+$ regulatory T cells suppress effector T cell proliferation. *Clin Immunol* **115:** 3–9. doi:10.1016/j.clim.2005.02.017

Efe O, Gassen RB, Morena L, Ganchiku Y, Al Jurdi A, Lape IT, Ventura-Aguiar P, LeGuern C, Madsen JC, Shriver Z, et al. 2024. A humanized IL-2 mutein expands Tregs and prolongs transplant survival in preclinical models. *J Clin Invest* **134:** e173107. doi:10.1172/JCI173107

Esensten JH, Muller YD, Bluestone JA, Tang Q. 2018. Regulatory T cell therapy for autoimmune and autoinflammatory diseases: the next frontier. *J Allergy Clin Immunol* **142:** 1710–1718. doi:10.1016/j.jaci.2018.10.015

Esplugues E, Huber S, Gagliani N, Hauser AE, Town T, Wan YY, O'Connor W, Rongvaux A, Van Rooijen N, Haberman AM, et al. 2011. Control of TH17 cells occurs in the small intestine. *Nature* **475:** 514–518. doi:10.1038/nature10228

Esterházy D, Canesso MCC, Mesin L, Muller PA, de Castro TBR, Lockhart A, ElJalby M, Faria AMC, Mucida D. 2019. Compartmentalized gut lymph node drainage dictates adaptive immune responses. *Nature* **569:** 126–130. doi:10.1038/s41586-019-1125-3

Ferreira LMR, Muller YD, Bluestone JA, Tang Q. 2019. Next-generation regulatory T cell therapy. *Nat Rev Drug Discov* **18:** 749–769. doi:10.1038/s41573-019-0041-4

Foster TP, Jacobsen LM, Bruggeman B, Salmon C, Hosford J, Chen A, Cintron M, Mathews CE, Wasserfall C, Brusko MA, et al. 2024. Low-dose antithymocyte globulin: a pragmatic approach to treating stage 2 type 1 diabetes. *Diabetes Care* **47:** 285–289. doi:10.2337/dc23-1750

Gambineri E, Torgerson TR, Ochs HD. 2003. Immune dysregulation, polyendocrinopathy, enteropathy, and X-linked inheritance (IPEX), a syndrome of systemic autoimmunity caused by mutations of FOXP3, a critical regulator of T-cell homeostasis. *Curr Opin Rheumatol* **15:** 430–435. doi:10.1097/00002281-200307000-00010

Garg G, Tyler JR, Yang JH, Cutler AJ, Downes K, Pekalski M, Bell GL, Nutland S, Peakman M, Todd JA, et al. 2012. Type 1 diabetes-associated *IL2RA* variation lowers IL-2 signaling and contributes to diminished $CD4^+CD25^+$ regulatory T cell function. *J Immunol* **188:** 4644–4653. doi:10.4049/jimmunol.1100272

Gearty SV, Dündar F, Zumbo P, Espinosa-Carrasco G, Shakiba M, Sanchez-Rivera FJ, Socci ND, Trivedi P, Lowe SW, Lauer P, et al. 2022. An autoimmune stem-like CD8 T cell population drives type 1 diabetes. *Nature* **602:** 156–161. doi:10.1038/s41586-021-04248-x

Gitelman SE, Gottlieb PA, Felner EI, Willi SM, Fisher LK, Moran A, Gottschalk M, Moore WV, Pinckney A, Keyes-Elstein L, et al. 2016. Antithymocyte globulin therapy for patients with recent-onset type 1 diabetes: 2 year results of a randomised trial. *Diabetologia* **59:** 1153–1161. doi:10.1007/s00125-016-3917-4

Gorus FK, Balti EV, Messaaoui A, Demeester S, Van Dalem A, Costa O, Dorchy H, Mathieu C, Van Gaal L, Keymeulen B, et al. 2017. Twenty-year progression rate to clinical onset according to autoantibody profile, age, and HLA-DQ genotype in a registry-based group of children and adults with a first-degree relative with type 1 diabetes. *Diabetes Care* **40:** 1065–1072. doi:10.2337/dc16-2228

Goto R, You S, Zaitsu M, Chatenoud L, Wood KJ. 2013. Delayed anti-CD3 therapy results in depletion of alloreactive T cells and the dominance of $Foxp3^+CD4^+$ graft infiltrating cells. *Am J Transplant* **13:** 1655–1664. doi:10.1111/ajt.12272

Grinberg-Bleyer Y, Baeyens A, You S, Elhage R, Fourcade G, Gregoire S, Cagnard N, Carpentier W, Tang Q, Bluestone J, et al. 2010. IL-2 reverses established type 1 diabetes in NOD mice by a local effect on pancreatic regulatory T cells. *J Exp Med* **207:** 1871–1878. doi:10.1084/jem.20100209

Haller MJ, Gitelman SE, Gottlieb PA, Michels AW, Rosenthal SM, Shuster JJ, Zou B, Brusko TM, Hulme MA, Wasserfall CH, et al. 2015. Anti-thymocyte globulin/G-CSF treatment preserves β cell function in patients with established type 1 diabetes. *J Clin Invest* **125:** 448–455. doi:10.1172/JCI78492

Haller MJ, Schatz DA, Skyler JS, Krischer JP, Bundy BN, Miller JL, Atkinson MA, Becker DJ, Baidal D, DiMeglio LA, et al. 2018. Low-dose anti-thymocyte globulin (ATG) preserves β-cell function and improves HbA_{1c} in new-onset type 1 diabetes. *Diabetes Care* **41:** 1917–1925. doi:10.2337/dc18-0494

Haller MJ, Long SA, Blanchfield JL, Schatz DA, Skyler JS, Krischer JP, Bundy BN, Geyer SM, Warnock MV, Miller JL, et al. 2019. Low-dose anti-thymocyte globulin preserves c-peptide, reduces HbA_{1c}, and increases regulatory to conventional T-cell ratios in new-onset type 1 diabetes: two-year clinical trial data. *Diabetes* **68:** 1267–1276. doi:10.2337/db19-0057

Henschel P, Landwehr-Kenzel S, Engels N, Schienke A, Kremer J, Riet T, Redel N, Iordanidis K, Saetzler V, John K, et al. 2023. Supraphysiological FOXP3 expression in human CAR-Tregs results in improved stability, efficacy, and safety of CAR-Treg products for clinical application. *J Autoimmun* **138:** 103057. doi:10.1016/j.jaut.2023.103057

Herold KC, Bundy BN, Long SA, Bluestone JA, DiMeglio LA, Dufort MJ, Gitelman SE, Gottlieb PA, Krischer JP, Linsley PS, et al. 2019. An anti-CD3 antibody, teplizumab, in relatives at risk for type 1 diabetes. *N Engl J Med* **381:** 603–613. doi:10.1056/NEJMoa1902226

Herppich S, Toker A, Pietzsch B, Kitagawa Y, Ohkura N, Miyao T, Floess S, Hori S, Sakaguchi S, Huehn J. 2019. Dynamic imprinting of the Treg cell-specific epigenetic signature in developing thymic regulatory T cells. *Front Immunol* **10:** 2382. doi:10.3389/fimmu.2019.02382

Hmida NB, Ahmed MB, Moussa A, Rejeb MB, Said Y, Kourda N, Meresse B, Abdeladhim M, Louzir H, Cerf-Bensussan N. 2012. Impaired control of effector T cells by regulatory T cells: a clue to loss of oral tolerance and autoimmunity in celiac disease? *Am J Gastroenterol* **107:** 604–611. doi:10.1038/ajg.2011.397

Hui E, Cheung J, Zhu J, Su X, Taylor MJ, Wallweber HA, Sasmal DK, Huang J, Kim JM, Mellman I, et al. 2017. T cell costimulatory receptor CD28 is a primary target for PD-1-mediated inhibition. *Science* **355:** 1428–1433. doi:10.1126/science.aaf1292

Husebye ES, Anderson MS, Kämpe O. 2018. Autoimmune polyendocrine syndromes. *N Engl J Med* **378:** 1132–1141. doi:10.1056/NEJMra1713301

Hyttinen V, Kaprio J, Kinnunen L, Koskenvuo M, Tuomilehto J. 2003. Genetic liability of type 1 diabetes and the onset age among 22,650 young Finnish twin pairs: a nationwide follow-up study. *Diabetes* **52:** 1052–1055. doi:10.2337/diabetes.52.4.1052

Iakovliev A, McGurnaghan SJ, Hayward C, Colombo M, Lipschutz D, Spiliopoulou A, Colhoun HM, McKeigue PM. 2023. Genome-wide aggregated trans-effects on risk of type 1 diabetes: a test of the "omnigenic" sparse effector hypothesis of complex trait genetics. *Am J Hum Genet* **110:** 913–926. doi:10.1016/j.ajhg.2023.04.003

Jacobsen LM, Diggins K, Blanchfield L, McNichols J, Perry DJ, Brant J, Dong X, Bacher R, Gersuk VH, Schatz DA, et al. 2023. Responders to low-dose ATG induce $CD4^+$ T cell exhaustion in type 1 diabetes. *JCI Insight* **8:** e161812. doi:10.1172/jci.insight.161812

Jamison BL, Neef T, Goodspeed A, Bradley B, Baker RL, Miller SD, Haskins K. 2019. Nanoparticles containing an insulin-ChgA hybrid peptide protect from transfer of autoimmune diabetes by shifting the balance between effector T cells and regulatory T cells. *J Immunol* **203:** 48–57. doi:10.4049/jimmunol.1900127

Jonuleit H, Schmitt E, Kakirman H, Stassen M, Knop J, Enk AH. 2002. Infectious tolerance: human $CD25^+$ regulatory T cells convey suppressor activity to conventional $CD4^+$ T helper cells. *J Exp Med* **196:** 255–260. doi:10.1084/jem.20020394

Kahan SM, Zajac AJ. 2019. Immune exhaustion: past lessons and new insights from lymphocytic choriomeningitis virus. *Viruses* **11:** 156. doi:10.3390/v11020156

Kalekar LA, Schmiel SE, Nandiwada SL, Lam WY, Barsness LO, Zhang N, Stritesky GL, Malhotra D, Pauken KE, Linehan JL, et al. 2016. $CD4^+$ T cell anergy prevents autoimmunity and generates regulatory T cell precursors. *Nat Immunol* **17:** 304–314. doi:10.1038/ni.3331

Kendal AR, Waldmann H. 2010. Infectious tolerance: therapeutic potential. *Curr Opin Immunol* **22:** 560–565. doi:10.1016/j.coi.2010.08.002

Kim GR, Choi JM. 2022. Current understanding of cytotoxic T lymphocyte antigen-4 (CTLA-4) signaling in T-cell biology and disease therapy. *Mol Cells* **45:** 513–521. doi:10.14348/molcells.2022.2056

Klein L, Kyewski B, Allen PM, Hogquist KA. 2014. Positive and negative selection of the T cell repertoire: what thymocytes see (and don't see). *Nat Rev Immunol* **14:** 377–391. doi:10.1038/nri3667

Klementowicz JE, Mahne AE, Spence A, Nguyen V, Satpathy AT, Murphy KM, Tang Q. 2017. Cutting edge: origins, recruitment, and regulation of $CD11c^+$ cells in inflamed islets of autoimmune diabetes mice. *J Immunol* **199:** 27–32. doi:10.4049/jimmunol.1601062

Krischer JP, Lynch KF, Schatz DA, Ilonen J, Lernmark Å, Hagopian WA, Rewers MJ, She JX, Simell OG, Toppari J, et al. 2015. The 6 year incidence of diabetes-associated autoantibodies in genetically at-risk children: the TEDDY study. *Diabetologia* **58:** 980–987. doi:10.1007/s00125-015-3514-y

Krummel MF, Allison JP. 1995. CD28 and CTLA-4 have opposing effects on the response of T cells to stimulation. *J Exp Med* **182:** 459–465. doi:10.1084/jem.182.2.459

Kuczma MP, Szurek EA, Cebula A, Ngo VL, Pietrzak M, Kraj P, Denning TL, Ignatowicz L. 2021. Self and microbiota-derived epitopes induce $CD4^+$ T cell anergy and conversion into $CD4^+$ $Foxp3^+$ regulatory cells. *Mucosal Immunol* **14:** 443–454. doi:10.1038/s41385-020-00349-4

Lawson JM, Tremble J, Dayan C, Beyan H, Leslie RD, Peakman M, Tree TI. 2008. Increased resistance to $CD4^+CD25^{hi}$ regulatory T cell-mediated suppression in patients with type 1 diabetes. *Clin Exp Immunol* **154:** 353–359. doi:10.1111/j.1365-2249.2008.03810.x

Létourneau S, van Leeuwen EM, Krieg C, Martin C, Pantaleo G, Sprent J, Surh CD, Boyman O. 2010. IL-2/anti-IL-2 antibody complexes show strong biological activity by avoiding interaction with IL-2 receptor α subunit CD25. *Proc Natl Acad Sci* **107:** 2171–2176. doi:10.1073/pnas.0909384107

Lewis JS, Stewart JM, Marshall GP, Carstens MR, Zhang Y, Dolgova NV, Xia C, Brusko TM, Wasserfall CH, Clare-Salzler MJ, et al. 2019. Dual-sized microparticle system for generating suppressive dendritic cells prevents and reverses type 1 diabetes in the nonobese diabetic mouse model. *ACS Biomater Sci Eng* **5:** 2631–2646. doi:10.1021/acsbiomaterials.9b00332

Li J, Tan J, Martino MM, Lui KO. 2018. Regulatory T-cells: potential regulator of tissue repair and regeneration. *Front Immunol* **9:** 585. doi:10.3389/fimmu.2018.00585

Lin A, Mack JA, Bruggeman B, Jacobsen LM, Posgai AL, Wasserfall CH, Brusko TM, Atkinson MA, Gitelman SE, Gottlieb PA, et al. 2021. Low-dose ATG/GCSF in established type 1 diabetes: a five-year follow-up report. *Diabetes* **70:** 1123–1129. doi:10.2337/db20-1103

Lio CW, Hsieh CS. 2008. A two-step process for thymic regulatory T cell development. *Immunity* **28:** 100–111. doi:10.1016/j.immuni.2007.11.021

Liu W, Putnam AL, Xu-Yu Z, Szot GL, Lee MR, Zhu S, Gottlieb PA, Kapranov P, Gingeras TR, de St Groth BF, et al. 2006. CD127 expression inversely correlates with FoxP3 and suppressive function of human $CD4^+$ T reg cells. *J Exp Med* **203:** 1701–1711. doi:10.1084/jem.20060772

Long SA, Cerosaletti K, Bollyky PL, Tatum M, Shilling H, Zhang S, Zhang ZY, Pihoker C, Sanda S, Greenbaum C, et al. 2010. Defects in IL-2R signaling contribute to diminished maintenance of FOXP3 expression in $CD4^+CD25^+$ regulatory T-cells of type 1 diabetic subjects. *Diabetes* **59:** 407–415. doi:10.2337/db09-0694

Long SA, Cerosaletti K, Wan JY, Ho JC, Tatum M, Wei S, Shilling HG, Buckner JH. 2011. An autoimmune-associated variant in PTPN2 reveals an impairment of IL-2R signaling in $CD4^+$ T cells. *Genes Immun* **12:** 116–125. doi:10.1038/gene.2010.54

Long SA, Rieck M, Sanda S, Bollyky JB, Samuels PL, Goland R, Ahmann A, Rabinovitch A, Aggarwal S, Phippard D, et al. 2012. Rapamycin/IL-2 combination therapy in patients with type 1 diabetes augments Tregs yet transiently impairs β-cell function. *Diabetes* **61:** 2340–2348. doi:10.2337/db12-0049

Lorenzon R, Ribet C, Pitoiset F, Aractingi S, Banneville B, Beaugerie L, Berenbaum F, Cacoub P, Champey J, Chazouilleres O, et al. 2024. The universal effects of low-dose interleukin-2 across 13 autoimmune diseases in a basket clinical trial. *J Autoimmun* **144:** 103172. doi:10.1016/j.jaut.2024.103172

Macian F. 2005. NFAT proteins: key regulators of T-cell development and function. *Nat Rev Immunol* **5:** 472–484. doi:10.1038/nri1632

Mahne AE, Klementowicz JE, Chou A, Nguyen V, Tang Q. 2015. Therapeutic regulatory T cells subvert effector T cell function in inflamed islets to halt autoimmune diabetes. *J Immunol* **194:** 3147–3155. doi:10.4049/jimmunol.1402739

Malchow S, Leventhal DS, Lee V, Nishi S, Socci ND, Savage PA. 2016. AIRE enforces immune tolerance by directing autoreactive T cells into the regulatory T cell lineage. *Immunity* **44:** 1102–1113. doi:10.1016/j.immuni.2016.02.009

Marek-Trzonkowska N, Myśliwiec M, Dobyszuk A, Grabowska M, Techmańska I, Juścińska J, Wujtewicz MA, Witkowski P, Młynarski W, Balcerska A, et al. 2012. Administration of $CD4^+CD25^{high}CD127^-$ regulatory T cells preserves β-cell function in type 1 diabetes in children. *Diabetes Care* **35:** 1817–1820. doi:10.2337/dc12-0038

Martin S, Wolf-Eichbaum D, Duinkerken G, Scherbaum WA, Kolb H, Noordzij JG, Roep BO. 2001. Development of type 1 diabetes despite severe hereditary B-cell deficiency. *N Engl J Med* **345:** 1036–1040. doi:10.1056/NEJMoa010465

McGovern J, Holler A, Thomas S, Stauss HJ. 2022. Forced Fox-P3 expression can improve the safety and antigen-specific function of engineered regulatory T cells. *J Autoimmun* **132:** 102888. doi:10.1016/j.jaut.2022.102888

Mhanna V, Fourcade G, Barennes P, Quiniou V, Pham HP, Ritvo PG, Brimaud F, Gouritin B, Churlaud G, Six A, et al. 2021. Impaired activated/memory regulatory T cell clonal expansion instigates diabetes in NOD mice. *Diabetes* **70:** 976–985. doi:10.2337/db20-0896

Michelson DA, Hase K, Kaisho T, Benoist C, Mathis D. 2022. Thymic epithelial cells co-opt lineage-defining transcription factors to eliminate autoreactive T cells. *Cell* **185:** 2542–2558.e18. doi:10.1016/j.cell.2022.05.018

Mikami N, Kawakami R, Chen KY, Sugimoto A, Ohkura N, Sakaguchi S. 2020. Epigenetic conversion of conventional T cells into regulatory T cells by CD28 signal deprivation. *Proc Natl Acad Sci* **117:** 12258–12268. doi:10.1073/pnas.1922600117

Miller CN, Proekt I, von Moltke J, Wells KL, Rajpurkar AR, Wang H, Rattay K, Khan IS, Metzger TC, Pollack JL, et al. 2018. Thymic tuft cells promote an IL-4-enriched medulla and shape thymocyte development. *Nature* **559:** 627–631. doi:10.1038/s41586-018-0345-2

Mohseni YR, Tung SL, Dudreuilh C, Lechler RI, Fruhwirth GO, Lombardi G. 2020. The future of regulatory T cell therapy: promises and challenges of implementing CAR technology. *Front Immunol* **11:** 1608. doi:10.3389/fimmu.2020.01608

Mohty M. 2007. Mechanisms of action of antithymocyte globulin: T-cell depletion and beyond. *Leukemia* **21:** 1387–1394. doi:10.1038/sj.leu.2404683

Nguyen H, Guyer P, Ettinger RA, James EA. 2021. Non-genetically encoded epitopes are relevant targets in autoimmune diabetes. *Biomedicines* **9:** 202. doi:10.3390/biomedicines9020202

Noorchashm H, Noorchashm N, Kern J, Rostami SY, Barker CF, Naji A. 1997. B-cells are required for the initiation of insulitis and sialitis in nonobese diabetic mice. *Diabetes* **46:** 941–946. doi:10.2337/diab.46.6.941

Noorchashm H, Lieu YK, Noorchashm N, Rostami SY, Greeley SA, Schlachterman A, Song HK, Noto LE, Jevnikar AM, Barker CF, et al. 1999. I-Ag7-mediated antigen presentation by B lymphocytes is critical in overcoming a checkpoint in T cell tolerance to islet β cells of nonobese diabetic mice. *J Immunol* **163:** 743–750. doi:10.4049/jimmunol.163.2.743

Obarorakpor N, Patel D, Boyarov R, Amarsaikhan N, Cepeda JR, Eastes D, Robertson S, Johnson T, Yang K, Tang Q, et al. 2023. Regulatory T cells targeting a pathogenic MHC class II: insulin peptide epitope postpone spontaneous autoimmune diabetes. *Front Immunol* **14:** 1207108. doi:10.3389/fimmu.2023.1207108

Ohkura N, Hamaguchi M, Morikawa H, Sugimura K, Tanaka A, Ito Y, Osaki M, Tanaka Y, Yamashita R, Nakano N, et al. 2012. T cell receptor stimulation-induced epigenetic changes and Foxp3 expression are independent and complementary events required for Treg cell development. *Immunity* **37:** 785–799. doi:10.1016/j.immuni.2012.09.010

Ou Q, Power R, Griffin MD. 2023. Revisiting regulatory T cells as modulators of innate immune response and inflammatory diseases. *Front Immunol* **14:** 1287465. doi:10.3389/fimmu.2023.1287465

Owen DL, Mahmud SA, Sjaastad LE, Williams JB, Spanier JA, Simeonov DR, Ruscher R, Huang W, Proekt I, Miller CN, et al. 2019a. Thymic regulatory T cells arise via two distinct developmental programs. *Nat Immunol* **20:** 195–205. doi:10.1038/s41590-018-0289-6

Owen DL, Sjaastad LE, Farrar MA. 2019b. Regulatory T cell development in the thymus. *J Immunol* **203:** 2031–2041. doi:10.4049/jimmunol.1900662

Pandiyan P, Zheng L, Ishihara S, Reed J, Lenardo MJ. 2007. $CD4^+CD25^+Foxp3^+$ regulatory T cells induce cytokine deprivation-mediated apoptosis of effector $CD4^+$ T cells. *Nat Immunol* **8:** 1353–1362. doi:10.1038/ni1536

Pasare C, Medzhitov R. 2003. Toll pathway-dependent blockade of $CD4^+CD25^+$ T cell-mediated suppression by dendritic cells. *Science* **299:** 1033–1036. doi:10.1126/science.1078231

Peluso I, Fantini MC, Fina D, Caruso R, Boirivant M, MacDonald TT, Pallone F, Monteleone G. 2007. IL-21 counteracts the regulatory T cell-mediated suppression of human $CD4^+$ T lymphocytes. *J Immunol* **178:** 732–739. doi:10.4049/jimmunol.178.2.732

Penaranda C, Tang Q, Bluestone JA. 2011. Anti-CD3 therapy promotes tolerance by selectively depleting pathogenic cells while preserving regulatory T cells. *J Immunol* **187:** 2015–2022. doi:10.4049/jimmunol.1100713

Pérol L, Lindner JM, Caudana P, Nunez NG, Baeyens A, Valle A, Sedlik C, Loirat D, Boyer O, Créange A, et al.

2016. Loss of immune tolerance to IL-2 in type 1 diabetes. *Nat Commun* **7:** 13027. doi:10.1038/ncomms13027

Pescovitz MD, Greenbaum CJ, Krause-Steinrauf H, Becker DJ, Gitelman SE, Goland R, Gottlieb PA, Marks JB, McGee PF, Moran AM, et al. 2009. Rituximab, B-lymphocyte depletion, and preservation of β-cell function. *N Engl J Med* **361:** 2143–2152. doi:10.1056/NEJMoa0904452

Peterson LB, Bell CJM, Howlett SK, Pekalski ML, Brady K, Hinton H, Sauter D, Todd JA, Umana P, Ast O, et al. 2018. A long-lived IL-2 mutein that selectively activates and expands regulatory T cells as a therapy for autoimmune disease. *J Autoimmun* **95:** 1–14. doi:10.1016/j.jaut.2018.10.017

Pieper T, Roth KDR, Glaser V, Riet T, Buitrago-Molina LE, Hagedorn M, Lieber M, Hust M, Noyan F, Jaeckel E, et al. 2023. Generation of chimeric antigen receptors against tetraspanin 7. *Cells* **12:** 1453. doi:10.3390/cells12111453

Pociot F, Akolkar B, Concannon P, Erlich HA, Julier C, Morahan G, Nierras CR, Todd JA, Rich SS, Nerup J. 2010. Genetics of type 1 diabetes: what's next. *Diabetes* **59:** 1561–1571. doi:10.2337/db10-0076

Putnam AL, Brusko TM, Lee MR, Liu W, Szot GL, Ghosh T, Atkinson MA, Bluestone JA. 2009. Expansion of human regulatory T-cells from patients with type 1 diabetes. *Diabetes* **58:** 652–662. doi:10.2337/db08-1168

Quandt Z, Young A, Perdigoto AL, Herold KC, Anderson MS. 2021. Autoimmune endocrinopathies: an emerging complication of immune checkpoint inhibitors. *Annu Rev Med* **72:** 313–330. doi:10.1146/annurev-med-050219-034237

Qureshi OS, Zheng Y, Nakamura K, Attridge K, Manzotti C, Schmidt EM, Baker J, Jeffery LE, Kaur S, Briggs Z, et al. 2011. *Trans*-endocytosis of CD80 and CD86: a molecular basis for the cell-extrinsic function of CTLA-4. *Science* **332:** 600–603. doi:10.1126/science.1202947

Raeber ME, Sahin D, Karakus U, Boyman O. 2023. A systematic review of interleukin-2-based immunotherapies in clinical trials for cancer and autoimmune diseases. *EBioMedicine* **90:** 104539. doi:10.1016/j.ebiom.2023.104539

Ramos EL, Dayan CM, Chatenoud L, Sumnik Z, Simmons KM, Szypowska A, Gitelman SE, Knecht LA, Niemoeller E, Tian W, et al. 2023a. Teplizumab and β-cell function in newly diagnosed type 1 diabetes. *N Engl J Med* **389:** 2151–2161. doi:10.1056/NEJMoa2308743

Ramos TL, Bolivar-Wagers S, Jin S, Thangavelu G, Simonetta F, Lin PY, Hirai T, Saha A, Koehn B, Su LL, et al. 2023b. Prevention of acute GVHD using an orthogonal IL-2/IL-2Rβ system to selectively expand regulatory T cells in vivo. *Blood* **141:** 1337–1352. doi:10.1182/blood.2022018440

Rewers M, Hyöty H, Lernmark Å, Hagopian W, She JX, Schatz D, Ziegler AG, Toppari J, Akolkar B, Krischer J, et al. 2018. The Environmental Determinants of Diabetes in the Young (TEDDY) study: 2018 update. *Curr Diab Rep* **18:** 136. doi:10.1007/s11892-018-1113-2

Ribas A, Wolchok JD. 2018. Cancer immunotherapy using checkpoint blockade. *Science* **359:** 1350–1355. doi:10.1126/science.aar4060

Rigby MR, DiMeglio LA, Rendell MS, Felner EI, Dostou JM, Gitelman SE, Patel CM, Griffin KJ, Tsalikian E, Gottlieb PA, et al. 2013. Targeting of memory T cells with alefacept in new-onset type 1 diabetes (T1DAL study): 12 month results of a randomised, double-blind, placebo-controlled phase 2 trial. *Lancet Diabetes Endocrinol* **1:** 284–294. doi:10.1016/S2213-8587(13)70111-6

Rigby MR, Harris KM, Pinckney A, DiMeglio LA, Rendell MS, Felner EI, Dostou JM, Gitelman SE, Griffin KJ, Tsalikian E, et al. 2015. Alefacept provides sustained clinical and immunological effects in new-onset type 1 diabetes patients. *J Clin Invest* **125:** 3285–3296. doi:10.1172/JCI81722

Riley JL, June CH. 2005. The CD28 family: a T-cell rheostat for therapeutic control of T-cell activation. *Blood* **105:** 13–21. doi:10.1182/blood-2004-04-1596

Rivera A, Chen CC, Ron N, Dougherty JP, Ron Y. 2001. Role of B cells as antigen-presenting cells in vivo revisited: antigen-specific B cells are essential for T cell expansion in lymph nodes and for systemic T cell responses to low antigen concentrations. *Int Immunol* **13:** 1583–1593. doi:10.1093/intimm/13.12.1583

Robertson CC, Inshaw JRJ, Onengut-Gumuscu S, Chen WM, Santa Cruz DF, Yang H, Cutler AJ, Crouch DJM, Farber E, Bridges SL, et al. 2021. Fine-mapping, trans-ancestral and genomic analyses identify causal variants, cells, genes and drug targets for type 1 diabetes. *Nat Genet* **53:** 962–971. doi:10.1038/s41588-021-00880-5

Rosenzwajg M, Churlaud G, Mallone R, Six A, Dérian N, Chaara W, Lorenzon R, Long SA, Buckner JH, Afonso G, et al. 2015. Low-dose interleukin-2 fosters a dose-dependent regulatory T cell tuned milieu in T1D patients. *J Autoimmun* **58:** 48–58. doi:10.1016/j.jaut.2015.01.001

Rosenzwajg M, Salet R, Lorenzon R, Tchitchek N, Roux A, Bernard C, Carel JC, Storey C, Polak M, Beltrand J, et al. 2020. Low-dose IL-2 in children with recently diagnosed type 1 diabetes: a phase I/II randomised, double-blind, placebo-controlled, dose-finding study. *Diabetologia* **63:** 1808–1821. doi:10.1007/s00125-020-05200-w

Sakaguchi S, Miyara M, Costantino CM, Hafler DA. 2010. $FOXP3^+$ regulatory T cells in the human immune system. *Nat Rev Immunol* **10:** 490–500. doi:10.1038/nri2785

Sakaguchi S, Mikami N, Wing JB, Tanaka A, Ichiyama K, Ohkura N. 2020. Regulatory T cells and human disease. *Annu Rev Immunol* **38:** 541–566. doi:10.1146/annurev-immunol-042718-041717

Salomon B, Lenschow DJ, Rhee L, Ashourian N, Singh B, Sharpe A, Bluestone JA. 2000. B7/CD28 costimulation is essential for the homeostasis of the $CD4^+CD25^+$ immunoregulatory T cells that control autoimmune diabetes. *Immunity* **12:** 431–440. doi:10.1016/S1074-7613(00)80195-8

Schenten D, Nish SA, Yu S, Yan X, Lee HK, Brodsky I, Pasman L, Yordy B, Wunderlich FT, Brüning JC, et al. 2014. Signaling through the adaptor molecule MyD88 in $CD4^+$ T cells is required to overcome suppression by regulatory T cells. *Immunity* **40:** 78–90. doi:10.1016/j.immuni.2013.10.023

Schneider A, Rieck M, Sanda S, Pihoker C, Greenbaum C, Buckner JH. 2008. The effector T cells of diabetic subjects are resistant to regulation via $CD4^+FOXP3^+$ regulatory T cells. *J Immunol* **181:** 7350–7355. doi:10.4049/jimmunol.181.10.7350

Setoguchi R, Hori S, Takahashi T, Sakaguchi S. 2005. Homeostatic maintenance of natural *Foxp3*$^+$ $CD25^+$ $CD4^+$

regulatory T cells by interleukin (IL)-2 and induction of autoimmune disease by IL-2 neutralization. *J Exp Med* **201:** 723–735. doi:10.1084/jem.20041982

Sharma P, Goswami S, Raychaudhuri D, Siddiqui BA, Singh P, Nagarajan A, Liu J, Subudhi SK, Poon C, Gant KL, et al. 2023. Immune checkpoint therapy—current perspectives and future directions. *Cell* **186:** 1652–1669. doi:10.1016/j.cell.2023.03.006

Silverman M, Kua L, Tanca A, Pala M, Palomba A, Tanes C, Bittinger K, Uzzau S, Benoist C, Mathis D. 2017. Protective major histocompatibility complex allele prevents type 1 diabetes by shaping the intestinal microbiota early in ontogeny. *Proc Natl Acad Sci* **114:** 9671–9676. doi:10.1073/pnas.1712280114

Sitrin J, Ring A, Garcia KC, Benoist C, Mathis D. 2013. Regulatory T cells control NK cells in an insulitic lesion by depriving them of IL-2. *J Exp Med* **210:** 1153–1165. doi:10.1084/jem.20122248

Sockolosky JT, Trotta E, Parisi G, Picton L, Su LL, Le AC, Chhabra A, Silveria SL, George BM, King IC, et al. 2018. Selective targeting of engineered T cells using orthogonal IL-2 cytokine-receptor complexes. *Science* **359:** 1037–1042. doi:10.1126/science.aar3246

Spanier JA, Fung V, Wardell CM, Alkhatib MH, Chen Y, Swanson LA, Dwyer AJ, Weno ME, Silva N, Mitchell JS, et al. 2023. Tregs with an MHC class II peptide-specific chimeric antigen receptor prevent autoimmune diabetes in mice. *J Clin Invest* **133:** e168601. doi:10.1172/JCI168601

Spence A, Purtha W, Tam J, Dong S, Kim Y, Ju CH, Sterling T, Nakayama M, Robinson WH, Bluestone JA, et al. 2018. Revealing the specificity of regulatory T cells in murine autoimmune diabetes. *Proc Natl Acad Sci* **115:** 5265–5270. doi:10.1073/pnas.1715590115

Stassen M, Schmitt E, Jonuleit H. 2004. Human $CD4^+CD25^+$ regulatory T cells and infectious tolerance. *Transplantation* **77:** S23–S25. doi:10.1097/00007890-200401151-00009

Sun H, Lee HS, Kim SH, Fernandes de Lima M, Gingras AR, Du Q, McLaughlin W, Ablack J, Lopez-Ramirez MA, Lagarrigue F, et al. 2023. IL-2 can signal via chemokine receptors to promote regulatory T cells' suppressive function. *Cell Rep* **42:** 112996. doi:10.1016/j.celrep.2023.112996

Tai X, Cowan M, Feigenbaum L, Singer A. 2005. CD28 costimulation of developing thymocytes induces Foxp3 expression and regulatory T cell differentiation independently of interleukin 2. *Nat Immunol* **6:** 152–162. doi:10.1038/ni1160

Tai X, Erman B, Alag A, Mu J, Kimura M, Katz G, Guinter T, McCaughtry T, Etzensperger R, Feigenbaum L, et al. 2013. Foxp3 transcription factor is proapoptotic and lethal to developing regulatory T cells unless counterbalanced by cytokine survival signals. *Immunity* **38:** 1116–1128. doi:10.1016/j.immuni.2013.02.022

Tang Q, Bluestone JA. 2008. The $Foxp3^+$ regulatory T cell: a jack of all trades, master of regulation. *Nat Immunol* **9:** 239–244. doi:10.1038/ni1572

Tang Q, Henriksen KJ, Boden EK, Tooley AJ, Ye J, Subudhi SK, Zheng XX, Strom TB, Bluestone JA. 2003. Cutting edge: CD28 controls peripheral homeostasis of $CD4^+CD25^+$ regulatory T cells. *J Immunol* **171:** 3348–3352. doi:10.4049/jimmunol.171.7.3348

Tang Q, Henriksen KJ, Bi M, Finger EB, Szot G, Ye J, Masteller EL, McDevitt H, Bonyhadi M, Bluestone JA. 2004. In vitro-expanded antigen-specific regulatory T cells suppress autoimmune diabetes. *J Exp Med* **199:** 1455–1465. doi:10.1084/jem.20040139

Tang Q, Adams JY, Tooley AJ, Bi M, Fife BT, Serra P, Santamaria P, Locksley RM, Krummel MF, Bluestone JA. 2006. Visualizing regulatory T cell control of autoimmune responses in nonobese diabetic mice. *Nat Immunol* **7:** 83–92. doi:10.1038/ni1289

Tang Q, Adams JY, Penaranda C, Melli K, Piaggio E, Sgouroudis E, Piccirillo CA, Salomon BL, Bluestone JA. 2008. Central role of defective interleukin-2 production in the triggering of islet autoimmune destruction. *Immunity* **28:** 687–697. doi:10.1016/j.immuni.2008.03.016

Tarbell KV, Yamazaki S, Olson K, Toy P, Steinman RM. 2004. $CD25^+$ $CD4^+$ T cells, expanded with dendritic cells presenting a single autoantigenic peptide, suppress autoimmune diabetes. *J Exp Med* **199:** 1467–1477. doi:10.1084/jem.20040180

Tenspolde M, Zimmermann K, Weber LC, Hapke M, Lieber M, Dywicki J, Frenzel A, Hust M, Galla M, Buitrago-Molina LE, et al. 2019. Regulatory T cells engineered with a novel insulin-specific chimeric antigen receptor as a candidate immunotherapy for type 1 diabetes. *J Autoimmun* **103:** 102289. doi:10.1016/j.jaut.2019.05.017

Todd JA, Bell JI, McDevitt HO. 1987. HLA-DQβ gene contributes to susceptibility and resistance to insulin-dependent diabetes mellitus. *Nature* **329:** 599–604. doi:10.1038/329599a0

Todd JA, Evangelou M, Cutler AJ, Pekalski ML, Walker NM, Stevens HE, Porter L, Smyth DJ, Rainbow DB, Ferreira RC, et al. 2016. Regulatory T cell responses in participants with type 1 diabetes after a single dose of interleukin-2: a non-randomised, open label, adaptive dose-finding trial. *PLoS Med* **13:** e1002139. doi:10.1371/journal.pmed.1002139

Tooley JE, Vudattu N, Choi J, Cotsapas C, Devine L, Raddassi K, Ehlers MR, McNamara JG, Harris KM, Kanaparthi S, et al. 2016. Changes in T-cell subsets identify responders to FcR-non-binding anti-CD3 mAb (teplizumab) in patients with type 1 diabetes. *Eur J Immunol* **46:** 230–241. doi:10.1002/eji.201545708

Toomer KH, Malek TR. 2018. Cytokine signaling in the development and homeostasis of regulatory T cells. *Cold Spring Harb Perspect Biol* **10:** a028597. doi:10.1101/cshperspect.a028597

Tran MT, Faridi P, Lim JJ, Ting YT, Onwukwe G, Bhattacharjee P, Jones CM, Tresoldi E, Cameron FJ, La Gruta NL, et al. 2021. T cell receptor recognition of hybrid insulin peptides bound to HLA-DQ8. *Nat Commun* **12:** 5110. doi:10.1038/s41467-021-25404-x

Trotta E, Bessette PH, Silveria SL, Ely LK, Jude KM, Le DT, Holst CR, Coyle A, Potempa M, Lanier LL, et al. 2018. A human anti-IL-2 antibody that potentiates regulatory T cells by a structure-based mechanism. *Nat Med* **24:** 1005–1014. doi:10.1038/s41591-018-0070-2

Tsai S, Shameli A, Yamanouchi J, Clemente-Casares X, Wang J, Serra P, Yang Y, Medarova Z, Moore A, Santamaria P. 2010. Reversal of autoimmunity by boosting memory-like autoregulatory T cells. *Immunity* **32:** 568–580. doi:10.1016/j.immuni.2010.03.015

Turley S, Poirot L, Hattori M, Benoist C, Mathis D. 2003. Physiological β cell death triggers priming of self-reactive T cells by dendritic cells in a type-1 diabetes model. *J Exp Med* **198:** 1527–1537. doi:10.1084/jem.20030966

VanDyke D, Iglesias M, Tomala J, Young A, Smith J, Perry JA, Gebara E, Cross AR, Cheung LS, Dykema AG, et al. 2022. Engineered human cytokine/antibody fusion proteins expand regulatory T cells and confer autoimmune disease protection. *Cell Rep* **41:** 111478. doi:10.1016/j.celrep.2022.111478

van Lummel M, Buis DTP, Ringeling C, de Ru AH, Pool J, Papadopoulos GK, van Veelen PA, Reijonen H, Drijfhout JW, Roep BO. 2019. Epitope stealing as a mechanism of dominant protection by HLA-DQ6 in type 1 diabetes. *Diabetes* **68:** 787–795. doi:10.2337/db18-0501

Voltarelli JC, Couri CE, Stracieri AB, Oliveira MC, Moraes DA, Pieroni F, Coutinho M, Malmegrim KC, Foss-Freitas MC, Simões BP, et al. 2007. Autologous nonmyeloablative hematopoietic stem cell transplantation in newly diagnosed type 1 diabetes mellitus. *JAMA* **297:** 1568–1576. doi:10.1001/jama.297.14.1568

Waldron-Lynch F, Henegariu O, Deng S, Preston-Hurlburt P, Tooley J, Flavell R, Herold KC. 2012. Teplizumab induces human gut-tropic regulatory cells in humanized mice and patients. *Sci Transl Med* **4:** 118ra12. doi:10.1126/scitranslmed.3003401

Walunas TL, Bakker CY, Bluestone JA. 1996. CTLA-4 ligation blocks CD28-dependent T cell activation. *J Exp Med* **183:** 2541–2550. doi:10.1084/jem.183.6.2541

Watanabe M, Lu Y, Breen M, Hodes RJ. 2020. B7-CD28 costimulation modulates central tolerance via thymic clonal deletion and Treg generation through distinct mechanisms. *Nat Commun* **11:** 6264. doi:10.1038/s41467-020-20070-x

Webster KE, Walters S, Kohler RE, Mrkvan T, Boyman O, Surh CD, Grey ST, Sprent J. 2009. In vivo expansion of T reg cells with IL-2-mAb complexes: induction of resistance to EAE and long-term acceptance of islet allografts without immunosuppression. *J Exp Med* **206:** 751–760. doi:10.1084/jem.20082824

Wen X, Yang J, James E, Chow IT, Reijonen H, Kwok WW. 2020. Increased islet antigen-specific regulatory and effector $CD4^+$ T cells in healthy individuals with the type 1 diabetes-protective haplotype. *Sci Immunol* **5:** eaax8767. doi:10.1126/sciimmunol.aax8767

Wiles TA, Delong T. 2019. HIPs and HIP-reactive T cells. *Clin Exp Immunol* **198:** 306–313. doi:10.1111/cei.13335

Wilhelm-Benartzi CS, Miller SE, Bruggraber S, Picton D, Wilson M, Gatley K, Chhabra A, Marcovecchio ML, Hendriks AEJ, Morobé H, et al. 2021. Study protocol: minimum effective low dose: anti-human thymocyte globulin (MELD-ATG): phase II, dose ranging, efficacy study of antithymocyte globulin (ATG) within 6 weeks of diagnosis of type 1 diabetes. *BMJ Open* **11:** e053669. doi:10.1136/bmjopen-2021-053669

Wohlfert EA, Clark RB. 2007. "Vive la résistance!"—the PI3K-Akt pathway can determine target sensitivity to regulatory T cell suppression. *Trends Immunol* **28:** 154–160. doi:10.1016/j.it.2007.02.003

Yeste A, Takenaka MC, Mascanfroni ID, Nadeau M, Kenison JE, Patel B, Tukpah AM, Babon JA, DeNicola M, Kent SC, et al. 2016. Tolerogenic nanoparticles inhibit T cell-mediated autoimmunity through SOCS2. *Sci Signal* **9:** ra61. doi:10.1126/scisignal.aad0612

You S, Belghith M, Cobbold S, Alyanakian MA, Gouarin C, Barriot S, Garcia C, Waldmann H, Bach JF, Chatenoud L. 2005. Autoimmune diabetes onset results from qualitative rather than quantitative age-dependent changes in pathogenic T-cells. *Diabetes* **54:** 1415–1422. doi:10.2337/diabetes.54.5.1415

Zhao LP, Skyler J, Papadopoulos GK, Pugliese A, Najera JA, Bondinas GP, Moustakas AK, Wang R, Pyo CW, Nelson WC, et al. 2022. Association of HLA-DQ heterodimer residues −18β and β57 with progression from islet autoimmunity to diabetes in the diabetes prevention trial-type 1. *Diabetes Care* **45:** 1610–1620. doi:10.2337/dc21-1628

Zheng Y, Chaudhry A, Kas A, de Roos P, Kim JM, Chu TT, Corcoran L, Treuting P, Klein U, Rudensky AY. 2009. Regulatory T-cell suppressor program co-opts transcription factor IRF4 to control T(H)2 responses. *Nature* **458:** 351–356. doi:10.1038/nature07674

Zieliński M, Żalińska M, Iwaszkiewicz-Grześ D, Gliwiński M, Hennig M, Jaźwińska-Curyłło A, Kamińska H, Sakowska J, Wołoszyn-Durkiewicz A, Owczuk R, et al. 2022. Combined therapy with $CD4^+$ $CD25^{high}CD127^-$ T regulatory cells and anti-CD20 antibody in recent-onset type 1 diabetes is superior to monotherapy: randomized phase I/II trial. *Diabetes Obes Metab* **24:** 1534–1543. doi:10.1111/dom.14723

Clinical Immunologic Interventions for the Treatment of Type 1 Diabetes: Challenges, Choice, and Timing of Immunomodulators

Danijela Tatovic and Colin Dayan

Division of Infection and Immunity, Cardiff University School of Medicine, Cardiff CF14 4XN, United Kingdom

Correspondence: dayancm@cardiff.ac.uk

Replacement insulin therapy has been the mainstay of type 1 diabetes mellitus (T1D) treatment ever since its introduction into clinical care more than 100 years ago. Despite advances in delivery methods, insulin remains a challenging medication. It is, therefore, not surprising that most people with T1D do not achieve optimal glycemic control and remain at risk of complications. The recent introduction of teplizumab as the first immunotherapy for T1D has ushered in an exciting era where the focus is shifted from metabolic replacement therapy with insulin to proactive disease-modifying treatments that prevent the loss of insulin secretory capacity. At least nine other clinical immunologic interventions have shown phase 2 trial efficacy in preserving β-cell function in T1D. To translate these findings to patient benefit, many changes are required. These include improvements in end points and trial design to accelerate drug development, changing the attitude of healthcare professionals toward novel strategies, and the development of effective screening programs to identify affected individuals in early-stage disease. This will enable a broad portfolio of β-cell preserving therapies to be approved, in turn allowing appropriate selection of immunomodulators tailored to an individual's response with an ultimate goal of "insulin-free T1D."

Type 1 diabetes mellitus (T1D) is caused by autoimmune-mediated destruction of the pancreatic β cells. The disease starts long before a clinical diagnosis is made and progresses to dependence on exogenous insulin with absolute or near-absolute insulin deficiency (Greenbaum et al. 2012; Oram et al. 2019, Powers 2021; Carr et al. 2022). Replacement insulin therapy has been the mainstay of T1D treatment ever since the introduction of insulin into clinical care more than 100 years ago (Mathieu et al. 2021; Russell-Jones and Herring 2021; Sims et al. 2021a; Tatovic and Dayan 2021). The discovery of insulin was undoubtedly a breakthrough as it meant that T1D ceased to be a fatal disease, but it converted T1D into a chronic disease. Despite significant advances in delivery methods, insulin remains arguably the single most complex and challenging medication in current medical practice. Achieving optimal glycemic control with insulin while avoiding hypoglycemia is estimated to involve up to 20 or more therapeutic decisions daily, including dose adjustments dependent not only on repeated blood glucose

Cite this article as *Cold Spring Harb Perspect Med* doi: 10.1101/cshperspect.a041597

measurements but also carbohydrate counting, and alterations for physical activity, stress, and intercurrent illness. It is therefore not surprising that most people with T1D (>70%) do not achieve optimal glycemic control with this approach (McKnight et al. 2015; Miller et al. 2015; Wasag et al. 2018; Foster et al. 2019; Anderzén et al. 2020; Van Loocke et al. 2021; Prigge et al. 2022; Holman et al. 2023; Sandy et al. 2024) and remain at risk of long-term complications, while at the same time frequently reporting high levels of "diabetes distress" (Hernar et al. 2024). This persisting unmet need in T1D management justifies efforts to develop clinical immunologic interventions in T1D that can modify the disease course and reduce, delay, or prevent the need for insulin.

THE CHALLENGES OF DEVELOPING DISEASE-MODIFYING THERAPIES FOR T1D

Insulin Therapy: a Blessing and a Curse

It is a striking observation that there are currently no approved disease-modifying therapies for new-onset clinical T1D, whereas other common autoimmune diseases, such as psoriasis, multiple sclerosis, rheumatoid arthritis, and inflammatory bowel disease, have adopted disease-modifying strategies more quickly with between 8 and 30 therapies already licensed. The availability of insulin as a replacement therapy, although clearly "a blessing," might also be considered a "curse" in this context, contributing to the delay in the development of clinical immunologic intervention therapies in T1D in three ways.

Firstly, the availability of insulin reduces the clinical urgency and apparent priority of developing alternative approaches as well as setting a high bar for safety. Secondly, insulin confounds the use of clinical end points in drug development. In cell-mediated autoimmune diseases, in general, we do not have a robust biomarker of the pharmacodynamics of the disease process itself and rely on clinical end points to guide drug development. Examples of clinical end points currently used in drug development include skin lesion counts (Psoriasis Area and Severity Index [PASI] score) in psoriasis, joint pain and inflammation scores (e.g., DAS 28, clinical disease activity index) in rheumatoid arthritis, magnetic resonance image (MRI) lesion count, annualized relapse rate, and the Expanded Disability Status Scale in multiple sclerosis and bowel symptoms scores (or tissue biopsies) in ulcerative colitis or Crohn's disease. Unfortunately, comparable clinical end points for T1D, such as average glucose levels, HbA1c, and hypoglycemia rates, are not reflections only of the loss of β-cell function but can also change as a result of alterations in adherence to insulin therapy, representing an additional challenge to drug development in T1D. This key issue is discussed in more detail in the next section. Thirdly, unlike most other autoimmune disease, T1D is clinically silent until a late stage, when an estimated 80% of the β cells have been destroyed. As a result, the "window" for intervention in clinical disease is short (~1–5 yr), before there is little clinically significant residual β-cell function. The population immediately available for clinical trials—individuals with new-onset disease—represents only ~2% of all patients with T1D. This extended "clinically silent" phase is similar to the situation in, for example, renal disease in which clinical symptoms are also a late manifestation, but the relatively low cost of replacement therapy with insulin as compared to renal replacement therapy is a further (financial) disincentive for drug development in T1D. An additional challenge that does not relate to the availability of insulin is that the disease is most active and rapidly progressive in children, especially under 5 years of age (Ismail et al. 2022). Regulatory authorities require proof of the likelihood of benefit as well as safety in adults before testing in children, especially very young children, adding extra time to drug development.

Outcome Assessments, Clinical, and Surrogate End Points in New-Onset (Stage 3) T1D

The clinically relevant outcomes recognized by regulatory authorities such as the Food and Drug Administration (FDA) for drug approvals in diabetes include long-term complications (e.g., nephropathy, retinopathy, cardiovascular disease, premature death) and acute complications (e.g., hypoglycemia, diabetic ketoacidosis). In view of the very long time required to develop such long-term complications, surrogate measures of glycemic control, which have been validated to be associated with these outcomes, are also accepted, notably HbA1c. In the context of disease-modifying therapies for T1D, these end points are problematic as they can also be modified by improvements in insulin therapy independent of β-cell preservation, and this is particularly relevant with the advent of highly effective hybrid closed-loop (artificial pancreas) insulin delivery systems (Crabtree et al. 2023).

The most relevant end point for disease-modifying therapies in established (stage 3) T1D currently is a measure of β-cell function, notably standardized meal-stimulated insulin C-peptide production, which uses a combination of glucose and amino acids as a stimulus. This end point is generally expressed as a time-normalized area under the curve (AUC) of C-peptide in a 2- or 4-hour mixed meal tolerance test (MMTT) referred to as the C-peptide AUC. C-peptide AUC declines in a broadly loglinear fashion in the first year after clinical diagnosis of T1D and is not affected by changes in insulin therapy (Bogun et al. 2020; Boughton et al. 2022).

Until recently, however, C-peptide levels were not accepted by the FDA or European Medicines Agency (EMA) as outcomes for drug approval as they do not directly impact on how a patient "feels, functions, or survives" but rather indirectly via glucose levels. A strong case that C-peptide levels nonetheless should represent a surrogate outcome marker for drug approval has been made by the T1D community following the collection of extensive data correlating C-peptide levels to clinical end points, and the situation is changing (Taylor et al. 2023; Latres et al. 2024).

A key issue is what is the lowest C-peptide level worth preserving in clinical trials and clinical practice is. It seems that even very low levels of C-peptide correlate well with less frequent hypoglycemic episodes. Analysis of the Diabetes Control and Complications Trial (DCCT) cohort indicated that individuals with stimulated C-peptide between 200 and 500 pmol/L had less hypoglycemia (The Diabetes Control and Complications Trial Research Group 1998). The subsequent follow-up of the same cohort (Epidemiology of Diabetes Interventions and Complications [EDIC] study 2015–2017), indicated that even lower C-peptide levels make a difference. Indeed, participants with residual C-peptide >30 pmol/L had substantially lower risk of hypoglycemia than people with undetectable C-peptide (<3 pmol/L) (Gubitosi-Klug et al. 2021). This was consistent with The Scottish Diabetes Research Network Type 1 Bioresource Study (SDRNT1BIO), where effects on the risk of serious hypoglycemic events followed a continuous relationship with C-peptide levels down to the lower limit of the detection test (3 pmol/L) (Jeyam et al. 2021).

On the other hand, meaningful prevention of microvascular complications probably requires higher C-peptide levels. This again dates back to the original DCCT where responders (defined as people with stimulated C-peptide levels of 200–500 pmol/L) had a lower rate of retinopathy in comparison to nonresponders (C-peptide <200 pmol/L) (The Diabetes Control and Complications Trial Research Group 1998). SDRNT1BIO showed a linear relationship between C-peptide and the incidence of retinopathy with no clear threshold (Jeyam et al. 2021).

At the high end of the spectrum is insulin independence, which according to data from the Clinical Islet Transplant Consortium (CITR) requires a much higher stimulated C-peptide of >970 pmol/L (Table 1; Baidal et al. 2023). Hence, the target C-peptide level in clinical trials and clinical practice depends on the clinical outcome, but even the less ambitious goal of avoiding undetectable C-peptide levels is anticipated to have a beneficial outcome on reducing the rate of severe hypoglycemic episodes. As we move higher up in the relationship continuum, we are more likely to observe a meaningful impact on complication prevention and further on to the "holy grail" of insulin independence.

Table 1. C-peptide values predictive for clinical benefits after islet transplants

Clinical outcome	C-peptide level (pmol/L) predicting clinical benefit	
	Fasting	MMTT stimulated
Absence of level 3 hypoglycemia (SHE)	70	120
HbA_{1c} <7.0%	150	800
HbA_{1c} ≤6.5%	310	800
HbA_{1c} <7.0% and absence of SHE	140	800
HbA_{1c} ≤6.5% and absence of SHE	310	800
Insulin independence	260	970
Absence of SHE, HbA_{1c} ≤6.5%, and insulin independence	330	970

Table reprinted from Latres et al. 2024, © 2024 by the American Diabetes Association.
(MMTT) Mixed meal tolerance test, (SHE) severe hypoglycemic event.

Note that trials of at least 6–12 months with 40–70 participants with very recent-onset clinical disease (typically recruited within 6–12 wk of diagnosis) are required for early phase studies to determine optimal dosing and provide the first evidence of efficacy. All too often, multiple doses or a wider population are not studied in the initial stages, and it is discovered late in phase 2 or 3 studies that the dose or target groups of patients were inappropriate, leading to unmet end points (Sherry et al. 2011; Ambery et al. 2014; Aronson et al. 2014).

Additional Challenges of Outcome Assessment in Early (Stage 1 or Stage 2) T1D

Three T1D stages have been defined (Couper et al. 2018; American Diabetes Association 2021). In stage 1, individuals are normoglycemic, but have two or more positive autoantibodies to β-cell antigens indicating active autoimmune process (Ziegler et al. 2013; Insel et al. 2015). In stage 2 that follows, individuals are still asymptomatic but have dysglycemia (Insel et al. 2015). Stage 3 is defined by glucose levels consistent with the ADA definition of diabetes, indicating that individuals now have a level of chronic hyperglycemia that eventually leads to the requirement for insulin replacement (American Diabetes Association 2021). While the use of AUC C-peptide represents a very valuable surrogate marker for drug development in late-stage clinical disease (stage 3 T1D), it is of less value in the early stages of the disease (stage 1 and stage 2) before insulin is required and indeed may show a paradoxical increase in stage 2 (Evans-Molina et al. 2018). This is likely due to two factors: Firstly, the early change in β-cell function comprises a delay in insulin release with the reduction in the early/first phase of secretion and a compensatory increase in the delayed secretion so that the overall AUC C-peptide changes little. Secondly, as β-cell function declines, the glucose rise during an oral glucose tolerance test is greater and this represents a more powerful stimulus to insulin release (Galderisi et al. 2023a; Martino et al 2024). As a result, to date, the outcome of intervention studies in stage 1 or stage 2 has been progression to the next metabolic stage (Herold et al. 2019; Libman et al. 2023; Russell et al. 2023). Unfortunately, this is slow requiring a minimum of 2 years of follow-up in stage 2 and longer in stage 1. There is therefore much interest in surrogate markers of early change in β-cell function. Markers that take into account the glucose rise during challenge testing as well as the C-peptide increase seem to perform better especially in stage 2 (e.g., index60). For stage 1, markers that can capture changes in first-phase insulin secretion (which occurs within 15 min of stimulation) are most valuable (e.g., the intravenous glucose tolerance test or modeling of glucose, C-peptide, and insulin with additional early sampling time points in the oral glucose tolerance test) (Keskinen et al. 2002; Galderisi et al.

2023a,b). The role of continuous glucose monitoring (CGM) as a marker of disease progression is currently being assessed. But without linkage to C-peptide, levels may not have greater discriminatory power (Ylescupidez et al. 2023a). The pros and cons of different metabolic outcome markers are summarized in Table 2.

Alternative markers of β-cell function have been explored, including levels of β-cell prohormones and exocrine enzymes. Proinsulin to C-peptide ratio (PI:C) shows some promise for this purpose as stressed β cells tend to release more proinsulin (Rodriguez-Calvo et al. 2017) and PI:C increases as individuals approach stage 3 (Sims et al. 2023). Interestingly and consistent with the maintenance of insulin production in early stages of the disease, a high PI:C ratio was linked to increases in absolute proinsulin rather than decreased C-peptide values in stage 2. In contrast, elevations of PI:C at the time of T1D diagnosis are more strongly linked to reductions in C-peptide (Watkins et al. 2016).

The Challenge of Demonstrating Longevity of Effect

To date, almost all disease-modifying therapies that appear to show promise in T1D appear to decline in their effect over time (Taylor et al. 2023). In some cases, this may be because treatment was only given for a limited time period and ongoing or repeated therapy is indicated (e.g., with golimumab or verapamil). In some, the effects declined despite repeated therapy (e.g., abatacept; Orban et al. 2014) and in others, continued therapy is either not part of the recommended dosing schedule (e.g., teplizumab and antithymocyte globulin [ATG]) or carries

Table 2. Comparison of strengths and weaknesses of biomarkers/end points at different stages of type 1 diabetes mellitus (T1D)

	Stage 1	Stage 2	Stage 3
HbA1c	Not applicable	Possible, not yet validated	Possible Confounded by insulin therapy Larger numbers required
Continuous glucose monitoring (CGM)	Not applicable	Possible, not yet validated	Possible Confounded by insulin therapy Larger numbers required
Insulin dose/kg	Not applicable	Not applicable	Possible ? Clinical importance Confounded by the intensity of glucose control
Insulin dose-adjusted glycated hemoglobin (IDAA1c)	Not applicable	Not applicable	Possible ? Clinical importance Large numbers required
Hypoglycemia	Not applicable	Not applicable	Confounded by insulin therapy Few events in early disease Large numbers required
Area under the curve (AUC) C-peptide	Not very sensitive	Confounded by glucose rise	Reliable, unconfounded Represents indirect (surrogate) clinical end point
Index60	? Untested	Valuable	Valuable—less reliable than AUC C-peptide
First-phase insulin release	Sensitive More invasive	? Sensitive More invasive	Not applicable (first-phase lost)
Advanced secretion and insulin sensitivity modeling	Under development	May not be better than index60	Not applicable

increased immunosuppressive risk (e.g., rituximab, alefacept). For disease-modifying therapies to be cost-effective and substantially improve quality of life and reduce the risk of long-term complications, the disease process needs to be halted altogether or at least substantially slowed for 5–10 years or more while still maintaining a favorable balance of benefit-to-risk ratio. This has been achieved in other autoimmune diseases with ongoing therapy. However, demonstrating this in T1D will require long-term ambitious projects spanning 5 or more years of continued follow-up and/or the use of combination therapies or changes in therapy to maintain benefit over time. This represents an additional challenge to the profitability of drug development programs that will need to be overcome for example by conditional regulatory approval with agreed postmarketing study programs of long-term follow-up.

IMMUNOTHERAPY APPROACHES

Although effective in preserving β-cell function (Bougnères et al. 1990; Jenner et al. 1992), generalized immunosuppression of the kind used in transplantation is not suitable for diabetes immunotherapy because of its adverse high-risk profile. Selective immunosuppression targeting specific cell subsets and cytokines represents a more favorable approach. Therapies that have demonstrated favorable effects so far in clinical trials are listed in Table 3 with mechanisms of action shown in Figure 1 (Tatovic et al. 2023). Note that for all these agents other than teplizumab, only data from small trials (phase 2) is available and maybe subject to error (Ylescupidez et al. 2023b).

The introduction of teplizumab into the clinical management of T1D in 2022 opened a new and exciting era and represents a paradigm change in the approach of treating T1D. Administration as a daily infusion over 2 weeks to people in stage 2 T1D delayed the need for insulin by almost 3 years (Herold et al. 2019; Sims et al. 2021b). However, while the plethora of immunotherapy targets already in clinical practice for other diseases opens numerous options, there are dilemmas for T1D: What are the right targets, timings, and doses for successful immunomodulation?

"Broad Target" Immunomodulators

Immunotherapies that initially showed success in preserving β-cell function have broader targets (Table 3). This is the case with targeting T cells (anti-CD3, ATG), B-cell deletion (anti-CD20), and reduction of circulating central and effector memory CD8 cells (alefacept). Teplizumab is an Fc-nonbinding monoclonal antibody targeting T cells through the T-cell receptor component CD3 (Herold et al. 2019) (this approach is discussed in more detail Chatenoud

Table 3. Summary of clinical interventions that have shown efficacy in clinical trials of preservation of β-cell function in type 1 diabetes mellitus (T1D) (see text for references)

Agent	Likely mechanism of action
Teplizumab/otelixizumab (anti-CD3)	Induction of an exhausted state in activated T cells
Alefacept (anti-CD2)	Depletion of T-effector memory cells
Low-dose antithymocyte globulin	Relative depletion of effector T cells versus T-regulator cells
Rituximab (anti-CD20)	Depletion of B cells
Abatacept (CTLA4-Ig)	Impaired T-cell activation
Golimumab/etanercept (anti-TNF)	Blockade of TNF-mediated β-cell stress
Imatinib (tyrosine kinase inhibitor)	Reduced β-cell stress, increased insulin sensitivity
Anti-IL-21 (in combination with liraglutide)	Reduced trafficking of CD8 T cells to the pancreas, reduced T follicular helper cell function
Verapamil	Reduced β-cell stress via the TXNIP pathway
Baricitinib (JAK 1/2 kinase inhibition)	Reduced MHC class I expression in β cells and CD8 T-cell activation

 Cite this article as *Cold Spring Harb Perspect Med* doi: 10.1101/cshperspect.a041597

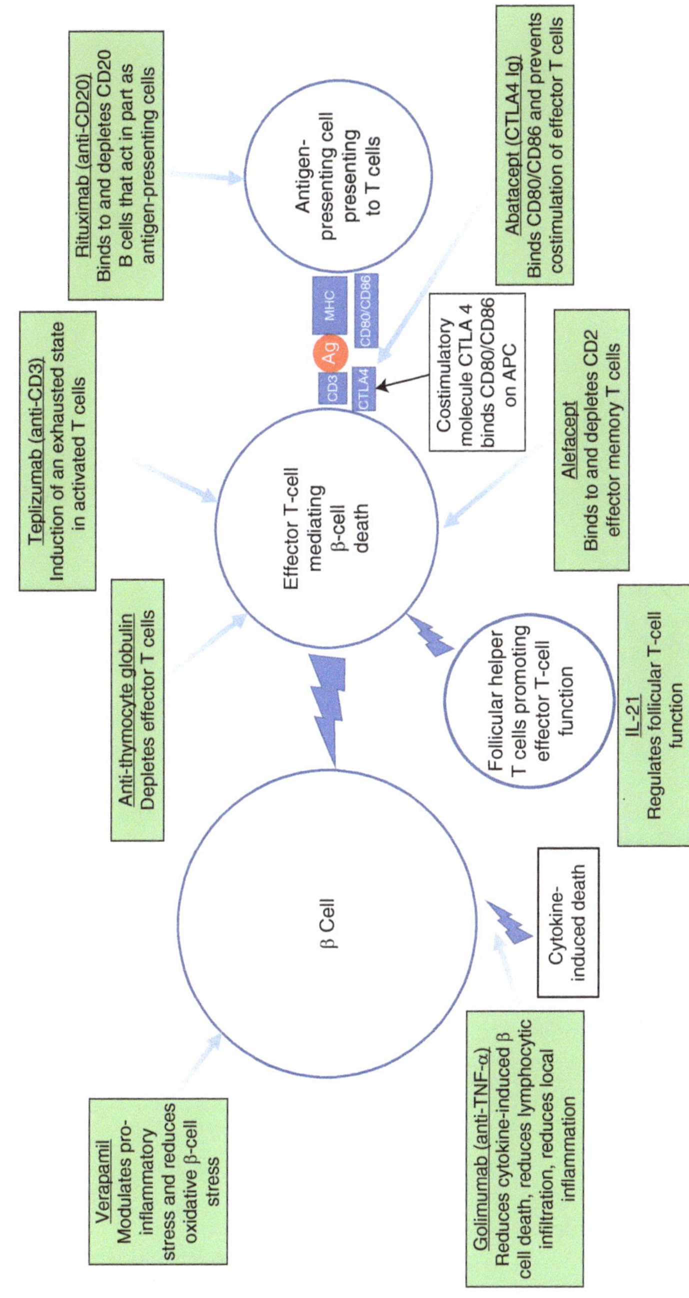

Figure 1. Different sites of action of clinical interventions to preserve β-cell function. (Ag) Antigen, (MHC) main histocompatibility complex. (Reprinted from Tatovic et al. 2023.)

et al. 2024). Low-dose ATG is an immunomodulatory agent that reduces $CD4^+$ T-effector cells, thus increasing memory $CD4^+$ cells while maintaining naive $CD8^+$ cells and most importantly having no significant effect on the T-regulatory cell compartment (Haller et al. 2019) in comparison to high-dose regimens (Gitelman et al. 2013). A recent study suggests that ATG induces an exhaustion phenotype in $CD4^+$ T cells in responders (Jacobsen et al. 2023). Rituximab addresses the autoimmunity in T1D from a different angle (i.e., by modulating the antigen presentation function of B cells through targeting their CD20 molecule) (Pescovitz et al. 2009). Alefacept binds CD2, which is expressed most prominently on $CD4^+$ and $CD8^+$ effector memory T cells, primarily responsible for autoimmune attack in T1D. It elicits a depletion of $CD4^+$ and $CD8^+$ central memory and effector memory T cells, while preserving T-regulatory cells (Rigby et al. 2015). Each of these immunotherapies has so far shown positive results by delaying C-peptide loss by 8.2–15.9 months in new-onset T1D (Ryden et al. 2013; Greenbaum et al. 2017). Selective targeting of the proinflammatory cytokine TNF with golimumab has proven to be effective in people with newly diagnosed T1D. At the end of the trial, mixed-meal-stimulated mean C-peptide levels were reduced by 18% in the golimumab group and by 51% in control (Quattrin et al. 2020). Only 43% of individuals receiving golimumab reached the definition of partial remission (defined as an insulin dose-adjusted glycated hemoglobin level score of ≤ 9) as compared to 7% in the placebo group. The effect appeared to be sustained in some people 1 year after treatment cessation (Rigby et al. 2023) and is consistent with earlier findings with etanercept (Mastrandrea et al. 2009).

The drawback with "broad target immunomodulators" is a higher level of immunosuppression and, in earlier cell-depleting therapies, problems with infusion reactions and cytokine release (Tatovic and Dayan 2021). Selective immunosuppression may therefore be a preferable choice in the long term. An exception to this may be treatments targeting an increase in regulatory T cells—these have yet to confirm benefit but are discussed in more detail in Muller et al. (2024).

"Precision" Immunomodulators

The ultimate goal is "precision" immunomodulation, which aims to target the specific pathway thought to be responsible for autoimmune attack in T1D, minimizing the degree of generalized immunosuppression and resulting in significant improvements in safety and tolerance. However, translating this approach to the clinic will require a better understanding of the effect of "precision immunomodulators" on the underlying immune mechanisms in T1D as well as rate-limiting elements of the autoimmune process.

One example is abatacept, a soluble CTLA-4 molecule fused with human IgG1. It increases CTLA-4 function and inhibits costimulation essential for T-cell activation. Studies of abatacept in people with new-onset T1D (Orban et al. 2010, 2011) and, recently, in individuals at risk of developing this disease (Russell et al. 2023) showed a modest effect on the preservation of β-cell function. A potential explanation for this limited impact is that abatacept treatment has a drawback; as well as targeting the T-effector cells that cause disease, it also decreases the homeostasis of T-regulatory cells.

The precision required for the right choice of immunomodulation also extends to determining the right dose of the agent, which may not necessarily translate from one autoimmune disease to another. This is very well reflected with treatment with low-dose interleukin 2 (IL-2). The standard regimen includes a 5-day induction phase with 1 million units/day followed by a maintenance dose of 1 million units every 2 weeks. This was proven to be effective in studies on a number of autoimmune diseases (Graßhoff et al. 2021). However, such doses did not show benefit in T1D (D Klatzmann, unpubl.). On the contrary, a lower dose of 0.2 million units/m^2 of body surface of IL-2 twice weekly in another study in T1D was more effective in preserving β-cell function (J Todd, unpubl.). This discrepancy can perhaps be explained if the ultra-low dose allows stimulation

Cite this article as *Cold Spring Harb Perspect Med* doi: 10.1101/cshperspect.a041597

solely of T-regulatory cells through their high-affinity IL-2 receptor (Yu et al. 2015) but has no effect on effector T cells. Additional "unexpected" effects, which may be favorable or unfavorable, need also to be taken into account in dose finding, such as increases in regulatory B cells (Inaba et al. 2023), CD56^{bright} natural killer (NK) cells, and mucosal-associated invariant T (MAIT) cells (Zhang et al. 2022). Similar critical dosing issues have been observed with other therapies, such anti-CD3 (Ambery et al. 2014) and ATG (Haller et al. 2019).

Another "precision" immunomodulator is ustekinumab, a monoclonal antibody that binds the shared p40 subunit of the IL-12 and IL-23 cytokines (Marwaha et al. 2021). These two cytokines play a key role in the development of T-helper 1 cells (interferon γ secreting) and T-helper 17 (IL-17 secreting) T cells, respectively (Patel and Kuchroo 2015). Although delayed, ustekinumab's effect on β-cell function in children and adolescents with newly diagnosed T1D (Tatovic et al. 2024) was evident (mixed-meal-stimulated mean C-peptide level in ustekinumab was 0.45 nmol/mol/L and 0.30 nmol/mol/L in control, i.e., 49% difference) at the end of the treatment period. The effect was to some extent comparable to some "broad" immunomodulators with the advantage of targeting only a pathogenic subset of Th17 T cells through low-risk IL-12/IL-23 inhibition without significant effect on the rest of the T-cell populations, but with resulting benefit on β-cell function.

An interesting example in the group of precision immunomodulators is anti-IL-21 monoclonal antibody that seemed to be effective in preserving endogenous insulin production only when used in combination with GLP-1 receptor agonist liraglutide in recent-onset T1D. Compared with placebo (ratio to baseline 0.61, 39% decrease), the decrease in MMTT-stimulated C-peptide concentration from baseline to week 54 was significantly smaller with combination treatment (0.90, 10% decrease), which was not seen with anti-IL-21 alone or liraglutide alone (von Herrath et al. 2021).

Antigen-based therapies are perhaps the cleanest approach to immunomodulation in T1D, but, so far, they have not been proven sufficiently effective to translate to clinical practice. (They are discussed in detail in Peakman and Santamaria 2024.)

Targeting β-Cell–Immune Systems Interactions

An alternative approach to improving precision is to target β-immune cell interactions. Three agents believed to act via this pathway, at least in part, have shown efficacy in clinical trials (see Table 3). The newest addition to this category is baricitinib inhibiting the JAK-STAT signaling pathway, which is downstream from type I and type II cytokine receptors. In this way, baricitinib blocks the action of proinflammatory cytokines that play an important role in the autoimmune destruction of β cells (Waibel et al. 2022). In a recent study in people with newly diagnosed T1D, baricitinib maintained endogenous insulin production over 12 months at baseline levels as opposed to placebo where loss was demonstrated (Waibel et al. 2023).

TIMING AND CHOICE OF IMMUNOMODULATION

Teplizumab opened the door for introducing immunotherapy for T1D into clinical practice, but we now need to keep this door wide open to allow the introduction of more agents. It is unlikely that immunotherapy for T1D will simply involve one-off "curative" treatment, as this has not been achieved in other autoimmune diseases. Instead, the approach will consist of the careful monitoring of autoimmune responses and repetitive interventions (either simultaneous or sequential). To achieve this, we need reliable immunological markers of efficacy to guide quick and efficient clinical trials that will lead to the translation to the clinic, despite all the limitations and difficulties in finding the right agent discussed above. Advanced trial designs may help in this regard (see next section).

Whatever is the choice of immunomodulation, the earlier we intervene the more β-cell function can be preserved. Although intervening in stage 3 can still lead to some β-cell preservation and metabolic improvement (Taylor et al. 2023), the greatest clinical benefit comes with the prevention of the need for insulin therapy for many years. This approach requires individuals in stage 1 and stage 2 T1D to be identified through family studies or population-based screening programs. These programs have been trialled in the research arena, where they addressed the issues of appropriate age for screening, follow-up of antibody-positive individuals, and optimal target population (Sims et al. 2022). Unfortunately, restricting screening to individuals with a family history of T1D, although convenient, will miss the majority of people in the early stages of T1D as ~90% of those who will present with new T1D do not have a positive family history (DiMeglio et al. 2018; Karges et al. 2021). Therefore, to identify individuals who would benefit from therapies to prevent T1D, those without a positive family history must also be identified. Data from public health screening in Bavaria indicate that the rate of multiple islet antibody positivity in children not known to have diabetes is 0.3% (Hummel et al. 2023).

The optimal choice of immunomodulation will probably also depend on the stage of the disease and the intensity of the autoimmune process that defines the rate of β-cell loss. This is very different in different people (Weiss et al. 2022). The group at the University of Exeter has described two distinct patterns of insulitis occurring in patients with recent-onset T1D, which they refer to as different "endotypes" (discussed in more detail in Herold and Krischer 2024). Patients diagnosed before age 7 display insulitis with a high $CD20^+$ cell infiltrate, while people diagnosed after the age of 13 have a histologically less aggressive disease with a lower frequency of $CD20^+$ cells (Leete et al. 2016). It remains to be established whether the latter group is a histological equivalent of the clinically recognized cohort of "slow progressors" who develop symptomatic disease late in life and decline slowly in insulin production (Long et al. 2018; Pöllänen et al. 2019). This suggests that some individuals may need only low-grade immunomodulation or none at all. On the other hand, those most in need of immunomodulation are the ones that will rapidly progress to near total insulin deficiency. A number of clinical and laboratory tools are available to help us identify those individuals. Age of diagnosis is one of the most striking determinants of rapid progression, with younger children progressing faster through stages of diabetes (Ylescupidez et al. 2023b). Genetics, defined by the Genetic Risk Score, plays an important role in determining risk (Greenbaum et al. 2019) and possibly also the rate of progression to T1D (Oram et al. 2016; Sharp et al. 2019; Ferrat et al. 2020). Taking this into account, we can postulate that the diagnosis of T1D in or shortly before stage 3 (when limited amount of rapidly declining β-cell function is available [Greenbaum et al. 2012]), or in younger children (irrespective of the T1D stage as they are likely to lose β-cell function rapidly) warrants the choice of "broad" immunomodulators to cover multiple potential pathways. Treatments such as teplizumab, which recently showed promising results even in stage 3 T1D (Ramos et al. 2023), would be suitable for this purpose. At this stage, when there is a race with time to preserve the small amount of β-cell function remaining, it is reasonable to also consider more aggressive simultaneous combinations of different agents. The choice of combinations will need to be based on a deep understanding of the pathophysiology on T1D to combine agents with complimentary activity. For instance, this can be achieved by targeting different immune cell subsets to achieve a balance between effector T cells and regulatory T cells or targeting different mechanistic pathways. In TN25, for example, rituximab-pvvr alone (targeting B cells) will be compared with rituximab plus abatacept (targeting B cells and T-cell activation—NCT03929601). An alternative approach is to combine a broad immunomodulator such as teplizumab with verapamil (a calcium channel blocker) that seems to preserve β-cell function in new-onset T1D (Ovalle et al. 2018) by reducing β-cell stress through the reduction in chromogranin A (Xu et al. 2022). In this way, the β cell is protected from stress while the immunomodulator addresses the autoimmune attack. Additional combinations with verapamil involving other immunotherapy agents, such as ATG and Golimumab, are being tested (ISRCTN45965456). Note that testing of combinations potentially requires large studies if placebo arms are also included, and advanced trial designs to increase the efficiency of use of trial subjects should be considered, see below (Anderson et al. 2022).

The excellent safety profile of "precision" immunomodulators, with little evidence of generalized immunosuppression, makes them attractive therapeutic candidates for earlier stages of T1D before clinical hyperglycemia when significant residual β-cell function allows certain flexibility. These stages require a careful balance between high safety profile agents (as they are given to a well individual) and highly efficient agents (to prevent further β-cell loss and insulin dependency). Agents that meet some of these criteria, certainly with their safety profile, were previously discussed (ustekinumab).

It is also reasonable to expect that some individuals will demonstrate an "escape" phenomenon from one agent, which will warrant a strategy with the combination of agents or a change to a different agent with the broader target, eliciting more substantive immunosuppression. This will be the approach if the disease progresses, and the affected individual is approaching stage 3 T1D.

ADVANCED TRIAL DESIGNS

The small numbers/difficulty in finding subjects for trials of disease-modifying agents in T1D coupled with the relatively long delay to clinical end points support the use of advanced trial designs such as platform, adaptive, and/or sequential multiple assignment randomized trials (SMART) to accelerate progress as used in oncology and COVID-19 (Berry et al. 2015; I-SPY COVID Consortium 2022; Park et al. 2022). Platform trials increase efficiency by including multiple interventions into a standard protocol with shared controls. Adaptive trials allow treatment arms to be dropped or new treatments introduced into a platform trial part way through the study following prespecified interim analysis criteria. SMART trials allow subjects who are failing in a treatment arm to be re-randomized to alternative therapies without having to recruit new subjects (Almirall et al. 2014). These designs are efficient in time and recruitment requirements. They generate a signal to decide which treatments or combinations of treatments to take forward but definitive studies such as placebo-controlled randomized trials or appropriately powered factorial-designed trials of combinations are required for confirmation (Anderson et al. 2022). The T1D plus trial combining verapamil with multiple immune modulatory against in stage 3 T1D represents an example of a platform rial design in T1D disease modification (ISRCTN45965456).

CONCLUSION

T1D is entering an exciting arena where the focus is shifted from metabolic replacement therapy with insulin to proactive disease-modifying treatments that prevent the loss of insulin secretory capacity. To reach this goal, many changes will need to be implemented. These include changing the attitude of healthcare professionals toward novel treatment strategies, the development of effective screening programs to identify affected individuals in early-stage disease, improvements in end points/biomarkers, and trial design to accelerate drug development and enable increasingly appropriate selection of immunomodulators tailored to an individual's needs and response (see Fig. 1). To achieve this and accelerate progress, pharmaceutical partners both from discovery/biotech and large pharma need to be engaged along with the voice of patients, families, and clinicians in emphasizing the value of moving toward "insulin-free T1D."

REFERENCES

**Reference is in this subject collection.*

Almirall D, Nahum-Shani I, Sherwood NE, Murphy SA. 2014. Introduction to SMART designs for the development of adaptive interventions: with application to weight loss research. *Transl Behav Med* **4:** 260–274. doi:10.1007/s13142-014-0265-0

Ambery P, Donner TW, Biswas N, Donaldson J, Parkin J, Dayan CM. 2014. Efficacy and safety of low-dose otelixizumab anti-CD3 monoclonal antibody in preserving C-peptide secretion in adolescent type 1 diabetes: DEFEND-2, a randomized, placebo-controlled, double-blind, multicentre study. *Diabet Med* **31:** 399–402. doi:10.1111/dme.12361

American Diabetes Association. 2021. Classification and diagnosis of diabetes: standards of medical care in diabetes-2021. *Diabetes Care* **44:** S15–S33. doi:10.2337/dc21-S002

Anderson RL, DiMeglio LA, Mander AP, Dayan CM, Linsley PS, Herold KC, Marinac M, Ahmed ST. 2022. Innovative designs and logistical considerations for expedited clinical development of combination disease-modifying treatments for type 1 diabetes. *Diabetes Care* **45:** 2189–2201. doi:10.2337/dc22-0308

Anderzén J, Hermann JM, Samuelsson U, Charalampopoulos D, Svensson J, Skrivarhaug T, Fröhlich-Reiterer E, Maahs DM, Akesson K, Kapellen T, et al. 2020. International benchmarking in type 1 diabetes: large difference in childhood HbA1c between eight high-income countries but similar rise during adolescence—a quality registry study. *Pediatr Diabetes* **21:** 621–627. doi:10.1111/pedi.13014

Aronson R, Gottlieb PA, Christiansen JS, Donner TW, Bosi E, Bode BW, Pozzilli P; DEFEND Investigator Group. 2014. Low-dose otelixizumab anti-CD3 monoclonal antibody DEFEND-1 study: results of the randomized phase III study in recent-onset human type 1 diabetes. *Diabetes Care* **37:** 2746–2754. doi:10.2337/dc13-0327

Baidal DA, Ballou CM, Rickels MR, Berney T, Pattou F, Payne EH, Barton FB, Alejandro R; CITR Investigators. 2023. Predictive value of C-peptide measures for clinical outcomes of β-cell replacement therapy in type 1 diabetes: report from the Collaborative Islet Transplant Registry (CITR). *Diabetes Care* **46:** 697–703. doi:10.2337/dc22-1155

Berry SM, Connor JT, Lewis RJ. 2015. The platform trial: an efficient strategy for evaluating multiple treatments. *JAMA* **313:** 1619–1620. doi:10.1001/jama.2015.2316

Bogun MM, Bundy BN, Goland RS, Greenbaum CJ. 2020. C-peptide levels in subjects followed longitudinally before and after type 1 diabetes diagnosis in TrialNet. *Diabetes Care* **43:** 1836–1842. doi:10.2337/dc19-2288

Boughton CK, Allen JM, Ware J, Wilinska ME, Hartnell S, Thankamony A, Randell T, Ghatak A, Besser REJ, Elleri D, et al. 2022. Closed-loop therapy and preservation of C-peptide secretion in type 1 diabetes. *N Engl J Med* **387:** 882–893. doi:10.1056/NEJMoa2203496

Bougnères PF, Landais P, Boisson C, Carel JC, Frament N, Boitard C, Chaussain JL, Bach JF. 1990. Limited duration of remission of insulin dependency in children with recent overt type I diabetes treated with low-dose cyclosporin. *Diabetes* **39:** 1264–1272. doi:10.2337/diab.39.10.1264

Carr ALJ, Inshaw JRJ, Flaxman CS, Leete P, Wyatt RC, Russell LA, Palmer M, Prasolov D, Worthington T, Hull B, et al. 2022. Circulating C-peptide levels in living children and young people and pancreatic β-cell loss in pancreas donors across type 1 diabetes disease duration. *Diabetes* **71:** 1591–1596. doi:10.2337/db22-0097

* Chatenoud L, Herold KC, Bach JF, Bluestone JA. 2024. The teplizumab saga: the challenge of not getting lost in clinical translation. *Cold Spring Harb Perspect Med* doi:10.1101/cshperspect.a041600

Couper JJ, Haller MJ, Greenbaum CJ, Ziegler AG, Wherrett DK, Knip M, Craig ME. 2018. ISPAD clinical practice consensus guidelines 2018: stages of type 1 diabetes in children and adolescents. *Pediatr Diabetes* **19:** 20–27. doi:10.1111/pedi.12734

Crabtree TSJ, Griffin TP, Yap YW, Narendran P, Gallen G, Furlong N, Cranston I, Chakera A, Philbey C, Karamat MA, et al. 2023. Hybrid closed-loop therapy in adults with type 1 diabetes and above-target HbA1c: a real-world observational study. *Diabetes Care* **46:** 1831–1838. doi:10.2337/dc23-0635

DiMeglio LA, Evans-Molina C, Oram RA. 2018. Type 1 diabetes. *Lancet* **391:** 2449–2462. doi:10.1016/S0140-6736(18)31320-5

Evans-Molina C, Sims EK, DiMeglio LA, Ismail HM, Steck AK, Palmer JP, Krischer JP, Geyer S, Xu P, Sosenko JM, et al. 2018. Β cell dysfunction exists more than 5 years before type 1 diabetes diagnosis. *JCI Insight* **3:** e120877. doi:10.1172/jci.insight.120877

Ferrat LA, Vehik K, Sharp SA, Lernmark Å, Rewers MJ, She JX, Ziegler AG, Toppari J, Akolkar B, Krischer JP, et al. 2020. A combined risk score enhances prediction of type 1 diabetes among susceptible children. *Nat Med* **26:** 1247–1255. doi:10.1038/s41591-020-0930-4

Foster NC, Beck RW, Miller KM, Clements MA, Rickels MR, DiMeglio LA, Maahs DM, Tamborlane WV, Bergenstal R, Smith E, et al. 2019. State of type 1 diabetes management and outcomes from the T1D exchange in 2016–2018. *Diabetes Technol Ther* **21:** 66–72. doi:10.1089/dia.2018.0384

Galderisi A, Carr ALJ, Martino M, Taylor P, Senior P, Dayan C. 2023a. Quantifying β cell function in the preclinical stages of type 1 diabetes. *Diabetologia* **66:** 2189–2199. doi:10.1007/s00125-023-06011-5

Galderisi A, Evans-Molina C, Martino M, Caprio S, Cobelli C, Moran A. 2023b. β-Cell function and insulin sensitivity in youth with early type 1 diabetes from a 2-hour 7-sample OGTT. *J Clin Endocrinol Metab* **108:** 1376–1386. doi:10.1210/clinem/dgac740

Gitelman SE, Gottlieb PA, Rigby MR, Felner EI, Willi SM, Fisher LK, Moran A, Gottschalk M, Moore WV, Pinckney A, et al. 2013. Antithymocyte globulin treatment for patients with recent-onset type 1 diabetes: 12-month results of a randomised, placebo-controlled, phase 2 trial. *Lancet Diabetes Endocrinol* **1:** 306–316. doi:10.1016/S2213-8587(13)70065-2

Graßhoff H, Comdühr S, Monne LR, Müller A, Lamprecht P, Riemekasten G, Humrich JY. 2021. Low-dose IL-2 therapy in autoimmune and rheumatic diseases. *Front Immunol* **12:** 648408. doi:10.3389/fimmu.2021.648408

Greenbaum CJ, Beam CA, Boulware D, Gitelman SE, Gottlieb PA, Herold KC, Lachin JM, McGee P, Palmer JP, Pescovitz MD, et al. 2012. Fall in C-peptide during first 2 years from diagnosis: evidence of at least two distinct phases from composite type 1 diabetes TrialNet data. *Diabetes* **61:** 2066–2073. doi:10.2337/db11-1538

Greenbaum C, Lord S, VanBuecken D. 2017. Emerging concepts on disease-modifying therapies in type 1 diabetes. *Curr Diab Rep* **17:** 119. doi:10.1007/s11892-017-0932-x

Greenbaum C, VanBuecken D, Lord S. 2019. Disease-modifying therapies in type 1 diabetes: a look into the future of diabetes practice. *Drugs* **79:** 43–61. doi:10.1007/s40265-018-1035-y

Gubitosi-Klug RA, Braffett BH, Hitt S, Arends V, Uschner D, Jones K, Diminick L, Karger AB, Paterson AD, Roshandel

D, et al. 2021. Residual β cell function in long-term type 1 diabetes associates with reduced incidence of hypoglycemia. *J Clin Invest* **131:** e143011. doi:10.1172/JCI143011

Haller MJ, Long SA, Blanchfield JL, Schatz DA, Skyler JS, Krischer JP, Bundy BN, Geyer SM, Warnock MV, Miller JL, et al. 2019. Low-dose anti-thymocyte globulin preserves C-peptide, reduces HbA1c, and increases regulatory to conventional T-cell ratios in new-onset type 1 diabetes: two-year clinical trial data. *Diabetes* **68:** 1267–1276. doi:10.2337/db19-0057

Hernar I, Cooper JG, Nilsen RM, Skinner TC, Strandberg RB, Iversen MM, Graue M, Ernes T, Løvaas KF, Madsen TV, et al. 2024. Diabetes distress and associations with demographic and clinical variables: a nationwide population-based registry study of 10,186 adults with type 1 diabetes in Norway. *Diabetes Care* **47:** 126–131. doi:10.2337/dc23-1001

* Herold KC, Krischer JP. 2024. The pathogenesis of type 1 diabetes. *Cold Spring Harb Perspect Med* doi:10.1101/cshperspect.a041623

Herold KC, Bundy BN, Long SA, Bluestone JA, DiMeglio LA, Dufort MJ, Gitelman SE, Gottlieb PA, Krischer JP, Linsley PS, et al. 2019. An anti-CD3 antibody, teplizumab, in relatives at risk for type 1 diabetes. *N Engl J Med* **381:** 603–613. doi:10.1056/NEJMoa1902226

Holman N, Woch E, Dayan C, Warner J, Robinson H, Young B, Elliott J. 2023. National trends in hyperglycemia and diabetic ketoacidosis in children, adolescents, and young adults with type 1 diabetes: a challenge due to age or stage of development, or is new thinking about service provision needed? *Diabetes Care* **46:** 1404–1408. doi:10.2337/dc23-0180

Hummel S, Carl J, Friedl N, Winkler C, Kick K, Stock J, Reinmüller F, Ramminger C, Schmidt J, Lwowsky D, et al. 2023. Children diagnosed with presymptomatic type 1 diabetes through public health screening have milder diabetes at clinical manifestation. *Diabetologia* **66:** 1633–1642. doi:10.1007/s00125-023-05953-0

Inaba A, Tuong ZK, Zhao TX, Stewart AP, Mathews R, Truman L, Sriranjan R, Kennet J, Saeb-Parsy K, Wicker L, et al. 2023. Low-dose IL-2 enhances the generation of IL-10-producing immunoregulatory B cells. *Nat Commun* **14:** 2071. doi:10.1038/s41467-023-37424-w

Insel RA, Dunne JL, Atkinson MA, Chiang JL, Dabelea D, Gottlieb PA, Greenbaum CJ, Herold KC, Krischer JP, Lernmark Å, et al. 2015. Staging presymptomatic type 1 diabetes: a scientific statement of JDRF, the Endocrine Society, and the American Diabetes Association. *Diabetes Care* **38:** 1964–1974. doi:10.2337/dc15-1419

Ismail HM, Cuthbertson D, Gitelman SE, Skyler JS, Steck AK, Rodriguez H, Atkinson M, Nathan BM, Redondo MJ, Herold KC, et al. 2022. The transition from a compensatory increase to a decrease in C-peptide during the progression to type 1 diabetes and its relation to risk. *Diabetes Care* **45:** 2264–2270. doi:10.2337/dc22-0167

I-SPY COVID Consortium. 2022. Clinical trial design during and beyond the pandemic: the I-SPY COVID trial. *Nat Med* **28:** 9–11. doi:10.1038/s41591-021-01617-x

Jacobsen LM, Bundy BN, Ismail HM, Clements M, Warnock M, Geyer S, Schatz DA, Sosenko JM. 2022. Index60 is superior to HbA1c for identifying individuals at high risk for type 1 diabetes. *J Clin Endocrinol Metab* **107:** 2784–2792. doi:10.1210/clinem/dgac440

Jacobsen LM, Diggins K, Blanchfield L, McNichols J, Perry DJ, Brant J, Dong X, Bacher R, Gersuk VH, Schatz DA, et al. 2023. Responders to low-dose ATG induce CD4$^+$ T cell exhaustion in type 1 diabetes. *JCI Insight* **8:** e161812. doi:10.1172/jci.insight.161812

Jenner M, Bradish G, Stiller C, Atkison P. 1992. Cyclosporin A treatment of young children with newly diagnosed type 1 (insulin-dependent) diabetes mellitus. London Diabetes Study Group. *Diabetologia* **35:** 884–888. doi:10.1007/BF00399937

Jeyam A, Colhoun H, McGurnaghan S, Blackbourn L, McDonald TJ, Palmer CNA, McKnight JA, Strachan MWJ, Patrick AW, Chalmers J, et al. 2021. Clinical impact of residual C-peptide secretion in type 1 diabetes on glycemia and microvascular complications. *Diabetes Care* **44:** 390–398. doi:10.2337/dc20-0567

Karges B, Prinz N, Placzek K, Datz N, Papsch M, Strier U, Agena D, Bonfig W, Kentrup H, Holl RW. 2021. A comparison of familial and sporadic type 1 diabetes among young patients. *Diabetes Care* **44:** 1116–1124. doi:10.2337/dc20-1829

Keskinen P, Korhonen S, Kupila A, Veijola R, Erkkilä S, Savolainen H, Arvilommi P, Simell T, Ilonen J, Knip M, et al. 2002. First-phase insulin response in young healthy children at genetic and immunological risk for type 1 diabetes. *Diabetologia* **45:** 1639–1648. doi:10.1007/s00125-002-0981-8

Latres E, Greenbaum CJ, Oyaski ML, Dayan CM, Colhoun HM, Lachin JM, Skyler JS, Rickels MR, Ahmed ST, Dutta S, et al. 2024. Evidence for C-peptide as a validated surrogate to predict clinical benefits in trials of disease-modifying therapies for type 1 diabetes. *Diabetes* **73:** 823–833. doi:10.2337/dbi23-0012

Leete P, Willcox A, Krogvold L, Dahl-Jørgensen K, Foulis AK, Richardson SJ, Morgan NG. 2016. Differential insulitic profiles determine the extent of β-cell destruction and the age at onset of type 1 diabetes. *Diabetes* **65:** 1362–1369. doi:10.2337/db15-1615

Libman I, Bingley PJ, Becker D, Buckner JH, DiMeglio LA, Gitelman SE, Greenbaum C, Haller MJ, Ismail HM, Krischer J, et al. 2023. Hydroxychloroquine in stage 1 type 1 diabetes. *Diabetes Care* **46:** 2035–2043. doi:10.2337/dc23-1096

Long AE, Wilson IV, Becker DJ, Libman IM, Arena VC, Wong FS, Steck AK, Rewers MJ, Yu L, Achenbach P, et al. 2018. Characteristics of slow progression to diabetes in multiple islet autoantibody-positive individuals from five longitudinal cohorts: the SNAIL study. *Diabetologia* **61:** 1484–1490. doi:10.1007/s00125-018-4591-5

Martino M, Galderisi A, Evans-Molina C, Dayan C. 2024. Revisiting the pattern of loss of β-cell function in preclinical type 1 diabetes. *Diabetes* **73:** 1769–1779. doi:10.2337/db24-0163

Marwaha AK, Chow S, Pesenacker AM, Cook L, Sun A, Long SA, Yang JHM, Ward-Hartstonge KA, Williams E, Domingo-Vila C, et al. 2021. A phase 1b open-label dose-finding study of ustekinumab in young adults with type 1 diabetes. *Immunother Adv* **2:** ltab022. doi:10.1093/immadv/ltab022

Mastrandrea L, Yu J, Behrens T, Buchlis J, Albini C, Fourtner S, Quattrin T. 2009. Etanercept treatment in children with new-onset type 1 diabetes: pilot randomized, placebo-controlled, double-blind study. *Diabetes Care* **32:** 1244–1249. doi:10.2337/dc09-0054

Mathieu C, Martens PJ, Vangoitsenhoven R. 2021. One hundred years of insulin therapy. *Nat Rev Endocrinol* **17:** 715–725. doi:10.1038/s41574-021-00542-w

McKnight JA, Wild SH, Lamb MJ, Cooper MN, Jones TW, Davis EA, Hofer S, Fritsch M, Schober E, Svensson J, et al. 2015. Glycaemic control of type 1 diabetes in clinical practice early in the 21st century: an international comparison. *Diabet Med* **32:** 1036–1050. doi:10.1111/dme.12676

Miller KM, Foster NC, Beck RW, Bergenstal RM, DuBose SN, DiMeglio LA, Maahs DM, Tamborlane WV, T1D Exchange Clinic Network. 2015. Current state of type 1 diabetes treatment in the U.S.: updated data from the T1D exchange clinic registry. *Diabetes Care* **38:** 971–978. doi:10.2337/dc15-0078

* Muller YD, Ho P, Bluestone JA, Tang Q. 2024. Rebalancing the immune system to treat type 1 diabetes. *Cold Spring Harb Perspect Med* doi:10.1101/cshperspect.a041599

Oram RA, Patel K, Hill A, Shields B, McDonald TJ, Jones A, Hattersley AT, Weedon MN. 2016. A type 1 diabetes genetic risk score can aid discrimination between type 1 and type 2 diabetes in young adults. *Diabetes Care* **39:** 337–344. doi:10.2337/dc15-1111

Oram RA, Sims EK, Evans-Molina C. 2019. β cells in type 1 diabetes: mass and function; sleeping or dead? *Diabetologia* **62:** 567–577. doi:10.1007/s00125-019-4822-4

Orban T, Farkas K, Jalahej H, Kis J, Treszl A, Falk B, Reijonen H, Wolfsdorf J, Ricker A, Matthews JB, et al. 2010. Autoantigen-specific regulatory T cells induced in patients with type 1 diabetes mellitus by insulin B-chain immunotherapy. *J Autoimmun* **34:** 408–415. doi:10.1016/j.jaut.2009.10.005

Orban T, Bundy B, Becker DJ, DiMeglio LA, Gitelman SE, Goland R, Gottlieb PA, Greenbaum CJ, Marks JB, Monzavi R, et al. 2011. Co-stimulation modulation with abatacept in patients with recent-onset type 1 diabetes: a randomised, double-blind, placebo-controlled trial. *Lancet* **378:** 412–419. doi:10.1016/S0140-6736(11)60886-6

Orban T, Bundy B, Becker DJ, DiMeglio LA, Gitelman SE, Goland R, Gottlieb PA, Greenbaum CJ, Marks JB, Monzavi R, et al. 2014. Costimulation modulation with abatacept in patients with recent-onset type 1 diabetes: follow-up 1 year after cessation of treatment. *Diabetes Care* **37:** 1069–1075. doi:10.2337/dc13-0604

Ovalle F, Grimes T, Xu G, Patel AJ, Grayson TB, Thielen LA, Li P, Shalev A. 2018. Verapamil and β cell function in adults with recent-onset type 1 diabetes. *Nat Med* **24:** 1108–1112. doi:10.1038/s41591-018-0089-4

Park JJH, Detry MA, Murthy S, Guyatt G, Mills EJ. 2022. How to use and interpret the results of a platform trial: users' guide to the medical literature. *JAMA* **327:** 67–74. doi:10.1001/jama.2021.22507

Patel DD, Kuchroo VK. 2015. Th17 cell pathway in human immunity: lessons from genetics and therapeutic interventions. *Immunity* **43:** 1040–1051. doi:10.1016/j.immuni.2015.12.003

* Peakman M, Santamaria P. 2024. Autoantigen-specific immunotherapies for the prevention and treatment of type 1 diabetes. *Cold Spring Harb Perspect Med* doi:10.1101/cshperspect.a041598

Pescovitz MD, Greenbaum CJ, Krause-Steinrauf H, Becker DJ, Gitelman SE, Goland R, Gottlieb PA, Marks JB, McGee PF, Moran AM, et al. 2009. Rituximab, B-lymphocyte depletion, and preservation of β-cell function. *N Engl J Med* **361:** 2143–2152. doi:10.1056/NEJMoa0904452

Pöllänen PM, Lempainen J, Laine AP, Toppari J, Veijola R, Ilonen J, Siljander H, Knip M. 2019. Characteristics of slow progression to type 1 diabetes in children with increased HLA-conferred disease risk. *J Clin Endocrinol Metab* **104:** 5585–5594. doi:10.1210/jc.2019-01069

Powers AC. 2021. Type 1 diabetes mellitus: much progress, many opportunities. *J Clin Invest* **131:** e142242. doi:10.1172/JCI142242

Prigge R, McKnight JA, Wild SH, Haynes A, Jones TW, Davis EA, Rami-Merhar B, Fritsch M, Prchla C, Lavens A, et al. 2022. International comparison of glycaemic control in people with type 1 diabetes: an update and extension. *Diabet Med* **39:** e14766. doi:10.1111/dme.14766

Quattrin T, Haller MJ, Steck AK, Felner EI, Li Y, Xia Y, Leu JH, Zoka R, Hedrick JA, Rigby MR, et al. 2020. Golimumab and β-cell function in youth with new-onset type 1 diabetes. *N Engl J Med* **383:** 2007–2017. doi:10.1056/NEJMoa2006136

Ramos EL, Dayan CM, Chatenoud L, Sumnik Z, Simmons KM, Szypowska A, Gitelman SE, Knecht LA, Niemoeller E, Tian W, et al. 2023. Teplizumab and β-cell function in newly diagnosed type 1 diabetes. *N Engl J Med* **389:** 2151–2161. doi:10.1056/NEJMoa2308743

Rigby MR, Harris KM, Pinckney A, DiMeglio LA, Rendell MS, Felner EI, Dostou JM, Gitelman SE, Griffin KJ, Tsalikian E, et al. 2015. Alefacept provides sustained clinical and immunological effects in new-onset type 1 diabetes patients. *J Clin Invest* **125:** 3285–3296. doi:10.1172/JCI81722

Rigby MR, Hayes B, Li Y, Vercruysse F, Hedrick JA, Quattrin T. 2023. Two-year follow-up from the T1GER study: continued off-therapy metabolic improvements in children and young adults with new-onset T1D treated with golimumab and characterization of responders. *Diabetes Care* **46:** 561–569. doi:10.2337/dc22-0908

Rodriguez-Calvo T, Zapardiel-Gonzalo J, Amirian N, Castillo E, Lajevardi Y, Krogvold L, Dahl-Jørgensen K, von Herrath MG. 2017. Increase in pancreatic proinsulin and preservation of β-cell mass in autoantibody-positive donors prior to type 1 diabetes onset. *Diabetes* **66:** 1334–1345. doi:10.2337/db16-1343

Russell WE, Bundy BN, Anderson MS, Cooney LA, Gitelman SE, Goland RS, Gottlieb PA, Greenbaum CJ, Haller MJ, Krischer JP, et al. 2023. Abatacept for delay of type 1 diabetes progression in stage 1 relatives at risk: a randomized, double-masked, controlled trial. *Diabetes Care* **46:** 1005–1013. doi:10.2337/dc22-2200

Russell-Jones D, Herring R. 2021. 100 years of physiology, discrimination and wonder. *Diabet Med* **38:** e14642. doi:10.1111/dme.14642

Ryden AK, Wesley JD, Coppieters KT, Von Herrath MG. 2013. Non-antigenic and antigenic interventions in type 1 diabetes. *Hum Vaccin Immunother* **10:** 838–846. doi:10.4161/hv.26890

Sandy JL, Tittel SR, Rompicherla S, Karges B, James S, Rioles N, Zimmerman AG, Fröhlich-Reiterer E, Maahs DM, Lanzinger S, et al. 2024. Demographic, clinical, management, and outcome characteristics of 8,004 young children with type 1 diabetes. *Diabetes Care* **47:** 660–667. doi:10.2337/dc23-1317

Sharp SA, Rich SS, Wood AR, Jones SE, Beaumont RN, Harrison JW, Schneider DA, Locke JM, Tyrrell J, Weedon MN, et al. 2019. Development and standardization of an improved type 1 diabetes genetic risk score for use in newborn screening and incident diagnosis. *Diabetes Care* **42:** 200–207. doi:10.2337/dc18-1785

Sherry N, Hagopian W, Ludvigsson J, Jain SM, Wahlen J, Ferry RJ, Bode B, Aronoff S, Holland C, Carlin D, et al. 2011. Teplizumab for treatment of type 1 diabetes (Protégé study): 1-year results from a randomised, placebo-controlled trial. *Lancet* **378:** 487–497. doi:10.1016/S0140-6736(11)60931-8

Sims EK, Carr ALJ, Oram RA, DiMeglio LA, Evans-Molina C. 2021a. 100 years of insulin: celebrating the past, present and future of diabetes therapy. *Nat Med* **27:** 1154–1164. doi:10.1038/s41591-021-01418-2

Sims EK, Bundy BN, Stier K, Serti E, Lim N, Long SA, Geyer SM, Moran A, Greenbaum CJ, Evans-Molina C, et al. 2021b. Teplizumab improves and stabilizes β cell function in antibody-positive high-risk individuals. *Sci Transl Med* **13:** eabc8980. doi:10.1126/scitranslmed.abc8980

Sims EK, Besser REJ, Dayan C, Geno Rasmussen C, Greenbaum C, Griffin KJ, Hagopian W, Knip M, Long AE, Martin F, et al. 2022. Screening for type 1 diabetes in the general population: a status report and perspective. *Diabetes* **71:** 610–623. doi:10.2337/dbi20-0054

Sims EK, Geyer SM, Long SA, Herold KC. 2023. High proinsulin ratio identifies individuals with stage 2 type 1 diabetes at high risk for progression to clinical diagnosis and responses to teplizumab treatment. *Diabetologia* **66:** 2283–2291. doi:10.1007/s00125-023-06003-5

Tatovic D, Dayan CM. 2021. Replacing insulin with immunotherapy: time for a paradigm change in type 1 diabetes. *Diabet Med* **38:** e14696. doi:10.1111/dme.14696

Tatovic D, Narendran P, Dayan CM. 2023. A perspective on treating type 1 diabetes mellitus before insulin is needed. *Nat Rev Endocrinol* **19:** 361–370. doi:10.1038/s41574-023-00837-0

Tatovic D, Marwaha A, Taylor P, Hanna SJ, Carter K, Cheung WY, Luzio S, Dunseath G, Hutchings HA, Holland G, et al. 2024. Ustekinumab for type 1 diabetes in adolescents: a multicenter, double-blind, randomized phase 2 trial. *Nat Med* **30:** 2657–2666. doi:10.1038/s41591-024-03115-2

Taylor PN, Collins KS, Lam A, Karpen SR, Greeno B, Walker F, Lozano A, Atabakhsh E, Ahmed ST, Marinac M, et al. 2023. C-peptide and metabolic outcomes in trials of disease modifying therapy in new-onset type 1 diabetes: an individual participant meta-analysis. *Lancet Diabetes Endocrinol* **11:** 915–925. doi:10.1016/S2213-8587(23)00267-X

The Diabetes Control and Complications Trial Research Group. 1998. Effect of intensive therapy on residual β-cell function in patients with type 1 diabetes in the diabetes control and complications trial. A randomized, controlled trial. *Ann Intern Med* **128:** 517–523. doi:10.7326/0003-4819-128-7-199804010-00001

Van Loocke M, Battelino T, Tittel SR, Prahalad P, Goksen D, Davis E, Casteels K; SWEET Study Group. 2021. Lower HbA1c targets are associated with better metabolic control. *Eur J Pediatr* **180:** 1513–1520. doi:10.1007/s00431-020-03891-2

von Herrath M, Bain SC, Bode B, Clausen JO, Coppieters K, Gaysina L, Gumprecht J, Hansen TK, Mathieu C, Morales C, et al. 2021. Anti-interleukin-21 antibody and liraglutide for the preservation of β-cell function in adults with recent-onset type 1 diabetes: a randomised, double-blind, placebo-controlled, phase 2 trial. *Lancet Diabetes Endocrinol* **9:** 212–224. doi:10.1016/S2213-8587(21)00019-X

Waibel M, Thomas HE, Wentworth JM, Couper JJ, MacIsaac RJ, Cameron FJ, So M, Krishnamurthy B, Doyle MC, Kay TW. 2022. Investigating the efficacy of baricitinib in new onset type 1 diabetes mellitus (BANDIT)-study protocol for a phase 2, randomized, placebo controlled trial. *Trials* **23:** 433. doi:10.1186/s13063-022-06356-z

Waibel M, Wentworth JM, So M, Couper JJ, Cameron FJ, MacIsaac RJ, Atlas G, Gorelik A, Litwak S, Sanz-Villanueva L, et al. 2023. Baricitinib and β-cell function in patients with new-onset type 1 diabetes. *N Engl J Med* **389:** 2140–2150. doi:10.1056/NEJMoa2306691

Wasag DR, Gregory JW, Dayan C, Harvey JN; Brecon Group. 2018. Excess all-cause mortality before age 30 in childhood onset type 1 diabetes: data from the Brecon Group Cohort in Wales. *Arch Dis Child* **103:** 44–48. doi:10.1136/archdischild-2016-312581

Watkins RA, Evans-Molina C, Terrell JK, Day KH, Guindon L, Restrepo IA, Mirmira RG, Blum JS, DiMeglio LA. 2016. Proinsulin and heat shock protein 90 as biomarkers of β-cell stress in the early period after onset of type 1 diabetes. *Transl Res* **168:** 96–106.e1. doi:10.1016/j.trsl.2015.08.010

Weiss A, Zapardiel-Gonzalo J, Voss F, Jolink M, Stock J, Haupt F, Kick K, Welzhofer T, Heublein A, Winkler C, et al. 2022. Progression likelihood score identifies substages of presymptomatic type 1 diabetes in childhood public health screening. *Diabetologia* **65:** 2121–2131. doi:10.1007/s00125-022-05780-9

Xu G, Grimes TD, Grayson TB, Chen J, Thielen LA, Tse HM, Li P, Kanke M, Lin TT, Schepmoes AA, et al. 2022. Exploratory study reveals far reaching systemic and cellular effects of verapamil treatment in subjects with type 1 diabetes. *Nat Commun* **13:** 1159. doi:10.1038/s41467-022-28826-3

Ylescupidez A, Speake C, Pietropaolo SL, Wilson DM, Steck AK, Sherr JL, Gaglia JL, Bender C, Lord S, Greenbaum CJ. 2023a. OGTT metrics surpass continuous glucose monitoring data for T1D prediction in multiple-autoantibody-positive individuals. *J Clin Endocrinol Metab* **109:** 57–67. doi:10.1210/clinem/dgad472

Ylescupidez A, Bahnson HT, O'Rourke C, Lord S, Speake C, Greenbaum CJ. 2023b. A standardized metric to enhance clinical trial design and outcome interpretation in type 1 diabetes. *Nat Commun* **14:** 7214. doi:10.1038/s41467-023-42581-z

Yu A, Snowhite I, Vendrame F, Rosenzwajg M, Klatzmann D, Pugliese A, Malek TR. 2015. Selective IL-2 responsiveness of regulatory T cells through multiple intrinsic mechanisms supports the use of low-dose IL-2 therapy in type 1 diabetes. *Diabetes* **64:** 2172–2183. doi:10.2337/db14-1322

Zhang JY, Hamey F, Trzupek D, Mickunas M, Lee M, Godfrey L, Yang JHM, Pekalski ML, Kennet J, Waldron-Lynch F, et al. 2022. Low-dose IL-2 reduces IL-21$^+$ T cell frequency and induces anti-inflammatory gene expression in type 1 diabetes. *Nat Commun* **13:** 7324. doi:10.1038/s41467-022-34162-3

Ziegler AG, Rewers M, Simell O, Simell T, Lempainen J, Steck A, Winkler C, Ilonen J, Veijola R, Knip M, et al. 2013. Seroconversion to multiple islet autoantibodies and risk of progression to diabetes in children. *JAMA* **309:** 2473–2479. doi:10.1001/jama.2013.6285

Autoantigen-Specific Immunotherapies for the Prevention and Treatment of Type 1 Diabetes

Mark Peakman[1] and Pere Santamaria[2,3]

[1]Immunology and Inflammation Research Therapeutic Area, Sanofi, Cambridge, Massachusetts 02141, USA

[2]Department of Microbiology, Immunology and Infectious Diseases, Snyder Institute for Chronic Diseases, Cumming School of Medicine, University of Calgary, Alberta T2N 4N1, Canada

[3]Institut D'Investigacions Biomèdiques August Pi i Sunyer, Barcelona 08036, Spain

Correspondence: mark.peakman@sanofi.com; psantama@ucalgary.ca

Type 1 diabetes (T1D) is driven by an immunologically complex, diverse, and self-sustaining immune response directed against tissue autoantigens, leading to loss or dysfunction of β cells. To date, the single approved immune intervention in T1D is based on a strategy that is similar to that used in other related autoimmune diseases, namely, the attenuation of immune cell activation. As a next-generation approach that is more focused on underlying mechanisms of loss of tolerance, antigen-specific immunotherapy is designed to establish or restore bystander immunoregulation in a highly tissue- and target-specific fashion. Here, we describe the basis for this alternative approach, which could also have potential for complementarity if used in combination with more conventional immune modulators, and highlight recent advances, knowledge gaps, and next steps in clinical development.

ANTIGEN-SPECIFIC VERSUS ANTIGEN NONSPECIFIC IMMUNE INTERVENTION IN AUTOIMMUNITY

Autoimmune diseases such as type 1 diabetes (T1D) are chronic pathological processes that affect 5%–7% of the population worldwide. They are driven by immunologically complex immune responses directed against tissue-specific or systemic autoantigens that culminate in tissue cell loss or dysfunction. In most autoimmune disorders, the autoreactive responses that sustain disease are targeted toward highly diverse antigenic repertoires, involving many epitopes on undefined numbers of autoantigens that expand as these diseases evolve (a phenomenon referred to as epitope and antigen spreading). Autoimmunity is not like allergies, in which the underlying immune responses focus on specific extrinsic molecules and use pathways (predominantly Th2) that have redundancy in defense against the pathogens commonly encountered in economically developed countries. It is quite the opposite; there is a high degree of immunological

Cite this article as *Cold Spring Harb Perspect Med* doi: 10.1101/cshperspect.a041598

and antigenic complexity in autoreactive immunity, and pathway responses show complete overlap with those that afford survival from microbial attack. These fundamental differences represent a barrier to the design and application of strategies to broadly suppress autoreactivity without impairing homeostatic immunity (Serra and Santamaria 2019). As a result, immune intervention in autoimmune disorders has so far almost exclusively relied upon non-disease-specific agents (i.e., targeting inflammatory mediators/receptors or immune cell signaling pathways) that attenuate autoimmune inflammation at the expense of increasing the risk of infections and malignancies, in addition to having other potential off-target adverse events. Importantly, since these approaches do not restore immune tolerance to self, they are not disease-modifying or curative and thus require chronic administration to achieve sustained efficacy.

In the face of this immunological and antigenic complexity, how could delivery of one or a few autoantigenic molecules possibly be able to broadly suppress polyspecific and polyfunctional autoreactivity? Clonal deletion of autoreactive T and/or B cells cannot restore immune tolerance (because new T- or B-cell specificities arising in primary lymphoid organs will continue to be recruited unless the therapy is continuously adapted); it is not a pharmacologically viable approach because numerous autoantigenic specificities (many of which remain to be defined) would need to be targeted. Instead, the answer to this conundrum may lie in work conducted in the field of immunoregulation over the last two decades, which has suggested that it might be possible to restore immune tolerance to self by inducing bystander immunoregulation. This approach increases the number and/or function of autoantigen-specific regulatory lymphocytes capable of linked suppression of immune responses to non-cognate autoantigenic targets at the site of autoimmune attack or draining lymphoid organs, while sparing the immune system at large. Therapeutic induction of linked/bystander immunoregulation thus has the potential to overcome the translational barrier to "a cure" imposed by the complexity of autoreactivity.

HISTORICAL PERSPECTIVE

The notion that the manipulated administration of an antigen in vivo can result in profound operational, immunological tolerance to the same target has been around for more than 50 years (Asherson and Barnes 1973). For an autoimmune disease such as T1D, in which the disease-driving process is focused on well-defined autoantigens and their interaction with specific T and B lymphocytes, exploiting antigen-induced tolerance as a potential treatment paradigm is clearly very appealing. The main theoretical advantage is the potential to control focal areas of islet inflammation without off-target, systemic immune suppression, at the same time focusing on the underlying pathology (impaired immune regulation) and leveraging natural immune-regulatory pathways that are hypothetically maintained beyond the treatment period. Realizing this potential in the clinic, however, has not been easy and few autoantigen-specific immunotherapy (ASI) approaches in autoimmune/inflammatory diseases have gone beyond phase I/II of clinical development. This contrasts with allergen immunotherapy, which also uses manipulated administration of antigen, and which has become a well-established clinical tool. It is timely, therefore, to review the progress of ASI in T1D, emphasizing any learnings from other fields in which antigen-focused therapies have already gained traction in the clinic, such as clinical allergy.

From a technological perspective, we are witnessing an exciting period of ASI innovation. As shown in Table 1, the field is moving beyond simple antigen administration to embrace DNA- and RNA-based delivery technologies, as well as sophisticated nanoparticle (NP) packaging that can include additional cargoes or externally presented human leukocyte antigen (HLA)/antigen complexes (Table 1). These potential advances for ASI are complemented by an increasingly sophisticated understanding of the immunological basis for induction and maintenance of tolerance, largely centered on the biology of regulatory T cells (Tregs) that are characterized by expression of CD4, high expression of the high-affinity interleukin (IL)-2 receptor CD25, and the

Table 1. Examples of different types of antigen-specific immunotherapy modalities developed for type 1 diabetes (T1D)

Modality	Advantages	Challenges	Examples
Recombinant antigen +/− adjuvant	Low technological complexity	Requires antigen processing to achieve sufficient peptide human leukocyte antigen (pHLA) density; antigen-processing/presenting cell not controlled; optimal route of administration may be intra–lymph node	GAD65-alum conjugate (Diamyd)
Synthetic peptide(s)	Achieves high molar doses; amenable to multiple epitope coverage; peptide(s) designed to match disease-relevant HLA types; avoids autoantibody interactions	Identification and selection of epitopes; achieving sufficient solubility/dose for selected epitopes; systemic versus local delivery	Single proinsulin peptide; insulin B chain multiple β-cell antigens/peptides (MultiPepT1De)
Modified peptide	Enhances tissue targeting; directs novel mechanism of action (MoA)	Limitation to size of cargo; linked suppression may be limited	Liver-targeting glycosylation signature conjugated to antigen (Anokion); inducer of antipathogenic cell cytotoxicity (Imcyse)
Nanoparticle (NP) encapsulation	Leverages natural scavenger receptor uptake and pro-tolerance effects; additional cargo optionality (e.g., rapamycin)	Selecting optimal particle size for biology and dosage	Poly(lactic-co-glycolic acid) (PLGA) NPs with various antigens (Cour) and with rapamycin (Selecta)
DNA-based delivery	Feasible for unstable or complex whole antigens; constructs contain immune-regulatory enhancers such as IL-10	Intramuscular route less well understood for antigen presentation	Single antigen (Tolerion); pre-proinsulin, TGF-β, IL-10, IL-2) (Novo Nordisk)
mRNA lipid NPs	Rapidly emerging technology; highly flexible delivery and cargoes	Impact of activation of damage-associated molecular patterns (DAMPs; e.g., nucleic acid sensors) in vivo to be determined	Preclinical at this stage; exemplified with myelin oligodendrocyte glycoprotein peptide in experimental autoimmune encephalomyelitis (EAE)
Peptide-HLA NPs	Precision therapy; drives Tr1 cell expansion and differentiation; promotes bystander effects	Intravenous route of administration required	Preclinical at this stage (Navacims, Parvus)

presence of the transcription factor FoxP3 and function to limit a range of immune effector cell types. Tregs are generated in the thymus for recognition of thymically available self-antigens (tTregs); they are also generated extrathymically in the periphery (pTregs). Antigen-specific immune regulation is also achieved by a $CD4^+$ T cell that is best characterized by secretion of the immune-suppressive cytokine IL-10 (T-regulatory type 1 [Tr1] cells; see below). This advance in understanding has highlighted the potential for the use of Tregs and Tr1 cells as antigen-specific, adoptive cell therapeutics and a number of early-stage efforts are focused in this direction, using, for example, chimeric antigen-receptor engineering to confer tissue regulation properties on ex vivo expanded cells, with the results of early clinical studies eagerly awaited.

AUTOANTIGEN-SPECIFIC IMMUNOTHERAPY: PROGRESS IN T1D

A small number of promising ASI candidates have progressed into clinical testing or are close to being evaluated in this setting (Table 1). As a general principle, antigen delivery for tolerance differs from antigen delivery to provoke an inflammatory response. For tolerance, proinflammatory adjuvants are not typically used; antigen is delivered in simple form in the absence of costimulation. Somewhat against this dogma has been the use of alum as an adjuvant with the hypothesis that it skews immune responses away from potentially pathogenic Th1 and Th17 pathway responses. Several studies have been conducted with the whole antigen GAD65 conjugated to alum (Ludvigsson 2022). A lack of efficacy (C-peptide preservation) following intradermal delivery was observed in pivotal phase 2 and 3 studies, but the approach has continued to undergo refinement. Currently, administration of GAD-alum via three intra–lymph node injections, with oral vitamin D supplementation (to promote a tolerance phenotype in antigen-presenting cells [APCs]), is planned in a phase 3 setting in newly diagnosed T1D patients with the HLA DR3-DQ2 haplotype (DIAGNODE-3), following findings of C-peptide preservation in this subset in a phase 2b trial, DIAGNODE-2, and in a larger meta-analysis of previous trials (Nowak et al. 2022). There is a mechanistic link that could explain preferential effects of GAD65 ASI in this HLA subset, since it is known to more frequently show a primary GAD65 autoantibody response, suggesting that GAD65 may exert an autoantigenic immunodominance in this group. The precise mechanism of action (MoA) of GAD65-alum in controlling T1D autoimmunity is not known: studies show that GAD-alum injection is followed by a rise in GAD65 antibody titers and induction of GAD-specific CD4 T cells with a distinctive bifunctionality (Th1/Th2), the biological implications of which are not yet resolved (Arif et al. 2020). Should this approach show clinical efficacy, it will raise the question of whether tolerance (defined as the absence of disease pathology in the absence of continued treatment) is always achieved with a "lack of a response" or whether there can also be states of "operational tolerance" in which modification of antigen-specific cell states or transdifferentiation (see below) is a critical component.

Primary and secondary prevention trials using insulin delivered via various routes of administration, including the oral route, have been unsuccessful (reviewed by Jacobsen and Schatz 2021). For example, in a recently completed randomized controlled trial, administration of oral insulin to children at risk for T1D, although safe, was not associated with a tolerogenic immune response to insulin (Assfalg et al. 2021). Antigen delivery to steady state (i.e., tolerogenic) dendritic cells (DCs) via anti-CD205 is another means to potentially induce antigen-specific T-cell tolerance (Kretschmer et al. 2005), but others have used this approach to elicit effector immune responses instead (Ngu et al. 2019). A further refinement of this approach is the harvesting and ex vivo induction of tolerogenic DCs, followed by antigen-pulsing and reinfusion (Nikolic et al. 2022), but the technical challenge of clinical translatability has seen a lack of progress beyond phase 1. Several additional strategies for insulin-based immunotherapy are at the preclinical stage. Antigen delivery to splenic APCs via erythrocytes loaded in vivo with antigens tethered to a glycophorin A–binding peptide could blunt the transfer of T1D to immunocompromised nonobese diabetic (NOD) mouse hosts by cognate T-cell receptor (TCR)-transgenic $CD4^+$ T cells, but this approach appears to operate via deletional tolerance rather than bystander immunoregulation (Kontos et al. 2013). A variation of this approach involves the use of sortase A to covalently bind autoantigens to tagged erythrocytes, which presumably operates through the same mechanism (Pishesha et al. 2017). Nanobody-antigen adducts that target all major histocompatibility complex (MHC) class II–expressing cells, including tolerogenic APCs in association with dexamethasone, have been reported to afford protection against various experimental autoimmune disease models including T1D (Pishesha et al. 2021). Others have used probiotic bacteria (*Lactococcus lactis*) to orally deliver proinsulin and IL-10 to the mucosal immune system. When combined with low-dose anti-CD3, this approach has been reported to reverse T1D in NOD mice (Takiishi et al. 2017).

In a broadening of the antigen-specific approach, a series of phase 1 studies using naturally processed and presented peptides of single or multiple β-cell-derived peptides has been conducted in stage 3 disease (including long-standing, recent-onset, and newly diagnosed) to examine tolerability, safety, and biomarker outcomes. In these small studies, clinical efficacy can only be hinted at, with some subjects showing stabilization of stimulated C-peptide (Alhadj Ali et al. 2017), but of greater interest has been the embedding of studies on pharmacodynamic (PD) biomarkers of immunological responses to drug. These analyses show that IL-10-producing CD4 T cells are induced against the therapeutically administered antigens and that there is increased expression of FoxP3 by Tregs, especially those expressing markers of activation (CD39, CD73) (Liu et al. 2022). It is not clear from these studies whether the IL-10-producing cells lie within the pool of $FoxP3^{hi}$ Tregs or are separate and reflect the Tr1 lineage. Indeed, in a preclinical model, the same group demonstrated that both PD effects can be observed, with the particular bias determined by the nature of the antigen delivered (Gibson et al. 2015). In a variation on peptide-based ASI approaches that induce tolerance via Treg effects, Imcyse uses modified epitopes that incorporate a thiol-disulfide oxidoreductase motif. Such epitopes have been reported to increase the strength of the pMHC/TCR interaction and induce $CD4^+$ cytolytic T cells (Carlier et al. 2012). A GAD65 peptide incorporating such a motif inhibited diabetes development in prediabetic NOD mice (Malek Abrahimians et al. 2016). The therapeutic effect is obtained when the cytotoxic effect is focused onto APCs presenting relevant self-peptides with this program expected to read out phase 2 data in stage 3 T1D in 2024.

In recent years, potential optimization strategies for ASI have emerged, including the use of multiple epitopes from multiple antigens discussed above, as well as the incorporation of enhancers that essentially work as adjuvants for tolerance induction. This innovation has been enabled by the exploitation of technology developments in the fields of NPs and nucleic acid–based therapeutics. The various experimental nanomedicines designed to treat autoimmune inflammation in different autoimmune disease models have been reviewed recently (Yang and Santamaria 2021, 2022).

A number of these approaches seek to deliver specific antigenic peptides to professional APCs, particularly DCs, while promoting their differentiation into tolerogenic APCs. As an example, although not yet undergoing development for T1D, Selecta has developed an NP approach in which rapamycin is co-delivered with antigen to promote tolerogenic differentiation of DCs that present the target antigen. This strategy is being used very effectively to control antidrug antibodies (ADAs), especially in enzyme therapies such as pegadricase for gout (Baraf et al. 2024). It will be important to establish whether similar approaches can go beyond limiting responses to neo-antigenic (drug) exposures, and also be used to address complex effector/memory responses that are already established in patients with T1D and other chronic autoimmune diseases. Other groups have used a similar approach in preclinical studies but deployed different NP scaffolds and immnoregulatory cytokines instead of rapamycin (i.e., TFG-β or IL-10) (Yang and Santamaria 2021, 2022). Poly(lactic-co-glycolic acid) (PLGA) microparticles loaded with three recombinant T1D-relevant autoantigens (insulin, chromogranin A, and GAD65) could inhibit T1D development in prediabetic NOD mice, although no antidiabetogenic properties were observed for PLGA particles delivering the individual antigens (Podojil et al. 2022). These compounds are being developed for clinical testing by Cour Pharma. Phosphatidylserine-containing liposomes loaded with an insulin peptide (Pujol-Autonell et al. 2015), as well as NPs carrying proinsulin and the aryl hydrocarbon receptor ligand ITE (to induce tolerogenic DCs) also inhibited the progression of T1D in NOD mice (Yeste et al. 2016). Subcutaneous administration of NPs delivering antisense oligonucleotides targeting mRNAs for CD80, CD86, and CD40 at sites anatomically proximal to the pancreas-draining lymph nodes reduced the expression of the corresponding costimulatory molecules on local APCs and suppressed T1D development. Although this was associated with the presence of increased frequencies of Tregs, addition of antigenic peptides into these compounds did not enhance their therapeutic efficacy (Engman et al. 2015). In a similar approach, subcutaneous delivery of large (50 µm) nonphagocytosable microparticles loaded with TGF-β and granulocyte-macrophage colony-stimulating factor (GM-CSF) and small NPs loaded with autoantigenic peptides (from insulin) and vitamin D3 (VD3) have been used to recruit DCs displaying a tolerogenic phenotype. This strategy reduced islet inflammation and induced transient reversal of hyperglycemia in newly diabetic NOD mice (Lewis et al. 2019). Although none of these approaches have been reported to induce expansions of antigen-specific Treg cells in wild-type mice, they may all operate by eliciting some form of immunoregulation, such as by promoting the formation of antigen-specific Treg cells from poised precursors in the absence of expansion. Nevertheless, since APCs have a short half-life, sustained induction and maintenance of operational tolerance by these compounds may require chronic administration. Systemic delivery of these compounds, particularly during chronic administration, may result in impairment of normal immune responses.

Emerging nucleic acid technologies can also address the need for inclusion of complex cargoes. An example is the development of a novel DNA plasmid expressing pre-proinsulin and a combination of immune-modulatory cytokines (TGF-β1, IL-10, and IL-2), which prevents autoimmune diabetes in NOD mice (Pagni et al. 2021) and is currently undergoing phase 1 testing for safety and tolerability (ClinicalTrials.gov Identifier: NCT04279613). In an earlier phase 1 study, intramuscular delivery of an insulin-encoding plasmid decreased the peripheral frequency of insulin-reactive $CD8^+$ T cells and preserved C-peptide levels in recently diagnosed T1D patients (Roep 2013). Other DNA vaccination strategies have sought to exploit the tolerogenic properties of the liver (Thomson and Knolle 2010; Akbarpour et al. 2015), although these have not progressed to the T1D clinic. Lipid NP delivery of mRNA is clearly another technology innovation that can be exploited for its multimodal delivery capability and which has, of course, been significantly de-risked as a therapeutic modality following the success of mRNA vaccines during the SARS-CoV-2 pandemic. Thus far, there is only preclinical development in this space, with the demonstration that systemic delivery of NP-formulated 1 methylpseudouridine-modified messenger RNA (m1Y mRNA) coding for the autoantigen myelin-oligodendrocyte promotes antigen presentation by splenic $CD11c^+$ APCs in the absence of costimulatory signals and suppresses disease in the extrinsic experimental autoimmune encephalomyelitis model (EAE) of multiple sclerosis (Krienke et al. 2021). Methylpseudouridine is a modified nucleoside that can be incorporated into mRNA to improve its stability and translation efficiency. It can also help prevent the activation of innate immune sensors that recognize foreign RNA, hence reduce an inflammatory response to the molecule. Notably, the treatment effect was associated with Treg generation and antagonism of effector T cells suggesting that a similar MoA is being exploited to that in play with "conventional" native ASI, although evidence for the antigenic specificity of the presumed Tregs was lacking. Nonetheless, this supports the generalized principle that antigen, delivered in whole or epitope form to certain APC compartments, may incite regulatory pathway programs involving Treg and Tr1 cell responses (Fig. 1A). A significant limitation of this and other studies using the EAE model to document therapeutic activity is that they often fail to demonstrate that treatment induces bystander immunoregulation. The antigen used in the drug formulation is the same as that used to induce disease, such that it is impossible to exclude clonal deletion of autoantigen-reactive T cells as the underlying MoA. Demonstration of therapeutic effects in spontaneous (hence polyantigenic and asynchronous) models of autoimmunity is essential. Where experimental models are used, the ability of treatment to suppress disease induced by immunization with a different antigen would be desirable.

A further innovation of ASI has been to deliver peptide–HLA complexes on NPs (pMHCII-NPs) (Tsai et al. 2010; Clemente-Casares et al. 2016; Singha et al. 2017) to achieve an artificial form of antigen presentation in the absence of any conventional costimulatory signals (Fig. 1B). This technology, exemplified as Navacims from Parvus Therapeutics, has shown considerable potential across preclinical models and is currently in development for several autoimmune indications. As noted below, this approach has exposed a novel MoA that is potentially relevant to other ASI strategies.

How ASI Works: Expansion and/or Formation of Antigen-Specific Tr1 Cells

The MoAs of the various ASI strategies described to date are, to a large extent, incompletely understood, but recent studies in mice treated with pMHCII-NPs have provided insights that are mechanistically relevant to other ASI approaches.

Early studies indicated that the MoA of peptide-HLA delivery with NPs operated through induction of antigen-specific Tr1 cell responses, similar to those reported for earlier approaches (see above). In an extension of this work, it has been demonstrated that the pMHC class II, NP-induced Tr1 cells derive from splenic T-follicular helper (Tfh) cells (Fig. 1B; Solé et al. 2023a, b). Despite a remarkably short circulating half-life (Yang et al. 2021), binding of these compounds to cognate TCRs on Tfh cells induces a rapid proliferative burst and immediate transdifferentiation into a polyclonal, yet monospecific pool of Tr1 cells that possess strong bystander immunoregulatory properties. As a result, the PD activity of these compounds is manifested by formation of relatively large pools of antigen-specific T cells that can be measured in peripheral (i.e., spleen and lymph nodes) and central (i.e., bone marrow) lymphoid organs as well as peripheral blood using pMHCII multimers. Detailed examination of the multimer$^+$ T-cell pools arising in response to therapy has indicated that they are exclusively composed of Tfh, terminally differentiated Tr1 cells, and a transitional Tr1-like subset, suggesting that these compounds selectively operate on Tfh cells (Solé et al. 2023b). Whereas mice lacking Tfh cells are completely refractory to the PD and therapeutic effects of these compounds, mice in which Tfh cells cannot transdifferentiate into Tr1 cells (a process driven by the transcription factor BLIMP-1, encoded by *Prdm1*), or in which the Tr1 cells cannot make IL-10 (in cell-specific conditional knockout mice) respond pharmacodynamically to treatment but the expanded T-cell pools cannot suppress disease (Solé et al. 2023b). Detailed examination of the transcriptional and epigenetic events underlying the Tfh-Tr1 transdifferentiation process harnessed by pMHCII-NPs (Navacims) has demonstrated that Tfh cells are epigenetically poised to become Tr1; that is, most of the Tr1 genes that are up-regulated by Tfh cells during transdifferentiation, including *Il10*, are already epigenetically marked for expression at the Tfh cell stage (i.e., have hypomethylated active enhancers around the locus) (Garnica et al. 2024). The antigen-specific Tr1 cells arising in response to treatment traffic and accumulating at sites of inflammation in response to chemokine gradients, undergo activation in situ by recognizing cognate pMHC on professional APCs, including DCs, resulting in the suppression of the DCs' proinflammatory and antigen-presentation properties (Fig. 2), as well as in the formation of IL-10-producing B-regulatory (Breg) cells (Clemente-Casares et al. 2016; Umeshappa et al. 2019, 2020). In autoimmune liver inflammation, treatment-induced Tr1 cells and Breg

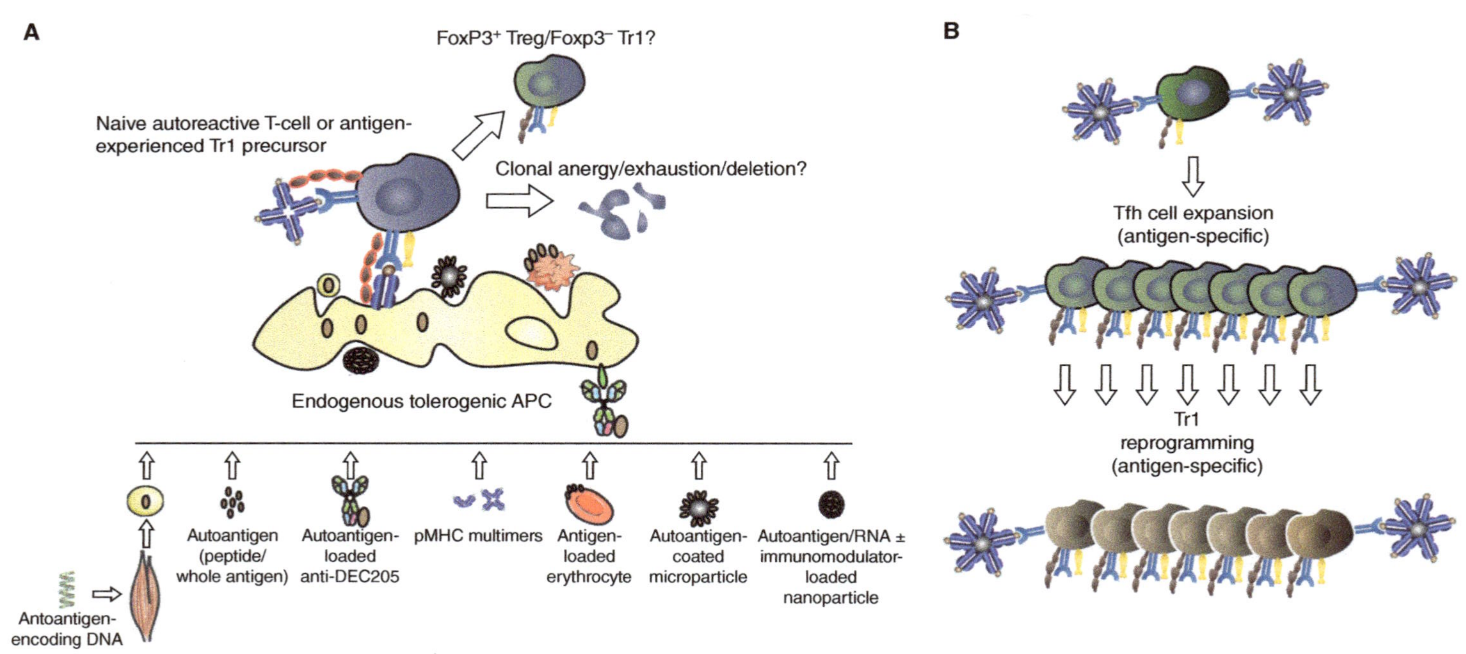

Figure 1. Schematic representation of the diverse approaches to antigen delivery and putative mechanism for action in antigen-specific immunotherapy. (*A*) Antigen delivery to tolerogenic antigen-presenting cells (APCs). Delivery approaches include antigen-encoding DNA, antigenic peptides, altered peptide ligands or whole antigens, antigens tethered to monoclonal antibodies (mAbs) against dendritic cell (DC) molecules, antigens tethered to immunomodulators and/or mAbs targeting major histocompatibility complex (MHC) molecules, peptide MHC (pMHC) multimers, antigen-loaded erythrocytes (ex vivo or in vivo), antigen-coated microparticles or nanoparticles (NPs) or micro/NPs loaded with antigen and immunomodulators, and autoantigen-loaded immature DCs. Tolerogenic APCs can trigger the functional inactivation (anergy) or deletion of cognate autoreactive T cells and/or promote Treg/Tr1 cell formation. (*B*) pMHC-based nanomedicines. NPs coated with disease-relevant pMHC class II complexes trigger the expansion of cognate T-follicular helper (Tfh) $CD4^+$ T cells and their immediate transdifferentiation into Tr1 cells.

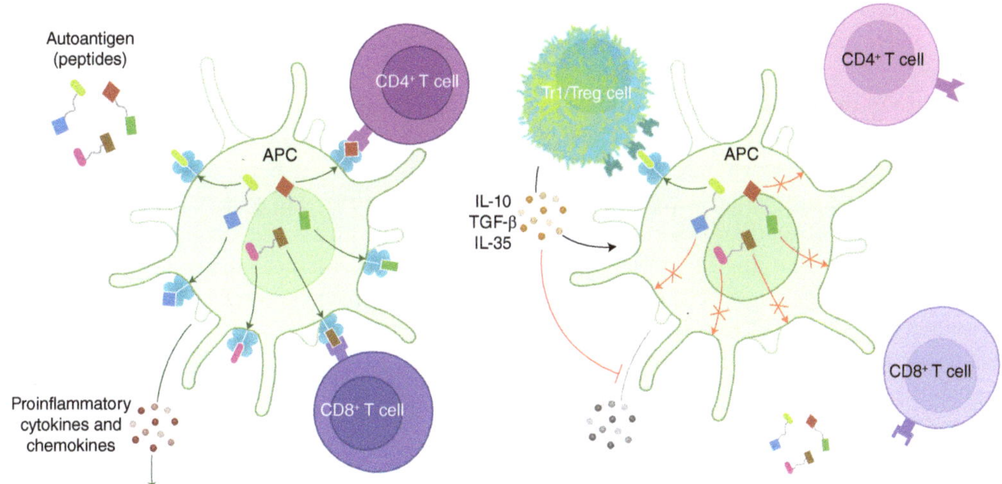

Figure 2. Bystander immunoregulation by autoantigen-specific regulatory T cells/T regulatory type 1 cells (Treg/Tr1). (*Left*) Autoantigen-loaded antigen-presenting cells (APCs) drive the recruitment and activation of numerous autoreactive $CD4^+$ and $CD8^+$ T-cell specificities to the site, which cause tissue damage and amplify a vicious cycle that evolves through epitope and antigen spreading, culminating in tissue destruction. (*Right*) Autoantigen-specific Treg/Tr1 cells suppress the APC-driven recruitment and activation of autoreactive T-cell effectors to the site by recognizing cognate peptide–HLA complexes (pMHCII) on the APC surface. A single Treg/Tr1 cell specificity can suppress the activation of T-cell specificities recognizing epitopes from other antigens that are also presented by the same APC.

cells cooperatively promote the recruitment of polymorphonuclear leukocytes and their differentiation into myeloid-derived suppressor-like cells (MDSCs) (Umeshappa et al. 2021). Collectively, these events promote the resolution of inflammation in a tissue- and disease-specific manner, without impairing normal immune responses to bacteria, viruses, or cancer.

The discovery of the Tfh-Tr1 transdifferentiation pathway suggests the possibility that other ASI approaches relying on chronic antigenic stimulation may harness it as well. Such approaches need not be preceded by an expansion of antigen-specific Tfh cells—this event, preceding the Tfh-Tr1 transdifferentiation step, appears to be a unique property of pMHCII-coated NPs. For example, I-A^{g7} dimers and tetramers displaying peptides derived from the T1D-relevant antigens GAD, insulin, or chromogranin A were reported to induce IL-10 expression in the absence of systemic expansion of cognate T cells in NOD mice (Li et al. 2009; Lin et al. 2010). Indeed, studies using α-galactosylceramide (αGalCer)/CD1d-coated NPs have established that these compounds can directly reprogram liver-resident invariant natural killer T cells (LiNKT) into a Tr1-like immunoregulatory NKT (iNKT)-cell subset (LiNKTR1) without inducing the proliferation of the precursors (Umeshappa et al. 2022). Likewise, the therapeutic success of repeated administration of autoantigenic peptides in T1D (see above) and allergens in allergy (Akdis and Akdis 2014) is often associated with generation of autoantigen- or allergen-specific IL-10-secreting Tregs, respectively. Following allergy immunotherapy, there is no obvious expansion of allergen-specific T-cell pools and thus it is conceivable that the preexisting high peripheral precursor frequency of allergen-specific T (and likely Tfh) cells in allergic individuals (Kwok et al. 2010) may facilitate the penetrance of the therapeutic effect of approaches that have otherwise been unsuccessful in autoimmunity.

It is therefore plausible that ASI approaches that do not elicit measurable expansions of antigen-specific Tr1 cells, unlike the case with pMHCII-NPs, directly reprogram cognate Tr1-

poised Tfh cells into Tr1 cell progeny, as is the case for LiNKT cells reprogrammed by αGalCer/CD1d-coated NPs. This could be investigated by examining whether experimental manipulation of key gatekeepers of the Tfh-Tr1 transdifferentiation pathway or selective abrogation of *Il10* expression in Tr1 cells interfere with the purported therapeutic activity of these other approaches. As noted above, mice lacking Tfh cells, mice carrying *Prdm1*-deficient Tfh cells (unable to transdifferentiate into Tr1 cells), or mice in which Tr1 cells cannot make IL-10 (by deleting *Il10* in transitional Tr1-like cells using Tbx21-Cre) are refractory to pMHCII-NP therapy (Solé et al. 2023b). Mirroring these outcomes in mice treated with ASI and other approaches suspected to induce immunoregulation would produce compelling evidence for or against the involvement of the Tfh-Tr1 pathway as an underlying MoA.

AUTOANTIGEN-SPECIFIC IMMUNOTHERAPY: CHALLENGES TO DEVELOPMENT IN T1D

It is perhaps worth noting that the obstacles to developing ASI for T1D go beyond the simple issue of selecting appropriate antigens and delivery modalities. At the preclinical evaluation stage, there is a paucity of appropriate (e.g., HLA transgenic) humanized models with which to obtain proof-of-efficacy, although innovations in this direction are emerging. Moreover, the clinical development pathway for T1D is highly challenging. It is typically focused on stage 3 disease, with proof-of-concept in terms of efficacy signals being required for deeper clinical investigations to phase 3 and beyond. Further aspects of the clinical development pathway include investigation of stage 3 adults (including for efficacy) before step-down in age to adolescents, children, and infants. This conflicts with the notion that ASI might work better in T1D at earlier disease stages (i.e., when inflammation is less overt, C-peptide reserve is greater and there has been less antigen- or epitope spreading). ASI might also, theoretically, work better in children and adolescents, in whom T1D pathogenesis has a greater contribution from autoantigens as drivers (as evidenced by the higher autoantibody prevalence and narrower HLA usage for antigen presentation compared with adults). There are also demanding registration end points at stage 3 (stabilization of C-peptide plus patient benefit such as reduced hyperglycemia), which can be especially difficult to surmount for therapies such as ASI that may require more time to achieve peak potency when compared with a more straightforward approach such as effector cell antagonism or cytokine blockade, which work relatively rapidly.

SAFETY OF ANTIGEN-SPECIFIC IMMUNOTHERAPY

As noted above, ASI approaches that rely on systemic delivery of antigens to APCs have the potential to suppress normal immune responses. For example, if delivery of antigen to systemic APCs includes delivery of an immunosuppressive/immunomodulatory agent, then APCs that are required for normal immune responses to antigens may be impaired. It is therefore imperative that this is investigated.

The ability of pMHCII-NP-induced Tr1 cells to suppress autoantigen-loaded APCs in mice may explain why they can spare normal immune responses to pathogens. It has been shown that suppression of disease by these compounds does not compromise immunity against viruses (vaccinia, influenza), bacteria (*Listeria* and *Staphylococcus aureus*), or metastatic (liver) allogeneic tumors (Umeshappa et al. 2019, 2020, 2021). Similar findings have been made in other studies (Alhadj Ali et al. 2017). The APCs that activate the local regulatory function of autoantigen-specific Tr1 cells must capture autoantigen shed from the tissue damaged by the autoimmune response. As a result, such APCs can only exist in sufficient numbers in the target organ and/or draining lymph nodes. The organ-distal APCs that orchestrate immune responses against foreign antigens will lack the autoantigenic epitopes targeted by the therapeutic Tr1 cells. Although there is a possibility that immunity to infections of the autoimmune-damaged tissue/organ may be compromised in the presence of autoantigen-specific Tr1 cells, it is more likely that the opposite will be true. That is, local replication of the infectious agent may overwhelm the antigen-

 Cite this article as *Cold Spring Harb Perspect Med* doi: 10.1101/cshperspect.a041598

presentation machinery of local APCs with pathogen-derived antigens, hence diluting autoantigenic pMHCII complexes on local APCs to levels below the threshold required for Tr1 cell activation, thus compromising their bystander immunoregulatory properties. Clearance of the pathogen would then allow these Tr1 cells to resume their immunoregulatory properties against autoimmune disease.

Another consideration is that systemic autoantigen delivery (i.e., peptides or antigens) has the theoretical potential to exacerbate disease by providing an excess of antigen to drive signal 1 in pathogenic T effector cells. In fact, disease exacerbation, at preclinical or clinical stages, has been seen only rarely, and usually has a rational explanation. One of the best-described examples of disease worsening, following the treatment of multiple sclerosis patients with a myelin basic protein-derived altered peptide ligand (Bielekova et al. 2000), is likely to have arisen due to the properties of the altered versus wild-type sequence. Hypersensitivity reactions have also been observed (Kappos et al. 2000), and the potential for exacerbation/hypersensitivity can be mitigated by careful clinical design, including dose escalation approaches. As discussed above, a precise understanding of the underlying MoAs will maximize the chances of success and minimize adverse events.

Understanding the relationship between pharmacokinetics and PDs, particularly for compounds other than mAbs, will help optimize dosing and minimize toxicity due to accumulation of the drug postdelivery. Off-target effects due to nonspecific accumulation and/or retention at nonintended tissues/organs, including kidney, lung, or liver, need also to be considered and ruled out in preclinical studies.

Immunogenicity is another factor that may require consideration, depending on the precise modality. Development of ADAs upon administration of the compounds may reduce the bioavailability of the drug or alter its PD and therapeutic activities. Minimizing the introduction of artificial epitopes in the final drug product and testing the consequences of ADAs on biological activity and safety are, therefore, a necessary component of drug development in this space.

BIOMARKERS OF ANTIGEN-SPECIFIC IMMUNOTHERAPY FOR SAFETY AND EFFICACY

Ideally, therapeutic effects of a given approach are associated with changes in immunological readouts that can be monitored, such as treatment-induced increases in the frequency of antigen-specific Treg cells in peripheral blood. The magnitude and persistence of these readouts may help guide the optimization of the magnitude and frequency of dosing during clinical testing, to increase the therapeutic index of the drug. Although several studies have reported increases in the relative frequencies of $Foxp3^+$ Treg cells, most studies did not examine (or report) on whether treatment specifically induced the expansion of antigen-specific Treg cells. As noted above, at least in the preclinical setting, pMHCII-NPs selectively induce the expansion of cognate Tr1 cells in the spleen and these cells then traffic to specific lymph nodes (as well as bone marrow) and inflamed tissues, through the circulation.

Antigen-specific T cells can currently be annotated using ELISPOT or via flow cytometry using multimeric reagents (tetramers, pentamers, dextramers, higher-order multimeric structures), but the general applicability of the latter will benefit from improvements in the sensitivity of detection, which remains relatively low for most ASI approaches where hypothetical Treg formation is not accompanied by an expansion phase.

Multiomic studies of bulk PBMCs or purified T-cell subsets (e.g., single-cell RNAseq, multiparametric mass cytometry) may or may not provide information on the therapeutic effects of treatment at the site of inflammation, but are unlikely to report antigen-specific effects, because the sensitivity of current assays is limited by the relatively low numbers of cells that can be analyzed.

KEY KNOWLEDGE GAPS

Incomplete understanding of the mechanisms responsible for the breakdown of self-tolerance in autoimmune diabetes development remains a limitation on our ability to rationally design approaches capable of restoring it, which is the ultimate goal of ASI. There is a general consensus that development of spontaneous autoimmunity, including T1D, in mice and humans is due to immune dysregulation. However, the specific sequence of events that trip the immune system into action against self, remain poorly understood, as does the real extent of antigen and epitope diversification that drives and sustains disease. A deeper understanding of the mechanistic underpinnings of pancreatic autoimmunity, including how environmental triggers, β-cell-intrinsic determinants of disease, genetic elements, and a dysregulated immune system, conspire to trigger and drive disease will continue to provide the insights required to design optimal ASI approaches. As discussed above, translation of these approaches will also benefit from the advancement of improved humanized mouse models that can spontaneously develop disease upon engraftment of complex human immune systems.

A number of ASI strategies seek to deliver disease-relevant autoantigens in various forms to tolerogenic APCs. Studies in experimental models of autoimmunity have provided proof-of-concept, but rigorous documentation of therapeutic activity in spontaneous models of established disease and in different genetic backgrounds are often lacking. This caveat is compounded by a limited understanding of the MoA, often relying on the outcomes of experimentation in reductionist or contrived systems (e.g., adoptive transfer of disease by TCR-transgenic T cells in immunocompromised hosts) that do not faithfully replicate the form of disease developed by wild-type animals. A number of ASI approaches appear to operate via various mechanisms, including clonal deletion, anergy, TCR down-regulation, cytokine deviation, and immunoregulation. There is some evidence that the weight of each of these mechanisms may be a function of other variables such as disease model, genetic background, dose, route of administration, TCR-binding avidity, and/or use of adjuvants/immunomodulators. In any case, it seems clear that the success of any ASI strategy in autoimmunity rests on its ability to induce bystander immunoregulation (i.e., the formation and/or expansion of autoantigen-specific Tregs that regulate in their immediate tissue environment where a breadth of autoantigens and epitopes are being co-presented). Demonstration of such properties is not trivial and not always adequately reported.

A general lack of biomarkers of PD activity that provide direct (qualitative and quantitative) information on the activation of targeted pathways responsible for therapeutic activity represents another limitation of most of the ASI strategies studied to date. Ideally, such PD effects should be measurable and amenable to measurement and monitoring. In the absence of such biomarkers, rationalization of dosing, treatment regimens, and duration or treatment become a significant challenge for clinical trial design.

COMPETING INTEREST STATEMENT

P.S. is founder, scientific officer and stockholder of Parvus Therapeutics. He is inventor on patents on pMHC-based nanomedicines and receives funding from the company. He also has a consulting agreement with Sanofi. M.P. is inventor on patents on HLA-peptide-based therapeutics and an employee of Sanofi.

ACKNOWLEDGMENTS

We thank the members of our laboratories for their contributions to some of the work reviewed herein. P.S.'s work was supported by Genome Canada and Genome Alberta (GAPP Program), the Canadian Institutes of Health Research (CIHR) (FDN-353029, PJT-479040, PJT-479038, FRN-168480 (with JDRF), DT4-179512), the Praespero Foundation, the ISCIII and FEDER (PIE14/00027, PI15/0797), and Ministerio de Ciencia e Innovación of Spain (MCIN; PID2021-125493OB-I00), Generalitat de Catalunya (SGR and CERCA Programmes).

REFERENCES

Akbarpour M, Goudy KS, Cantore A, Russo F, Sanvito F, Naldini L, Annoni A, Roncarolo MG. 2015. Insulin B chain 9–23 gene transfer to hepatocytes protects from type 1 diabetes by inducing Ag-specific FoxP3$^+$ Tregs. *Sci Transl Med* **7:** a281. doi:10.1126/scitranslmed.aaa3032

Akdis CA, Akdis M. 2014. Mechanisms of immune tolerance to allergens: role of IL-10 and Tregs. *J. Clin Invest* **124:** 4678–4680. doi:10.1172/JCI78891

Alhadj Ali M, Liu YF, Arif S, Tatovic D, Shariff H, Gibson VB, Yusuf N, Baptista R, Eichmann M, Petrov N, et al. 2017. Metabolic and immune effects of immunotherapy with proinsulin peptide in human new-onset type 1 diabetes. *Sci Transl Med* **9:** eaaf7779. doi:10.1126/scitranslmed.aaf7779

Arif S, Gomez-Tourino I, Kamra Y, Pujol-Autonell I, Hanton E, Tree T, Melandri D, Hull C, Wherrett DK, Beam C, et al. 2020. GAD-alum immunotherapy in type 1 diabetes expands bifunctional Th1/Th2 autoreactive CD4 T cells. *Diabetologia* **63:** 1186–1198. doi:10.1007/s00125-020-05130-7

Asherson GL, Barnes RM. 1973. Classification of immunological unresponsiveness and tolerance. *Proc R Soc Med* **66:** 468–471.

Assfalg R, Knoop J, Hoffman KL, Pfirrmann M, Zapardiel-Gonzalo JM, Hofelich A, Eugster A, Weigelt M, Matzke C, Reinhardt J, et al. 2021. Oral insulin immunotherapy in children at risk for type 1 diabetes in a randomised controlled trial. *Diabetologia* **64:** 1079–1092. doi:10.1007/s00125-020-05376-1

Baraf HSB, Khanna PP, Kivitz AJ, Strand V, Choi HK, Terkeltaub R, Dalbeth N, DeHaan W, Azeem R, Traber PG, et al. 2024. The COMPARE head-to-head, randomised-controlled trial of SEL-212 (pegadricase plus rapamycin-containing nanoparticle, ImmTOR) versus pegloticase for refractory gout. *Rheumatology (Oxford)* **63:** 1058–1067. doi:10.1093/rheumatology/kead333

Bielekova B, Goodwin B, Richert N, Cortese I, Kondo T, Afshar G, Gran B, Eaton J, Antel J, Frank JA, et al. 2000. Encephalitogenic potential of the myelin basic protein peptide (amino acids 83-99) in multiple sclerosis: results of a phase II clinical trial with an altered peptide ligand. *Nat Med* **6:** 1167–1175. doi:10.1038/80516

Carlier VA, VanderElst L, Janssens W, Jacquemin MG, Saint-Remy JM. 2012. Increased synapse formation obtained by T cell epitopes containing a CxxC motif in flanking residues convert CD4$^+$ T cells into cytolytic effectors. *PLoS ONE* **7:** e45366. doi:10.1371/journal.pone.0045366

Clemente-Casares X, Blanco J, Ambalavanan P, Yamanouchi J, Singha S, Fandos C, Tsai S, Wang J, Garabatos N, Izquierdo C, et al. 2016. Expanding antigen-specific regulatory networks to treat autoimmunity. *Nature* **530:** 434–440. doi:10.1038/nature16962

Engman C, Wen Y, Meng WS, Bottino R, Trucco M, Giannoukakis N. 2015. Generation of antigen-specific Foxp3$^+$ regulatory T-cells in vivo following administration of diabetes-reversing tolerogenic microspheres does not require provision of antigen in the formulation. *Clin Immunol* **160:** 103–123. doi:10.1016/j.clim.2015.03.004

Garnica J, Sole P, Yamanouchi J, Moro J, Mondal D, Fandos C, Serra P, Santamaria P. 2024. T-follicular helper cells are epigenetically poised to transdifferentiate into T-regulatory type-1 cells. *eLife* doi:10:7554/eLife.97665

Gibson VB, Nikolic T, Pearce VQ, Demengeot J, Roep BO, Peakman M. 2015. Proinsulin multi-peptide immunotherapy induces antigen-specific regulatory T cells and limits autoimmunity in a humanized model. *Clin Exp Immunol* **182:** 251–260. doi:10.1111/cei.12687

Jacobsen LM, Schatz DA. 2021. Insulin immunotherapy for pretype 1 diabetes. *Curr Opin Endocrinol Diabetes Obes* **28:** 390–396. doi:10.1097/MED.0000000000000648

Kappos L, Comi G, Panitch H, Oger J, Antel J, Conlon P, Steinman L. 2000. Induction of a non-encephalitogenic type 2T helper-cell autoimmune response in multiple sclerosis after administration of an altered peptide ligand in a placebo-controlled, randomized phase II trial. The Altered Peptide Ligand in Relapsing MS Study Group. *Nat Med* **6:** 1176–1182. doi:10.1038/80525

Kontos S, Kourtis IC, Dane KY, Hubbell JA. 2013. Engineering antigens for in situ erythrocyte binding induces T-cell deletion. *Proc Natl Acad Sci* **110:** E60–E68. doi:10.1073/pnas.1216353110

Kretschmer K, Apostolou I, Hawiger D, Khazaie K, Nussenzweig MC, von Boehmer H. 2005. Inducing and expanding regulatory T cell populations by foreign antigen. *Nat Immunol* **6:** 1219–1227. doi:10.1038/ni1265

Krienke C, Kolb L, Diken E, Streuber M, Kirchhoff S, Bukur T, Akilli-Öztürk Ö, Kranz LM, Berger H, Petschenka J, et al. 2021. A noninflammatory mRNA vaccine for treatment of experimental autoimmune encephalomyelitis. *Science* **371:** 145–153. doi:10.1126/science.aay3638

Kwok WW, Roti M, Delong JH, Tan V, Wambre E, James EA, Robinson D. 2010. Direct ex vivo analysis of allergen-specific CD4$^+$ T cells. *J. Allergy Clin Immunol* **125:** 1407–1409.e1. doi:10.1016/j.jaci.2010.03.037

Lewis JS, Stewart JM, Marshall GP, Carstens MR, Zhang Y, Dolgova NV, Xia C, Brusko TM, Wasserfall CH, Clare-Salzler MJ, et al. 2019. Dual-Sized microparticle system for generating suppressive dendritic cells prevents and reverses type 1 diabetes in the nonobese diabetic mouse model. *ACS Biomater Sci Eng* **5:** 2631–2646. doi:10.1021/acsbiomaterials.9b00332

Li L, Yi Z, Wang B, Tisch R. 2009. Suppression of ongoing T cell-mediated autoimmunity by peptide-MHC class II dimer vaccination. *J Immunol* **183:** 4809–4816. doi:10.4049/jimmunol.0901616

Lin M, Stoica-Nazarov C, Surls J, Kehl M, Bona C, Olsen C, Brumeanu TD, Casares S. 2010. Reversal of type 1 diabetes by a new MHC II-peptide chimera: "single-epitope-mediated suppression" to stabilize a polyclonal autoimmune T-cell process. *Eur J Immunol* **40:** 2277–2288. doi:10.1002/eji.200940094

Liu YF, Powrie J, Arif S, Yang JHM, Williams E, Khatri L, Joshi M, Lhuillier L, Fountoulakis N, Smith E, et al. 2022. Immune and metabolic effects of antigen-specific immunotherapy using multiple β-cell peptides in type 1 diabetes. *Diabetes* **71:** 722–732. doi:10.2337/db21-0728

Ludvigsson J. 2022. Glutamic acid decarboxylase immunotherapy for type 1 diabetes. *Curr Opin Endocrinol Diabetes Obes* **29:** 361–369. doi:10.1097/MED.0000000000000748

Malek Abrahimians E, Vander Elst L, Carlier VA, Saint-Remy JM. 2016. Thioreductase-containing epitopes inhibit the development of type 1 diabetes in the NOD mouse model. *Front Immunol* **7:** 67. doi:10.3389/fimmu.2016.00067

Ngu LN, Nji NN, Ambada GE, Sagnia B, Sake CN, Tchadji JC, Njambe Priso GD, Lissom A, Tchouangueu TF, Manga Tebit D, et al. 2019. In vivo targeting of protein antigens to dendritic cells using anti-DEC-205 single chain antibody improves HIV Gag specific CD4$^+$ T cell responses protecting from airway challenge with recombinant vaccinia-gag virus. *Immun Inflamm Dis* **7:** 55–67. doi:10.1002/iid3.151

Nikolic T, Suwandi JS, Wesselius J, Laban S, Joosten AM, Sonneveld P, Mul D, Aanstoot HJ, Kaddis JS, Zwaginga JJ, et al. 2022. Tolerogenic dendritic cells pulsed with islet antigen induce long-term reduction in T-cell autoreactivity in type 1 diabetes patients. *Front Immunol* **13:** 1054968. doi:10.3389/fimmu.2022.1054968

Nowak C, Lind M, Sumnik Z, Pelikanova T, Nattero-Chavez L, Lundberg E, Rica I, Martínez-Brocca MA, Ruiz de Adana M, Wahlberg J, et al. 2022. Intralymphatic GAD-Alum (Diamyd) improves glycemic control in type 1 diabetes with HLA DR3-DQ2. *J Clin Endocrinol Metab* **107:** 2644–2651. doi:10.1210/clinem/dgac343

Pagni PP, Chaplin J, Wijaranakula M, Wesley JD, Granger J, Cracraft J, O'Brien C, Perdue N, Kumar V, Li S, et al. 2021. Multicomponent plasmid protects mice from spontaneous autoimmune diabetes. *Diabetes* **71:** 157–169. doi:10.2337/db21-0327

Pishesha N, Bilate AM, Wibowo MC, Huang NJ, Li Z, Deshycka R, Bousbaine D, Li H, Patterson HC, Dougan SK, et al. 2017. Engineered erythrocytes covalently linked to antigenic peptides can protect against autoimmune disease. *Proc Natl Acad Sci* **114:** 3157–3162. doi:10.1073/pnas.1701746114

Pishesha N, Harmand T, Smeding LY, Ma W, Ludwig LS, Janssen R, Islam A, Xie YJ, Fang T, McCaul N, et al. 2021. Induction of antigen-specific tolerance by nanobody-antigen adducts that target class-II major histocompatibility complexes. *Nat Biomed Eng* **5:** 1389–1401. doi:10.1038/s41551-021-00738-5

Podojil JR, Genardi S, Chiang MY, Kakade S, Neef T, Murthy T, Boyne MT II, Elhofy A, Miller SD. 2022. Tolerogenic immune-modifying nanoparticles encapsulating multiple recombinant pancreatic β cell proteins prevent onset and progression of type 1 diabetes in nonobese diabetic mice. *J Immunol* **209:** 465–475. doi:10.4049/jimmunol.2200208

Pujol-Autonell I, Serracant-Prat A, Cano-Sarabia M, Ampudia RM, Rodriguez-Fernandez S, Sanchez A, Izquierdo C, Stratmann T, Puig-Domingo M, Maspoch D, et al. 2015. Use of autoantigen-loaded phosphatidylserine-liposomes to arrest autoimmunity in type 1 diabetes. *PLoS ONE* **10:** e0127057. doi:10.1371/journal.pone.0127057

Roep BO. 2013. Immune intervention therapy in type 1 diabetes: safety first. *Lancet Diabetes Endocrinol* **1:** 263–265. doi:10.1016/S2213-8587(13)70124-4

Serra P, Santamaria P. 2019. Antigen-specific therapeutic approaches for autoimmunity. *Nat Biotechnol* **37:** 238–251. doi:10.1038/s41587-019-0015-4

Singha S, Shao K, Yang Y, Clemente-Casares X, Solé P, Clemente A, Blanco J, Dai Q, Song F, Liu SW, et al. 2017. Peptide–MHC-based nanomedicines for autoimmunity function as T-cell receptor microclustering devices. *Nat Nanotechnol* **12:** 701–710. doi:10.1038/nnano.2017.56

Solé P, Parras D, Yamanouchi J, Garnica J, Garabatos N, Moro J, Montaño J, Mondal D, Fandos C, Yang Y, et al. 2023a. Transcriptional re-programming of insulin B-chain epitope-specific T-follicular helper cells into anti-diabetogenic T-regulatory type-1 cells. *Front Immunol* **14:** 1177722. doi:10.3389/fimmu.2023.1177722

Solé P, Yamanouchi J, Garnica J, Uddin MM, Clarke R, Moro J, Garabatos N, Thiessen S, Ortega M, Singha S, et al. 2023b. A T follicular helper cell origin for T regulatory type 1 cells. *Cell Mol Immunol* **20:** 489–511. doi:10.1038/s41423-023-00989-z

Takiishi T, Cook DP, Korf H, Sebastiani G, Mancarella F, Cunha JP, Wasserfall C, Casares N, Lasarte JJ, Steidler L, et al. 2017. Reversal of diabetes in NOD mice by clinical-grade proinsulin and IL-10-secreting *Lactococcus lactis* in combination with low-dose anti-CD3 depends on the induction of Foxp3-positive T cells. *Diabetes* **66:** 448–459. doi:10.2337/db15-1625

Thomson AW, Knolle PA. 2010. Antigen-presenting cell function in the tolerogenic liver environment. *Nat Rev Immunol* **10:** 753–766. doi:10.1038/nri2858

Tsai S, Shameli A, Yamanouchi J, Clemente-Casares X, Wang J, Serra P, Yang Y, Medarova Z, Moore A, Santamaria P. 2010. Reversal of autoimmunity by boosting memory-like autoregulatory T cells. *Immunity* **32:** 568–580. doi:10.1016/j.immuni.2010.03.015

Umeshappa CS, Singha S, Blanco J, Shao K, Nanjundappa RH, Yamanouchi J, Parés A, Serra P, Yang Y, Santamaria P. 2019. Suppression of a broad spectrum of liver autoimmune pathologies by single peptide-MHC-based nanomedicines. *Nat Commun* **10:** 2150. doi:10.1038/s41467-019-09893-5

Umeshappa CS, Mbongue J, Singha S, Mohapatra S, Yamanouchi J, Lee JA, Nanjundappa RH, Shao K, Christen U, Yang Y, et al. 2020. Ubiquitous antigen-specific T regulatory type 1 cells variably suppress hepatic and extrahepatic autoimmunity. *J Clin Invest* **130:** 1823–1829. doi:10.1172/JCI130670

Umeshappa CS, Solé P, Surewaard BGJ, Yamanouchi J, Mohapatra S, Uddin MM, Clarke R, Ortega M, Singha S, Mondal D, et al. 2021. Liver-specific T regulatory type-1 cells program local neutrophils to suppress hepatic autoimmunity via CRAMP. *Cell Rep* **34:** 108919. doi:10.1016/j.celrep.2021.108919

Umeshappa CS, Solé P, Yamanouchi J, Mohapatra S, Surewaard BGJ, Garnica J, Singha S, Mondal D, Cortés-Vicente E, D'Mello C, et al. 2022. Re-programming mouse liver-resident invariant natural killer T cells for suppressing hepatic and diabetogenic autoimmunity. *Nat Commun* **13:** 3279. doi:10.1038/s41467-022-30759-w

Yang Y, Santamaria P. 2021. Evolution of nanomedicines for the treatment of autoimmune disease: from vehicles for drug delivery to inducers of bystander immunoregulation. *Adv Drug Deliv Rev* **176:** 113898. doi:10.1016/j.addr.2021.113898

Yang Y, Santamaria P. 2022. Antigen-specific nanomedicines for the treatment of autoimmune disease: target cell types, mechanisms and outcomes. *Curr Opin Biotechnol* **74:** 285–292. doi:10.1016/j.copbio.2021.12.012

Yang Y, Ellestad KK, Singha S, Uddin MM, Clarke R, Mondal D, Garabatos N, Solé P, Fandos C, Serra P, et al. 2021. Extremely short bioavailability and fast pharmacodynamic effects of pMHC-based nanomedicines. *J Control Release* **338:** 557–570. doi:10.1016/j.jconrel.2021.08.043

Yeste A, Takenaka MC, Mascanfroni ID, Nadeau M, Kenison JE, Patel B, Tukpah AM, Babon JA, DeNicola M, Kent SC, et al. 2016. Tolerogenic nanoparticles inhibit T cell-mediated autoimmunity through SOCS2. *Sci Signal* **9:** ra61. doi:10.1126/scisignal.aad0612

The Teplizumab Saga: The Challenge of Not Getting Lost in Clinical Translation

Lucienne Chatenoud,[1] Kevan C. Herold,[2] Jean-François Bach,[1] and Jeffrey A. Bluestone[3]

[1]Université Paris Cité, CNRS, INSERM, Institut Necker Enfants Malades-INEM, Paris 75015, France

[2]Departments of Immunobiology and Internal Medicine, Yale University, New Haven, Connecticut 06511, USA

[3]Sonoma Biotherapeutics, South San Francisco, California 09080, USA

Correspondence: lucienne.chatenoud@inserm.fr; kevan.herold@yale.edu; jbluestone@sonomabio.com

In November 2022, teplizumab became the first drug approved to delay the course of any autoimmune disease and to change the course of type 1 diabetes (T1D) since the discovery of insulin. The path to its approval took more than 30 years with both successes and failures along the way that would have normally led to its abandonment in other circumstances. Development of the drug was based on studies in preclinical models and parallels efforts in transplantation. From a series of innovative adaptations in response to issues related to adverse events and immunogenicity, humanized Fc receptors (FcR) nonbinding antibodies were developed with improved clinical outcomes and safety as well as new mechanisms. Importantly, as a result of these developments, teplizumab has been able to achieve efficacy over extended periods of time without global immune suppression. The approval of teplizumab represents a significant first step toward achieving escape from T1D and, in the future, reversal of the disease.

On November 17, 2022, the Food and Drug Administration (FDA) announced the approval of a CD3 antibody, Tzield (teplizumab), for the prevention of insulin-dependent type 1 diabetes (T1D) (www.fda.gov/news-events/press-announcements/fda-approves-first-drug-can-delay-onset-type-1-diabetes). Teplizumab is the first immunotherapy on the market for T1D, one of the most common chronic diseases of childhood, a veritable scourge whose incidence continues to rise at a dizzying pace, and in ever younger children (Bach 2002, 2018; Lawrence et al. 2014; Fazeli Farsani et al. 2016; Rami-Merhar et al. 2020; Gregory et al. 2022). This was the "happy ending" to a long scientific and medical adventure spanning more than 30 years.

It has been known since the 1970s that insulin-dependent T1D is an autoimmune disease when it was discovered that the serum of patients suffering from this condition contained autoantibodies directed against the β cells of the islets of Langerhans (Bottazzo et al. 1974, 2017). Also, the pioneering work of George Eisenbarth in the mid-1980s suggested that autoimmune diabetes was a chronic disease evolving for many years before the advent of hyperglycemia and insulin dependency (Nerup et al. 1974; Eisenbarth et al. 1985; Soeldner et al. 1985;

Cite this article as *Cold Spring Harb Perspect Med* doi: 10.1101/cshperspect.a041600

Srikanta et al. 1985). Susceptibility to T1D was inherited, and the progression of the autoimmune attack of β cells could be detected in siblings of diabetic patients by the measure of β-cell-specific autoantibodies (Nerup et al. 1974; Eisenbarth et al. 1985; Soeldner et al. 1985; Srikanta et al. 1985). Multiple β-cell autoantibody specificities were identified (directed against insulin, glutamic acid decarboxylase [GAD], the IA2 antigen, a phosphatase, and a zinc transporter ZnT8) and data from the TrialNet Pathway to Prevention Study show that β-cell dysfunction may precede diabetes diagnosis by more than 5 years in a subset of autoantibody-positive individuals (Evans-Molina et al. 2018).

The paradigm of T1D progression has evolved to distinguish three main stages based on the detection of β-cell autoantibodies and dysglycemia. In stage 1, individuals are normoglycemic, but the autoimmune response is triggered as indicated by the presence of two or more anti-β-cell autoantibodies; the 5-year and 10-year risks of insulin dependency are ~44% and ~70%, respectively (Ziegler et al. 2013). Stage 2 also includes individuals with two or more anti-β-cell autoantibodies but whose loss of β-cell mass has progressed, leading to glucose intolerance or dysglycemia; the 5-year risk of insulin dependency is ~75%, and the lifetime risk is higher (Krischer et al. 2022). The advent of hyperglycemia marks the beginning of stage 3 with possible ketoacidosis and, in all cases, insulin dependence.

Knowledge of the intimate mechanisms of the autoimmune reaction that causes the disease has benefited greatly from access to a remarkable animal model of spontaneous autoimmune diabetes, the nonobese diabetic (NOD) mouse (Makino et al. 1980). These mice develop insulin-dependent diabetes comparable in many respects to that of humans. In these mice, it is possible to follow the progression of insulitis (i.e., islet infiltration by mononuclear cells, lymphocytes, and macrophages) (Anderson and Bluestone 2005). The NOD mouse has also shown that the disease can be transferred from a diabetic mouse to a recipient mouse using purified T lymphocytes (Wicker et al. 1986; Bendelac et al. 1987; Anderson and Bluestone 2005).

Given the central role played by T lymphocytes in the pathogenesis of the disease, it became logical to try to act on these lymphocytes to slow or halt the progression of diabetes. However, during the past three decades, we have also learned that the β-cell autoimmune response is tuned by fine regulatory mechanisms, mostly provided by regulatory T lymphocytes, which are now well characterized (Salomon et al. 2000; Anderson and Bluestone 2005; You et al. 2007, 2008). Thus, attempts to induce sustained tolerance have ultimately meant shifting the balance from pathogenicity to regulation. Initially, broad immune suppressives that targeted T cells, such as cyclosporine (Granelli-Piperno et al. 1988, 1990), were tested in clinical trials as a treatment for T1D (Feutren et al. 1986; Canadian 1988). In patients with recent-onset hyperglycemia (≤6 wk), cyclosporine treatment led to clinically significant remission (i.e., insulin independency) in a significantly higher percentage of patients than in placebo-treated patients (Feutren et al. 1986; Canadian 1988). However, the effect was only observed during drug treatment with disease relapsing upon a decrease in dosage or cessation of treatment (Feutren et al. 1986; Canadian 1988). The cyclosporine trials proved that remission of hyperglycemia in T1D was possible thanks to effective targeting of the immune system, presumably T lymphocytes. Nonetheless, the use of cyclosporine as a routine treatment of T1D was inconceivable, given the toxicity profile and long-term consequences of lifelong treatment, especially to young T1D patients for whom a palliative therapy, insulin, was available.

This led to the conviction that any immunotherapy had to be extremely safe and, in an ideal solution, would be able to induce "paralysis" of the anti-islet autoimmune response without altering immune responses as a whole. In fact, this paralysis or immune tolerance is the hallmark of any healthy individual whose immune system does not react pathogenically against "self" tissues. The work of Monaco et al. (1965) in the 1960s, in mouse allograft models, showed that specific paralysis to donor alloantigens was induced by a short course of polyclonal antilymphocyte sera, without impairing unrelated immune responses. A similar transplant tolerance was induced with T-cell-specific monoclonal antibodies (mAbs), in particular, CD4-specific mAbs alone (Pearson et al. 1992), combination of CD4 and CD8 (Qin et al. 1989, 1993), or CD3 mAbs (Nicolls et al. 1993). The challenges in the treatment of T1D were greater as the aim was not to induce tolerance at the time of first antigen exposure but rather to restore tolerance to β-cell autoantigens, which had been disrupted by autoimmunity. In addition to the challenge of rebalancing a dysregulated immune response, there were additional challenges due to clear genetic predisposition.

THE HISTORY OF CD3 AS A TARGET FOR IMMUNE MODULATION

It all began in 1975 when Cesar Milstein and George Kohler published a brief communication in *Nature* that described the production of mAb from the fusion of mouse B lymphocytes to a myeloma cell (Köhler and Milstein 1975). This technology was exploited when Gideon Goldstein, working in the Ortho Pharmaceutical Company (now Johnson and Johnson) with Patrick Kung, produced a series of hybridomas secreting mAbs directed at a number of molecules expressed by human lymphocytes (Kung et al. 1979). Mice were immunized with human thymocytes and the antibody-producing cells of their spleens were fused with mouse myeloma cells. The very first fusions resulted in an amazing number of major anti-T-cell antibody specificities. The laboratory notebook read OKT1, OKT2, OKT3, OKT4, OKT5, OKT6, OKT7, OKT8.... O stood for *Ortho*, K for *Kung*, and T for *T lymphocytes*. OKT3 was determined to be the first anti-CD3 antibody, which was designated by a Human Leukocyte Differentiation Antigen Workshop. This was an international effort to use antibodies to define individual proteins based on "clusters of differentiation" (CD). The workshop went on to show that these first mAbs recognized fundamental T lymphocyte markers we still use today (OKT4, CD4; OKT8, and CD8).

Given his long-standing interest in immunomodulation and pharmaceutical development, Goldstein was quick to consider the therapeutic application of the T-cell-specific mAb Ortho and Kung had produced. OKT3 was chosen first because it recognized all mature T lymphocytes in the blood and in the primary lymphoid organs, spleen, and lymph nodes. The question was then for which indication should OKT3 be developed? The answer was obvious in 1980—organ transplantation. Acute renal allograft rejection was a major problem, occurring very early, within 3 months from implantation of the cadaver kidney. In 1980, the only drugs available for transplanted patients were corticosteroids, azathioprine, and in some centers polyclonal antilymphocyte serum (ALS). Cyclosporine was just making its appearance with the first patients treated (Calne et al. 1978). So, it was only natural that the OKT3 antibody was entrusted to kidney transplant centers. The first, in Boston, headed by Paul Russell and Benedict Cosimi, developed trials aimed at reversal of acute rejection episodes that frequently occurred within the first 6 months of transplantation (Cosimi et al. 1981a,b; Ortho Multicenter Transplant Study Group 1985). At Hôpital Necker–Enfants Malades, a group headed by Henri Kreis explored the ability of OKT3 to prevent acute renal allograft rejection (Vigeral et al. 1986; Debure et al. 1988). The strong immunosuppressive capacity of OKT3 was appreciated from the very first treated patients. Amazingly in the first seven patients who received OKT3 as the only immunosuppressant treated for 14 consecutive days after the transplant surgery, allograft function was preserved as long as significant levels of OKT3 were present in the circulation (Chatenoud et al. 1986; Vigeral et al. 1986). Unfortunately, after 5–7 days of treatment, a humoral response directed to OKT3 idiotypic determinants was generated resulting in clearance of the therapeutic monoclonal, which led to rapid allograft rejection that could only be reversed by the addition of conventional immunosuppressants (Vigeral et al. 1986).

So, what was the rationale for the clinical use of OKT3? Certainly, it recognized circulating T lymphocytes, a good candidate to replace ALS. OKT3 inhibited a mixed lymphocyte reaction in vitro, a surrogate of allograft rejection. But when the first patients were injected with OKT3 in 1981, the precise molecular target had not yet been identified. When the target became clear a few years later after the T-cell receptor (TCR) was identified, it was determined that OKT3 recognized CD3ε, a nonpolymorphic subunit of the human TCR complex (Meuer et al. 1983; Leo et al. 1987; Clevers et al. 1988). At the time, the rationale to treat transplant patients with OKT3 was not based on a molecular definition or mechanism of action. It was more intuition, excellent research with the tools available at the time, excellent experience in how to convert a laboratory product into a drug that could be administered to patients, and, last but not least, an overwhelming clinical need.

OKT3 APPROVAL IN ORGAN TRANSPLANTATION: STRENGTHS AND WEAKNESSES

Based on the results of a randomized clinical trial, in 1986, OKT3 (Ortho Multicenter Transplant Study Group 1985) (muromonab-CD3) became the first mAb approved in the clinic by the FDA (Orthoclone OKT3 by Janssen-Cilag; Ecker et al. 2015) for treatment of kidney followed by liver and heart transplantation (Gilbert et al. 1987; Renlund et al. 1989; Woodle et al. 1991a,b; Farges et al. 1994) and in the pediatric setting (Goldstein et al. 1987; Woodle et al. 1991a,b; Niaudet et al. 1993).

What were the strengths of OKT3? Definitely, the immunosuppressive activity of OKT3 in transplantation was truly remarkable. Interestingly, OKT3-induced immunosuppression occurred in the absence of long-lasting T-cell depletion that occurred with polyclonal ALS. Although there was a rapid lymphocytopenia observed in the blood 10–30 min after the first OKT3 injection, it was reversible within 2–3 days following the end of treatment (Cosimi et al. 1981a,b; Chatenoud et al. 1986; Vigeral et al. 1986; Debure et al. 1988). The lymphocytopenia was in great part due to marginalization of blood lymphocytes, secondary to activation of endothelial cells by the cytokines released after the first OKT3 injection (see below). Among these were tumor necrosis factor (TNF) and interferon (IFN)-γ-induced adhesion molecules (i.e., ICAM-1 and VCAM-1) on endothelial cells, explaining the lymphocytopenia (Bemelman et al. 1995; Buysmann et al. 1996a,b). In fact, studies that looked at cell depletion in lymph nodes suggested even less depletion within tissues.

What were the weaknesses of OKT3? Certainly, two major consequences of OKT3 treatment resulted in limited usefulness of mAb therapy and ultimately withdrawal from the market. The first was cytokine release syndrome (CRS) defined at the time as "flu-like," that included high fever, gastrointestinal symptoms (diarrhea, vomiting), and, in the most severe cases, acute lung edema requiring intensive care (Abramowicz et al. 1989; Chatenoud et al. 1989, 1990). Follow-up of OKT3-treated patients showed that the CRS was transient and occurred during the first two to three injections of OKT3 as a consequence of its mitogenic activity (Abramowicz et al. 1989; Chatenoud et al. 1989, 1990; Ellenhorn et al. 1990). This toxicity associated with these first injections, even under the cover of other immunosuppressive agents, limited the broad applicability of the drug to other immune diseases, such as autoimmunity, where the immune system was most active, and this degree of toxicity was deemed unacceptable. The second concern with OKT3 therapy was the immunogenicity of the murine immunoglobulin, which included anti-idiotypic antibodies that could rapidly and completely neutralize OKT3. The immunogenicity and CRS issues could be, at least partially, ameliorated with the coadministration of conventional immunosuppressants, an alternative that could easily be applied in clinical transplantation, but represented a major obstacle for an extension of OKT3 to other clinical settings such as autoimmunity.

Therefore, it appeared essential to access fundamental and preclinical research tools, going back from the patient's bedside to the bench. In doing so, as described below, the pathophysiological basis of both the CRS and the immunization was dissected and, very rapidly, second-generation antibodies were created by genetic engineering, which at the time had dramatically evolved. These modified versions of OKT3 had been designed to replace OKT3 but this did not happen since Johnson and Johnson made a strategic decision to stop their mAb programs. In 2010, Orthoclone OKT3 was withdrawn from the market.

Who lost out? Certainly, the development of the next generation of CD3 mAbs, and other mAbs, were very significantly delayed. In retrospect, this was a very sad situation for an immunotherapy that may have activities far beyond immunosuppression, and whose field of application successfully extended from transplantation to autoimmunity. The development of OKT3 was certainly an important example from which lessons were learned. Suffice it to say that, contrary to what some had predicted, therapeutic mAbs now constitute a major class of new drugs currently experiencing explosive market growth.

PRECLINICAL MODELS ADVANCE NEXT-GENERATION ANTI-CD3 MABS

By the end of the 1980s, there was a pressing need to develop robust mouse experimental models to investigate more thoroughly the pathophysiology of the OKT3-related side effects and to find effective ways of circumventing them. The first hindrance had been the species specificity of anti-T-cell mAb in general and CD3-specific mAbs in particular. OKT3 did not cross-react with the respective mouse molecule, CD3ε. The case of OKT3 was particularly striking, since among nonhuman primates it cross-reacted only with chimpanzee T lymphocytes. Importantly, while rat mAbs that were specific for several mouse T-cell markers such as CD4 and CD8 were made, producing the first mouse CD3ε-specific mAb was a real challenge. It took 5 years after the first patient was treated with OKT3 for Leo et al. (1987) to generate the first antimouse CD3 mAb, 145-2C11. It required more than 100 fusions, switching to Armenian hamsters as immunization hosts, and screening over 10,000 tissue culture wells to identify this mAb. From that moment on, things accelerated dramatically; mechanistic studies and experimental models were developed providing results that highly impacted what happened next.

In mice as in the clinic, treatment with 145-2C11 led to rapid cytokine production within 30 minutes to 4 hours following the injection in a dose-dependent manner. This included high levels of TNF-α, IFN-γ, interleukin (IL)-2, IL-3, GM-CSF, and CSF (Hirsch et al. 1989; Ferran et al. 1990a,b, 1991). Mouse studies also demonstrated that T lymphocytes were the major source of these early produced cytokines, including TNF-α (Ferran et al. 1994). This is relevant because TNF-α is upstream in the cascade of released cytokines and its neutralization completely blocked the transcription of other cytokines (Ferran et al. 1994) and the biological effect of the mAb (Ferran et al. 1994). The use of anti-TNF-α was tested in the clinic as well. The addition of anti-TNF-α led to a better tolerated OKT3 treatment in transplant patients having received a single injection of anti-TNF-α before the first dose (CB006, Celltech) (Charpentier et al. 1992).

A better understanding of the cellular and molecular basis of activating properties and CRS in mouse studies enabled the development of next-generation CD3 mAbs. First, the mitogenic effect of the CD3 mAbs in vivo could be shown to be eliminated when bivalent $F(ab')_2$ fragments of 145-2C11 were used (Hirsch et al. 1990) stressing the importance of receptor cross-linking through Fc receptors (FcRs). In addition, the use of "FcR nonbinding" CD3 mAbs led to a better understanding of mechanism of action of the drug. Mouse studies showed that FcR binding of CD3 mAbs did not induce massive T-cell depletion as initially demonstrated in patients treated with OKT3 (see above). Injection of FcR nonbinding 145-2C11 did not eliminate high proportions of $CD4^+$ and $CD8^+$ T lymphocytes in the spleen and lymph nodes. During treatment, these T cells lost expression of surface CD3/TCR due to antigenic modulation as observed with OKT3 on human T cells (Chatenoud et al. 1982; Hirsch et al. 1988, 1989, 1990, 1991; Hughes et al. 1994). A series of functional and biochemical studies showed that when T cells interacted with the bivalent agent, downstream signaling was quite distinct from the mitogenic agents. Studies by Hirsch et al. (1990) and later Smith and Bluestone showed that $F(ab')_2$ fragments of antimurine CD3 mAb (145-2C11) retained the immune modulatory features of the whole mAb but without the same activating features. The $F(ab')_2$ fragments failed to induce the highly phosphorylated form of ζ(p23) and tyrosine phosphorylation of ZAP-70 and LCK tyrosine kinases. The consequences of these novel biochemical signals resulted in a decrease in downstream NFAT transcription factor activation and led to selective depletion and inactivation of effector T cells, so-called T-cell anergy at the time, while keeping the naive T cells and Tregs largely unscathed (Smith et al. 1997). Unexpectedly, the reduction in mitogenic activity also had a major impact on 145-2C11 immunogenicity (Hirsch et al. 1990). Mice treated with $F(ab')_2$ fragments of 145-2C11 showed a significantly decreased antimAb response (Hirsch et al. 1990).

Murine models also enabled study of the drug in various immunopathological situations. Investigators demonstrated a significant delay of rejection in fully mismatched skin transplants in mice treated with a short course of 145-2C11, mirroring the immunosuppressive effect of OKT3 in organ transplantation (Hirsch et al. 1990). Crucially, this therapeutic effect was fully preserved with the better tolerated $F(ab')_2$ fragments of the 145-2C11 antibody (Hirsch et al. 1990). Therapeutic effectiveness was also shown in models of induced autoimmunity. Treatment of mice with $F(ab')_2$ fragments of the 145-2C11 delayed the onset and reduced the severity of arthritis in DBA/1 mice immunized with type II collagen. Although autoantibody production was not affected, IL-2 and IFN-γ-producing Th1 cells harvested from the lymph nodes of treated mice were hyporesponsive to autoantigen stimulation (Hughes et al. 1994). In a model of streptozotocin-induced autoimmune diabetes in CD1 mice, a short treatment with $F(ab')_2$ fragments of 145-2C11 significantly reduced hyperglycemia (Herold et al. 1992).

At the same time, the NOD mouse model was made available to different laboratories worldwide (Makino et al. 1980). This model enabled preclinical studies that were relevant to new-onset human T1D. Beginning at 10 weeks of age, NOD mice were closely monitored for the appearance of glycosuria and, as soon as it appeared, mice treated for only 5 consecutive days with low doses of FcR-binding or FcR-nonbinding 145-2C11 displayed rapid remission of diabetes (Chatenoud et al. 1992, 1994, 1997). These results were somewhat expected since this treatment regimen delayed rejection of mismatched skin allografts for 1–2 months (Campos et al. 1993). However, autoimmune diabetes was reversed throughout the life of the majority of treated mice. Mice in remission retained normal immune responses to foreign antigens (i.e., alloantigens or infectious antigens) (Chatenoud et al. 1994; Chatenoud and Bluestone 2007; Chatenoud 2010). It was therefore possible to restore β-cell tolerance to autoantigens in NOD mice by treating with a short course of CD3 antibody that impacted immunoregulation and apoptosis of autoantigen-activated T cells (Belghith et al. 2003; Chatenoud and Bluestone 2007; Perruche et al. 2008). Another surprise was that the treatment was effective only in a particular therapeutic window once active destruction of β cells was ongoing. In fact, young NOD mice with incipient insulitis (4 wk of age) or peripheral nondestructive insulitis (8 wk of age) were insensitive to treatment. Response to CD3-specific antibody treatment was observable beginning at 12 weeks of age, when invasive insulitis and β-cell destruction started and was the more significant with the advent of hyperglycemia (Chatenoud et al. 1997; Chatenoud and Bluestone 2007; Chatenoud 2010). These results were most important as it provided a path to development of a human therapy that would be transformative as it could lead to long-term tolerance in the absence of the side effects, immunosuppression, and immunogenicity seen with OKT3. That said, no one could have predicted the adventure it would lead to.

SECOND-GENERATION ANTI-CD3 ANTIBODY—THE BIRTH OF TEPLIZUMAB

The preclinical findings provided a basis for further development of CD3 mAbs with mutations

 Cite this article as *Cold Spring Harb Perspect Med* doi: 10.1101/cshperspect.a041600

in the Ig heavy chain to eliminate binding to the FcR, change its activation properties, and prevent complement activation, while retaining immune effects even at lower dosing levels (Alegre et al. 1994; Woodle et al. 1998; Richards et al. 1999; Xu et al. 2000; Hale et al. 2010). This had immediate implications for R.W. Johnson Pharmaceutical Research Institute's (RWJPRI, a part of Ortho Pharmaceutical Corp.) efforts to generate a next-generation OKT3 and greatly impacted the design of the engineered Fc-mutated CD3 antibodies coupled with their efforts to "humanize" the OKT3 mAb by engrafting the complementarity-determining regions (CDRs) onto a human Ig backbone. In a series of studies, FcR nonbinding variants of OKT3, including F$(ab')_2$ fragments of the drug, were shown to have similar qualities as the modified form of 145-2C11 (Woodle et al. 1991a,b). Next, studies were initiated to determine whether mutants could be generated in the Fc portion of the antibody while preserving pharmacokinetics, and a stability decision was made to make two amino acid changes in the human IgG1 isotype at positions 234 and 235. The resultant antibody did not bind human FcR or trigger T cells similar to the F$(ab')_2$ fragments (Woodle et al. 1992). It is important to note that during the same period, Waldmann and colleagues determined, based on preclinical mouse studies, that elimination of Fc receptor binding obviated the mitogenic activity of a rat antimouse CD3 mAb. In addition, they generated an aglycosylated FcR nonbinding form of a different antihuman CD3 mAb having many of the same properties as the FcR nonbinding OKT3 (Bolt et al. 1993; Routledge et al. 1995).

The efforts by RWJPRI and the Bluestone laboratory resulted in the first humanized FcR nonbinding anti-CD3 Ab tested in humans, called hOKT3γ1(Ala-Ala) or, more recently, teplizumab. The first trials were conducted in patients who had undergone solid organ transplant (renal and renal/pancreas) but were experiencing allograft rejection. In the phase I trial, the drug was given (with glucocorticoids) at a starting dose of 5 mg with doubling daily to reach a target serum trough level of 1000 ng/mL, which has been shown to provide complete CD3 binding and saturation in vitro. There were minimal first-dose reactions and the treatment resulted in rapid reversal of rejection. There were elevated levels of serum IL-10 but no IL-2 after the first dose. The pharmacokinetic analysis showed a half-life of 142 ± 32 h. (Woodle et al. 1998, 1999).

Subsequently, Utset et al. (2002) performed a phase I/II open label clinical trial of teplizumab in eight patients with psoriatic arthritis in four dosing protocols. The drug was given in a dose-ascending manner over 2–6 days. They found improvement in 6/7 patients at day 30 with two patients having sustained improvement to day 90. Unfortunately, beginning in the mid-1990s, Ortho had decided not to pursue the development of teplizumab, and the drug was transferred to Centocor. However, during this time, the drug continued to be pursued in academic laboratories. It was then that Herold and colleagues, building on the preclinical efforts in Paris and Chicago using the mouse NOD model of spontaneous diabetes and preventing induction of diabetes with low doses of streptozotocin, respectively, set in motion plans to conduct a phase II trial with teplizumab in patients with stage 3 (Insel et al. 2015) new-onset T1D (Herold et al. 2002). A single 12- or 14-day course of the drug was given. The trial was conducted as an in-patient dose escalation study, starting at very low doses and reaching plateau doses that were slightly lower than those used to treat transplant rejection (Cosimi et al. 1981a,b). The initial publication, reporting on the first 24 randomized patients, showed significant improvement in stimulated C-peptide responses to a mixed meal at 12 months after drug treatment. There was also reduced HbA1c levels and insulin doses in the drug-treated versus control patients. It was clear from that trial there were effects of treatment on $CD8^+$ T cells since the ratio of CD4/CD8 T cells decreased in drug-treated clinical responders that were defined as maintaining C-peptide responses at year 1 within 7.5% of the baseline response. Subsequent studies showed that the $CD8^+$ T cells isolated after drug treatment produced IL-10, suggesting a potential suppressive activity induced by the teplizumab treatment. Enrollment and the follow-up in this trial was expanded ($n = 42$), which showed persistent improvement in C-peptide 2 years after a single-treatment course (Herold et al. 2013a,b).

Around the same time, Keymeulen et al. (2005, 2010a,b) reported the results from a randomized placebo-controlled trial of ChAglyCD3 (otelixizumab), the chimeric FcR nonbinding CD3 mAb that was developed by Waldmann and colleagues (Bolt et al. 1993). In the otelixizumab trial, a short 1-week treatment with the drug resulted in reduced requirement for insulin, lasting at least 18 months. However, neutralizing antibodies were detected in a significant proportion of patients by days 22–29, although there were no adverse clinical effects associated with the antidrug antibody responses or effects on pharmacokinetics of the drug (Hale et al. 2010; Alkemade et al. 2011). Importantly, the study showed that recall immunity was not significantly affected, demonstrating some selectivity for the biologic effects. All of the patients in this trial were Epstein–Barr Virus (EBV) seropositive at enrollment, and some of the otelixizumab-treated patients showed an increase in EBV viral loads with symptoms of mononucleosis. These signs and symptoms rapidly resolved once the T cells returned to the circulation (Keymeulen et al. 2010a,b).

Unlike the murine studies, the single-drug course at diagnosis did not lead to permanent remission with either antihuman CD3 mAb. Although the stimulated C-peptide levels were significantly higher in the drug-treated versus control groups in the studies with both mAbs, there was a decline with time. These observations prompted a study by the Immune Tolerance Network testing two courses of teplizumab using a new drug product and dosing regimen that entailed four ascending doses followed by 10 days of plateau dosing. In that randomized open label trial (ITN027AI, AbATE) (Herold et al. 2009), the drug was first administered within 100 days after diagnosis and again after 1 year. At 2 years, there was significant improvement in drug-treated ($n = 52$) versus control patients ($n = 25$) in stimulated C-peptide responses, as well as insulin use. The clinical responders from this trial were defined as those in whom the stimulated C-peptide responses were higher than all of the control patients at the primary end point at year 2. With an analysis of RNAseq from peripheral blood cells, Long et al. (2016) showed a relationship between induction of $EOMES^{+}KLRG1^{+}TIGIT^{+}CD8^{+}$ T cells with drug treatment and identified these cells as biomarkers of clinical responders. These features suggested "partial exhaustion," which was subsequently shown by reduced production of IFN-γ and TNF when they were stimulated ex vivo. This phenotype was reminiscent of the effects observed using the $F(ab')_2$ fragments of 145-2C11 mAb in mouse studies. A follow-up trial (Delay) that enrolled patients with significant residual levels of β-cell function (i.e., a stimulated level of $\geq$0.2 pmol/mL) even after the new onset period also showed improvement in C-peptide 1 year after treatment, although the results were not as robust as when the drug was given at the time of diagnosis (Herold et al. 2013a,b).

For development, a Biotech/Pharma partner was needed for teplizumab. It was then that Macrogenics licensed teplizumab and committed to a phase 3 trial in new-onset stage 3 patients. The Protégé trial, a phase 3 randomized placebo-controlled study was conducted in collaboration with Lilly. The patients older than age 8 years and within 100 days of diagnosis of T1D were randomized in a 1:1:1:1 proportion to the "full" 14-day course of teplizumab, 14 days of 1/3 of the dose each day, 1/3 of the 14 days of dosing with full dose, or placebo. The drug was given at enrollment and again at 6 months. Unlike other trials, the primary end point used was a comparison of the frequency of individuals with HbA1c <6.5% who were using <0.5 U/kg/d of insulin at year 1. This primary end point was not met, but C-peptide responses to a mixed meal were significantly improved in the full dose regimen compared to placebo with even greater differences at year 2. Those who enrolled within 6 weeks of diagnosis were <18 and from the United States showed the most robust responses of stimulated C-peptide when treated with teplizumab. However, given the failure to meet the complex primary end point, Lilly dropped the drug from their portfolio and Macrogenics struggled to raise funds to repeat the study. At about the same time, a lower dosing regimen of otelixizumab was tested (DEFEND-1) and it also failed to meet its primary end point (Aronson et al. 2014). This dose selection was designed to avoid any of the EBV reactivation that had occurred in the previous study. The lower dose regimens in Protégé and DEFEND-1 were safe but did not show significant benefit. So, had the development of CD3 mAbs reached the end of the line?

THE REBIRTH OF TEPLIZUMAB IN PREDIABETIC STAGE 2 T1D INDIVIDUALS

In an effort to understand the natural history of T1D, samples from nondiabetic relatives of patients with two or more positive autoantibodies were used to demonstrate that these individuals were at increased risk of developing T1D. In fact, within this group of individuals showing signs of deterioration in glucose tolerance (i.e., dysglycemia), the risk for diagnosis with clinical T1D was 75% in 5 years. Furthermore, ongoing investigations of these patients suggested loss of β-cell function even though they did not have clinical signs of disease. These observations created an opportunity to test whether teplizumab might delay or prevent the clinical diagnosis of T1D in this high-risk group. NIDDK TrialNet developed and commenced the TN10 trial of teplizumab treatment before the results of the Protégé study. Patients with stage 2 T1D (i.e., those who had at least 2+ autoantibodies and dysglycemia but who had not been diagnosed with stage 3 T1D) were enrolled. A total of 76 patients were randomized to a single 14-day course of teplizumab or placebo and then followed for progression to clinical diagnosis, stage 3 T1D. The drug was administered in an outpatient setting. The primary end point was a comparison of the median time to diagnosis with stage 3 T1D in the two treatment arms. The trial took an extended period (8 yr) to enroll and follow the participants until there were a sufficient number of new diagnoses for the time to event analysis. But perhaps that was a hint of efficacy since the modeling suggested that half the high-risk individuals would develop disease within 5 years. Because of the time required, the NIDDK/TrialNet decided to reduce the overall size of the trial. The study design was modified midway to require a 60% effect size to identify a significant difference in the primary outcome—a more robust effect size than had been achieved in the prior stage 3 T1D trials.

When the trial finally reached its end point, the data overwhelmed expectations. The median time to diagnosis of stage 3 T1D was delayed significantly, from 24.4 months in the placebo group to 48.4 months in the teplizumab group (Fig. 1; Herold et al. 2019). A follow-up analysis showed a significant delay from 27.1 to 59.6 months (Sims et al. 2021). The safety experience in the TN10 and previous trials was similar. The drug was administered in an outpatient setting. Transient lymphopenia occurred in 75%–80% of patients with a nadir after the first full dose of teplizumab, but the lymphocyte count increased even with ongoing drug administration. There were symptoms of mild cytokine release in up to 20% of patients with the first doses of the drug that were managed with ibuprofen, antihistamines, or acetaminophen. Transient liver function abnormalities occurred in ∼1/4 of patients. About 1/3 of patients developed a maculopapular rash after day 5 that resolved spontaneously after dosing was completed. EBV reactivation occurred in ∼45% of the patients who were EBV seropositive before drug treatment but resolved in all cases and was infrequently symptomatic.

By this time, teplizumab had been handed off to a fifth company, Provention Bio. They had already decided to rerun the phase 3 trial in stage 3 new-onset patients (PROTECT). But, with the completion of the TN10 trial Provention Bio, submitted a biologics license application (BLA) for approval of its use for delay of the diagnosis of stage 3 T1D in patients with stage 2 disease. The data used for evaluating the efficacy of drug treatment included an integrated analysis from five clinical trials, including the investigator-initiated studies. The efficacy analysis included data from the five trials ($n = 375$ treated with teplizumab and 234 placebo treated or control patients). An integrated analysis with these data showed highly robust improvement in

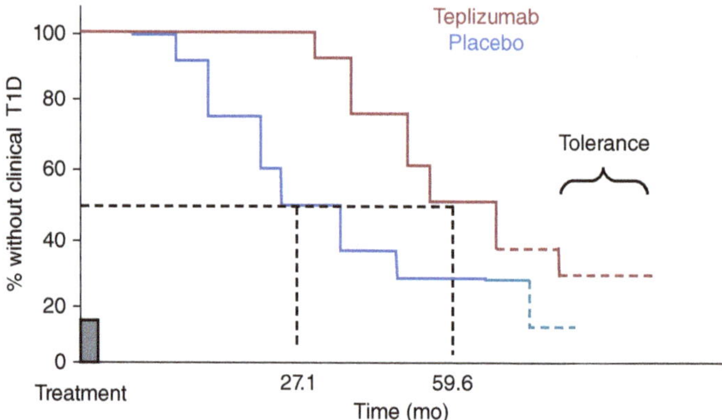

Figure 1. Representation of the outcome of the teplizumab prevention trial that was done by NIDDK type 1 diabetes (T1D) TrialNet. After a median follow-up of 24.5 months, stage 3 T1D was diagnosed in 47 participants (22 of 44 in the teplizumab arm and 25 of 32 in the placebo arm). (Figure based on data from Sims et al. 2021.)

C-peptide responses at 1 and 2 years after treatment as well as reduced use of exogenous insulin at the two time points (Herold et al. 2023). The advisory panel review and subsequent analysis of the data led to approval of teplizumab in November 2022 for delaying the onset of stage 3 T1D in at-risk individuals with stage 2 disease. The authorization represented approval of the first drug to change the course of T1D since the discovery of insulin 100 years prior and the first drug approved for delay of any autoimmune disease.

Finally, following the approval of teplizumab for at-risk individuals, the results from the Provention Bio PROTECT trial, a randomized, placebo-controlled phase 3 trial of children and adolescents with new-onset stage 3 T1D, became available (Ramos et al. 2023). This trial enrolled children within 6 weeks of diagnosis. The drug or placebo was administered at enrollment and again at 6 months, although, because of COVID, some patients received their second course at month 12 rather than 6. The primary end point was a comparison of stimulated C-peptide responses 18 months after enrollment with new-onset stage 3 T1D. This trial met its clinical end point showing improved C-peptide responses. In the PROTECT study, the investigators were successful in treating according to the American Diabetes Association (ADA) Standards of Care, matching HbA1c levels in the two study arms. However, to achieve similar HbA1c levels, the doses of insulin that were required were lower in the teplizumab-treated patients. In addition, in a sensitivity analysis, the frequency of clinically higher-grade hypoglycemic events was significantly reduced. Collectively, these data indicated that teplizumab treatment not only reduced the decline in C-peptide over 18 months but also improved clinical parameters, including significant hypoglycemia, which is the most common complication of insulin therapy. Based on the results of this trial, as well as all the other clinical data accumulated over the last 22 years, Sanofi (who bought Provention Bio) is currently working toward further development. Among pending challenges are the improvement of the mode of delivery of teplizumab and the dosing regimen, characterizing immunologic and/or metabolic markers to define the optimum therapeutic window, and the pricing. Unfortunately, all recently developed agents and technologies have come at a high cost.

SO, WHERE DO WE GO FROM HERE?

The road for teplizumab has been long and hard but there has been a great deal learned along the way that should propel the field for the future, not only in the treatment of T1D but other autoimmune diseases (Fig. 2). First, we have

Cite this article as *Cold Spring Harb Perspect Med* doi: 10.1101/cshperspect.a041600

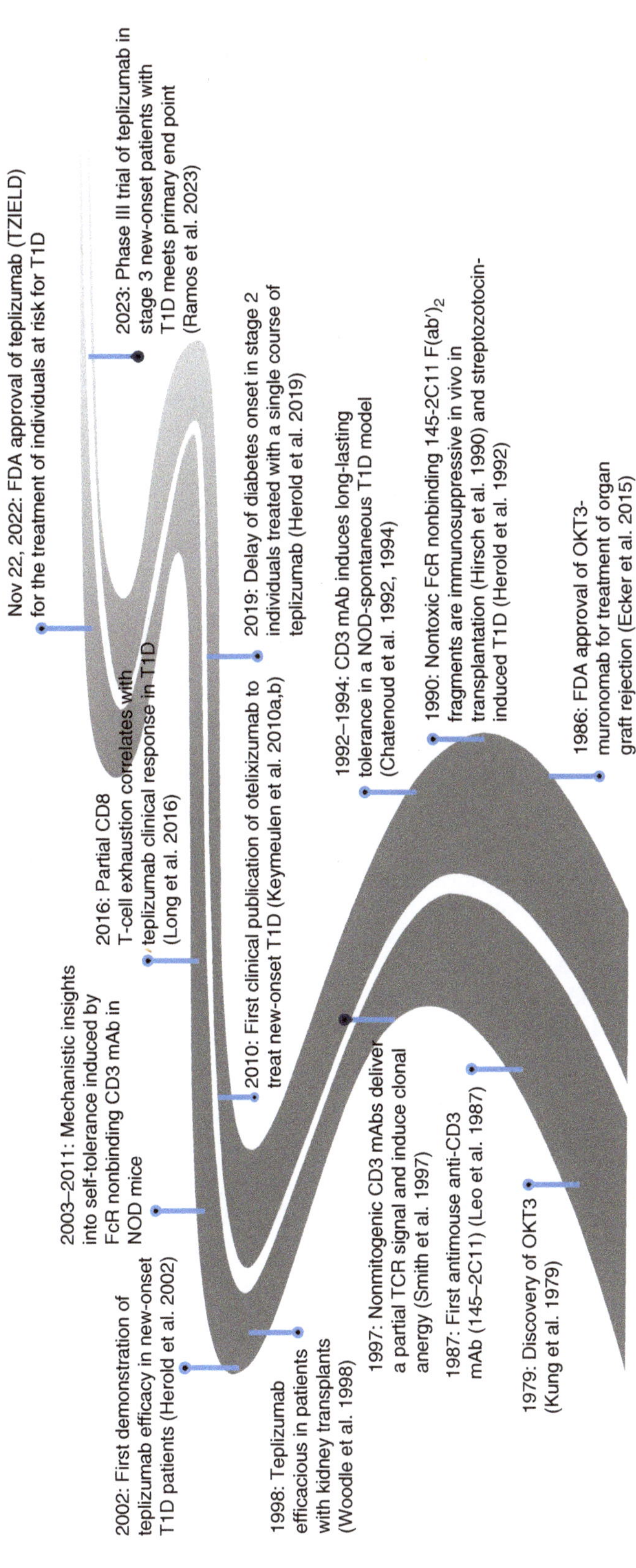

Figure 2. Traveling the teplizumab road.

learned that one can achieve long-term tolerance with a single 2-week treatment. In fact, there are many patients from the TN10 trial that are now 8–10 years out after receiving the drug, versus very few in the placebo group. This supports the concept of dominant immune regulation. Although not detailed in this article, other articles in this collection highlight the possible role of Treg cells in this process and note that teplizumab treatment preserves Tregs. Other regulatory cells may also play an important role in long-term tolerance, such as the IL-10-producing $CD8^+$ T cells or the partially exhausted T cells observed in treated patients. Second, the success of these studies supports the potential for new trials that can combine teplizumab with other agents, perhaps targeting another arm of the immune system or targeting the repair and regeneration of islet cells. Although it may be possible to genetically engineer these cells to escape immunity, it is equally likely that a combination with teplizumab could obviate any autoimmune destruction. Finally, the results of these decades of work give some hope that persistence can pay off. We live in a Biotech/Pharma community that has little patience for taking the long road. Partly, this is an economic issue, where investors and shareholders are looking for quick profits. But it is also the nature of science that the pipeline of new ideas is constantly being translated into novel medicines, often pushing aside the "outdated" approaches. Had it not been the support of a village, including small companies, investors, investigators, the National Institutes of Health (NIH), philanthropy, and those scientists who toil in the laboratory every day, teplizumab would not be helping patients live a disease-free life for some time now, with the expectation that ongoing investigations will extend their escape from clinical T1D. All authors participated equally to the saga.

REFERENCES

Abramowicz D, Schandene L, Goldman M, Crusiaux A, Vereerstraeten P, De Pauw L, Wybran J, Kinnaert P, Dupont E, Toussaint C. 1989. Release of tumor necrosis factor, interleukin-2, and γ-interferon in serum after injection of OKT3 monoclonal antibody in kidney transplant recipients. *Transplantation* **47:** 606–608. doi:10.1097/00007890-198904000-00008

Alegre ML, Peterson LJ, Xu D, Sattar HA, Jeyarajah DR, Kowalkowski K, Thistlethwaite JR, Zivin RA, Jolliffe L, Bluestone JA. 1994. A non-activating "humanized" anti-CD3 monoclonal antibody retains immunosuppressive properties in vivo. *Transplantation* **57:** 1537–1543. doi:10.1097/00007890-199457110-00001

Alkemade GM, Hilbrands R, Vandemeulebroucke E, Pipeleers D, Waldmann H, Mathieu C, Keymeulen B, Roep BO. 2011. Preservation of recall immunity in anti-CD3-treated recent onset type 1 diabetes patients. *Diabetes Metab Res Rev* **27:** 925–927. doi:10.1002/dmrr.1273

Anderson MS, Bluestone JA. 2005. The NOD mouse: a model of immune dysregulation. *Annu Rev Immunol* **23:** 447–485. doi:10.1146/annurev.immunol.23.021704.115643

Aronson R, Gottlieb PA, Christiansen JS, Donner TW, Bosi E, Bode BW, Pozzilli P. 2014. Low-dose otelixizumab anti-CD3 monoclonal antibody DEFEND-1 study: results of the randomized phase III study in recent-onset human type 1 diabetes. *Diabetes Care* **37:** 2746–2754. doi:10.2337/dc13-0327

Bach JF. 2002. The effect of infections on susceptibility to autoimmune and allergic diseases. *N Engl J Med* **347:** 911–920. doi:10.1056/NEJMra020100

Bach JF. 2018. The hygiene hypothesis in autoimmunity: the role of pathogens and commensals. *Nat Rev Immunol* **18:** 105–120. doi:10.1038/nri.2017.111

Belghith M, Bluestone JA, Barriot S, Mégret J, Bach JF, Chatenoud L. 2003. TGF-β-dependent mechanisms mediate restoration of self-tolerance induced by antibodies to CD3 in overt autoimmune diabetes. *Nat Med* **9:** 1202–1208. doi:10.1038/nm924

Bemelman FJ, Buysmann S, Yong SL, van Diepen FN, Schellekens PT, ten Berge RJ. 1995. Biphasic granulocytopenia after administration of the first dose of OKT3. *J Lab Clin Med* **126:** 571–579.

Bendelac A, Carnaud C, Boitard C, Bach JF. 1987. Syngeneic transfer of autoimmune diabetes from diabetic NOD mice to healthy neonates. Requirement for both $L3T4^+$ and $Lyt\text{-}2^+$ T cells. *J Exp Med* **166:** 823–832. doi:10.1084/jem.166.4.823

Bolt S, Routledge E, Lloyd I, Chatenoud L, Pope H, Gorman SD, Clark M, Waldmann H. 1993. The generation of a humanized, non-mitogenic CD3 monoclonal antibody which retains in vitro immunosuppressive properties. *Eur J Immunol* **23:** 403–411. doi:10.1002/eji.1830230216

Bottazzo GF, Florin-Christensen A, Doniach D. 1974. Islet-cell antibodies in diabetes mellitus with autoimmune polyendocrine deficiencies. *Lancet* **2:** 1279–1283. doi:10.1016/S0140-6736(74)90140-8

Bottazzo GF, Florin-Christensen A, Doniach D. 2017. Pillars article: Islet-cell antibodies in diabetes mellitus with autoimmune polyendocrine deficiencies. *Lancet.* 1974. 304: 1279–1283. *J Immunol* **199:** 3014–3018. doi:10.4049/jimmunol.1701303

Buysmann S, Bemelman FJ, Schellekens PT, van Kooyk Y, Figdor CG, ten Berge IJ. 1996a. Activation and increased expression of adhesion molecules on peripheral blood lymphocytes is a mechanism for the immediate lymphocytopenia after administration of OKT3. *Blood* **87:** 404–411. doi:10.1182/blood.V87.1.404.404

Buysmann S, van Diepen FN, Surachno S, Pals ST, ten Berge RJ. 1996b. Increased dermal expression of ICAM-1 and VCAM-1 after administration of OKT3 in man. *Clin Nephrol* **46:** 84–91.

Calne RY, Thiru S, McMaster P, Craddock GN, White DJ, Evans DJ, Dunn DC, Pentlow BD, Rolles K. 1978. Cyclosporin A in patients receiving renal allografts from cadaver donors. *J Am Soc Nephrol* **9:** 1751–1756. doi:10.1681/ASN.V991751

Campos HH, Bach JF, Chatenoud L. 1993. Devising murine models to better adapt clinical protocols: sequential low-dose treatment with anti-CD3 and anti-CD4 monoclonal antibodies to prevent fully mismatched allograft rejection. *Transplant Proc* **25:** 798–799.

Canadian European Randomized Control Trial Group. 1988. Cyclosporin-induced remission of IDDM after early intervention. Association of 1 yr of cyclosporin treatment with enhanced insulin secretion. *Diabetes* **37:** 1574–1582. doi:10.2337/diab.37.11.1574

Charpentier B, Hiesse C, Lantz O, Ferran C, Stephens S, O'Shaugnessy D, Bodmer M, Benoit G, Bach JF, Chatenoud L. 1992. Evidence that antihuman tumor necrosis factor monoclonal antibody prevents OKT3-induced acute syndrome. *Transplantation* **54:** 997–1002. doi:10.1097/00007890-199212000-00011

Chatenoud L. 2010. Immune therapy for type 1 diabetes mellitus—what is unique about anti-CD3 antibodies? *Nat Rev Endocrinol* **6:** 149–157. doi:10.1038/nrendo.2009.275

Chatenoud L, Bluestone JA. 2007. CD3-specific antibodies: a portal to the treatment of autoimmunity. *Nat Rev Immunol* **7:** 622–632. doi:10.1038/nri2134

Chatenoud L, Baudrihaye MF, Kreis H, Goldstein G, Schindler J, Bach JF. 1982. Human in vivo antigenic modulation induced by the anti-T cell OKT3 monoclonal antibody. *Eur J Immunol* **12:** 979–982. doi:10.1002/eji.1830121116

Chatenoud L, Baudrihaye MF, Chkoff N, Kreis H, Goldstein G, Bach JF. 1986. Restriction of the human in vivo immune response against the mouse monoclonal antibody OKT3. *J Immunol* **137:** 830–838. doi:10.4049/jimmunol.137.3.830

Chatenoud L, Ferran C, Reuter A, Legendre C, Gevaert Y, Kreis H, Franchimont P, Bach JF. 1989. Systemic reaction to the anti-T-cell monoclonal antibody OKT3 in relation to serum levels of tumor necrosis factor and interferon-γ [corrected]. *N Engl J Med* **320:** 1420–1421. doi:10.1056/NEJM198905253202117

Chatenoud L, Ferran C, Legendre C, Thouard I, Merite S, Reuter A, Gevaert Y, Kreis H, Franchimont P, Bach JF. 1990. In vivo cell activation following OKT3 administration. Systemic cytokine release and modulation by corticosteroids. *Transplantation* **49:** 697–702. doi:10.1097/00007890-199004000-00009

Chatenoud L, Thervet E, Primo J, Bach JF. 1992. Remission of established disease in diabetic NOD mice induced by anti-CD3 monoclonal antibody. *C R Acad Sci III* **315:** 225–228.

Chatenoud L, Thervet E, Primo J, Bach JF. 1994. Anti-CD3 antibody induces long-term remission of overt autoimmunity in nonobese diabetic mice. *Proc Natl Acad Sci* **91:** 123–127. doi:10.1073/pnas.91.1.123

Chatenoud L, Primo J, Bach JF. 1997. CD3 antibody-induced dominant self tolerance in overtly diabetic NOD mice. *J. Immunol* **158:** 2947–2954. doi:10.4049/jimmunol.158.6.2947

Clevers H, Alarcon B, Wileman T, Terhorst C. 1988. The T cell receptor/CD3 complex: a dynamic protein ensemble. *Annu Rev Immunol* **6:** 629–662. doi:10.1146/annurev.iy.06.040188.003213

Cosimi AB, Burton RC, Colvin RB, Goldstein G, Delmonico FL, Laquaglia MP, Tolkoff-rubin N, Rubin RH, Herrin JT, Russell PS. 1981a. Treatment of acute renal allograft rejection with OKT3 monoclonal antibody. *Transplantation* **32:** 535–539. doi:10.1097/00007890-198112000-00018

Cosimi AB, Colvin RB, Burton RC, Rubin RH, Goldstein G, Kung PC, Hansen WP, Delmonico FL, Russell PS. 1981b. Use of monoclonal antibodies to T-cell subsets for immunologic monitoring and treatment in recipients of renal allografts. *N Engl J Med* **305:** 308–314. doi:10.1056/NEJM198108063050603

Debure A, Chkoff N, Chatenoud L, Lacombe M, Campos H, Noël LH, Goldstein G, Bach JF, Kreis H. 1988. One-month prophylactic use of OKT3 in cadaver kidney transplant recipients. *Transplantation* **45:** 546–553. doi:10.1097/00007890-198803000-00009

Ecker DM, Jones SD, Levine HL. 2015. The therapeutic monoclonal antibody market. *MAbs* **7:** 9–14. doi:10.4161/19420862.2015.989042

Eisenbarth GS, Srikanta S, Fleischnick E, Ganda OP, Jackson RA, Brink SJ, Soeldner JS, Yunis EJ, Alper C. 1985. Progressive autoimmune β cell insufficiency: occurrence in the absence of high-risk HLA alleles DR3, DR4. *Diabetes Care* **8:** 477–480. doi:10.2337/diacare.8.5.477

Ellenhorn JD, Woodle ES, Ghobreal I, Thistlethwaite JR, Bluestone JA. 1990. Activation of human T cells in vivo following treatment of transplant recipients with OKT3. *Transplantation* **50:** 608–612. doi:10.1097/00007890-199010000-00016

Evans-Molina C, Sims EK, DiMeglio LA, Ismail HM, Steck AK, Palmer JP, Krischer JP, Geyer S, Xu P, Sosenko JM. 2018. Β cell dysfunction exists more than 5 years before type 1 diabetes diagnosis. *JCI Insight* **3:** e120877. doi:10.1172/jci.insight.120877

Farges O, Ericzon BG, Bresson-Hadni S, Lynch SV, Höckerstedt K, Houssin D, Galmarini D, Faure JL, Baldauf C, Bismuth H. 1994. A randomized trial of OKT3-based versus cyclosporine-based immunoprophylaxis after liver transplantation. Long-term results of a European and Australian multicenter study. *Transplantation* **58:** 891–898. doi:10.1097/00007890-199410270-00006

Fazeli Farsani S, Souverein PC, van der Vorst MM, Knibbe CA, Herings RM, de Boer A, Mantel-Teeuwisse AK. 2016. Increasing trends in the incidence and prevalence rates of type 1 diabetes among children and adolescents in the Netherlands. *Pediatr Diabetes* **17:** 44–52. doi:10.1111/pedi.12232

Ferran C, Dy M, Merite S, Sheehan K, Schreiber R, Leboulenger F, Landais P, Bluestone J, Bach JF, Chatenoud L. 1990a. Reduction of morbidity and cytokine release in anti-CD3 MoAb-treated mice by corticosteroids. *Transplantation* **50:** 642–648. doi:10.1097/00007890-199010000-00023

Ferran C, Sheehan K, Dy M, Schreiber R, Merite S, Landais P, Noel LH, Grau G, Bluestone J, Bach JF, et al. 1990b. Cytokine-related syndrome following injection of anti-CD3 monoclonal antibody: further evidence for transient in vivo T cell activation. *Eur J Immunol* **20:** 509–515. doi:10.1002/eji.1830200308

Ferran C, Dy M, Sheehan K, Schreiber R, Grau G, Bluestone J, Bach JF, Chatenoud L. 1991. Cascade modulation by anti-tumor necrosis factor monoclonal antibody of interferon-γ, interleukin 3 and interleukin 6 release after triggering of the CD3/T cell receptor activation pathway. *Eur J Immunol* **21:** 2349–2353. doi:10.1002/eji.1830211009

Ferran C, Dautry F, Mérite S, Sheehan K, Schreiber R, Grau G, Bach JF, Chatenoud L. 1994. Anti-tumor necrosis factor modulates anti-CD3-triggered T cell cytokine gene expression in vivo. *J Clin Invest* **93:** 2189–2196. doi:10.1172/JCI117215

Feutren G, Papoz L, Assan R, Vialettes B, Karsenty G, Vexiau P, Du Rostu H, Rodier M, Sirmai J, Lallemand A, et al. 1986. Cyclosporin increases the rate and length of remissions in insulin-dependent diabetes of recent onset. Results of a multicentre double-blind trial. *Lancet* **2:** 119–124. doi:10.1016/S0140-6736(86)91943-4

Gilbert EM, Dewitt CW, Eiswirth CC, Renlund DG, Menlove RL, Freedman LA, Herrick CM, Gay WA, Bristow MR. 1987. Treatment of refractory cardiac allograft rejection with OKT3 monoclonal antibody. *Am J Med* **82:** 202–206. doi:10.1016/0002-9343(87)90056-8

Goldstein G, Kremer AB, Barnes L, Hirsch RL. 1987. OKT3 monoclonal antibody reversal of renal and hepatic rejection in pediatric patients. *J Pediatr* **111:** 1046–1050. doi:10.1016/S0022-3476(87)80054-9

Granelli-Piperno A, Keane M, Steinman RM. 1988. Evidence that cyclosporine inhibits cell-mediated immunity primarily at the level of the T lymphocyte rather than the accessory cell. *Transplantation* **46:** 53S–60S. doi:10.1097/00007890-198808001-00011

Granelli-Piperno A, Nolan P, Inaba K, Steinman RM. 1990. The effect of immunosuppressive agents on the induction of nuclear factors that bind to sites on the interleukin 2 promoter. *J Exp Med* **172:** 1869–1872. doi:10.1084/jem.172.6.1869

Gregory GA, Robinson TIG, Linklater SE, Wang F, Colagiuri S, de Beaufort C, Donaghue KC, Magliano DJ, Maniam J, Orchard TJ, et al. 2022. Global incidence, prevalence, and mortality of type 1 diabetes in 2021 with projection to 2040: a modelling study. *Lancet Diabetes Endocrinol* **10:** 741–760. doi:10.1016/S2213-8587(22)00218-2

Hale G, Rebello P, Al Bakir I, Bolam E, Wiczling P, Jusko WJ, Vandemeulebroucke E, Keymeulen B, Mathieu C, Ziegler AG, et al. 2010. Pharmacokinetics and antibody responses to the CD3 antibody otelixizumab used in the treatment of type 1 diabetes. *J Clin Pharmacol* **50:** 1238–1248. doi:10.1177/0091270009356299

Herold KC, Bluestone JA, Montag AG, Parihar A, Wiegner A, Gress RE, Hirsch R. 1992. Prevention of autoimmune diabetes with nonactivating anti-CD3 monoclonal antibody. *Diabetes* **41:** 385–391. doi:10.2337/diab.41.3.385

Herold KC, Hagopian W, Auger JA, Poumian Ruiz E, Taylor L, Donaldson D, Gitelman SE, Harlan DM, Xu D, Zivin RA, et al. 2002. Anti-CD3 monoclonal antibody in new-onset type 1 diabetes mellitus. *N Engl J Med* **346:** 1692–1698. doi:10.1056/NEJMoa012864

Herold KC, Gitelman S, Greenbaum C, Puck J, Hagopian W, Gottlieb P, Sayre P, Bianchine P, Wong E, Seyfert-Margolis V, et al. 2009. Treatment of patients with new onset Type 1 diabetes with a single course of anti-CD3 mAb Teplizumab preserves insulin production for up to 5 years. *Clin Immunol* **132:** 166–173. doi:10.1016/j.clim.2009.04.007

Herold KC, Gitelman SE, Ehlers MR, Gottlieb PA, Greenbaum CJ, Hagopian W, Boyle KD, Keyes-Elstein L, Aggarwal S, Phippard D, et al. 2013a. Teplizumab (anti-CD3 mAb) treatment preserves C-peptide responses in patients with new-onset type 1 diabetes in a randomized controlled trial: metabolic and immunologic features at baseline identify a subgroup of responders. *Diabetes* **62:** 3766–3774. doi:10.2337/db13-0345

Herold KC, Gitelman SE, Willi SM, Gottlieb PA, Waldron-Lynch F, Devine L, Sherr J, Rosenthal SM, Adi S, Jalaludin MY, et al. 2013b. Teplizumab treatment may improve C-peptide responses in participants with type 1 diabetes after the new-onset period: a randomised controlled trial. *Diabetologia* **56:** 391–400. doi:10.1007/s00125-012-2753-4

Herold KC, Bundy BN, Long SA, Bluestone JA, DiMeglio LA, Dufort MJ, Gitelman SE, Gottlieb PA, Krischer JP, Linsley PS, et al. 2019. An anti-CD3 antibody, teplizumab, in relatives at risk for type 1 diabetes. *N Engl J Med* **381:** 603–613. doi:10.1056/NEJMoa1902226

Herold KC, Gitelman SE, Gottlieb PA, Knecht LA, Raymond R, Ramos EL. 2023. Teplizumab: a disease-modifying therapy for type 1 diabetes that preserves β-cell function. *Diabetes Care* **46:** 1848–1856. doi:10.2337/dc23-0675

Hirsch R, Eckhaus M, Auchincloss HJR, Sachs DH, Bluestone JA. 1988. Effects of in vivo administration of anti-T3 monoclonal antibody on T cell function in mice. I: Immunosuppression of transplantation responses. *J Immunol* **140:** 3766–3772. doi:10.4049/jimmunol.140.11.3766

Hirsch R, Gress RE, Pluznik DH, Eckhaus M, Bluestone JA. 1989. Effects of in vivo administration of anti-CD3 monoclonal antibody on T cell function in mice. II: In vivo activation of T cells. *J Immunol* **142:** 737–743. doi:10.4049/jimmunol.142.3.737

Hirsch R, Bluestone JA, De Nenno L, Gress RE. 1990. Anti-CD3 F(ab′)2 fragments are immunosuppressive in vivo without evoking either the strong humoral response or morbidity associated with whole mAb. *Transplantation* **49:** 1117–1123. doi:10.1097/00007890-199006000-00018

Hirsch R, Archibald J, Gress RE. 1991. Differential T cell hyporesponsiveness induced by in vivo administration of intact or F(ab′)2 fragments of anti-CD3 monoclonal antibody. F(ab′)2 fragments induce a selective T helper dysfunction. *J Immunol* **147:** 2088–2093. doi:10.4049/jimmunol.147.7.2088

Hughes C, Wolos JA, Giannini EH, Hirsch R. 1994. Induction of T helper cell hyporesponsiveness in an experimental model of autoimmunity by using nonmitogenic anti-CD3 monoclonal antibody. *J Immunol* **153:** 3319–3325. doi:10.4049/jimmunol.153.7.3319

Insel RA, Dunne JL, Atkinson MA, Chiang JL, Dabelea D, Gottlieb PA, Greenbaum CJ, Herold KC, Krischer JP, Lernmark Å, et al. 2015. Staging presymptomatic type 1 diabetes: a scientific statement of JDRF, the Endocrine Society, and the American Diabetes Association. *Diabetes Care* **38:** 1964–1974. doi:10.2337/dc15-1419

Keymeulen B, Vandemeulebroucke E, Ziegler AG, Mathieu C, Kaufman L, Hale G, Gorus F, Goldman M, Walter M, Candon S, et al. 2005. Insulin needs after CD3-antibody therapy in new-onset type 1 diabetes. *N Engl J Med* **352:** 2598–2608. doi:10.1056/NEJMoa043980

Keymeulen B, Candon S, Fafi-Kremer S, Ziegler A, Leruez-Ville M, Mathieu C, Vandemeulebroucke E, Walter M, Crenier L, Thervet E, et al. 2010a. Transient Epstein–Barr virus reactivation in CD3 monoclonal antibody-treated patients. *Blood* **115:** 1145–1155. doi:10.1182/blood-2009-02-204875

Keymeulen B, Walter M, Mathieu C, Kaufman L, Gorus F, Hilbrands R, Vandemeulebroucke E, Van de Velde U, Crenier L, De Block C, et al. 2010b. Four-year metabolic outcome of a randomised controlled CD3-antibody trial in recent-onset type 1 diabetic patients depends on their age and baseline residual β cell mass. *Diabetologia* **53:** 614–623. doi:10.1007/s00125-009-1644-9

Köhler G, Milstein C. 1975. Continuous cultures of fused cells secreting antibody of predefined specificity. *Nature* **256:** 495–497. doi:10.1038/256495a0

Krischer JP, Liu X, Lernmark Å, Hagopian WA, Rewers MJ, She JX, Toppari J, Ziegler AG, Akolkar B; TEDDY Study Group. 2022. Predictors of the initiation of islet autoimmunity and progression to multiple autoantibodies and clinical diabetes: the TEDDY Study. *Diabetes Care* **45:** 2271–2281. doi:10.2337/dc21-2612

Kung P, Goldstein G, Reinherz EL, Schlossman SF. 1979. Monoclonal antibodies defining distinctive human T cell surface antigens. *Science* **206:** 347–349. doi:10.1126/science.314668

Lawrence JM, Imperatore G, Dabelea D, Mayer-Davis EJ, Linder B, Saydah S, Klingensmith GJ, Dolan L, Standiford DA, Pihoker C, et al. 2014. Trends in incidence of type 1 diabetes among non-Hispanic white youth in the U.S., 2002–2009. *Diabetes* **63:** 3938–3945. doi:10.2337/db13-1891

Leo O, Foo M, Sachs DH, Samelson LE, Bluestone JA. 1987. Identification of a monoclonal antibody specific for a murine T3 polypeptide. *Proc Natl Acad Sci* **84:** 1374–1378. doi:10.1073/pnas.84.5.1374

Long SA, Thorpe J, DeBerg HA, Gersuk V, Eddy J, Harris KM, Ehlers M, Herold KC, Nepom GT, Linsley PS. 2016. Partial exhaustion of CD8 T cells and clinical response to teplizumab in new-onset type 1 diabetes. *Sci Immunol* **1:** eaai7793. doi:10.1126/sciimmunol.aai7793

Makino S, Kunimoto K, Muraoka Y, Mizushima Y, Katagiri K, Tochino Y. 1980. Breeding of a non-obese, diabetic strain of mice. *Exp Anim* **29:** 1–13. doi:10.1538/expanim1978.29.1_1

Meuer SC, Acuto O, Hussey RE, Hodgdon JC, Fitzgerald KA, Schlossman SF, Reinherz EL. 1983. Evidence for the T3-associated 90K heterodimer as the T-cell antigen receptor. *Nature* **303:** 808–810. doi:10.1038/303808a0

Monaco AP, Wood ML, Russell PS. 1965. Adult thymectomy: effect on recovery from immunologic depression in mice. *Science* **149:** 432–435. doi:10.1126/science.149.3682.432

Nerup J, Platz P, Andersen OO, Christy M, Lyngsøe J, Poulsen JE, Ryder LP, Nielsen LS, Thomsen M, Svejgaard A. 1974. HL-A antigens and diabetes mellitus. *Lancet* **2:** 864–866. doi:10.1016/S0140-6736(74)91201-X

Niaudet P, Jean G, Broyer M, Chatenoud L. 1993. Anti-OKT3 response following prophylactic treatment in paediatric kidney transplant recipients. *Pediatr Nephrol* **7:** 263–267. doi:10.1007/BF00853215

Nicolls MR, Aversa GG, Pearce NW, Spinelli A, Berger MF, Gurley KE, Hall BM. 1993. Induction of long-term specific tolerance to allografts in rats by therapy with an anti-CD3-like monoclonal antibody. *Transplantation* **55:** 459–468. doi:10.1097/00007890-199303000-00001

Ortho Multicenter Transplant Study Group. 1985. A randomized clinical trial of OKT3 monoclonal antibody for acute rejection of cadaveric renal transplants. *N Engl J Med* **313:** 337–342. doi:10.1056/NEJM198508083130601

Pearson TC, Madsen JC, Larsen CP, Morris PJ, Wood KJ. 1992. Induction of transplantation tolerance in adults using donor antigen and anti-CD4 monoclonal antibody. *Transplantation* **54:** 475–483. doi:10.1097/00007890-199209000-00018

Perruche S, Zhang P, Liu Y, Saas P, Bluestone JA, Chen W. 2008. CD3-specific antibody-induced immune tolerance involves transforming growth factor-β from phagocytes digesting apoptotic T cells. *Nat Med* **14:** 528–535. doi:10.1038/nm1749

Qin SX, Cobbold S, Benjamin R, Waldmann H. 1989. Induction of classical transplantation tolerance in the adult. *J Exp Med* **169:** 779–794. doi:10.1084/jem.169.3.779

Qin S, Cobbold SP, Pope H, Elliott J, Kioussis D, Davies J, Waldmann H. 1993. "Infectious" transplantation tolerance. *Science* **259:** 974–977. doi:10.1126/science.8094901

Rami-Merhar B, Hofer SE, Fröhlich-Reiterer E, Waldhoer T, Fritsch M. 2020. Time trends in incidence of diabetes mellitus in Austrian children and adolescents <15 years (1989–2017). *Pediatr Diabetes* **21:** 720–726. doi:10.1111/pedi.13038

Ramos EL, Dayan CM, Chatenoud L, Sumnik Z, Simmons KM, Szypowska A, Gitelman SE, Knecht LA, Niemoeller E, Tian W, et al. 2023. Teplizumab and β-cell function in newly diagnosed type 1 diabetes. *N Engl J Med* **389:** 2151–2161. doi:10.1056/NEJMoa2308743

Renlund DG, O'Connell JB, Gilbert EM, Hammond ME, Burton NA, Jones KW, Karwande SV, Doty DB, Menlove RL, Herrick CM, et al. 1989. A prospective comparison of murine monoclonal CD-3 (OKT3) antibody-based and equine antithymocyte globulin-based rejection prophylaxis in cardiac transplantation. Decreased rejection and less corticosteroid use with OKT3. *Transplantation* **47:** 599–605. doi:10.1097/00007890-198904000-00007

Richards J, Auger J, Peace D, Gale D, Michel J, Koons A, Haverty T, Zivin R, Jolliffe L, Bluestone JA. 1999. Phase I evaluation of humanized OKT3: toxicity and immunomodulatory effects of hOKT3γ4. *Cancer Res* **59:** 2096–2101.

Routledge EG, Falconer ME, Pope H, Lloyd IS, Waldmann H. 1995. The effect of aglycosylation on the immunogenicity of a humanized therapeutic CD3 monoclonal antibody. *Transplantation* **60:** 847–853. doi:10.1097/00007890-199510270-00015

Salomon B, Lenschow DJ, Rhee L, Ashourian N, Singh B, Sharpe A, Bluestone JA. 2000. B7/CD28 costimulation is essential for the homeostasis of the $CD4^+$ $CD25^+$ immunoregulatory T cells that control autoimmune diabetes. *Immunity* **12:** 431–440. doi:10.1016/S1074-7613(00)80195-8

Sims EK, Bundy BN, Stier K, Serti E, Lim N, Long SA, Geyer SM, Moran A, Greenbaum CJ, Evans-Molina C, et al. 2021. Teplizumab improves and stabilizes β cell function in antibody-positive high-risk individuals. *Sci Transl Med* **13:** eabc8980. doi:10.1126/scitranslmed.abc8980

Smith JA, Tso JY, Clark MR, Cole MS, Bluestone JA. 1997. Nonmitogenic anti-CD3 monoclonal antibodies deliver a partial T cell receptor signal and induce clonal anergy. *J Exp Med* **185:** 1413–1422. doi:10.1084/jem.185.8.1413

Soeldner JS, Tuttleman M, Srikanta S, Ganda OP, Eisenbarth GS. 1985. Insulin-dependent diabetes mellitus and autoimmunity: islet-cell autoantibodies, insulin autoantibodies, and β-cell failure. *N Engl J Med* **313:** 893–894. doi:10.1056/NEJM198510033131417

Srikanta S, Ganda OP, Rabizadeh A, Soeldner JS, Eisenbarth GS. 1985. First-degree relatives of patients with type I diabetes mellitus. islet-cell antibodies and abnormal insulin secretion. *N Engl J Med* **313:** 461–464. doi:10.1056/NEJM198508223130801

Utset TO, Auger JA, Peace D, Zivin RA, Xu D, Jolliffe L, Alegre ML, Bluestone JA, Clark MR. 2002. Modified anti-CD3 therapy in psoriatic arthritis: a phase I/II clinical trial. *J Rheumatol* **29:** 1907–1913.

Vigeral P, Chkoff N, Chatenoud L, Campos H, Lacombe M, Droz D, Goldstein G, Bach JF, Kreis H. 1986. Prophylactic use of OKT3 monoclonal antibody in cadaver kidney recipients. Utilization of OKT3 as the sole immunosuppressive agent. *Transplantation* **41:** 730–733. doi:10.1097/00007890-198606000-00013

Wicker LS, Miller BJ, Mullen Y. 1986. Transfer of autoimmune diabetes mellitus with splenocytes from nonobese diabetic (NOD) mice. *Diabetes* **35:** 855–860. doi:10.2337/diab.35.8.855

Woodle ES, Thistlethwaite JR, Ghobrial IA, Jolliffe LK, Stuart FP, Bluestone JA. 1991a. OKT3 F(ab′)2 fragments—retention of the immunosuppressive properties of whole antibody with marked reduction in T cell activation and lymphokine release. *Transplantation* **52:** 354–360. doi:10.1097/00007890-199108000-00033

Woodle ES, Thistlethwaite JR Jr, Emond JC, Whitington PF, Black DD, Aran PP, Baker AL, Stuart FP, Broelsch CE. 1991b. OKT3 therapy for hepatic allograft rejection. Differential response in adults and children. *Transplantation* **51:** 1207–1212. doi:10.1097/00007890-199106000-00012

Woodle ES, Thistlethwaite JR, Jolliffe LK, Zivin RA, Collins A, Adair JR, Bodmer M, Athwal D, Alegre ML, Bluestone JA. 1992. Humanized OKT3 antibodies: successful transfer of immune modulating properties and idiotype expression. *J Immunol* **148:** 2756–2763. doi:10.4049/jimmunol.148.9.2756

Woodle ES, Bluestone JA, Zivin RA, Jolliffe LK, Auger J, Xu D, Thistlethwaite JR. 1998. Humanized, nonmitogenic OKT3 antibody, huOKT3γ(Ala-Ala): initial clinical experience. *Transplant Proc* **30:** 1369–1370. doi:10.1016/S0041-1345(98)00278-4

Woodle ES, Xu D, Zivin RA, Auger J, Charette J, O'laughlin R, Peace D, Jollife LK, Haverty T, Bluestone JA, et al. 1999. Phase I trial of a humanized, Fc receptor nonbinding OKT3 antibody, huOKT3γ1(Ala-Ala) in the treatment of acute renal allograft rejection. *Transplantation* **68:** 608–616. doi:10.1097/00007890-199909150-00003

Xu D, Alegre ML, Varga SS, Rothermel AL, Collins AM, Pulito VL, Hanna LS, Dolan KP, Parren PW, Bluestone JA, et al. 2000. In vitro characterization of five humanized OKT3 effector function variant antibodies. *Cell Immunol* **200:** 16–26. doi:10.1006/cimm.2000.1617

You S, Leforban B, Garcia C, Bach JF, Bluestone JA, Chatenoud L. 2007. Adaptive TGF-β-dependent regulatory T cells control autoimmune diabetes and are a privileged target of anti-CD3 antibody treatment. *Proc Natl Acad Sci* **104:** 6335–6340. doi:10.1073/pnas.0701171104

You S, Alyanakian MA, Segovia B, Damotte D, Bluestone J, Bach JF, Chatenoud L. 2008. Immunoregulatory pathways controlling progression of autoimmunity in NOD mice. *Ann NY Acad Sci* **1150:** 300–310. doi:10.1196/annals.1447.046

Ziegler AG, Rewers M, Simell O, Simell T, Lempainen J, Steck A, Winkler C, Ilonen J, Veijola R, Knip M, et al. 2013. Seroconversion to multiple islet autoantibodies and risk of progression to diabetes in children. *JAMA* **309:** 2473–2479. doi:10.1001/jama.2013.6285

Advances in Islet Transplantation and the Future of Stem Cell–Derived Islets to Treat Diabetes

Timothy J. Kieffer,[1,2] Corinne A. Hoesli,[3,4] and A.M. James Shapiro[5,6,7]

[1]Department of Cellular and Physiological Sciences, Life Sciences Institute, School of Biomedical Engineering; [2]Department of Surgery, The University of British Columbia, Vancouver V6T1Z3, British Columbia, Canada

[3]Department of Chemical Engineering; [4]Associate Member, Department of Biomedical Engineering, McGill University, Montreal H3A 0C5, Québec, Canada

[5]Clinical Islet Transplant Program; [6]Department of Surgery; [7]Alberta Diabetes Institute, University of Alberta, Edmonton T6G2E1, Alberta, Canada

Correspondence: tim.kieffer@ubc.ca

β-Cell replacement for type 1 diabetes (T1D) can restore normal glucose homeostasis, thereby eliminating the need for exogenous insulin and halting the progression of diabetes complications. Success in achieving insulin independence following transplantation of cadaveric islets fueled academic and industry efforts to develop techniques to mass produce β cells from human pluripotent stem cells, and these have now been clinically validated as an alternative source of regulated insulin production. Various encapsulation strategies are being pursued to contain implanted cells in a retrievable format, and different implant sites are being explored with some strategies reaching clinical studies. Stem cell lines, whether derived from embryonic sources or reprogrammed somatic cells, are being genetically modified for designer features, including immune evasiveness to enable implant without the use of chronic immunosuppression. Although hurdles remain in optimizing large-scale manufacturing, demonstrating efficacy, durability, and safety, products containing stem cell–derived β cells promise to provide a potent treatment for insulin-dependent diabetes.

Healthy glucose homeostasis relies upon the coordinated secretion of insulin and glucagon from a few milliliters of endocrine cells in the pancreas located within the islets of Langerhans (islets). Inadequate production of insulin by the islet β cells results in diabetes and the inability to effectively utilize glucose. The 1921 discovery of insulin by Frederick Banting, Charles Best, James Collip, and John Macleod has been lifesaving for millions suffering from diabetes. Advancements in insulin formulations and delivery techniques coupled with sophisticated glucose monitoring technologies have improved the ability to artificially control blood glucose levels and thereby reduce the progression of diabetes-associated complications, but they remain burdensome and unmatched in terms of the precision accomplished by our biological systems (Latres et al. 2019). Whole pancreas transplant or portal infusion of purified pancreatic islets can restore healthy glucose metabolism and entirely eliminate the need for exogenous insulin administra-

Cite this article as *Cold Spring Harb Perspect Med* doi: 10.1101/cshperspect.a041624

tion, but is severely limited by the reliance upon relatively scarce cadaveric tissue as well as the requirement for chronic immunosuppression to prevent graft rejection and recurrent autoimmunity against β cells. Here, we review progress to generate unlimited quantities of implantable insulin-producing islet cells from human pluripotent stem cells (PSCs), approaches to enhance cell engraftment, and efforts underway to protect the cells from immune rejection in the absence of immunosuppression drugs.

EVOLUTION OF ISLET CELL TRANSPLANTATION

Recently, the University of Alberta celebrated the 25th anniversary of the first Edmonton Protocol transplant of human allogeneic islets injected intraportally into a schoolteacher with intractable recurrent hypoglycemia whose health was deemed unsafe to teach his class. Since then, the team has carried out 765 intraportal islet cell transplants in 327 patients with unstable forms of type 1 diabetes (T1D) in Edmonton, Canada. How did we get to this single-center milestone?

A pathologist from St. Louis, MO, Paul E. Lacy, began work to extract rodent islets with collagenase enzymes initially for physiologic study, and out of curiosity transplanted these in rats in 1972 (Ballinger and Lacy 1972). In the following year, Reckard and Barker reversed diabetes in rats that were induced with the β-cell toxin streptozotocin, by intraperitoneal transplant of isolated rat islets (Reckard et al. 1973), and Lacy's group found that transplanting islets into the portal vein successfully reversed diabetes, whereas subcutaneous or intraperitoneal implantation failed (Kemp et al. 1973). Camillo Ricordi, a young surgeon working with Paul Lacy, later discovered an intriguing means to extract large numbers of human islets in a chamber containing a screen and a handful of marbles in a closed system that recirculated collagenase until the islets were liberated (Ricordi et al. 1989). The addition of density gradient purification steps, more consistent high-quality recombinant collagenase, and advances in islet culture led to highly standardized protocols for human islet cell transplantation. The process is still crude, however, and the late pioneer transplant surgeon Professor Sir Roy Calne reflected when he came to watch islet isolations in our center that the process was rather like "digging for potatoes in the dark."

David Scharp and Paul Lacy reported the first patient to achieve insulin independence in 1990 in an islet-after-kidney transplant recipient who received 800,000 islet equivalents (IEQ) into the portal vein (Scharp et al. 1990). The cells were rejected by the end of the first month, which was not highlighted in the report. Up until 1999, there had been almost 300 attempts to transplant islets in patients with T1D, with fewer than 8% resulting in sustained insulin independence. The vast majority of these failed rapidly due to poor islet quality, inadequate protection from allograft rejection, and exposure to traditional immunosuppressants, which cause insulin resistance (high-dose corticosteroids) or are toxic to β cells (high-dose calcineurin inhibitors). Recurrence of autoimmune islet destruction from difficult-to-eradicate recalcitrant, primed memory T cells remained an ever-present challenge, as first highlighted in living donor segmental pancreas transplants carried out between identical twins (human leucocyte antigen [HLA] identical) by Sibley and Sutherland (Sibley et al. 1985). Even today, we are uncertain how much or what type of immunosuppression will best eliminate the risk of recurrent autoimmunity in transplanted islets.

On March 11, 1999 in Edmonton, a schoolteacher with T1D and severe hypoglycemia received a first transplant of 376,838 IEQ that resulted in a 50% decrease in exogenous insulin, and resolution of hypoglycemic events. An infusion of a further 361,577 IEQ from a second donor a month later (total 9407 IEQ/kg) resulted in sustained insulin independence. Immunosuppression consisted of the combination of low-dose tacrolimus combined with high-dose sirolimus (a new immunosuppressive drug at that time, known from experimental study to augment insulin release from transplanted islets). Induction T-cell-directed therapy was given with an anti-IL2R antibody (daclizumab) and no corticosteroids were given. A total of seven patients were treated in a similar manner, all of whom were rendered insulin-independent for periods up to 15 months

(Shapiro et al. 2000). The Edmonton Protocol was replicated to variable degree by 10 international centers participating in a trial supported through the Immune Tolerance Network (Shapiro et al. 2006). Although high rates of insulin independence were observed in the first 2 years posttransplant, it soon became apparent that insulin independence was gradually lost in a proportion of subjects by 5 years posttransplant (Ryan et al. 2005). The decrement in islet function was atypical for acute rejection in most cases as sustained C-peptide secretion was maintained—often sufficient to prevent the recurrence of hypoglycemia. This decrement is presumed to be related to recurrent autoimmunity or to islet burnout from hyperstressed marginal grafts. However, the exact etiology remains unknown as sufficient interpretation of histopathology within the portal tracts of the liver has not been possible.

Two multicenter trials were conducted by the National Institutes of Health (NIH) in islet-alone (CIT-07) and islet-after-kidney (CIT-06) T1D patients, with a view to securing a biological license application (BLA) for islet manufacture from the Food and Drug Administration (FDA) in the United States (Hering et al. 2016; Markmann et al. 2021). The design of these trials was based on refinements in immune suppression described by Hering et al. (2005) in Minnesota, where T-cell depletion induction was given using thymoglobulin (6 mg/kg) together with tacrolimus and sirolimus. The use of etanercept, a TNF-α blocking antibody (50 mg iv pretransplant, and 25 mg s.c. on days 3, 7, and 10) was found to markedly improve islet engraftment and long term survival (Hering et al. 2023). Both the CIT-06 and CIT-7 trials successfully met their primary endpoints of safety, protection against risk of hypoglycemia, and target improvement in HbA1c below 7%. Approximately $100 million was invested in these trials by the NIH, yet almost a decade later the FDA has not granted a BLA to any of the participating centers. This has led to considerable frustration among the U.S. centers where isolated human islets are treated as a "drug" rather than a cellular or organ-transplant-derived product (Witkowski et al. 2021). However, the FDA did grant a BLA in 2023 to a not-for-profit company based in Chicago, IL (Donislecel) for a human allogeneic islet product (Lantidra)—the only group able to meet the stringent FDA requirements to date. This situation contrasts sharply with their neighbors in Canada where Heath Canada approved the manufacture of human islets for transplant in April 2001. Similar approvals were subsequently obtained in the United Kingdom (National Institutes of Healthcare Excellence [NICE]), Switzerland–France (as part of the GRAGIL network), Italy, and Australia.

Controlled Trials and Long-Term Outcomes of Islet Transplantation

Adding to the successful outcomes of the two FDA-registration trials (CIT-06 and -07), a prospective, crossover cohort study comparing intensive medical therapy to islet transplantation was completed in Vancouver, Canada, and showed significant improvement in glycemic control (HbA1c 6.6% ± 0.7 in the islet group vs. 7.5% ± 0.9 in the insulin-treated controls; $P < 0.01$). Also noted was reduced decline in renal function despite exposure to calcineurin inhibitors, and reduced progression of retinopathy and neuropathy (Warnock et al. 2008). A European trial randomized 50 patients to insulin versus immediate islet transplant and found marked improvement in metabolic outcomes (Lablanche et al. 2018).

The 20-year outcomes after islet transplantation in 255 subjects treated in Edmonton were reported in 2022 (Marfil-Garza et al. 2022). Seventy-nine percent of patients were able to achieve insulin independence after a median of two islet infusions. Twenty-year patient survival was 75%, and graft survival (C-peptide >0.3 ng/mL and protection from hypoglycemia) was 50%. Rates of complete insulin independence diminished to 75% by year 1, 62% by year 2, 32% by year 5, and 23% by year 10. Interestingly, two subjects were still insulin-independent beyond 20 years (the longest published experience), one of whom with their original transplanted graft and no subsequent top-ups. Multivariate analysis showed that the combination of anakinra (a human IL-1 receptor recombinant antagonist protein) and etanercept improved islet engraftment and long-term survival by a factor of 7.5 times—a finding that had previously been demonstrated in mice (McCall et al. 2012). This long-term data, together with reports from other centers, including Miami (Lemos et al. 2021), continue to support the notion that islet transplantation is a relatively safe procedure and that with intensive monitoring and expert management, the long-term risks from chronic immunosuppression are justified —at least in patients at high risk for recurrent hypoglycemia, glycemic lability, or accelerated end-stage diabetes-related complications. In Canada, active islet transplantation programs in Edmonton, Vancouver, Montreal, and Toronto have all been approved for reimbursement by provincial health agencies based on analyses of costs associated with standard-of-care, considering the reduction in severe hypoglycemic events after islet transplants.

RISKS AND POTENTIAL WAYS AROUND THE NEED FOR IMMUNOSUPPRESSION, AND CONTROL OF RECURRENT AUTOIMMUNITY

Systemic side effects of chronic immune suppression are well recognized and have been observed repeatedly in all clinical trials of islet transplantation to date. Risks of malignancy, opportunistic infection, posttransplant lymphoproliferative disorder (PTLD), renal impairment mouth ulceration, tremor, and hyperlipidemia may be included on a long list of undesirable effects. This is the principal reason why islet cell transplantation is currently not offered to children, or to those with less severe forms of T1D. If immune suppression could be lowered, or ideally eliminated entirely, this would completely alter the risk-benefit equation for treatment using cell-based therapies in diabetes. Immunological tolerance has been demonstrated repeatedly in small animal models since early landmark studies (Billingham et al. 1953). Robust tolerance has readily been attained in multiple rodent models of islet transplantation, and replicated using potent induction in large animal primate models (Singh et al. 2019). The need for profound myeloablation in some studies, with the generation of macrochimerism using bone marrow transplantation has been one strategy to render immunological nonresponsiveness, but the approach is both harsh and risky; probably far more so than chronic immune suppression.

Recent advances in ex vivo expansion of polyclonal or chimeric antigen receptor regulatory T cells (Tregs) have renewed interest in a cell-based approach to immune regulation in an approach that potentially could reduce or eliminate the need for chronic immunosuppression (Tang and Bluestone 2006; Ho et al. 2024). Notably, approaches are being developed to generate functional antigen-specific Tregs from PSCs, with the ability to generate an Ag-specific immunosuppressive response (Haque et al. 2016; MacDonald et al. 2022). The impact of Tregs in mitigating recurrent autoimmunity in patients with T1D could be a critical step forward in markedly improving the long-term durable benefit of cell replacement in diabetes.

An Fc-non-binding antibody (humanized anti-CD3, hOKT3g1; Ala–Ala) approved by the FDA in 2022 under the generic name teplizumab, was first developed in Dr Jeffrey Bluestone's laboratory >30 years ago. This antibody was tested by Hering et al. (2004) in islet transplantation with excellent early single-donor engraftment outcomes. Teplizumab was later shown in trials conducted through TrialNET to delay the onset of clinical symptoms (stage 3) in T1D in adults and children aged 8 and older by a median of 24 months when first reported in 2019 (Herold et al. 2019). A recent phase 3 placebo-controlled RCT from Ramos et al. in the PROTECT study found that two 12-day courses of teplizumab in children and adolescents with newly diagnosed T1D maintained a significant and clinically meaningful peak C-peptide level ≥0.2 pmol/mL in 94.9% of cases as compared to 79.2% in controls (95% CI 67.7–87.4) by week 78. Antibodies such as teplizumab and future more effective variants, given even earlier in the course of T1D (including at-risk subjects) could halt progression to diabetes, thus obviating the need for cell replacement therapy. Where diabetes has progressed, islet cell therapy combined with these protective antibodies could substantially improve the long-term protective benefit of cell transplantation by more effectively and directly controlling the risk of autoimmunity.

 Cite this article as *Cold Spring Harb Perspect Med* doi: 10.1101/cshperspect.a041624

PLURIPOTENT STEM CELLS TO MANUFACTURE ISLETS ON DEMAND

The clinical validation of islet cell replacement fueled efforts to identify islet sources that do not rely upon cadaveric organs. PSCs are attractive in this regard, because they have the inherent ability to self-renew via replication as well as form every cell type in the body, including insulin-producing β cells. Embryonic stem cells (ESCs) were isolated from donated blastocysts unused after in vitro fertilization by Thomson et al. (1998) and demonstrated to be capable of extensive expansion while still maintaining the developmental potential to form derivatives of the endoderm, mesoderm, and ectoderm germ layers. Political bans on generating new lines and funding their use in academic laboratories for ethical reasons curtailed research for many years but guidelines and regulations now define what is deemed acceptable use, albeit still lacking in consensus around the world. Another major milestone in the PSC field came in 2006 when Takahashi and Yamanaka reported the generation of induced PSCs (iPSCs) by reprogramming murine somatic cells through activation of pluripotency-promoting genes (Takahashi and Yamanaka 2006). The following year, the same group accomplished this with human cells (Takahashi et al. 2007), as did a team led by James Thomson (Yu et al. 2007), thereby providing a less controversial alternative to ESCs. Both ESCs and iPSCs have the potential to serve as a source from which to manufacture vast quantities of islets to treat diabetes.

A few years after the isolation of ESCs, Assady et al. (2001) reported spontaneous in vitro differentiation in human ESC cultures that included the generation of cells with characteristics of insulin-producing β cells, validating ESCs as a possible source for cell replacement therapy in diabetes. While academic research with human ESCs was curtailed in the United States, the California company ViaCyte (first Cythera, then Novocell) used ESCs they had generated to develop strategies for the directed and controlled differentiation down the pancreatic lineage, with a plan to commercialize a stem cell–derived product for the treatment of diabetes. The approach they used was to mimic natural pancreatic development, triggering key pathways that had been identified through decades of basic research with model organisms such as zebrafish and mice. Informed by these developmental biology studies, the team developed a ~2-week, five-stage culture protocol to convert hESCs through to islet endocrine cells (D'Amour et al. 2006). They started with WNT3a and activin A to drive nodal signaling to promote the formation of definitive endoderm, marked by expression of SOX17. Removal of activin A at stage 2 plus the addition of FGF10 and the hedgehog-signaling inhibitor KAAD-cyclopamine facilitated the transition of the cells toward the gut-tube fate based on observed increases in the levels of the hepatocyte nuclear factors (HNFs) HNF1β and HNF4α. Proximal foregut marked by the expression of the transcription factors PDX1 and HNF6 was formed in stage 3 by the addition of retinoic acid and then the posterior-foregut endoderm cells were transitioned toward the endocrine lineage in stage 4, marked by the induction of NKX6.1, with the addition of the Notch pathway inhibitor DAPT and the GLP-1 receptor agonist exendin-4. Additionally, a subset of the cells expressed the master regulator of endocrine commitment, NEUROG3, and in stage 5, the addition of insulin-like growth factor 1, and hepatocyte growth factor (HGF) further enhanced differentiation efficiencies toward endocrine cells. The final stage 5 cells were immature, largely polyhormonal, and more functionally like fetal islets with limited glucose-stimulated insulin secretion and incomplete proinsulin processing. Nevertheless, the work was widely embraced as clear evidence of the potential of this approach and a solid foundation for others to build upon.

Russ et al. (2015) found that removing cyclopamine and Noggin supplementation from the stage 3 media (leaving only retinoic acid) and removing Noggin supplementation from the stage 4 media (leaving EFG and KGF) reduced the early induction of NGN3, thereby decreasing the percentage of insulin/glucagon copositive cells that formed. Through a kinase inhibitor screen, Rezania et al. (2011) identified ALK5 inhibition as a potent inducer of endocrine hormone expression, likely via up-regulation of the transcription factors NEUROD and NGN3.

Thus, in stage 4, inhibition of TGFβ signaling using ALK5 inhibitor, as well as Notch signaling using DAPT, progressed cells toward a pancreatic endocrine phenotype. The transition of pancreatic progenitors from 2D planar culture into spheroids in 3D suspension enhances the development of functional islet endocrine cells (Rezania et al. 2014; Takeuchi et al. 2014). Moreover, through a small molecule and growth factor screen, Rezania identified R428, a selective inhibitor of the tyrosine kinase receptor AXL, as an inducer of the transcription factor MAFA, key to promoting the maturation of β cells. Thyroid hormone (T3) was also found to induce MAFA and maturation of β cells, consistent with prior evidence that it promotes β-cell maturation in rats (Aguayo-Mazzucato et al. 2013), and *N*-acetylcysteine (*N*-Cys) was added to the culture promote maintenance of nuclear MAFA. Collectively, the inclusion of *N*-Cys, the AXL inhibitor, the ALK5 inhibitor, and T3 boosted the maturation of stem cell–derived endocrine cells, although the resulting β cells were still immature when compared to donor-derived human islets (Rezania et al. 2014). Balboa et al. (2022) achieved enhanced β-cell function from their stem cell–derived islets in part by incorporating the antiproliferative aurora kinase inhibitor (ZM447439) in the final stage of culture as well as prolonging the culture period for more than 9 weeks in total. Thus, it is now possible to reliably convert human PSCs to islets with cytoarchitecture and functionality approaching those of adult primary islets, which is a remarkable achievement.

EFFECTS OF THE TRANSPLANTATION ENVIRONMENT ON PSC-DERIVED GRAFT FUNCTION

While remarkable progress has been made toward producing functional islets from PSCs, high-resolution transcriptional analysis indicates that the maturation of the β cells achieved in vitro remains incomplete, and stem cell–derived β cells made with current protocols possess a unique transcriptional profile characterized by the persistent expression and activation of progenitor and neural-biased gene networks (Schmidt et al. 2024). Moreover, several weeks post-engraftment in immunodeficient mice, a plethora of transcriptomic changes occur indicating continued maturation (Balboa et al. 2022; Augsornworawat et al. 2023). While the in vitro derivation of β cells from PSCs that faithfully replicate bona fide β cells is desirable for mechanistic studies of cell function, disease modeling, and drug screening, it may not be required for the development of a successful cell replacement therapy for diabetes, given that the cultivated cells seem capable of maturing in vivo post-implant. Moreover, it seems that once cells reach the pancreatic endoderm cell (PEC) stage, characterized by the coexpression of PDX1 and NKX6.1, they are fully capable of completing differentiation and maturation in vivo. This notion is supported by earlier work showing functional islet generation from the implant of human fetal pancreas as early as ∼9 weeks gestation (Hayek and Beattie 1997; Castaing et al. 2001). Indeed, there is compelling evidence that several months following implant, stem cell–derived PECs further differentiate into mature cell types producing insulin and glucagon, capable of ameliorating hyperglycemia and weight loss in diabetic mice (Shim et al. 2007; Kroon et al. 2008; Rezania et al. 2012). Clinically, the delay in attaining function post-implant would require patients to carefully monitor blood glucose levels and adjust exogenous insulin dosing accordingly as the implanted cells ramp up insulin production and take over glycemic control; this would be acceptable if the end result is insulin freedom. Put simply, for a person living with diabetes for several decades, it is almost inconsequential that it might take some months for the cells to mature and become fully functional.

One consideration with the use of PECs as a cell replacement product for diabetes is how the implant environment may impact the trajectory of the immature cells on route to becoming islets (Saber and Kieffer 2024). For instance, when implanting hESC-derived PECs in rodents, differential bias to the formation of β cells versus α cells was observed in rats compared to mice and the cells developed glucose-developed glucose-stimulated insulin secretion faster in the rats (Bruin et al. 2015). Given the impact of thyroid hormone on islet cell maturation (Aguayo-Mazzucato et al. 2013; Rezania et al. 2014), Bruin et al. assessed PEC maturation in animals with abnormal thyroid hormone levels. Chronic hypothyroidism resulted in severely blunted basal human C-peptide secretion, impaired glucose-stimulated insulin secretion, and elevated plasma glucagon levels associated with a graft bias to α cells over β cells compared to euthyroid mice (Bruin et al. 2016). A hyperglycemic environment enhanced the differentiation of hESC-derived PECs into glucose-responsive insulin-producing cells in mice (Bruin et al. 2013) and, interestingly, PECs matured faster in female than male mice (Saber et al. 2018). Additionally, the implant site can influence the differentiation of PECs. Saber et al. (2023) noted quicker achievement of glucose-stimulated insulin secretion when PECs were implanted subcutaneously within macroencapsulation devices compared to under the kidney capsule or in the gonadal fat pad, as well as less cyst formation. There is also evidence that mechanical signals impact the expression of key pancreatic and endocrine transcription factors (Nair et al. 2019; Hogrebe et al. 2020; Tran et al. 2020a,b), which likely impacts cell fate decisions both pre- and post-implantation. Nevertheless, it remains to be determined what factors in the recipient may influence the endocrine specification and function of hPSC-derived cells in humans, although recent clinical studies suggest thyroid hormone levels may impact graft development (Ramzy et al. 2024).

While there are potential caveats with implanting cells that are not fully differentiated, pancreatic progenitors may offer significant advantages as a product relative to fully matured endocrine cells (Iworima et al. 2021). Cell-based therapies are incredibly complex and expensive to manufacture at large scale; any steps that shorten the duration of culture can significantly reduce labor and material costs. Aside from taking significantly less time to produce, the yield of progenitors is also much greater than that of endocrine cells, as the cells are proliferative during the initial stages of differentiation to pancreatic progenitors, whereas significant cell losses typically occur during the later stages. PEC may also have advantages when it comes to cell survival post-implant. As discussed below, a major hurdle to overcome for successful cell therapy is rapid cell loss during engraftment. There is a metabolic shift from glycolysis during the initial stages of pancreatic progenitor formation to oxidative phosphorylation as the endocrine cells form (Iworima et al. 2024) and pancreatic progenitors have lower oxygen consumption rates than matured endocrine cells (Pepper et al. 2017; Nair et al. 2019). This relative metabolic quiescence in PECs could facilitate survival in the hypoxic implant environment before adequate vascularization supplies the cells.

TRANSPLANT SITES

Interestingly, now, 50 years since the studies of Kemp and Lacy demonstrated the portal vein as a functional site for islet engraftment in rodents, this site has been hard to beat in patients. There is still no large series of patients rendered insulin-free through cell transplantation using any alternative site. When comparing the intraportal hepatic site of islet engraftment in patients with T1D with extrahepatic sites including omentum (Baidal et al. 2017; Pellicciaro et al. 2017), subgastric mucosal, and subcutaneous, an odds ratio of successful islet engraftment of over 1700 times in favor of the portal site was obtained (Verhoeff et al. 2022). In theory, the portal site has many drawbacks—the instant blood-mediated inflammatory reaction (IBMIR) associated with innate immune destruction of about half of any transplant cell load; the risk of portal venous thrombosis; exposure to high portal levels of toxic immunosuppressants; an active phagocytic immune environment; and, in the context of future stem cell–derived potentially proliferative cell transplant populations, the islets are relatively irretrievable (without major surgery). These factors have to be balanced against the marked ischemia and risk of failed engraftment in the subcutaneous and other sites. The impact of these factors can depend on the oxygen consumption rates and other attributes of the cell source. While adult human islets do not survive in humans following subcutaneous implant (Verhoeff et al. 2022) nor thrive within planar macroencapsulation devices designed for the subcutaneous implant (theracytes), human fetal pancreatic islet-like cell clusters survived, replicated, and acquired a level of glucose-responsive insulin secretion sufficient to ameliorate hyperglycemia in diabetic mice (Lee et al. 2009). Moreover, efficient survival and differentiation of human ESC-derived PECs can occur in a macroencapsulation device in mice, yielding glucose-responsive insulin-producing cells capable of reversing diabetes and retaining function for at least 1 year (Bruin et al. 2013; Rezania et al. 2013; Motté et al. 2014; Robert et al. 2018).

ENGINEERING TAILORED CELL TRANSPLANTATION SITES—ENCAPSULATION AND BEYOND

The idea that islets could be immobilized in polymers or devices that would offer protection from the immune system emerged in the 1980s (Lim and Sun 1980). Broadly, immunoprotective encapsulation devices aim to create a size exclusion barrier between the graft and components of the immune system. In the context of PSC-derived grafts, even if the material is not immunoprotective, the encapsulation device can improve graft containment and retrievability to reduce risks to the recipient.

Researchers new to the field may not be aware of the roller coaster ride of breakthroughs and hurdles that have paved the way toward current encapsulation approaches. Microencapsulation relies on islet immobilization in <2 mm diameter microbeads, leading to hundreds of thousands of beads per patient, whereas macroencapsulation opts for immobilization of hundreds of thousands of IEQ in one or a few devices per patient. In terms of publications, microencapsulation strategies have historically dominated research efforts (>6000 Pubmed hits vs. 213 for "microencapsulation"). Allogeneic (Soon-Shiong et al. 1993; Duvivier-Kali et al. 2001) or xenogeneic (Omer et al. 2003; Calafiore et al. 2004) islets encapsulated in alginate microbeads normalize blood glucose levels in animal models of T1D (Sun et al. 1996; Dufrane et al. 2010). Survival of microencapsulated islets for several months has also been reported in nonhuman primates (Cardona et al. 2006; Dufrane et al. 2006; Bochenek et al. 2018; Safley et al. 2020). Early reports of long-term microencapsulated human islet survival and in some cases improved glycemic control in T1D recipients without immunosuppression have not been broadly replicated (Soon-Shiong 1999; Calafiore et al. 2006; Elliott et al. 2007; Tuch et al. 2009). While the higher surface area/volume ratio of microencapsulation is a significant advantage over macroencapsulation, the challenge of ensuring batch-to-batch and capsule-to-capsule consistency, as well as the difficulty in the retrieval of all the capsules if adverse events occur, can pose challenges for regulatory approval. Commercial efforts have centered mainly on macroencapsulation approaches such as pouches, sheets, or even vascular grafts (Scharp and Marchetti 2014; Moeun et al. 2019). Primary islets within macroencapsulation devices such as fibers (Gentile et al. 1998), sheets (Storrs et al. 2001; Dufrane et al. 2010), or pouches (Bruce et al. 2004; Martinson et al. 2010) can reestablish glycemic control in rodents (Lacy et al. 1991; Lanza et al. 1991; Storrs et al. 2001; Dufrane et al. 2010; Lamb et al. 2011; Kumagai-Braesch et al. 2013; Agulnick et al. 2015), dogs (Storrs et al. 2001), and nonhuman primates (Dufrane et al. 2010). Some devices are permissive to vascularization but by the same token either require the need for immunosuppression or the use of genetically modified grafts that are not rejected. One such example is Viacyte's PEC-Direct device, further described below. With long-standing evidence that encapsulation devices can be both safe and effective in animal models of T1D, why has this not yet been replicated in the clinic? Encapsulation strategies—whether immunoprotective or not—create a barrier not only to immune cells or higher-risk graft cells, but also hinder complete graft integration with recipient tissues. This leads to several key limitations but also opportunities for innovation (Fig. 1).

Fibrosis

Polymeric materials used for islet immobilization or encapsulation, while creating a physical barrier between the graft and components of the immune system, will interact with physiological fluids and proteins. Rapid adsorption of proteins onto these polymers occurs both in contact with protein-containing cell culture medium (Wargenau et al. 2019) and post-implantation. The amount and conformation of proteins will vary depending on material hydrophilicity, chemistry, and topography. In turn, this will impact the type of cells recruited and their reaction to the foreign body. The macro-

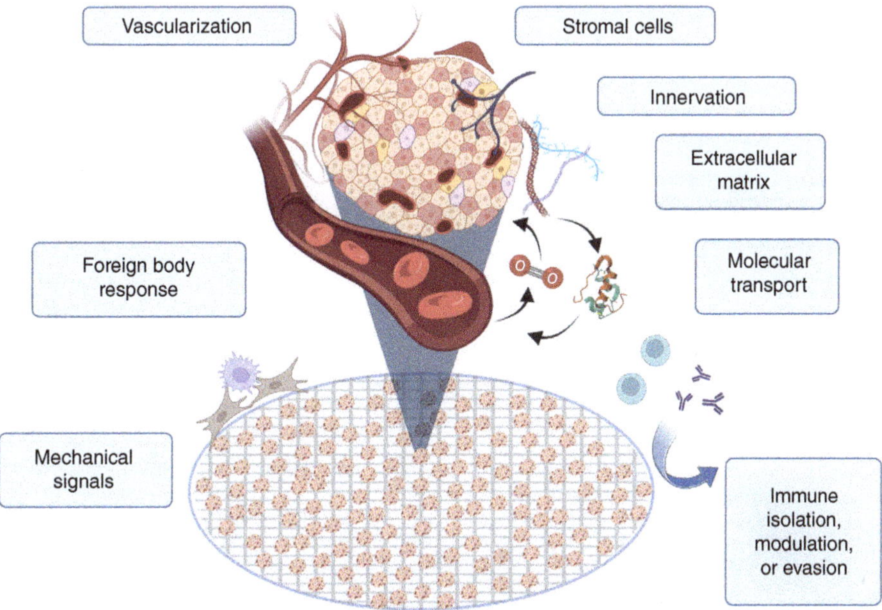

Figure 1. Engineering extrahepatic transplantation and encapsulation sites for stem cell–derived islets. Engineered sites may mimic some but not all attributes of the native islet niche, including vasculature (and paracrine signals), innervation, and surrounding extracellular matrix components and stromal cells. Some of these components can be artificially introduced, for example by grafting extracellular matrix-derived peptides onto polymeric scaffolds, or by cotransplanting vascular cell subsets. Device and/or genetic engineering strategies may allow immune isolation, modulation, or evasion. Devices can trigger foreign body responses, but these can be modulated through materials engineering or strategies such as the controlled release of anti-inflammatory agents. Mechanical stimuli from polymers or surrounding cells may also impact cell fate decisions. Ultimately, cell survival and effective molecular transport—particularly of oxygen and insulin—are key to graft efficacy. Insulin source: PDB 3I40. (Figure generated with BioRender, biorender.com.)

phages, foreign body giant cells, myofibroblasts, and other cells recruited can wall off the implant and create an oxygen sink at the device surface. The foreign body reaction observed in humans can differ from preclinical models and can vary with small changes in material surface properties or graft status. Potential ways forward to reduce fibrotic responses are changes to device shape (Veiseh et al. 2015), surface topography, and material chemistry (King et al. 2003; Vegas et al. 2016), including chemical surface modifications (Vaithilingam et al. 2014; Hu and de Vos 2019).

Molecular Transport

By hindering direct contact with vasculature, encapsulation devices also change the kinetics by which molecules such as oxygen or growth factors are transported to the graft, and by which insulin reaches the circulation. Oxygen supply is particularly problematic because of its low solubility in water as compared to other nutrients. Arterial oxygen concentration values are ~4.4 mg/L (~100 mmHg partial pressure), while the oxygen consumption rate of human islets is ~100 nmol min^{-1} mg DNA^{-1} (~37 mg O_2 min^{-1} L^{-1} assuming 6 pg DNA and 10 µm diameter β cells) (Papas et al. 2007). Therefore, if one were to suspend islets at 10% volume in a closed vessel with oxygen at 100 mmHg partial pressure, it would take ~1 min for all of the oxygen to be consumed. The surface area of sheet-based devices required to adequately oxygenate primary human islet grafts while avoiding defects in insulin secretion has been estimated to be on the order of 1 m^3 (Papas et al. 2016). Higher oxygen partial pressure at the device interface, integration of oxygen-releasing materials (Coronel et al. 2019), lower oxygen consumption rates, higher graft cell resilience to hypoxic conditions, and to some extent higher oxygen diffusion coefficient through the encapsulation material all reduce the required surface area. Bulk fluid motion—either through blood flow provided internally or within device compartments, or through other fluid circulation, will be more efficient and yield more compact designs (Song et al. 2017, 2019; Yang et al. 2021; Fernandez et al. 2022). This is not only important for oxygen but also for effective insulin transport. A device with an oxygenation compartment tested in patients by Beta O_2 Technologies showed outstanding islet survival but required daily gas refilling and resulted in little detectable circulating C-peptide levels (Carlsson et al. 2017). It will be hard to engineer a better solution than dense networks of capillaries to irrigate highly metabolically active endocrine cells such as occurs within the native pancreatic islets. Hybrid solutions, which address the time delay between islet implantation and vascularization, may offer a compromise between engineered extrahepatic sites and tissue integration.

Biomechanical Signals

Plastics, hydrogels, and other polymers used to manufacture devices may not appropriately mimic the mechanical properties of the native islet extracellular environment. Extracellular matrix components present within and at the surface of native islets may be absent. Growth factors, which interact with these extracellular matrix proteins may be presented differently to the islets. Finally, interactions with blood vessels and innervation may be absent or insufficient to replicate the native islet architecture. For immunoprotective devices that do not permit immune cell entry or graft cell egress, perfusion by capillaries as is the case for native islets (Carlsson et al. 2017) will not be possible. As noted above, cell-impermeable encapsulation devices can nevertheless control glycemic levels in diabetic animal models, and hence the requirement for direct islet vascularization and innervation to achieve long-term insulin independence, or a significant reduction in insulin requirements, may not be absolute.

Adaptive Rejection and Recurrent Autoimmunity

While most immunoprotective encapsulation devices aim to block access by immune cells such as T cells, smaller potentially harmful molecules can pass through. While the role of autoantibodies as a mediator of β-cell death remains to be elucidated (Bottazzo et al. 1974), it is not inconceivable that antibodies targeting islet surface antigens could recruit complement proteins and lead to islet cell death. Antigens can also reach antigen-presenting cells outside the graft, which may increase local inflammatory signals and the production of cytokines that are harmful to the islets. Chemically modified polymers and controlled release strategies offer the opportunity to create immune-regulatory materials that induce anti-inflammatory or tolerogenic responses (Skoumal et al. 2019; Hu et al. 2021).

Beyond fundamental considerations such as oxygenation or insulin transport, the wide array of device materials and geometries being tested leads to an additional problem—comparability between studies. To advance the field and avoid previous pitfalls, it will be important to understand not only differences in outcomes (e.g., graft survival, C-peptide levels) but why differences arose versus in previous studies. To allow more direct comparison between preclinical and clinical data, as well as between device designs and materials, it has been proposed that more uniform quality control and reporting should be applied. For example, surface characteristics such as surface charge/zeta potential, surface chemical composition, and surface roughness should be reported for different devices (Rokstad et al. 2014). When it comes to oxygen or insulin transport, engineering principles ranging from the simplest (e.g., use of dimensionless numbers to estimate diffusive vs. bulk oxygen transport) to the most complex (finite element models of oxygen and insulin transport) will facilitate comparisons. Extrapolating models beyond the range of input data sets can be problematic even with simple and well-defined systems. Even the most cunning engineering designs may not succeed in translating positive findings obtained in young mice with gossamer thin tissue planes to adult humans with heterologous immunity and vascular impairment from chronic damage from diabetes.

CLINICAL TRIALS WITH ENCAPSULATED PSC-DERIVED PANCREATIC GRAFTS

Encapsulated PECs

A major milestone in the field was the 2014 approval by the FDA for clinical testing of ViaCyte's human ESC-derived PECs for patients with T1D and glycemic lability. This was a prospective, open-label phase 1/2 trial with the primary end points of studying the safety, tolerability, and efficacy of their "VC-01" product consisting of their PECs loaded within their version of the Theracyte device ("Encaptra," combination termed "PEC-Encap"; clinicaltrials.gov identifier: NCT02239354). The team developed a scalable suspension format culture system to produce PECs through a 2-week, four-stage differentiation protocol under GMP conditions followed by cell cryopreservation (Schulz et al. 2012). As the first of its kind with human ESC-based products, regulators were comforted by the fact that the subcutaneously inserted Encaptra devices could be monitored by ultrasound to detect any unanticipated expansion, and were retrievable. However, while the product was tolerated and led to few complications, unlike preclinical studies in mice there was poor cell survival within the Encaptra devices in patients as a result of a strong foreign body response (Henry et al. 2018). To bolster cell survival, ViaCyte modified the Encaptra with portals allowing direct vascularization of the cells within, but as a result requiring chronic immunosuppression to prevent graft rejection. Nevertheless, the device is still able to contain the cell aggregates and can be readily removed in the event of concerns related to the generation of off-target cells. A clinical trial testing this device/PEC cell combination (called PEC-Direct) was launched in 2017 (clinicaltrials.gov identifier: NCT03163511). There were no severe graft-related adverse events, and there was no evidence of teratoma formation or off-target cell differentiation into nonpancreatic lineage based on ultrasound examination of graft expansion and detailed pathologist review (Ramzy et al. 2021). Surviving cells with markers of mature β cells (e.g., insulin, islet amyloid polypeptide, MAFA) were located within retrieved devices 35–57 weeks post-implant, albeit only in isolated pockets and less abundant than glucagon immunoreactive cells (Ramzy et al. 2021). The primary end point of meal-responsive C-peptide production was met in a subset of patients though the results were highly heterogeneous with C-peptide levels of <0.01 pM up to 50 pM (Ramzy et al. 2021; Shapiro et al. 2021). Generally, plasma levels of C-peptide of at least 100 pM are considered as a threshold for metabolic significance (Rickels et al. 2018) and no improvement in glycemic control or reduction in exogenous insulin requirements could be firmly attributed to the implants (Ramzy et al. 2021; Shapiro et al. 2021). Subsequent patients in this trial were given twofold to threefold higher cell doses (8–10 devices). Three of 10 patients with undetectable baseline C-peptide achieved levels ≥100 pM from month 6 onward that correlated with improved glucose control measures and reduced insulin dosing, providing the first evidence of a glucose-controlling effect of the cell implant (Keymeulen et al. 2023). The patient with the highest C-peptide (230 pM), characteristic of an intermediate functional state of β cells (Rickels et al. 2020) increased glycemic time-in-range (71–180 mg/dL) from 55% to 85% at month 12 while daily insulin doses decreased by as much as 44% between month 6 and month 12 (Keymeulen et al. 2023). The cause of the variability among patients was not resolved but clearly, the poor survival of the implanted PECs needs to be addressed. Even in the patient with the highest C-peptide levels, analysis of a retrieved device at month 6 indicated β-cell mass at 4% of the initial cell mass, indicating substantial improvements are needed to promote better cell survival and differentiation to β cells (Keymeulen et al. 2023). Nevertheless, these important clinical studies demonstrate the feasibility of achieving glucose control by stem cell–generated β cells in a retrievable device placed subcutaneously in patients with T1D.

Encapsulated PSC-Derived Islets

In 2023, the company Vertex initiated their phase 1/2 single arm, open-label study in patients with

T1D with their implantable macroencapsulation disc device containing their stem cell–derived islets (differentiated beyond the PECs used by ViaCyte) called VX-264 (clinicaltrials.gov identifier: NCT05791201). The discs are implanted in the properitoneal space. As the device does not permit direct vascularization of the cell product, it is being used without chronic immunosuppression. At the time of writing, no results have been released from this trial. VX-264 uses the same stem cell–derived pancreatic islet cells as in their VX-880 program, under evaluation for safety, tolerability, and efficacy of the cells in participants with T1D and impaired awareness of hypoglycemia and severe hypoglycemia (ClinicalTrials.gov Identifier: NCT04786262). As VX-880 mimics the Edmonton Protocol with an intraportal infusion of the stem cell–generated islets, the patients require immunosuppression. Initial communicated results from the VX-880 trial were encouraging; all six patients treated with VX-880 cells produced endogenous insulin (C-peptide) and had improved glycemic control, with two eventually entirely eliminating exogenous insulin use, yet maintaining HbA1c values of 5.3% and 6.0% (Reichman et al. 2023; Vertex 2023 Press Release). However, earlier this year, Vertex announced a pause on the trial following the death of two patients out of a total of 14 dosed thus far, both said to be unrelated to VX-880 (Vertex 2024 Press Release). Until the findings from the investigations are released, it is unclear what impact these tragic deaths will have on the future of cell therapy approaches for T1D.

UNIVERSAL GRAFTS THAT EVADE AUTOIMMUNE REJECTION

Vertex has also disclosed plans to generate gene-engineered cells designed to evade immune-mediated destruction so they can be infused without chronic immunosuppression. The concept of producing a PSC line that can become a universal source of "off-the-shelf" differentiated cells for allogenic cell therapy is highly attractive, but also presents with additional safety concerns when contemplated for delivery without means of cell retrieval or elimination. Thus, efforts are underway to develop layers of safety such as the incorporation of drug-inducible safety switches that if triggered, can eliminate the implanted cells (Lanza et al. 2019). Harding and colleagues overexpressed a combination of eight factors in human ESCs: *CCL21* to disrupt dendritic cell migration, *PD-L1*, *FASL*, *HLA-G*, and *SERPINB9* to target and/or protect against T-cell and NK-cell attack, and *CD47*, *CD200*, and *MFGE8* to target monocytes and macrophages (Harding et al. 2024). Differentiated progeny from these cells (e.g., endothelial cells and retinal pigment epithelium) did not activate allogeneic human peripheral blood mononuclear cells or their inflammatory responses. The authors also demonstrated the ability to trigger the death of any dividing cells by incorporation of a safety switch consisting of a transcriptional link between the "suicide gene" herpes simplex virus thymidine kinase (*HSV-TK*) and a cell-division gene (*CDK1*) that can be triggered by administration of clinically approved prodrug ganciclovir (Liang et al. 2018; Harding et al. 2024). As an alternative approach, Hu et al. (2024) recently demonstrated the ability to generate hypoimmune nonhuman primate islets devoid of HLA classes I and II that could engraft and take over control of blood glucose in an immunocompetent diabetic allogenic recipient A transfection-based approach with CRISPR-Cas9 was used in primary islets isolated from multiple rhesus macaque pancreas donors to disrupt HLA class I expression by knocking out the accessory chain β-2-microglobulin (*B2M*) and HLA class II expression by targeting its transcriptional master regulator, *CIITA*, while *CD47* was delivered by lentivirus to provide protection from the innate immune response. Importantly, after achieving diabetes reversal for ~200 days in the absence of immunosuppression, the authors were able to trigger the destruction of the engineered islets in vivo using a CD47-targeting strategy; cells in which CD47 is blocked are recognized as MHC classes I and II double-negative and thereby susceptible to attack by NK cells and macrophages. When given several doses of anti-CD47 IgG4 antibody, the animal became C-peptide negative and hyperglycemia resumed, supporting the ability to noninvasively remove the majority of the graft at will (Hu et al. 2024). The world's first test with a stem cell product that was gene-edited for immune evasiveness and enhanced cell fitness was initiated in 2023 by ViaCyte in partnership with CRISPR Therapeutics. That trial (NCT05565248), called VCTX211, examines the safety, tolerability, and efficacy of hESCs with two gene knockouts (*B2M*, *TXNIP*) and four insertions (*PD-L1*, *HLA-E*, *TNFAIP3*, *MANF*) differentiated to PEC, and contained within PEC-Direct devices that are implanted subcutaneously into subjects with T1D, without chronic immunosuppression (clinicaltrials.gov identifier: NCT05565248). The knockout of B2M disrupts the cell surface expression of HLA-I to eliminate T-cell-mediated rejection, supplemented by knockin of programmed death-ligand 1 (PD-L1), and the expression of HLA-E to dampen the natural killer (NK) cell response to cells that are otherwise "missing self." TNFAIP3 (A20) knockin may also facilitate graft acceptance and protection from cytokine-induced apoptosis, while thioredoxin interacting protein (TXNIP) knockout is designed to protect the cells from oxidative and ER stress, and mesencephalic astrocyte-derived neurotrophic factor (MANF) knockin may protect β cells from inflammatory stress. Whether the edits achieve immune evasiveness and promote graft survival has not yet been disclosed, but the interpretation is predicted to be challenging given the known cell survival limitations of the macroencapsulation devices used in that study.

WHERE DO PSC GRAFTS AND DEVICES FOR DIABETES THERAPY GO FROM HERE?

Several inflection points can be anticipated over the next few years as we continue to advance toward optimized PSC-derived grafts for diabetes. A major goal in the field remains determining the best approach to reduce or eliminate the need for immunosuppression—whether it be through genetic engineering, physical barriers, immunomodulatory materials engineering, or a combination thereof. An important consideration is this in practice may not have to be all or none—a strategy that markedly lowers immunosuppressive exposure could dramatically lower the potential patient risk. It is also important to determine whether direct graft vascularization will be needed. Direct vascularization better reflects the native islet environment, with signals from the vasculature driving pancreatic progenitor differentiation and supporting mature islet function (Ranjan et al. 2009). Accelerating vascularization through cotransplantation of vascular cell subsets, which may be preassembled is a promising avenue to limit early hypoxic islet losses (Kang et al. 2012; Borg et al. 2014; Vlahos et al. 2017; Takahashi et al. 2018; Song et al. 2019; Forbes et al. 2020; Aghazadeh et al. 2021). As a result of such approaches, significantly lower islet doses may be needed to achieve therapeutic effects—reducing costs and constraints on encapsulation device sizing. Prevascularization strategies could further improve engraftment, potentially even in sites with low endogenous oxygen levels such as subcutaneous transplants (Vlahos et al. 2021). A prevascularized Cell Pouch system developed by Sernova was tested clinically with human islets but the engrafted islet mass was insufficient to result in detectable graft function or impact glycemic control (Gala-Lopez et al. 2016; Colton and Weir 2017). Work to improve this strategy is ongoing (Sernova June 2023 Press Release). Pepper and colleagues obtained encouraging results in mice with a prevascularized, subcutaneous site created by temporary placement of a medically approved vascular access catheter, both with islets (Pepper et al. 2015) and PSC-derived PECs (Pepper et al. 2017). In follow-up work, the team demonstrated that a preformed subcutaneous cavity could support the implant of a geometrically matching islet-encapsulation device consisting of a twisted nylon surgical thread coated with an islet-seeded alginate hydrogel (Wang et al. 2023). This neovascularized cavity led to the sustained reversal of diabetes in immunocompetent syngeneic, allogeneic, and xenogeneic mouse models of diabetes, and implant procedures were optimized in Göttingen minipigs. A recently initiated clinical trial (ClinicalTrials.gov Identifier: NCT05073302) of the prevascularization technique will prove extremely informative in guiding the further optimization and clinical translation of this approach. One can also envision creating predetermined perfused vascular geometries through technologies such as 3D printing (Gurlin et al. 2021; Moeun et al. 2023a,b), but regulatory considerations around

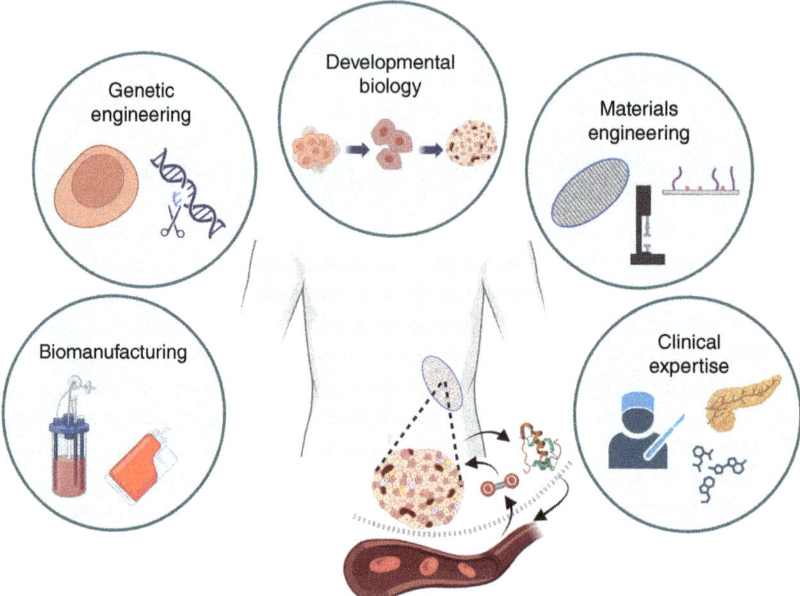

Figure 2. Convergence of technologies toward a durable cellular treatment for type 1 diabetes. Synergy between several disciplines is needed to develop engineered solutions for the safe and efficacious delivery of stem cell-derived insulin-producing cell grafts in extrahepatic sites.

aseptic tissue handling and reproducibility would have to be addressed. We predict that approaches with fewer steps and components will likely be preferred upon refinement of existing technologies. Once first-in-human technologies have shown safety and efficacy, it is likely that a competitive landscape will lead to several alternative products with a drive toward cost-efficient and clinically simpler/safer solutions.

CONCLUSION

Diabetes therapy has evolved in step with medical revolutions—from the discovery of insulin to its synthesis using recombinant DNA and islet transplantation. The convergence of several technologies—from induced PSCs to gene-editing tools, differentiation protocols, clinical experience with islet transplants, as well as advances in bioprocessing and tissue engineering—has led to the promise of the next step toward a durable treatment for T1D (Fig. 2). Successful cellular therapy without the need for immunosuppression in people with T1D would demonstrate that, indeed, artificial organs can be tailor-made. Like insulin, which opened the door toward industrialized production of recombinant proteins, bioreactor-made PSC-derived islets transplanted in engineered environments could demonstrate the feasibility of laboratory-made artificial organs and pave the way to next-generation cell-based therapies.

COMPETING INTEREST STATEMENT

T.J.K. previously served as Chief Scientific Officer (CSO) for ViaCyte (2021–2022), as a consultant for Sigilon, had a contract research agreement with Aspect Biosystems, and served as CSO for Fractyl Health during the preparation of this manuscript. C.A.H. is CSO of Cellterix Biomedical as well as Capcyte Biotherapeutics, both spinoff companies from her laboratory at McGill. A.M.J.S. served as a consultant for ViaCyte (up to 2023), Vertex Inc., Betalin Therapeutics, and Aspect Biosystems Inc.

ACKNOWLEDGMENTS

T.J.K. has received support for research on this topic from the JDRF, the Canadian Stem Cell

Network, the Canadian Institutes for Health Research (CIHR), Diabetes Canada, Genome BC, and the National Institutes of Health (NIH). C.A.H. holds the Tier 2 Canada Research Chair in Cellular Therapy Bioprocess Engineering, and has received support for this work from Diabetes Québec, JDRF, NSERC, CIHR, FRQNT, Médicament Québec and Diabetes Canada, and is supported by several research networks including the Quebec Cell, Tissue and Gene Therapy Network—ThéCell; the Research Network on Cardiometabolic Health, Diabetes, and Obesity (CMDO); PROTEO—The Quebec Network for Research on Protein Function; and the CQMF/QCAM—Quebec Center for Advanced Materials. A.M.J.S. is supported through a Tier 1 Canada Research Chair, and through grant support from the JDRF, the Canadian Stem Cell Network, the CIHR, the Diabetes Research Institute Foundation of Canada (DRIFCan), and the University Hospital Foundation.

REFERENCES

Aghazadeh Y, Poon F, Sarangi F, Wong FTM, Khan ST, Sun X, Hatkar R, Cox BJ, Nunes SS, Nostro MC. 2021. Microvessels support engraftment and functionality of human islets and hESC-derived pancreatic progenitors in diabetes models. *Cell Stem Cell* **28:** 1936–1949.e8. doi:10.1016/j.stem.2021.08.001

Aguayo-Mazzucato C, Zavacki AM, Marinelarena A, Hollister-Lock J, El Khattabi I, Marsili A, Weir GC, Sharma A, Larsen PR, Bonner-Weir S. 2013. Thyroid hormone promotes postnatal rat pancreatic β-cell development and glucose-responsive insulin secretion through MAFA. *Diabetes* **62:** 1569–1580. doi:10.2337/db12-0849

Agulnick AD, Ambruzs DM, Moorman MA, Bhoumik A, Cesario RM, Payne JK, Kelly JR, Haakmeester C, Srijemac R, Wilson AZ, et al. 2015. Insulin-producing endocrine cells differentiated in vitro from human embryonic stem cells function in macroencapsulation devices in vivo. *Stem Cells Transl Med* **4:** 1214–1222. doi:10.5966/sctm.2015-0079

Assady S, Maor G, Amit M, Itskovitz-Eldor J, Skorecki KL, Tzukerman M. 2001. Insulin production by human embryonic stem cells. *Diabetes* **50:** 1691–1697. doi:10.2337/diabetes.50.8.1691

Augsornworawat P, Hogrebe NJ, Ishahak M, Schmidt MD, Marquez E, Maestas MM, Veronese-Paniagua DA, Gale SE, Miller JR, Velazco-Cruz L, et al. 2023. Single-nucleus multi-omics of human stem cell-derived islets identifies deficiencies in lineage specification. *Nat Cell Biol* **25:** 904–916. doi:10.1038/s41556-023-01150-8

Baidal DA, Ricordi C, Berman DM, Alvarez A, Padilla N, Ciancio G, Linetsky E, Pileggi A, Alejandro R. 2017. Bioengineering of an intraabdominal endocrine pancreas. *N Engl J Med* **376:** 1887–1889. doi:10.1056/NEJMc1613959

Balboa D, Barsby T, Lithovius V, Saarimäki-Vire J, Omar-Hmeadi M, Dyachok O, Montaser H, Lund PE, Yang M, Ibrahim H, et al. 2022. Functional, metabolic and transcriptional maturation of human pancreatic islets derived from stem cells. *Nat Biotechnol* **40:** 1042–1055. doi:10.1038/s41587-022-01219-z

Ballinger WF, Lacy PE. 1972. Transplantation of intact pancreatic islets in rats. *Surgery* **72:** 175–186.

Billingham RE, Brent L, Medawar PB. 1953. Actively acquired tolerance' of foreign cells. *Nature* **172:** 603–606. doi:10.1038/172603a0

Bochenek MA, Veiseh O, Vegas AJ, McGarrigle JJ, Qi M, Marchese E, Omami M, Doloff JC, Mendoza-Elias J, Nourmohammadzadeh M, et al. 2018. Alginate encapsulation as long-term immune protection of allogeneic pancreatic islet cells transplanted into the omental bursa of macaques. *Nat Biomed Eng* **2:** 810–821. doi:10.1038/s41551-018-0275-1

Borg DJ, Weigelt M, Wilhelm C, Gerlach M, Bickle M, Speier S, Bonifacio E, Hommel A. 2014. Mesenchymal stromal cells improve transplanted islet survival and islet function in a syngeneic mouse model. *Diabetologia* **57:** 522–531. doi:10.1007/s00125-013-3109-4

Bottazzo GF, Florin-Christensen A, Doniach D. 1974. Islet-cell antibodies in diabetes mellitus with autoimmune polyendocrine deficiencies. *Lancet* **304:** 1279–1283. doi:10.1016/S0140-6736(74)90140-8

Bruce AT, Bruce L, Nilsson B, Korsgren O. 2004. Bioartificial implant and its use and method of reducing the risk for formation of connective tissue after implantation. National Center for Biotechnology Information. PubChem Patent Summary for US-2006263405-A1. https://pubchem.ncbi.nlm.nih.gov/patent/US-2006263405-A1. Accessed May 30, 2024.

Bruin JE, Rezania A, Xu J, Narayan K, Fox JK, O'Neil JJ, Kieffer TJ. 2013. Maturation and function of human embryonic stem cell-derived pancreatic progenitors in macroencapsulation devices following transplant into mice. *Diabetologia* **56:** 1987–1998. doi:10.1007/s00125-013-2955-4

Bruin JE, Asadi A, Fox JK, Erener S, Rezania A, Kieffer TJ. 2015. Accelerated maturation of human stem cell-derived pancreatic progenitor cells into insulin-secreting cells in immunodeficient rats relative to mice. *Stem Cell Reports* **5:** 1081–1096. doi:10.1016/j.stemcr.2015.10.013

Bruin JE, Saber N, O'Dwyer S, Fox JK, Mojibian M, Arora P, Rezania A, Kieffer TJ. 2016. Hypothyroidism impairs human stem cell-derived pancreatic progenitor cell maturation in mice. *Diabetes* **65:** 1297–1309. doi:10.2337/db15-1439

Calafiore R, Basta G, Luca G, Calvitti M, Calabrese G, Racanicchi L, Macchiarulo G, Mancuso F, Guido L, Brunetti P. 2004. Grafts of microencapsulated pancreatic islet cells for the therapy of diabetes mellitus in non-immunosuppressed animals. *Biotechnol Appl Biochem* **39:** 159–164. doi:10.1042/BA20030151

Calafiore R, Basta G, Luca G, Lemmi A, Montanucci MP, Calabrese G, Racanicchi L, Mancuso F, Brunetti P. 2006. Microencapsulated pancreatic islet allografts into nonimmunosuppressed patients with type 1 diabetes: first two cases. *Diabetes Care* **29:** 137–138. doi:10.2337/diacare.29.01.06.dc05-1270

Cardona K, Korbutt GS, Milas Z, Lyon J, Cano J, Jiang W, Bello-Laborn H, Hacquoil B, Strobert E, Gangappa S, et al. 2006. Long-term survival of neonatal porcine islets in non-human primates by targeting costimulation pathways. *Nat Med* **12:** 304–306. doi:10.1038/nm1375

Carlsson PO, Espes D, Sedigh A, Rotem A, Zimmermann B, Grinberg H, Goldman T, Barkai U, Avni Y, Westermark GT, et al. 2018. Transplantation of macroencapsulated human islets within the bioartificial pancreas βAir to patients with type 1 diabetes mellitus. *Am J Transplant* **18:** 1735–1744. doi:10.1111/ajt.14642

Castaing M, Peault B, Basmaciogullari A, Casal I, Czernichow P, Scharfmann R. 2001. Blood glucose normalization upon transplantation of human embryonic pancreas into β-cell-deficient SCID mice. *Diabetologia* **44:** 2066–2076. doi:10.1007/s001250100012

ClinicalTrials.gov. 2021. A safety, tolerability, and efficacy study of VX-880 in participants with type 1 diabetes. Sponsor: Vertex Pharmaceuticals Incorporated. Identifier: NCT04786262. https://clinicaltrials.gov/study/NCT04786262

ClinicalTrials.gov. 2023. Device-less technique in islet transplantation. Sponsor: University of Alberta. Identifier: NCT05073302. https://classic.clinicaltrials.gov/ct2/show/NCT05073302

Colton CK, Weir GC. 2017. Commentary—a hard lesson about transplanting islets into prevascularized devices. *CellR4* **5:** e2251.

Coronel MM, Liang JP, Li Y, Stabler CL. 2019. Oxygen generating biomaterial improves the function and efficacy of β cells within a macroencapsulation device. *Biomaterials* **210:** 1–11. doi:10.1016/j.biomaterials.2019.04.017

D'Amour KA, Bang AG, Eliazer S, Kelly OG, Agulnick AD, Smart NG, Moorman MA, Kroon E, Carpenter MK, Baetge EE. 2006. Production of pancreatic hormone-expressing endocrine cells from human embryonic stem cells. *Nat Biotechnol* **24:** 1392–1401. doi:10.1038/nbt1259

Dufrane D, Goebbels RM, Saliez A, Guiot Y, Gianello P. 2006. Six-month survival of microencapsulated pig islets and alginate biocompatibility in primates: proof of concept. *Transplantation* **81:** 1345–1353. doi:10.1097/01.tp.0000208610.75997.20

Dufrane D, Goebbels RM, Gianello P. 2010. Alginate macroencapsulation of pig islets allows correction of streptozotocin-induced diabetes in primates up to 6 months without immunosuppression. *Transplantation* **90:** 1054–1062. doi:10.1097/TP.0b013e3181f6e267

Duvivier-Kali VF, Omer A, Parent RJ, O'Neil JJ, Weir GC. 2001. Complete protection of islets against allorejection and autoimmunity by a simple barium-alginate membrane. *Diabetes* **50:** 1698–1705. doi:10.2337/diabetes.50.8.1698

Elliott RB, Escobar L, Tan PL, Muzina M, Zwain S, Buchanan C. 2007. Live encapsulated porcine islets from a type 1 diabetic patient 9.5 yr after xenotransplantation. *Xenotransplantation* **14:** 157–161. doi:10.1111/j.1399-3089.2007.00384.x

Fernandez SA, Champion KS, Danielczak L, Gasparrini M, Paraskevas S, Leask RL, Hoesli CA. 2022. Engineering vascularized islet macroencapsulation devices: an in vitro platform to study oxygen transport in perfused immobilized pancreatic β cell cultures. *Front Bioeng Biotechnol* **10:** 884071. doi:10.3389/fbioe.2022.884071

Forbes S, Bond AR, Thirlwell KL, Burgoyne P, Samuel K, Noble J, Borthwick G, Colligan D, McGowan NWA, Lewis PS, et al. 2020. Human umbilical cord perivascular cells improve human pancreatic islet transplant function by increasing vascularization. *Sci Transl Med* **12:** eaan5907. doi:10.1126/scitranslmed.aan5907

Gala-Lopez B, Pepper AR, Dinyari P, Malcolm AJ, Kin T, Pawlick R, Senior PA, Shapiro AMJ. 2016. Subcutaneous clinical islet transplantation in a prevascularized subcutaneous pouch—preliminary experience. *CellR4* **4:** e2132.

Gentile FTW, Winn SR, Lysaght M, Baurmeister U, Wechs F, Rottger H. 1998. Bioartificial organ containing cells encapsulated in a permselective polyether suflfone membrane. CytoTherapeutics, Inc., Lincoln, RI. https://patents.google.com/patent/US5837234A/en

Gurlin RE, Giraldo JA, Latres E. 2021. 3D bioprinting and translation of β cell replacement therapies for type 1 diabetes. *Tissue Eng Part B Rev* **27:** 238–252. doi:10.1089/ten.TEB.2020.0192

Haque M, Song J, Fino K, Sandhu P, Song X, Lei F, Zheng S, Ni B, Fang D, Song J. 2016. Stem cell-derived tissue-associated regulatory T cells ameliorate the development of autoimmunity. *Sci Rep* **6:** 20588. doi:10.1038/srep20588

Harding J, Vintersten-Nagy K, Yang H, Tang JK, Shutova M, Jong ED, Lee JH, Massumi M, Oussenko T, Izadifar Z, et al. 2024. Immune-privileged tissues formed from immunologically cloaked mouse embryonic stem cells survive long term in allogeneic hosts. *Nat Biomed Eng* **8:** 427–442. doi:10.1038/s41551-023-01133-y

Hayek A, Beattie GM. 1997. Processing, storage and experimental transplantation of human fetal pancreatic cells. *Ann Transplant* **2:** 46–54.

Henry RR, Pettus J, Wilensky J, Shapiro J, Senior PA, Roep B, Wang R, Kroon EJ, Scott M, D'Amour KA, et al. 2018. Initial clinical evaluation of VC-01TM combination product—a stem cell-derived islet replacement for type 1 diabetes (T1D). *Diabetes* **67:** 138-OR. doi:10.2337/db18-138-OR

Hering BJ, Kandaswamy R, Harmon JV, Ansite JD, Clemmings SM, Sakai T, Paraskevas S, Eckman PM, Sageshima J, Nakano M, et al. 2004. Transplantation of cultured islets from two-layer preserved pancreases in type 1 diabetes with anti-CD3 antibody. *Am J Transplant* **4:** 390–401. doi:10.1046/j.1600-6143.2003.00351.x

Hering BJ, Kandaswamy R, Ansite JD, Eckman PM, Nakano M, Sawada T, Matsumoto I, Ihm SH, Zhang HJ, Parkey J, et al. 2005. Single-donor, marginal-dose islet transplantation in patients with type 1 diabetes. *J Am Med Assoc* **293:** 830–835. doi:10.1001/jama.293.7.830

Hering BJ, Clarke WR, Bridges ND, Eggerman TL, Alejandro R, Bellin MD, Chaloner K, Czarniecki CW, Goldstein JS, Hunsicker LG, et al. 2016. Phase 3 trial of transplantation of human islets in type 1 diabetes complicated by severe hypoglycemia. *Diabetes Care* **39:** 1230–1240. doi:10.2337/dc15-1988

Hering BJ, Ballou CM, Bellin MD, Payne EH, Kandeel F, Witkowski P, Alejandro R, Rickels MR, Barton FB. 2023. Factors associated with favourable 5 year outcomes in islet transplant alone recipients with type 1 diabetes complicated by severe hypoglycaemia in the Collaborative Islet

Transplant Registry. *Diabetologia* **66:** 163–173. doi:10.1007/s00125-022-05804-4

Herold KC, Bundy BN, Long SA, Bluestone JA, DiMeglio LA, Dufort MJ, Gitelman SE, Gottlieb PA, Krischer JP, Linsley PS, et al. 2019. An anti-CD3 antibody, teplizumab, in relatives at risk for type 1 diabetes. *N Engl J Med* **381:** 603–613. doi:10.1056/NEJMoa1902226

Ho P, Cahir-McFarland E, Fontenot JD, Lodie T, Nada A, Tang Q, Turka LA, Bluestone JA. 2024. Harnessing regulatory T cells to establish immune tolerance. *Sci Transl Med* **16:** eadm8859. doi:10.1126/scitranslmed.adm8859

Hogrebe NJ, Augsornworawat P, Maxwell KG, Velazco-Cruz L, Millman JR. 2020. Targeting the cytoskeleton to direct pancreatic differentiation of human pluripotent stem cells. *Nat Biotechnol* **38:** 460–470. doi:10.1038/s41587-020-0430-6

Hu S, de Vos P. 2019. Polymeric approaches to reduce tissue responses against devices applied for islet-cell encapsulation. *Front Bioeng Biotechnol* **7:** 134. doi:10.3389/fbioe.2019.00134

Hu S, Martinez-Garcia FD, Moeun BN, Burgess JK, Harmsen MC, Hoesli CA, de Vos P. 2021. An immune regulatory 3D-printed alginate-pectin construct for immunoisolation of insulin producing β-cells. *Mater Sci Eng C Mater Biol Appl* **123:** 112009. doi:10.1016/j.msec.2021.112009

Hu X, White K, Young C, Olroyd AG, Kievit P, Connolly AJ, Deuse T, Schrepfer S. 2024. Hypoimmune islets achieve insulin independence after allogeneic transplantation in a fully immunocompetent non-human primate. *Cell Stem Cell* **31:** 334–340.e5. doi:10.1016/j.stem.2024.02.001

Iworima DG, Rieck S, Kieffer TJ. 2021. Process parameter development for the scaled generation of stem cell-derived pancreatic endocrine cells. *Stem Cells Transl Med* **10:** 1459–1469. doi:10.1002/sctm.21-0161

Iworima DG, Baker RK, Ellis C, Sherwood C, Zhan L, Rezania A, Piret JM, Kieffer TJ. 2024. Metabolic switching, growth kinetics and cell yields in the scalable manufacture of stem cell-derived insulin-producing cells. *Stem Cell Res Ther* **15:** 1. doi:10.1186/s13287-023-03574-3

Kang S, Park HS, Jo A, Hong SH, Lee HN, Lee YY, Park JS, Jung HS, Chung SS, Park KS. 2012. Endothelial progenitor cell cotransplantation enhances islet engraftment by rapid revascularization. *Diabetes* **61:** 866–876. doi:10.2337/db10-1492

Kemp CB, Knight MJ, Scharp DW, Ballinger WF, Lacy PE. 1973. Effect of transplantation site on the results of pancreatic islet isografts in diabetic rats. *Diabetologia* **9:** 486–491. doi:10.1007/BF00461694

Keymeulen B, De Groot K, Jacobs-Tulleneers-Thevissen D, Thompson DM, Bellin MD, Kroon EJ, Daniels M, Wang R, Jaiman M, Kieffer TJ, et al. 2023. Encapsulated stem cell-derived β cells exert glucose control in patients with type 1 diabetes. *Nat Biotechnol* doi:10.1038/s41587-023-02055-5

King A, Strand B, Rokstad AM, Kulseng B, Andersson A, Skjåk-Bræk G, Sandler S. 2003. Improvement of the biocompatibility of alginate/poly-L-lysine/alginate microcapsules by the use of epimerized alginate as a coating. *J Biomed Mater Res A* **64A:** 533–539. doi:10.1002/jbm.a.10276

Kroon E, Martinson LA, Kadoya K, Bang AG, Kelly OG, Eliazer S, Young H, Richardson M, Smart NG, Cunningham J, et al. 2008. Pancreatic endoderm derived from human embryonic stem cells generates glucose-responsive insulin-secreting cells in vivo. *Nat Biotechnol* **26:** 443–452. doi:10.1038/nbt1393

Kumagai-Braesch M, Jacobson S, Mori H, Jia X, Takahashi T, Wernerson A, Flodström-Tullberg M, Tibell A. 2013. The TheraCyte™ device protects against islet allograft rejection in immunized hosts. *Cell Transplant* **22:** 1137–1146. doi:10.3727/096368912X657486

Lablanche S, Vantyghem MC, Kessler L, Wojtusciszyn A, Borot S, Thivolet C, Girerd S, Bosco D, Bosson JL, Colin C, et al. 2018. Islet transplantation versus insulin therapy in patients with type 1 diabetes with severe hypoglycaemia or poorly controlled glycaemia after kidney transplantation (TRIMECO): a multicentre, randomised controlled trial. *Lancet Diabetes Endocrinol* **6:** 527–537. doi:10.1016/S2213-8587(18)30078-0

Lacy PE, Hegre OD, Gerasimidi-Vazeou A, Gentile FT, Dionne KE. 1991. Maintenance of normoglycemia in diabetic mice by subcutaneous xenografts of encapsulated islets. *Science* **254:** 1782–1784. doi:10.1126/science.1763328

Lamb M, Storrs R, Li S, Liang O, Laugenour K, Dorian R, Chapman D, Ichii H, Imagawa D, Foster C, et al. 2011. Function and viability of human islets encapsulated in alginate sheets: in vitro and in vivo culture. *Transplant Proc* **43:** 3265–3266. doi:10.1016/j.transproceed.2011.10.028

Lanza RP, Butler DH, Borland KM, Staruk JE, Faustman DL, Solomon BA, Muller TE, Rupp RG, Maki T, Monaco AP, et al. 1991. Xenotransplantation of canine, bovine, and porcine islets in diabetic rats without immunosuppression. *Proc Natl Acad Sci* **88:** 11100–11104. doi:10.1073/pnas.88.24.11100

Lanza R, Russell DW, Nagy A. 2019. Engineering universal cells that evade immune detection. *Nat Rev Immunol* **19:** 723–733. doi:10.1038/s41577-019-0200-1

Latres E, Finan DA, Greenstein JL, Kowalski A, Kieffer TJ. 2019. Navigating two roads to glucose normalization in diabetes: automated insulin delivery devices and cell therapy. *Cell Metab* **29:** 545–563. doi:10.1016/j.cmet.2019.02.007

Lee SH, Hao E, Savinov AY, Geron I, Strongin AY, Itkin-Ansari P. 2009. Human β-cell precursors mature into functional insulin-producing cells in an immunoisolation device: implications for diabetes cell therapies. *Transplantation* **87:** 983–991. doi:10.1097/TP.0b013e31819c86ea

Lemos JRN, Baidal DA, Ricordi C, Fuenmayor V, Alvarez A, Alejandro R. 2021. Survival after islet transplantation in subjects with type 1 diabetes: twenty-year follow-up. *Diabetes Care* **44:** e67–e68. doi:10.2337/dc20-2458

Liang Q, Monetti C, Shutova MV, Neely EJ, Hacibekiroglu S, Yang H, Kim C, Zhang P, Li C, Nagy K, et al. 2018. Linking a cell-division gene and a suicide gene to define and improve cell therapy safety. *Nature* **563:** 701–704. doi:10.1038/s41586-018-0733-7

Lim F, Sun AM. 1980. Microencapsulated islets as bioartificial endocrine pancreas. *Science* **210:** 908–910. doi:10.1126/science.6776628

MacDonald KN, Salim K, Levings MK. 2022. Manufacturing next-generation regulatory T-cell therapies. *Curr Opin Biotechnol* **78:** 102822. doi:10.1016/j.copbio.2022.102822

Marfil-Garza BA, Imes S, Verhoeff K, Hefler J, Lam A, Dajani K, Anderson B, O'Gorman D, Kin T, Bigam D, et al. 2022.

Pancreatic islet transplantation in type 1 diabetes: 20-year experience from a single-centre cohort in Canada. *Lancet Diabetes Endocrinol* **10:** 519–532. doi:10.1016/S2213-8587(22)00114-0

Markmann JF, Rickels MR, Eggerman TL, Bridges ND, Lafontant DE, Qidwai J, Foster E, Clarke WR, Kamoun M, Alejandro R, et al. 2021. Phase 3 trial of human islet-after-kidney transplantation in type 1 diabetes. *Am J Transplant* **21:** 1477–1492. doi:10.1111/ajt.16174

Martinson L, Green C, Kroon E, Agulnick A, Kelly O, D'amour K, Baetge EE. 2010. Encapsulation of pancreatic cells derived from human pluripotent stem cells. U.S. patent US10272179B2. https://patents.google.com/patent/US10272179B2/en

McCall M, Pawlick R, Kin T, Shapiro AM. 2012. Anakinra potentiates the protective effects of etanercept in transplantation of marginal mass human islets in immunodeficient mice. *Am J Transplant* **12:** 322–329. doi:10.1111/j.1600-6143.2011.03796.x

Moeun BN, Ling SD, Gasparinni M, Rutman A, Negi S, Paraskevas S, Hoesli CA. 2019. Islet encapsulation: a long-term treatment for type 1 diabetes. In *Encyclopedia of tissue engineering and regenerative medicine* (ed. Reis RL), pp. 217–231. Academic, London.

Moeun BN, Fernandez SA, Collin S, Lescot T, Fortin MA, Ruel J, Bégin-Drolet A, Leask R, Hoesli CA. 2023a. Improving the 3D printability of sugar glass to engineer sacrificial vascular templates. *3D Print Addit Manuf* **10:** 869–886. doi:10.1089/3dp.2021.0147

Moeun BN, Rahimnejad M, Brassard JA, Paraskevas S, Leask R, Lerouge S, Hoesli CA. 2023b. Vascularizing a human-scale bioartificial pancreas using sacrificial embedded 3D printing into self-healing alginate. *Transplantation* **107:** 60. doi:10.1097/01.tp.0000994068.03911.8e

Motté E, Szepessy E, Suenens K, Stangé G, Bomans M, Jacobs-Tulleneers-Thevissen D, Ling Z, Kroon E, Pipeleers D. 2014. Composition and function of macroencapsulated human embryonic stem cell-derived implants: comparison with clinical human islet cell grafts. *Am J Physiol Endocrinol Metab* **307:** E838–E846. doi:10.1152/ajpendo.00219.2014

Nair GG, Liu JS, Russ HA, Tran S, Saxton MS, Chen R, Juang C, Li ML, Nguyen VQ, Giacometti S, et al. 2019. Recapitulating endocrine cell clustering in culture promotes maturation of human stem-cell-derived β cells. *Nat Cell Biol* **21:** 263–274. doi:10.1038/s41556-018-0271-4

Omer A, Duvivier-Kali VF, Trivedi N, Wilmot K, Bonner-Weir S, Weir GC. 2003. Survival and maturation of microencapsulated porcine neonatal pancreatic cell clusters transplanted into immunocompetent diabetic mice. *Diabetes* **52:** 69–75. doi:10.2337/diabetes.52.1.69

Papas KK, Colton CK, Nelson RA, Rozak PR, Avgoustiniatos ES, Scott WE III, Wildey GM, Pisania A, Weir GC, Hering BJ. 2007. Human islet oxygen consumption rate and DNA measurements predict diabetes reversal in nude mice. *Am J Transplant* **7:** 707–713. doi:10.1111/j.1600-6143.2006.01655.x

Papas KK, Avgoustiniatos ES, Suszynski TM. 2016. Effect of oxygen supply on the size of implantable islet-containing encapsulation devices. *Panminerva Med* **58:** 72–77.

Pellicciaro M, Vella I, Lanzoni G, Tisone G, Ricordi C. 2017. The greater omentum as a site for pancreatic islet transplantation. *CellR4 Repair Replace Regen Reprogram* **5:** e2410.

Pepper AR, Gala-Lopez B, Pawlick R, Merani S, Kin T, Shapiro AM. 2015. A prevascularized subcutaneous device-less site for islet and cellular transplantation. *Nat Biotechnol* **33:** 518–523. doi:10.1038/nbt.3211

Pepper AR, Pawlick R, Bruni A, Wink J, Rafiei Y, O'Gorman D, Yan-Do R, Gala-Lopez B, Kin T, MacDonald PE, et al. 2017. Transplantation of human pancreatic endoderm cells reverses diabetes post transplantation in a prevascularized subcutaneous site. *Stem Cell Reports* **8:** 1689–1700. doi:10.1016/j.stemcr.2017.05.004

Ramzy A, Thompson DM, Ward-Hartstonge KA, Ivison S, Cook L, Garcia RV, Loyal J, Kim PTW, Warnock GL, Levings MK, et al. 2021. Implanted pluripotent stem-cell-derived pancreatic endoderm cells secrete glucose-responsive C-peptide in patients with type 1 diabetes. *Cell Stem Cell* **28:** 2047–2061.e5. doi:10.1016/j.stem.2021.10.003

Ramzy A, Saber N, Bruin JE, Thompson DM, Kim PTW, Warnock GL, Kieffer TJ. 2024. Thyroid hormone levels correlate with the maturation of implanted pancreatic endoderm cells in patients with type 1 diabetes. *J Clin Endocrinol Metab* **109:** 413–423. doi:10.1210/clinem/dgad499

Ranjan AK, Joglekar MV, Hardikar AA. 2009. Endothelial cells in pancreatic islet development and function. *Islets* **1:** 2–9. doi:10.4161/isl.1.1.9054

Reckard CR, Ziegler MM, Barker CF. 1973. Physiological and immunological consequences of transplanting isolated pancreatic islets. *Surgery* **74:** 91–99.

Reichman TW, Ricordi C, Naji A, Markmann JF, Perkins BA, Wijkstrom M, Paraskevas S, Bruinsma B, Marigowda G, Shih JL, et al. 2023. Glucose-dependent insulin production and insulin-independence in type 1 diabetes from stem cell-derived, fully differentiated islet cells—updated data from the VX-880 clinical trial. *Diabetes* **72**. doi:10.2337/db23-836-P

Rezania A, Riedel MJ, Wideman RD, Karanu F, Ao Z, Warnock GL, Kieffer TJ. 2011. Production of functional glucagon-secreting α-cells from human embryonic stem cells. *Diabetes* **60:** 239–247. doi:10.2337/db10-0573

Rezania A, Bruin JE, Riedel MJ, Mojibian M, Asadi A, Xu J, Gauvin R, Narayan K, Karanu F, O'Neil JJ, et al. 2012. Maturation of human embryonic stem cell-derived pancreatic progenitors into functional islets capable of treating pre-existing diabetes in mice. *Diabetes* **61:** 2016–2029. doi:10.2337/db11-1711

Rezania A, Bruin JE, Xu J, Narayan K, Fox JK, O'Neil JJ, Kieffer TJ. 2013. Enrichment of human embryonic stem cell-derived NKX6.1-expressing pancreatic progenitor cells accelerates the maturation of insulin-secreting cells in vivo. *Stem Cells* **31:** 2432–2442. doi:10.1002/stem.1489

Rezania A, Bruin JE, Arora P, Rubin A, Batushansky I, Asadi A, O'Dwyer S, Quiskamp N, Mojibian M, Albrecht T, et al. 2014. Reversal of diabetes with insulin-producing cells derived in vitro from human pluripotent stem cells. *Nat Biotechnol* **32:** 1121–1133. doi:10.1038/nbt.3033

Rickels MR, Stock PG, de Koning EJP, Piemonti L, Pratschke J, Alejandro R, Bellin MD, Berney T, Choudhary P, Johnson PR, et al. 2018. Defining outcomes for β-cell replacement therapy in the treatment of diabetes: a consensus report on the Igls criteria from the IPITA/EPITA opinion leaders workshop. *Transpl Int* **31:** 343–352. doi:10.1111/tri.13138

Rickels MR, Evans-Molina C, Bahnson HT, Ylescupidez A, Nadeau KJ, Hao W, Clements MA, Sherr JL, Pratley RE, Hannon TS, et al. 2020. High residual C-peptide likely contributes to glycemic control in type 1 diabetes. *J Clin Invest* **130:** 1850–1862. doi:10.1172/JCI134057

Ricordi C, Lacy PE, Scharp DW. 1989. Automated islet isolation from human pancreas. *Diabetes* **38** (Suppl 1)**:** 140–142. doi:10.2337/diab.38.1.S140

Robert T, De Mesmaeker I, Stangé GM, Suenens KG, Ling Z, Kroon EJ, Pipeleers DG. 2018. Functional β cell mass from device-encapsulated hESC-derived pancreatic endoderm achieving metabolic control. *Stem Cell Reports* **10:** 739–750. doi:10.1016/j.stemcr.2018.01.040

Rokstad AM, Lacík I, de Vos P, Strand BL. 2014. Advances in biocompatibility and physico-chemical characterization of microspheres for cell encapsulation. *Adv Drug Deliv Rev* **67–68:** 111–130. doi:10.1016/j.addr.2013.07.010

Russ HA, Parent AV, Ringler JJ, Hennings TG, Nair GG, Shveygert M, Guo T, Puri S, Haataja L, Cirulli V, et al. 2015. Controlled induction of human pancreatic progenitors produces functional β-like cells in vitro. *EMBO J* **34:** 1759–1772. doi:10.15252/embj.201591058

Ryan EA, Paty BW, Senior PA, Bigam D, Alfadhli E, Kneteman NM, Lakey JR, Shapiro AM. 2005. Five-year follow-up after clinical islet transplantation. *Diabetes* **54:** 2060–2069. doi:10.2337/diabetes.54.7.2060

Saber N, Kieffer TJ. 2024. *Pluripotent stem cell therapy for diabetes*, pp. 67–83. Springer, New York.

Saber N, Bruin JE, O'Dwyer S, Schuster H, Rezania A, Kieffer TJ. 2018. Sex differences in maturation of human embryonic stem cell–derived β cells in mice. *Endocrinology* **159:** 1827–1841. doi:10.1210/en.2018-00048

Saber N, Ellis CE, Iworima DG, Baker RK, Rezania A, Kieffer TJ. 2023. The impact of different implantation sites and sex on the differentiation of human pancreatic endoderm cells into insulin-secreting cells in vivo. *Diabetes* **72:** 590–598. doi:10.2337/db22-0692

Safley SA, Kenyon NS, Berman DM, Barber GF, Cui H, Duncanson S, De Toni T, Willman M, De Vos P, Tomei AA, et al. 2020. Microencapsulated islet allografts in diabetic NOD mice and nonhuman primates. *Eur Rev Med Pharmacol Sci* **24:** 8551–8565.

Scharp DW, Marchetti P. 2014. Encapsulated islets for diabetes therapy: history, current progress, and critical issues requiring solution. *Adv Drug Deliv Rev* **67–68:** 35–73. doi:10.1016/j.addr.2013.07.018

Scharp DW, Lacy PE, Santiago JV, McCullough CS, Weide LG, Falqui L, Marchetti P, Gingerich RL, Jaffe AS, Cryer PE, et al. 1990. Insulin independence after islet transplantation into type I diabetic patient. *Diabetes* **39:** 515–518. doi:10.2337/diab.39.4.515

Schmidt MD, Ishahak M, Augsornworawat P, Millman JR. 2024. Comparative and integrative single cell analysis reveals new insights into the transcriptional immaturity of stem cell-derived β cells. *BMC Genomics* **25:** 105. doi:10.1186/s12864-024-10013-x

Schulz TC, Young HY, Agulnick AD, Babin MJ, Baetge EE, Bang AG, Bhoumik A, Cepa I, Cesario RM, Haakmeester C, et al. 2012. A scalable system for production of functional pancreatic progenitors from human embryonic stem cells. *PLoS ONE* **7:** e37004. doi:10.1371/journal.pone.0037004

Sernova June 2023 Press Release. Sernova announces positive updated interim phase 1/2 clinical data for the Cell Pouch System™ at American Diabetes Association 83rd Scientific Sessions. https://www.sernova.com/press/release/?id=374

Shapiro AM, Lakey JR, Ryan EA, Korbutt GS, Toth E, Warnock GL, Kneteman NM, Rajotte RV. 2000. Islet transplantation in seven patients with type 1 diabetes mellitus using a glucocorticoid-free immunosuppressive regimen. *N Engl J Med* **343:** 230–238. doi:10.1056/NEJM200007273430401

Shapiro AM, Ricordi C, Hering BJ, Auchincloss H, Lindblad R, Robertson RP, Secchi A, Brendel MD, Berney T, Brennan DC, et al. 2006. International trial of the Edmonton protocol for islet transplantation. *N Engl J Med* **355:** 1318–1330. doi:10.1056/NEJMoa061267

Shapiro AMJ, Thompson D, Donner TW, Bellin MD, Hsueh W, Pettus J, Wilensky J, Daniels M, Wang RM, Brandon EP, et al. 2021. Insulin expression and C-peptide in type 1 diabetes subjects implanted with stem cell-derived pancreatic endoderm cells in an encapsulation device. *Cell Rep Med* **2:** 100466. doi:10.1016/j.xcrm.2021.100466

Shim JH, Kim SE, Woo DH, Kim SK, Oh CH, McKay R, Kim JH. 2007. Directed differentiation of human embryonic stem cells towards a pancreatic cell fate. *Diabetologia* **50:** 1228–1238. doi:10.1007/s00125-007-0634-z

Sibley RK, Sutherland DE, Goetz F, Michael AF. 1985. Recurrent diabetes mellitus in the pancreas iso- and allograft. A light and electron microscopic and immunohistochemical analysis of four cases. *Lab Invest* **53:** 132–144.

Singh A, Ramachandran S, Graham ML, Daneshmandi S, Heller D, Suarez-Pinzon WL, Balamurugan AN, Ansite JD, Wilhelm JJ, Yang A, et al. 2019. Long-term tolerance of islet allografts in nonhuman primates induced by apoptotic donor leukocytes. *Nat Commun* **10:** 3495. doi:10.1038/s41467-019-11338-y

Skoumal M, Woodward KB, Zhao H, Wang F, Yolcu ES, Pearson RM, Hughes KR, García AJ, Shea LD, Shirwan H. 2019. Localized immune tolerance from FasL-functionalized PLG scaffolds. *Biomaterials* **192:** 271–281. doi:10.1016/j.biomaterials.2018.11.015

Song S, Blaha C, Moses W, Park J, Wright N, Groszek J, Fissell W, Vartanian S, Posselt AM, Roy S. 2017. An intravascular bioartificial pancreas device (iBAP) with silicon nanopore membranes (SNM) for islet encapsulation under convective mass transport. *Lab Chip* **17:** 1778–1792. doi:10.1039/C7LC00096K

Song W, Chiu A, Wang LH, Schwartz RE, Li B, Bouklas N, Bowers DT, An D, Cheong SH, Flanders JA, et al. 2019. Engineering transferrable microvascular meshes for subcutaneous islet transplantation. *Nat Commun* **10:** 4602. doi:10.1038/s41467-019-12373-5

Soon-Shiong P. 1999. Treatment of type I diabetes using encapsulated islets. *Adv Drug Deliv Rev* **35:** 259–270. doi:10.1016/S0169-409X(98)00076-3

Soon-Shiong P, Feldman E, Nelson R, Heintz R, Yao Q, Yao Z, Zheng T, Merideth N, Skjak-Braek G, Espevik T, et al. 1993. Long-term reversal of diabetes by the injection of immunoprotected islets. *Proc Natl Acad Sci* **90:** 5843–5847. doi:10.1073/pnas.90.12.5843

Storrs R, Dorian R, King SR, Lakey J, Rilo H. 2001. Preclinical development of the Islet sheet. *Ann NY Acad Sci* **944:** 252–266. doi:10.1111/j.1749-6632.2001.tb03837.x

Sun Y, Ma X, Zhou D, Vacek I, Sun AM. 1996. Normalization of diabetes in spontaneously diabetic cynomologus monkeys by xenografts of microencapsulated porcine islets without immunosuppression. *J Clin Invest* **98:** 1417–1422. doi:10.1172/JCI118929

Takahashi K, Yamanaka S. 2006. Induction of pluripotent stem cells from mouse embryonic and adult fibroblast cultures by defined factors. *Cell* **126:** 663–676. doi:10.1016/j.cell.2006.07.024

Takahashi K, Tanabe K, Ohnuki M, Narita M, Ichisaka T, Tomoda K, Yamanaka S. 2007. Induction of pluripotent stem cells from adult human fibroblasts by defined factors. *Cell* **131:** 861–872. doi:10.1016/j.cell.2007.11.019

Takahashi Y, Sekine K, Kin T, Takebe T, Taniguchi H. 2018. Self-condensation culture enables vascularization of tissue fragments for efficient therapeutic transplantation. *Cell Rep* **23:** 1620–1629. doi:10.1016/j.celrep.2018.03.123

Takeuchi H, Nakatsuji N, Suemori H. 2014. Endodermal differentiation of human pluripotent stem cells to insulin-producing cells in 3D culture. *Sci Rep* **4:** 4488. doi:10.1038/srep04488

Tang Q, Bluestone JA. 2006. Regulatory T-cell physiology and application to treat autoimmunity. *Immunol Rev* **212:** 217–237. doi:10.1111/j.0105-2896.2006.00421.x

Thomson JA, Itskovitz-Eldor J, Shapiro SS, Waknitz MA, Swiergiel JJ, Marshall VS, Jones JM. 1998. Embryonic stem cell lines derived from human blastocysts. *Science* **282:** 1145–1147. doi:10.1126/science.282.5391.1145

Tran R, Moraes C, Hoesli CA. 2020a. Controlled clustering enhances PDX1 and NKX6.1 expression in pancreatic endoderm cells derived from pluripotent stem cells. *Sci Rep* **10:** 1190. doi:10.1038/s41598-020-57787-0

Tran R, Moraes C, Hoesli CA. 2020b. Developmentally-inspired biomimetic culture models to produce functional islet-like cells from pluripotent precursors. *Front Bioeng Biotechnol* **8:** 583970. doi:10.3389/fbioe.2020.583970

Tuch BE, Keogh GW, Williams LJ, Wu W, Foster JL, Vaithilingam V, Philips R. 2009. Safety and viability of microencapsulated human islets transplanted into diabetic humans. *Diabetes Care* **32:** 1887–1889. doi:10.2337/dc09-0744

Vaithilingam V, Kollarikova G, Qi M, Larsson R, Lacik I, Formo K, Marchese E, Oberholzer J, Guillemin GJ, Tuch BE. 2014. Beneficial effects of coating alginate microcapsules with macromolecular heparin conjugates-in vitro and in vivo study. *Tissue Eng Part A* **20:** 324–334. doi:10.1089/ten.tea.2013.0254

Vegas AJ, Veiseh O, Doloff JC, Ma M, Tam HH, Bratlie K, Li J, Bader AR, Langan E, Olejnik K, et al. 2016. Combinatorial hydrogel library enables identification of materials that mitigate the foreign body response in primates. *Nat Biotechnol* **34:** 345–352. doi:10.1038/nbt.3462

Veiseh O, Doloff JC, Ma M, Vegas AJ, Tam HH, Bader AR, Li J, Langan E, Wyckoff J, Loo WS, et al. 2015. Size- and shape-dependent foreign body immune response to materials implanted in rodents and non-human primates. *Nat Mater* **14:** 643–651. doi:10.1038/nmat4290

Verhoeff K, Marfil-Garza BA, Sandha G, Cooper D, Dajani K, Bigam DL, Anderson B, Kin T, Lam A, O'Gorman D, et al. 2022. Outcomes following extrahepatic and intraportal pancreatic islet transplantation: a comparative cohort study. *Transplantation* **106:** 2224–2231. doi:10.1097/TP.0000000000004180

Vertex 2023 Press Release. Vertex presents new data from VX-880 phase 1/2 clinical trial at the American Diabetes Association 82nd Scientific Sessions. https://investors.vrtx.com/news-releases/news-release-details/vertex-presents-positive-vx-880-results-ongoing-phase-12-study

Vertex 2024 Press Release. Vertex provides pipeline and business updates in advance of upcoming investor meetings. https://investors.vrtx.com/news-releases/news-release-details/vertex-provides-pipeline-and-business-updates-advance-upcoming

Vlahos AE, Cober N, Sefton MV. 2017. Modular tissue engineering for the vascularization of subcutaneously transplanted pancreatic islets. *Proc Natl Acad Sci* **114:** 9337–9342. doi:10.1073/pnas.1619216114

Vlahos AE, Talior-Volodarsky I, Kinney SM, Sefton MV. 2021. A scalable device-less biomaterial approach for subcutaneous islet transplantation. *Biomaterials* **269:** 120499. doi:10.1016/j.biomaterials.2020.120499

Wang LH, Marfil-Garza BA, Ernst AU, Pawlick RL, Pepper AR, Okada K, Epel B, Viswakarma N, Kotecha M, Flanders JA, et al. 2023. Inflammation-induced subcutaneous neovascularization for the long-term survival of encapsulated islets without immunosuppression. *Nat Biomed Eng* doi:10.1038/s41551-023-01145-8

Wargenau A, Fekete N, Beland AV, Sabbatier G, Bowden OM, Boulanger MD, Hoesli CA. 2019. Protein film formation on cell culture surfaces investigated by quartz crystal microbalance with dissipation monitoring and atomic force microscopy. *Colloids Surf B Biointerfaces* **183:** 110447. doi:10.1016/j.colsurfb.2019.110447

Warnock GL, Thompson DM, Meloche RM, Shapiro RJ, Ao Z, Keown P, Johnson JD, Verchere CB, Partovi N, Begg IS, et al. 2008. A multi-year analysis of islet transplantation compared with intensive medical therapy on progression of complications in type 1 diabetes. *Transplantation* **86:** 1762–1766. doi:10.1097/TP.0b013e318190b052

Witkowski P, Philipson LH, Kaufman DB, Ratner LE, Abouljoud MS, Bellin MD, Buse JB, Kandeel F, Stock PG, Mulligan DC, et al. 2021. The demise of islet allotransplantation in the United States: a call for an urgent regulatory update. *Am J Transplant* **21:** 1365–1375. doi:10.1111/ajt.16397

Yang K, O'Cearbhaill ED, Liu SS, Zhou A, Chitnis GD, Hamilos AE, Xu J, Verma MKS, Giraldo JA, Kudo Y, et al. 2021. A therapeutic convection-enhanced macroencapsulation device for enhancing β cell viability and insulin secretion. *Proc Natl Acad Sci* **118:** e2101258118. doi:10.1073/pnas.2101258118

Yu J, Vodyanik MA, Smuga-Otto K, Antosiewicz-Bourget J, Frane JL, Tian S, Nie J, Jonsdottir GA, Ruotti V, Stewart R, et al. 2007. Induced pluripotent stem cell lines derived from human somatic cells. *Science* **318:** 1917–1920. doi:10.1126/science.1151526

Index

C

D

E

H

I

J

K

L

M

N

O

P

Q

R

S

T

U

V

Z

www.ingramcontent.com/pod-product-compliance
Lightning Source LLC
Chambersburg PA
CBHW040138200326
41458CB00025B/6308
* 9 7 8 1 6 2 1 8 2 5 0 7 4 *